The Substance Abuse Handbook

The Substance Abuse Handbook

Pedro Ruiz, M.D.

Professor and Vice Chair
Department of Psychiatry and Behavioral Sciences
The University of Texas Medical School
Houston, Texas

Eric C. Strain, M.D.

Professor
Department of Psychiatry and Behavioral Sciences
Johns Hopkins University School of Medicine
Baltimore, Maryland

John G. Langrod, A.C.S.W., C.A.S.A.C., L.C.S.W.R., Ph.D.

Director of Admissions and Evaluation
Division of Substance Abuse
Albert Einstein College of Medicine of Yeshiva University
Bronx, New York

Wolters Kluwer | Lippincott Williams & Wilkins
Health
Philadelphia · Baltimore · New York · London
Buenos Aires · Hong Kong · Sydney · Tokyo

Publisher: Charles W. Mitchell
Managing Editor: Sirkka Howes Bertling
Project Manager: Jennifer Harper
Senior Manufacturing Manager: Benjamin Rivera
Associate Director of Marketing: Adam Glazer
Creative Director: Doug Smock
Production Services: International Typesetting and Composition
Printer: Data Reproductions Corporation

© 2007 by Lippincott Williams & Wilkins, a Wolters Kluwer business
530 Walnut Street
Philadelphia, PA 19106
www.LWW.com

Printed in the USA

Library of Congress Cataloging-in-Publication Data

Ruiz, Pedro, 1936-
  The substance abuse handbook / Pedro Ruiz, Eric C. Strain, John G.
Langrod.
        p. ; cm.
  Companion to: Substance abuse: a comprehensive textbook / editors, Joyce
H. Lowinson . . . [et al.]. 4th ed. 2005.
  Includes bibliographical references.
  ISBN-13: 978-0-7817-6045-4
  ISBN-10: 0-7817-6045-3
  1. Substance abuse—Handbooks, manuals, etc.   I. Strain, Eric C.   II.
Langrod, John.   III. Substance abuse.   IV. Title.
  [DNLM: 1. Substance-Related Disorders.   2. Behavior, Addictive. WM 270
R935s 2007]
  RC564.15.R85 2007
  616.86—dc22
                                                              2006100520

Care has been taken to confirm the accuracy of the information presented and to describe generally accepted practices. However, the authors, editors, and publisher are not responsible for errors or omissions or for any consequences from application of the information in this book and make no warranty, expressed or implied, with respect to the currency, completeness, or accuracy of the contents of the publication. Application of this information in a particular situation remains the professional responsibility of the practitioner.

The authors, editors, and publisher have exerted every effort to ensure that drug selection and dosage set forth in this text are in accordance with current recommendations and practice at the time of publication. However, in view of ongoing research, changes in government regulations, and the constant flow of information relating to drug therapy and drug reactions, the reader is urged to check the package insert for each drug for any change in indications and dosage and for added warnings and precautions. This is particularly important when the recommended agent is a new or infrequently employed drug.

Some drugs and medical devices presented in this publication have Food and Drug Administration (FDA) clearance for limited use in restricted research settings. It is the responsibility of health care providers to ascertain the FDA status of each drug or device planned for use in their clinical practice.

The publisher has made every effort to trace copyright holders for borrowed material. If they have inadvertently overlooked any, they will be pleased to make the necessary arrangements at the first opportunity.

To purchase additional copies of this book, call our customer service department at (800) 638-3030 or fax orders to (301) 223-2320. International customers should call (301) 223-2300. Lippincott Williams & Wilkins customer service representatives are available from 8:30 am to 6:30 pm, EST, Monday through Friday, for telephone access. Visit Lippincott Williams & Wilkins on the Internet: http://www.lww.com.

10 9 8 7 6 5 4 3 2 1

Preface

This handbook was conceived and created as a practical companion book to the fourth edition of *Substance Abuse: A Comprehensive Textbook*, published by Lippincott Williams & Wilkins in 2005. It was clear to us that mental health professionals working in the field of addiction, primary care practitioners, students, residents, and trainees, as well as medical practitioners and counselors at large needed a clinically oriented handbook that focused on the most essential aspects of addictive disorders and their treatment. In creating this handbook our goal was very ambitious. We wanted to offer the field the most authoritative, clinically oriented information on the subject of substance use, abuse, and dependence, with emphasis on diagnosis, treatment, and prevention. We also wanted to create a handbook that could be useful to all disciplines involved, directly or indirectly, in the addiction field.

The addiction field continues to change and evolve. Currently, we are better able than ever to understand the biologic, psychologic, behavioral, and sociocultural aspects of addictive disorders and conditions. New treatments and modes of intervention are being continuously developed. Today, the treatment of patients with addictive disorders and conditions can be very rewarding and effective. Addiction patients who are able to control their use and abuse of addictive substances are often some of the most gratifying people to see in our daily clinical practices. These types of clinical experiences were a further stimulus for us to produce this handbook.

The handbook includes 11 sections. The first addresses the etiologic factors that are determinants of abuse and dependence behavior. The second section covers all relevant substances of abuse; the third discusses important topics related to compulsive and addictive behaviors. The fourth section is dedicated to evaluation and diagnostic classifications, including laboratory procedures, and the fifth focuses on treatment modalities. Section VI reviews the management of associated medical conditions. The seventh section covers relevant issues pertaining to the life cycle; the eighth emphasizes special addictive issues among women. Section IX underlines key addictive areas among special groups and special treatment settings, and Section X reviews relevant models of prevention. The final section discusses important training and educational aspects within the addiction field. Our hope is that all clinically relevant areas covered in these 11 sections will be of benefit for clinicians at large.

Finally, we take this opportunity to thank and show appreciation to all the persons who made possible the publication of this handbook. First, we thank all the expert authors of the fourth edition of *Substance Abuse: A Comprehensive Textbook*. Second, we thank the editorial staff of Lippincott Williams & Wilkins, especially Charles W. Mitchell, Executive Editor, who provided the guidance and support needed to bring this handbook to reality. Third, we thank Marie O. Gonzales-Arms, who worked very hard to make the publication of this handbook possible. Fourth, we show appreciation to our spouses, Angela Ruiz, Grace Serafini, and Susan Langrod, who tolerated with good cheer time away from them while we worked on this project, and who also understood the relevance of this contribution to the addiction field. Fifth and most importantly, we extend our sincere gratitude to the patients who suffer or have suffered from addictive disorders and conditions. These patients taught us over many years the complexities of addictive disorders and associated conditions. Their lessons have been invaluable to us and we will eternally be grateful to them.

Pedro Ruiz
Eric C. Strain
John G. Langrod

Contents

Section I

ETIOLOGIC FACTORS

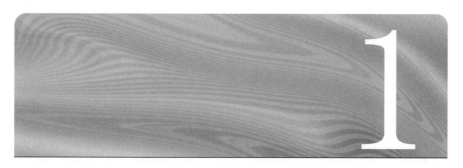

DETERMINANTS OF SUBSTANCE ABUSE AND DEPENDENCE

The reasons different persons use drugs can vary enormously, and the circumstances that lead to drug initiation versus continued use are likely to be different. Broadly, the determinants of drug use can be grouped into factors associated with the environment (sociocultural), and factors unique to the individual (genetic, neurobiologic, psychologic). However, these divisions are somewhat artificial, and no single factor accounts for the use of a drug. Rather, it is a complex interaction of social, cultural, biologic, and psychologic factors that determine drug use. Each of these topics is important in understanding the disorder, and in treating the patient.

Genetic Factors in the Risk for Substance Use Disorders

This section reviews evidence for genetic factors contributing to the risk of alcohol use disorders, using as an illustration one type of abused substance for which there is substantial evidence of genetic predisposition. The next section then briefly addresses the evidence for a genetic component to abuse of other substances.

Family, Twin, and Adoption Studies of Alcoholism

The basic design for family studies of any complex illness is to compare the risk for developing the disorder in relatives of probands (individuals manifesting the phenotype or trait) with the rate for relatives of control groups or for the general population. Numerous studies have found that rates of alcoholism are substantially higher in relatives of alcoholics than in relatives of nonalcoholics, with children of alcoholics demonstrating a four- to fivefold increased risk for developing the disorder. This increased risk appears to be relatively specific for alcoholism. However, familial aggregation might also reflect the shared social and developmental influences of being raised in the same environment by biologic parents.

Research with twins evaluates the relative contributions of genetic and environmental factors by comparing concordance rates for illness in pairs of monozygotic versus dizygotic twins. The twin study design allows researchers to estimate the contribution of genetic and environmental effects on the individual's susceptibility to alcoholism. Identical twin pairs who share all of their genes should show higher concordance rates for gene-transmitted disorders than should fraternal twin pairs, who generally share only half their genes. Environmentally influenced disorders should show no difference between monozygotic and dizygotic twin pairs so long as both types of twins were exposed to the same childhood environment.

Several major twin studies have directly addressed the concordance rates for alcoholism in identical versus fraternal twins. These studies have shown that the concordance rate for alcoholism in male monozygotic pairs was greater than that for dizygotic twins. Although results in women were initially less consistent, larger studies of female twins have generally found a similar relationship as that initially identified in males.

Perhaps the most convincing way to separate genetic from environmental effects is to study individuals who were separated soon after birth from their biologic relatives and who were raised by nonrelative adoptive parents. This can be done through classical adoption studies or through a half-sibling approach. Regarding the half-sibling approach, subjects who had a biologic parent with severe alcohol problems were significantly more likely to have alcoholism themselves than if a surrogate parent was alcoholic.

Genetically Mediated Markers of Alcoholism

Molecular Genetic Studies

Recent efforts have targeted identifying genes that influence susceptibility to alcoholism. Briefly, this involves the meticulous dissection of deoxyribonucleic acid (DNA) into specific nucleotide (e.g., the building blocks of DNA) patterns called markers or microsatellites. Such markers are then analyzed to determine whether there is *linkage* between the marker and the phenotype (i.e., the marker is transmitted along with the disease in families) or whether there is an *association* between the polymorphism and the phenotype (i.e., a given marker allele is more common among those individuals with the disease in a population). A number of candidate genes for alcohol dependence have been proposed.

Alcohol dehydrogenase (ADH) and aldehyde dehydrogenase (ALDH) are the major enzymes involved in the degradation of ethanol. Studies show that allelic variants of ADH and ALDH genes play an important role in influencing the metabolism of alcohol and that these polymorphisms are associated with the risk for developing alcohol dependence.

ALDH is the major enzyme that catabolizes acetaldehyde in the liver and other organs. Family 2 genes (ALDH 2) have been the most well studied genes regarding an association with alcohol dependence. This family of genes encodes mitochondrial enzymes that oxidize acetaldehyde. ALDH 2 has a deficient allelic variant (ALDH 2*2), when compared with the wild-type of ALDH 2 (ALDH 2*1). The ALDH 2*2 variant gene is found in approximately 50% of the Asian population. Individuals with the ALDH 2*2 variant typically experience aversive responses (e.g., facial flushing, tachycardia, and a burning sensation in the stomach) to alcohol consumption as a result of the accumulation of acetaldehyde. Several studies demonstrate the protective effect of ALDH 2*2 gene carriers from developing alcohol dependence.

The association between polymorphisms in ADH genes (located on chromosome 4) and alcohol dependence is not as robust as for ALDH genes. The variant allele ADH 2*2 (also known as the ADH1B*2 allele) encodes a high-activity enzyme involved in the oxidation of ethanol to acetaldehyde. Interestingly, it has been found that having the combination of the ADH 2*2 and ALDH 2*2 gene variants was associated with the lowest risk for alcoholism.

There also is evidence that an allele of the D2 dopamine receptor (DRD2) may be implicated in severe cases of alcoholism, although not all studies support this relationship. Interestingly, there is also some evidence to implicate the DRD2 gene in other substance use disorders, leading some investigators to label it a potential "reward gene."

γ-Aminobutyric acid (GABA) receptor genes, which encode the $GABA_A$ and $GABA_B$ receptors that bind GABA (the major inhibitory neurotransmitter in the human brain), have also been identified as promising candidate genes for alcoholism. *In vitro* studies have found that ethanol potentiates GABAergic neurotransmission, and preclinical studies in experimental animals have determined that GABA plays an important role in brain-depressant behavioral effects of alcohol.

Serotonin dysfunction has been repeatedly implicated in both preclinical and clinical studies examining vulnerability for alcoholism. As a result, a growing number of studies have evaluated candidate genes that encode various components (i.e., the serotonin transporter and serotonin receptor subtypes that modulate serotonergic neurotransmission) of the serotonergic system. There is controversial support for an association between alcoholism and genetic polymorphisms on chromosome 17 that encode the serotonin transporter.

In summary it is clear is that many genes likely influence the vulnerability for alcoholism and that different combinations of genes are likely to be more or less salient for each endophenotype associated with the disorder. Certain genes (e.g., ALDH 2*2) may provide protection against developing serious alcohol-related problems, whereas others (e.g., the DRD2 gene) might predispose certain individuals to alcoholism and other substance use disorders.

Genetic Influences in Other Drug Dependencies

As is the case with alcohol, there is also evidence of genetic factors for a variety of other abused substances. Although not as extensively studied as alcohol, data do support a genetic component for nicotine, cocaine, opioid, and cannabis dependence.

With respect to nicotine use, adoption and twin studies provide support for a genetic component (although the role of environment in smoking interacts with genetic vulnerability). Both past and current cigarette smokers have been found to have a significantly higher prevalence of the A1 allele of the DRD2 than do nonsmoking controls, suggesting a genetic propensity mediated by the dopamine (DA) receptor (although not all studies have found this association). There is some evidence for involvement of the genes encoding the serotonin transporter, and the protein involved with serotonin synthesis as well. Other possible genetic factors that may either increase the risk of developing nicotine dependence or protect against developing this disorder include genes for the CYP2D6 enzyme (which metabolizes nicotine) and for nicotinic acetylcholine receptors.

There is relatively limited information available about genetic variants affecting DA transporter function and cocaine dependence in humans. There is some evidence that the dopamine D3 (DRD3) receptor gene may play a modest role in the susceptibility to cocaine dependence, although such findings have not been consistent.

The μ-opioid receptor is one of several opioid receptors and is the primary site of drug action. A polymorphism at position 118 (A118G) of the μ-receptor gene has been found that changes the ability of the receptor to bind opioid ligands, especially β-endorphin. It has been suggested that this single-nucleotide polymorphism may be implicated in the development or protection from opioid addiction. However, not all studies have been able to replicate this association.

Twin studies of cannabis use in both males and females provide evidence for a genetic component to use of this drug. There are at least two cannabinoid receptors: CB1 primarily located in the central nervous system (CNS), and CB2 located strictly in the periphery. Studies on the relationships among substance use disorders and genetic variants in the cannabinoid receptor gene (CNR1) have, to date, provided conflicting results.

In summary, genetic factors can play an important role in the initiation and persistence of substance dependence. The search for candidate genes that contribute to the risk of developing and maintaining substance use disorders is still in its early stages. The task of identifying such genes is made more arduous because it is likely that variation in substance-dependence susceptibility results not only from genotypic differences and environmental influences, but also from their interactions. Thus, genetic factors are background sources of variance that can be minimized or exaggerated by environmental factors before the phenotype (substance dependence) can be expressed.

Brain-Reward Mechanisms

Although there is substantial evidence that genetic vulnerability plays an important role in determining drug use, it is important to understand and appreciate the reward mechanisms in the brain that mediate drug use. The acute enhancement of brain-reward mechanisms appears to be the single essential pharmacologic commonality of abusable substances. This section addresses various aspects of this unifying conception of the neural nature of the positive reinforcement engendered by self-administration of abusable substances.

Self-administration of Abusable Substances by Laboratory Animals

Abusable substances can be self-administered by laboratory animals using the intravenous, intramuscular, intraperitoneal, and intracerebral routes, as well as oral, intragastric, and inhalation routes. Animals will self-administer abusable substances in the absence of tolerance, physical dependence, withdrawal, or, indeed, any prior history of drug taking. This shows that drug-taking behavior cannot be explained simply in terms of the ability of abusable drugs to ameliorate withdrawal discomfort. As with human substance abuse, drug self-administration in laboratory animals is profoundly influenced by the subject's previous experience with drugs and by the environmental context in which the drug administration takes place.

By and large the substances that are voluntarily self-administered by laboratory animals are the same ones that humans also voluntarily self-administer, and by and large the same drugs that are eschewed by animals are also eschewed by humans. In addition, virtually all adequately studied abusable substances enhance brain-stimulation reward or lower brain-reward thresholds in the mesotelencephalic DA system. Finally, virtually all adequately studied abusable substances enhance basal neuronal firing or basal neurotransmitter release in reward-relevant brain circuits.

Underlying Neurobiology of Drug Reward: Electrical Self-stimulation of Brain-reward Circuits

To study electrical brain-stimulation reward, animals are first surgically implanted with chronic indwelling intracranial stimulating electrodes in specific brain loci, allowed to recover from the surgery, and then trained to self-administer the rewarding electrical stimulation by bar pressing or lever pressing in a standard operant chamber. Acquisition of lever pressing for brain-stimulation reward is very rapid, with high asymptotic operant levels. Electrical brain-stimulation reward is one of the most powerful rewards known to biology, rivaled only by the reward engendered by the most powerful self-administered drugs (e.g., cocaine). The few human studies of electrical stimulation of brain-reward areas confirm this, with the human experience one of intense subjective pleasure or euphoria.

Numerous studies have shown that brain reward is, in fact, critically dependent on the functional integrity of DA neurotransmission within the mesotelencephalic DA systems, with the mesolimbic DA system constituting a particularly important focal point within these brain-reward systems. Compellingly, DA blockade mimics the effect of decreasing the electrical intensity of the rewarding brain stimulation. However, the original supposition of many researchers that electrical brain-stimulation reward directly activates the DA fibers of the medial forebrain bundle appears contrary to the preponderance of evidence.

It has been clear that the majority of *first-stage* non-DA medial forebrain bundle reward neurons conduct their pleasure/reward neural signals caudally along axons projecting from the area of the lateral hypothalamus to the ventral tegmental area. This has led to the hypothesis that a majority of *first-stage* reward neurons arise rostral to the lateral hypothalamus and send their descending neuronal projections to the ventral tegmental area. To test this hypothesis, several research groups studied the role of descending medial forebrain bundle neurons in electrical brain stimulation reward by damaging their various nuclei of origin. Lesions of a number of the descending inputs to the medial forebrain bundle have been found to not degrade the reward efficacy of medial forebrain bundle electrical brain-stimulation reward.

In addition, it is now clear that a *third-stage* reward pathway does exist, carrying the pleasure/reward neural signal beyond the nucleus accumbens, that is, beyond the mesolimbic DA terminal loci to which the *second-stage* DA caudorostrally conducting medial forebrain bundle reward neurons project. This third-stage pathway uses the endogenous opioid peptide enkephalin as its primary neurotransmitter and projects anatomically to the ventral pallidum. Anatomic mapping and tracing studies show clearly that a major efferent pathway for nucleus accumbens output signals projects to the ventral pallidum, and that this pathway is enkephalinergic. This nucleus accumbens output pathway is known to be critical for expression of reward-related and incentive-related behaviors.

Intracranial Microinjection of Abusable Substances

A direct way to study the neuroanatomy of drug-induced reward is to meld intracranial microinjection technology with the self-administration paradigm, so that animals are allowed to work for direct intracranial self-administration of abusable substances into discrete brain loci. For example, animals will voluntarily self-administer microinjections of amphetamine into the nucleus accumbens and prefrontal cortex. Similarly, cocaine is voluntarily self-administered into the prefrontal cortex. Morphine is self-administered into the ventral tegmental area, lateral hypothalamus, and nucleus accumbens, all of which are either nuclei or terminal projection loci of the mesolimbic DA system, but not into other brain sites. Ethanol is self-administered into the ventral tegmental area, but—provocatively—only by animals with a genetic predisposition to high oral ethanol self-administration and not by animals with a genetic predisposition to ethanol abstinence. Phencyclidine is self-administered into the nucleus accumbens, and within that structure, preferentially self-administered into the "shell" subportion of nucleus accumbens.

An important theme in such intracranial microinjection studies, already alluded to, is the ability of such approaches to yield data showing which brain loci are responsible for the initiation of each separate and individual pharmacologic action of any given abusable substance. So, for example, the analgesic effect of opiates is mediated by local action on opioid peptidergic circuits within the periaqueductal and periventricular gray matter of the brainstem, the thermoregulatory effect by action in the preoptic area, whereas the rewarding effects appear mediated by action on the nuclei, tracts, and terminal projection loci of the mesolimbic DA system. Physical dependence on opiates has been shown by microinjection studies to be mediated by action on brainstem loci anatomically distinct and far removed from the mesolimbic DA loci mediating opiate-induced reward.

In Vivo Brain Chemistry Measurements during Administration of Abusable Substances

In Vivo Brain Microdialysis Studies

Using *in vivo* brain microdialysis, it has been shown that cocaine produces a robust enhancement of extracellular DA in the neostriatal and nucleus accumbens terminal projection areas of the reward-relevant mesotelencephalic DA system. This enhancement of the time course of DA is more pronounced in the nucleus accumbens than in other forebrain DA loci, and is dose dependent. Amphetamine also produces a robust enhancement of extracellular DA in reward-relevant neostriatal and nucleus accumbens DA terminal projection areas as measured by *in vivo* microdialysis, with stronger effect in the nucleus accumbens than in other forebrain DA loci. When the amphetamine is microinjected directly into the DA reward loci, instead of administered systemically, the enhancing effect on extracellular DA is extremely strong.

Morphine also produces robust dose-dependent enhancement of extracellular DA in reward-relevant neostriatal and nucleus accumbens DA terminal loci as measured by *in vivo* microdialysis. This effect is duplicated by other μ-opiate receptor agonists, including methadone, levorphanol, and fentanyl, and is antagonized by low-dose naloxone and by the irreversible μ-receptor antagonist β-funaltrexamine.

Nicotine enhances extracellular DA levels in both nucleus accumbens and neostriatum, with more pronounced effects in nucleus accumbens. Muscarinic cholinergic agonists and antagonists are without effect on DA efflux in forebrain reward loci. The enhancing effect of nicotine on DA efflux is blocked by 5-hydroxytryptamine-3 (5-HT$_3$) antagonists. Alcohol also enhances extracellular DA levels in both nucleus accumbens and neostriatum with more pronounced effects in nucleus accumbens. This effect of alcohol is dose dependent; low and moderate doses enhance DA efflux whereas the highest dose produces a biphasic effect—initial inhibition of DA release followed (as the high dose begins to wear off) by facilitation of DA efflux. The abusable dissociative anesthetic phencyclidine also enhances extracellular DA levels in both nucleus accumbens and neostriatum after either systemic administration or local intracranial microinjection, with preferential effects in the nucleus accumbens. Barbiturates, including pentobarbital, phenobarbital, and barbital, enhance extracellular DA levels in both nucleus accumbens and neostriatum, with more pronounced effects in nucleus accumbens. This effect of barbiturates is dose dependent; low doses enhance DA efflux, whereas high doses inhibit it. Δ^9-Tetrahydrocannabinol, the psychoactive constituent of Marijuana and hashish, also enhances extracellular DA levels in nucleus accumbens, neostriatum, and medial prefrontal cortex—all DA terminal fields of the reward-relevant mesotelencephalic DA system.

Within the nucleus accumbens, drugs of abuse (cocaine, amphetamine, morphine) preferentially increase extracellular DA in the "shell" subportion of nucleus accumbens as compared to the "core" subportion, congruent with the suggestion that the shell subportion of nucleus accumbens is specialized for mediating brain-reward functions.

Dopaminergic Brain-Reward System and Increased Vulnerability to Drug-Taking Behavior

Dopamine Reward Synapse and Modulatory Mechanisms Acting on the Dopamine Reward System

The first-stage neurons of the reward system appear to originate within the anterior bed nuclei of the medial forebrain bundle, and project caudally within the medial forebrain bundle in a moderately fast conducting, myelinated, heavily collateralized and diffuse neural system, of unknown neurotransmitter type(s), to synapse within the somatodendritic zone of DA cell bodies in the ventral tegmental area. These DA neurons of the ventral tegmental area constitute the second-stage neurons of the reward system. The ventral tegmental area that gives rise to these second-stage DA reward neurons is heavily innervated, and neurophysiologically modulated, by numerous synaptic inputs including GABAergic, glutamatergic, serotonergic, noradrenergic, opioid peptidergic, cholecystokinergic, and neurotensinergic neural systems. The second-stage DA reward neurons project rostrally within the medial forebrain bundle to synapse in the nucleus accumbens. These second-stage DA reward neurons constitute a critical locus for the addictive pharmacologic actions of abusable substances. Within the region of their axonal terminal projections in the nucleus accumbens, these second-stage reward neurons are heavily innervated, and neurophysiologically modulated, by numerous synaptic inputs. The most crucial reward synapses within the nucleus accumbens may be defined by their intra-accumbens locations and their synaptic connectivities—that is, within the accumbens shell, in reward-relevant synaptic plexuses containing an opioid–DA axoaxonic link, a DA–opioid presynaptic–postsynaptic link, and neural inputs from limbic cortex and amygdala. From the nucleus accumbens, additional third-stage reward-relevant neurons, some of them opioid peptidergic or GABAergic, appear to carry the reward signal further, to or via the ventral pallidum. The profuse, complex, and reciprocal neural interconnections between the ventral tegmental area, nucleus accumbens, ventral pallidum, amygdala, and bed nuclei of the medial forebrain bundle appear to be critically involved in regulating the functional set point for hedonic tone. In all of this complex neuronal computational machinery, the DA link between ventral tegmental area and nucleus accumbens seems central and crucial for drug-induced alterations in hedonic tone.

The drug-sensitive DA second-stage component of the reward circuitry appears to be under the modulatory control of a wide variety of other neural systems, including GABAergic, glutamatergic, serotonergic, noradrenergic, and neuropeptide neurotransmitter and neuromodulatory mechanisms, and theoretically an even wider variety of transsynaptic modulatory influences on the brain-reward systems are possible. It appears that the functioning of the reward system can be altered by directly manipulating these other neurotransmitter systems that synaptically interconnect with the DA substrates, as well as by manipulating the DA substrates directly.

Dopamine Reward Mechanisms: Chronic Administration and Withdrawal

In contrast to the clear-cut and agreed-on effects of acute administration of addicting drugs on brain-reward mechanisms, the effects of chronic administration of abuse-prone drugs on reward mechanisms are less clear-cut. With respect to neurochemical indices, a clear difference appears to exist between the effects of continuous administration and the effects of intermittent low-dose treatment, which presumably produces intermittent phasic stimulation. With intermittent low doses of psychostimulants (cocaine, amphetamines), "reverse tolerance" or "sensitization" of DA overflow in forebrain reward loci is seen upon subsequent psychostimulant rechallenge. Similar sensitization of DA overflow in forebrain-reward loci has been reported for opiates and many other classes of abused drugs. With chronic continuous or intermittent high-dose psychostimulant treatment, decreased DA synthesis is seen, as well as, in withdrawal from such dose regimens, depletion of basal extracellular DA in such brain-reward loci as nucleus accumbens. When cocaine is administered to emulate human "binges," decreased basal and cocaine-stimulated DA levels are reported. Reward-related functional and behavioral sequelae have also been reported. With continuous treatment or intermittent treatment with high doses, acute tolerance to the rewarding effects of cocaine develops, and withdrawal from the continuous intoxication produced by frequent low-dose cocaine or amphetamine produces elevations in brain-stimulation reward thresholds.

In opiate withdrawal from chronic dosing regimens (either abstinence withdrawal or precipitated withdrawal), a pattern of decreased DA levels in forebrain reward loci (particularly nucleus accumbens) similar to that seen in withdrawal from continuous or high-dose intermittent psychostimulant administration is seen. Opiate self-administration increases significantly in withdrawal, and the increase correlates with severity of withdrawal. Significantly, the neural mechanisms underlying this withdrawal-produced presumptive negative hedonic tone or dysphoria may involve the nucleus accumbens, just as the acute–drug-induced positive hedonic tone may.

Very importantly, because DA depletion, unlike other withdrawal symptoms, offers a withdrawal symptom common to psychostimulants, opiates, and ethanol, it may offer a long-sought common denominator for addiction.

In summary, it appears that abusable substances have two fundamental commonalities: (a) that they are voluntarily self-administered by nonhuman mammals, and (b) that they acutely enhance brain-reward mechanisms. The reward circuits of the brain, upon which abusable substances act to enhance brain reward, include first-stage, second-stage, and third-stage components. Complex reciprocal neural interconnections between the first-stage, second-stage, and third-stage reward neurons also appear to be importantly involved in regulating the functional set point for hedonic tone, and (at least in laboratory animals) manipulating these neural interconnections can alter drug-taking behavior. Perturbations in the neural substrates of the DA reward system may be capable of altering vulnerability to drug-taking behavior. Relapse to drug-seeking or drug-taking behavior triggered by re-exposure to a drug appears to involve reactivation of DA reward-linked substrates. The subjective experience of drug craving itself may also involve activation of DA reward-linked substrates. A clinically relevant derivative of such considerations is that pharmacotherapeutic interventions to alter drug reward, drug craving, or even pre-existing drug vulnerabilities could conceivably target an exceedingly wide range of neurotransmitter systems that synaptically modulate the reward circuitry.

Sociocultural Issues

Substance use takes place within a sociocultural environment that mediates which substances are available, their desirability, and their acceptability. Accordingly, the drugs to which persons are exposed and their reactions to them are strongly influenced by the person's place in society. This section describes sociocultural processes that underlie the emergence and course of drug use.

Multiple Social Crises in the Inner City

During the 1970s, but especially in the 1980s and 1990s, American cities experienced a continued catastrophic decline in manufacturing and other labor-intensive industries that provide unskilled "working-class" jobs with steady employment and low but adequate incomes. When new jobs were created, they tended to require advanced education, or were in service industries paying a near-minimum wage. In addition, costs for housing rose, while funds for subsidized housing were reduced. The end result has been the marginalization of working-class and middle-class people, white and minority.

Important shifts also occurred in family structure, particularly among minorities. The proportion of African American children living in mother-only families increased from 30% to 51% between 1970 and 1985. Almost 90% of African American children will experience poverty if the family is headed by a single woman younger than age 30 years. Other crises compounded difficulties faced by inner-city residents and low-income persons. The Personal Responsibility and Work Opportunity Reconciliation Act of 1996 mandated that people receiving welfare be required to work 35 hours a week. Many welfare recipients found opportunities for employment, when available, rarely paid much more than welfare. Health care and preventive health clinic services were cut back. Youth recreation and service programs were reduced. State mental health institutions released large numbers of clients into communities with marginal support services. Transfer payments, such as home relief, Temporary Assistance to Needy Families (TANF), and Supplemental Security Income (SSI), declined in purchasing power.

A sizable proportion of inner-city households can be categorized as severely distressed—not simply experiencing a few temporary social problems, but enduring the impact of multiple and continual social crises. In such households, income from legal employment is usually unstable and insufficient to pay for rent, food, and clothing. Transfer payments are inadequate. Only a few people in the family or kin network can support adequate housing. Family or kin without housing or shelter descend continuously upon such households, sleeping and eating "free" to themselves but at high cost to the householder's budget. Youths growing up in such households do poorly in marginal inner-city schools. The household head is frequently a maternal figure. She is likely to be a grandmother or older aunt to the children. Economic contributions to the family by the children's father or male partners of the household's head are rare. At various times, family members or kin experience serious illness, mental health problems, drug or alcohol abuse, jail or prison, child abuse or neglect, or death. Although households with multiple problems are most numerous and persistent in the inner cities and ghettos of major American cities, households throughout American society experience similar problems.

Individuals from severely distressed households routinely come to the attention of various social programs, including drug treatment. As adults, these persons often need "habilitation" rather than "rehabilitation."

Natural History of Recent Drug Eras

Overall, widespread use of illicit drugs emerged in the 1960s as the first members of the baby boom came of age and developed their own distinctive subcultural identities with associated behaviors. Since then, evolving tastes in the face of a changing sociohistorical context have led to distinct nationwide drug eras. These drug eras are identified as historical periods during which a new drug or "innovative" mode of use (e.g., heroin use, or crack use as an innovative mode of cocaine administration) becomes institutionalized within segments of the population. Typically, four phases to a drug era can be distinguished. First is the *incubation phase* in which some "pioneers" begin use, refine innovations, and develop relatively standard patterns of use or selling practices. This usually takes place within a highly specific social context as the "in" thing to do. The *expansion phase* occurs when the pioneers "initiate" or "turn on" larger numbers of users to the new drug or mode of consumption. The *plateau phase* occurs when most of those at highest risk for becoming regular users have had the opportunity to do so, leading to a leveling of the overall prevalence. Subsequently, a steady flow of new initiates continues as many adolescents choose to use whichever drug is currently popular. The *decline phase* represents a shift in a drug's popularity, especially among adolescents as proportionately fewer of them even try the drug. Nevertheless, because many older users of a specific drug/modality will persist in their habits, the overall prevalence of use declines only slowly with time.

Impact of Drug Use on Public Agencies

Drug Treatment

During the late 1970s in New York City approximately 25,000 admissions (90% for heroin) for drug abuse treatment occurred annually. The number of heroin admissions declined to about 15,000 in 1991, and increased modestly through the 1990s to about 23,000 in 2001. Beginning in 1984, cocaine as the primary drug of abuse at admission began to increase substantially; it rose from about 2,000 in 1983, to more than 8,000 in 1986, to 13,000 in 1991, to 17,000 in 1997, to 14,000 in 2001. Most cocaine admissions were for crack abuse. Virtually all drug treatment programs indicate that they routinely cannot admit the many crack abusers who seek help. At drug-free residential and outpatient programs, approximately 80% of admissions listed cocaine or crack as the primary drug of abuse.

The 1990s and early 2000s also experienced a large influx of marijuana/blunt users into drug treatment programs. Treatment admissions for marijuana increased steadily from about 1,000 in 1991 to 13,000 in 2001. Most marijuana/blunt users do not voluntarily seek drug treatment, but are referred by the criminal justice system as an alternative to incarceration. Although referred by courts, only modest proportions of marijuana/blunt users actually enroll and even fewer are retained in drug treatment.

Criminal Justice System

The public and politicians demanded a harsh approach to reducing drug use and the open-air markets. In New York City (as elsewhere), police developed special task forces to "crack down" on crack dealers. The number of heroin arrests increased from about 17,000 in 1987, to 24,000 in 1990, to 33,000 in 1994. Cocaine and crack arrests nearly doubled from 28,600 in 1986 to 54,000 in 1989, and then declined to 40,200 in 1995 and to 32,000 in 2001. Heroin-related arrests increased from 24,000 in 1991 to 38,000 in 1995, but declined to about 33,000 in 2000. Marijuana-related arrests soared from about 5,000 in 1991 to 60,000 in 2000.

Much of the growth in criminal justice populations is a result of convictions for drug crimes. The proportion of drug offenders rose from 8% to 26% between 1980 and 1994. Especially in federal prisons, the proportion serving sentences for drug crimes increased from 25% to 60%. A careful analysis of this increase indicated that much of the increase was a consequence of mandatory sentences imposed on crack sellers.

In 1989, 25% of all young African American males were under criminal justice supervision (jail, prison, parole, or probation); this figure reached 33% in 1994, and 46% in 2001 (an additional 16% were Hispanics). Most data show that minorities are disproportionately arrested and incarcerated for drug offenses. Popular support for the "incarceration" solution to the crack and drug problem proved very expensive. In 1980, the nation's corrections (jail and prison) costs were about $9 billion; this rose to $49 billion by 2001.

Public Health System

Heroin and crack abuse continue to have a substantial impact on the public health and social service delivery system. The number of emergency room mentions for heroin in New York declined slightly in the early 1980s, rose to about 5,000 per year in the last years of the 1980s, but then doubled to about 10,000 in 1995, and remained relatively constant through 2001. The number of cocaine-related emergency room mentions, however, increased much more dramatically from 1,324 in 1981, to 3,102 in 1984, to 14,925 in 1989, with further increases to about 20,000 in the period 1992 through 1998, but declined to about 14,000 in the period 1999 through 2001.

The acquired immune deficiency syndrome (AIDS) epidemic is directly linked to the heroin epidemic. The numerous heroin addicts who shared needles and routinely went to shooting galleries in the 1970s and 1980s became major carriers and transmitters of human immunodeficiency virus (HIV) and AIDS. Thousands have died from AIDS-related illnesses. Along the way, they transmit HIV to their sexual partners and, among women, transmit HIV to their children.

In summary, drug abuse and its attendant problems are embedded within a complex evolving sociocultural context. The illicit drug-of-choice changes over time. More centrally, the impact of drug use in a person's life is strongly mediated by the person's social position. Illicit drug abuse is associated with particularly widespread devastation in disadvantaged inner-city communities. Members of these communities have limited social capital and resources to draw upon. Consequently, drug use often leads these persons into contact with the criminal justice system, leads them to public drug treatment programs, and complicates their family's relationship with public welfare programs. This comorbidity of drug abuse with other social problems suggests that the negative impact of illicit drug use and, possibly, the use itself might be reduced by addressing broader social problems.

Psychodynamics

This final section adopts a psychodynamic perspective, one that examines the inner emotional terrain and the psychologic organization and structures of an individual, to explore the psychologic compulsion to use and become dependent on addictive drugs.

Contemporary Theories of Psychoanalysis

Recent psychoanalytic understanding of addictive vulnerability has drawn on advances in contemporary psychoanalysis, which places emphasis on developmental, structural (ego/self), and object relations theory, as well as the centrality of affects. Addicted individuals, if asked, frequently indicate that their pursuit and use of drugs make them feel "normal," "calm," "relaxed," "alive," "energized," and "not anxious—overwhelmed—[or] out of control." What contemporary psychodynamic theorists draw from clinical experience suggests that substance use is an attempt at self-correction. In one view of this, addictive behaviors become a special adaptation to compensate for inadequate or overdrawn defenses to regulate relationships, sense of self/self-respect, intense emotions, and compulsive/impulsive behaviors. Contemporary theory attempts to unravel the psychodynamic underpinnings of the suffering entailed in substance use.

It has been suggested that narcotics are used adaptively by narcotic addicts to compensate for defects in affect defense, particularly against feelings of rage, shame, and abandonment. Narcotics act to reverse regressive states and serve to counteract the disorganizing influences of rage and aggression on the ego. Further expansion of these views led to a "self-medication" hypothesis, which focused on the use of heroin and cocaine dependence as an attempt to alleviate emotional suffering. Addicts, for the most part, do not choose drugs randomly to alleviate the painful affect states. Rather, drugs are chosen because an individual discovers a specific psychopharmacologic action, which helps alleviate the individual's suffering.

For example, pain-relieving properties of the opiates help users modulate disturbing, rageful feelings that are the source of much suffering in their lives, feelings that may originate in past experiences in which they were victims, perpetrators, or both. Sedative–hypnotics can help tense, emotionally restricted individuals to experience walled-off affect and to overcome related fears concerning closeness, dependency, and intimacy. Cocaine can help overcome feelings of fatigue and the depletion states associated with depression or boredom, and persons with high energy may be attracted to cocaine because it increases feelings of self-esteem and frustration tolerance or augments a preferred hyperactive style and amplifies feelings of self-sufficiency.

An alternative understanding is that addiction is a response to feelings of helplessness that are experienced by addicts as a narcissistic injury. In this view, addiction is an active behavior that reverses the feeling of helplessness and restores a sense of internal power by controlling and regulating one's affective state. At the same time, addictive behavior is an expression of the narcissistic rage that inevitably accompanies such states of helplessness. The action of using a drug is seen as a displacement or substitution for more direct action to correct the addict's helplessness and express the addict's rage. When addictive behavior is seen as the expression of an idea that must be acted on (the enraged impulse to reassert mastery against helplessness) and as an action that must be taken in displacement because of the need to ward off the direct expression of this feeling, then addiction can be understood to be a subset of compulsions. This hypothesis is significant because it suggests the treatability of addictions with a psychodynamic approach that has been accepted for many years for compulsions. This view also allows many compulsions to be better understood as true addictions. In considering the implications of this hypothesis for treatment, the therapist can reframe the impulse for the patient as a healthy drive for mastery of helplessness, but displaced. The drive can be seen as "a drive for life" that can help alleviate the feelings of shame and helplessness that are painful for the abuser.

Yet another conceptualization of drug use is that it is an artificial affective defense, suggestive of a primary phobia. The compulsive search of the addict for the addictive object is a mirror image of the usual avoidant behavior of the phobic. This external addictive object serves as a narcissistic protector against the primary phobia, becoming highly overvalued. Internally, a defense of narcissism is developed that is experienced by others as ruthlessness and coldness, and who then punish the addict's perceived haughtiness with humiliation and shame. Splitting, fragmentation, and massive depersonalization can occur. The limiting functioning of the superego is experienced as restricting and suffocating, re-enacting the primary phobia. The protecting self-care functions of the superego are pathologized into new constricting structures.

Self-Regulatory Deficiencies

A main framework for understanding substance abuse emphasizes self-regulatory deficiencies, encompassing deficits in self-care, self-development and self-esteem, self–object relationships, and affects. The ego must serve as a signal and guide in protecting the self against realistic, external dangers and against instability and chaos in internal emotional life. It follows that many substance abusers, as a consequence of deficits in self-regulation, experience painful and confusing emotions, troubled behaviors, poor self-esteem, stormy relationships, or isolated existences.

Many patients who are drug dependent show a disregard of possible dangers to their well-being, including the use of abusive substances. The addict's disregard of self is not primarily the result of unconscious motivations of self-destructiveness, but results from a lack of early development internalization of key parenteral features such as caring. Many problems in self-care are apparent in the histories of substance abusers prior to the use of a drug or subsequently after long periods of abstinence.

Deficits in self-development and self-esteem in substance abusers may cause major problems in relationships. They can be experts in disguising their needs for nurturance, although these needs can be excessive. They may be at the mercy of their significant other or external world to supply self-esteem, but at the same time may be paralyzed in asking for validation. They tend to go to extremes, totally depending on and being subservient to the other, or isolating themselves.

Deficits in affect tolerance have an important relationship to the craving for drugs or alcohol. Substance abusers' problems with affect regulation have been described as being too porous, allowing the contents (e.g., rage and anger) to pour out uncontrollably; overly restrictive and sealed, thus constricting experiences and communication; or depleted, resulting in emptiness. Another developmental line involves the desomatization of affects. Affects that are experienced only as physiologic experiences are overwhelming and experienced as very dangerous. The use of drugs is seen as an attempt to shore up the defense against re-experiencing the chaos of traumatic feelings that occurred preverbally. The continued pattern of working into an unbearable state drives the person to search for a substance that will give relief.

In attempting to understand why a user continues, beyond physiologic factors, despite chronic suffering from their abuse (physical deterioration, psychologic regression, and an internal world of chaos), it has been speculated that the abuser feels some means of control in the active behavior of using. Thus the suffering experienced from the drug or alcohol is more bearable because it is something the user understands and controls. Thus, the vulnerabilities of affect tolerance exhibited by addicts may involve attempts to block feelings, not connect their affect with cognition, and therefore not feel at all, or be frozen without fantasy or metaphor.

Conclusion

The psychology of substance abuse, as formulated from a psychodynamic perspective, focuses on understanding addictions as adaptive attempts to alleviate emotional suffering and repair self-regulatory deficiencies. Treatment emphasizes the development of an understanding of the emotional factors that lie behind and produce addiction as a restorative response. This is fostered by mutual understanding of the addict's suffering, gradual toleration, and modulation of painful feelings; learning of psychologic skills to care for and nurture the self; and the adoption of a reality not based on childhood illusions. Our greatest source of knowledge is our patients. We learn by listening attentively to the uniqueness of their stories.

Suggested Readings

Dick DM, Foroud T. Candidate genes for alcohol dependence: a review of genetic evidence from human studies. *Alcohol Clin Exp Res.* 2003;27(5):868–879.

Director L. The value of relational psychoanalysis in the treatment of chronic drug and alcohol use. *Psychoanal Dialog.* 2002;12:551–579.

Gardner EL. Brain-reward mechanisms. In: Lowinson JH, Ruiz P, Millman RB, et al., eds. *Substance abuse: a comprehensive textbook*, 4th ed. Philadelphia: Lippincott Williams & Wilkins; 2005:48–97.

Gardner EL. What we have learned about addiction from animal models of drug self-administration. *Am J Addict.* 2000;9(4):285–313.

Johnson BD, Golub A, Dunlap E. The rise and decline of hard drugs, drug markets and violence in New York City. In: Blumstein A, Wallman J, eds. *The crime drop in America*. New York: Cambridge; 2000:164–206.

Johnson BD, Golub A. Sociocultural issues. In: Lowinson JH, Ruiz P, Millman RB, et al., eds. *Substance abuse: a comprehensive textbook*, 4th ed. Philadelphia: Lippincott Williams & Wilkins; 2005:107–120.

Khantzian EJ, Dodes L, Brehm NM. Psychodynamics. In: Lowinson JH, Ruiz P, Millman RB, et al., eds. *Substance abuse: a comprehensive textbook*, 4th ed. Philadelphia: Lippincott Williams & Wilkins; 2005:97–107.

Khantzian EJ. Reflections on group treatments as corrective experiences for addictive vulnerability. *Int J Group Psychother.* 2001;51:11–20.

Lin SW, Anthenelli RM. Genetic factors in the risk for substance use disorders. In: Lowinson JH, Ruiz P, Millman RB, et al., eds. *Substance abuse: a comprehensive textbook*, 4th ed. Philadelphia: Lippincott Williams & Wilkins; 2005:33–47.

Section II

SUBSTANCES OF ABUSE

2

ALCOHOL

Alcoholism is one of the most costly diseases afflicting persons in the United States today. The circumstances that lead to compulsive alcohol intake are complex and include psychosocial, environmental, genetic, and neurobiologic factors. During the past decade, neurobiology has made tremendous advances in our understanding of the actions of alcohol on the brain. However, key questions regarding the precise sites of alcohol action remain unanswered. Notable discoveries are that alcohol, like other drugs of abuse, increases the firing and dopamine release of ventral tegmental area (VTA) dopamine neurons. This action is likely critical for the reinforcing aspects of alcohol, but the neurochemical and biophysical mechanisms responsible for this effect remain to be elucidated. The reductionist approach of searching for alcohol-sensitive synaptic receptors has been successful, and the ligand-gated ion channels, that is, γ-aminobutyric acid A (GABA$_A$), glycine, N-methyl-D-aspartic acid (NMDA), 5-hydroxytryptamine-3 (5-HT$_3$), and nicotinic acetylcholine (nACh) receptors, have emerged as likely sites of alcohol action. However, the molecular mechanisms by which alcohol affects the function of these receptors are not clear. There is considerable evidence that protein phosphorylation either determines or modifies the actions of alcohol on some of these receptors, but questions regarding alcohol interactions with protein kinases and phosphatases remain. Furthermore, in addition to the voltage-gated ion channels, G protein–coupled receptor systems have also been shown to be sensitive to alcohol. Now that these actions of alcohol have been identified in isolated systems, the challenge is to determine which sites are important for specific electrophysiologic and behavioral actions of alcohol.

It is evident that alcoholism is not a homogeneous disease but consists of subtypes, each with varying degrees of biologic and psychosocial antecedents. Standardized nomenclatures, such as the *Diagnostic and Statistical Manual of Mental Disorders*, 4th edition, text revision (DSM-IV-TR), define the core features of alcoholism, which encompass the concepts of tolerance, withdrawal, and reinstatement after a period of abstinence. The DSM-IV-TR is widely used throughout the world, and the term *alcohol dependence* is used in favor of *alcoholism* to remove emphasis on the individual but instead focus on the concept of disease.

Epidemiology

Alcoholism is a major cause of morbidity and mortality in the United States and worldwide. Globally, the disease impact of alcoholism is greatest in regions with the highest per capita consumption, such as Latin America, and is smallest in regions like the Middle East where drinking levels are relatively low. In the United States, there are 8 million individuals dependent on alcohol. An additional 5.6 million American citizens abuse alcohol. Not only is the disease prevalence for alcoholism high, but it also tends to run in families. In all, alcohol abuse costs the nation about $185 billion per annum—more than $600 for every man, woman, and child living in the United States.

Alcoholism is associated with a range of physical and mental disorders. Perhaps the best-known disease associated with alcoholism is liver cirrhosis. In the United States, about 900,000 individuals have liver cirrhosis; of these, more than 20,000 die each year. Approximately 33% of all cases of liver cirrhosis are associated with alcohol abuse or dependence. Cancer of the oropharynx, the prevalence of which is associated with the extent of tissue exposure to alcohol, is on the increase. Local gastrointestinal effects of alcohol include chronic gastritis, and excessive drinking increases the risk of both rectal and pancreatic cancer. Women receiving hormone replacement therapy who drink may be at increased risk of breast cancer; however, it does not appear that alcohol intake is associated with prostate or endometrial cancers.

Mental disorders appear to be commonly associated with alcohol dependence; however, it is often difficult to determine which is the primary or preceding disorder. The risk of mental disease appears to be correlated with the amount of alcohol consumed, and the intake of more than 29 drinks per week can double the risk of mental disease. Individuals with affective and anxiety disorders have high rates of alcohol dependence. For example, rates of alcohol dependence are as high as 60% among those with bipolar disorder. Excessive drinking undoubtedly aggravates concurrent Alzheimer or multi-infarct dementia. Nevertheless, in practice, it is often difficult to differentiate these dementias from a supervening or underlying alcohol dementia.

Excessive and binge drinking episodes increase the risk of a multitude of injuries that can occur from the operation of heavy machinery, vehicle accidents, fires, and falls. No level of drinking can be considered "safe" because the risk of injury correlates predictably with the amount of alcohol-related performance impairment. Aggressive behavior and related traumatic injuries also become more likely if alcohol is consumed 6 hours or less prior to the incident.

In general, mortality rates increase when drinking levels rise. Interestingly, there appears to be a protective effect of light or moderate drinking on the development of coronary heart disease; hence, mortality rates for abstainers approach those of heavy drinkers.

Drinking through the Ages and Natural History

In recent times, there has been no improvement in the epidemic patterns of underage drinking, even though there appears to have been a slight decrease in alcohol consumption among those older than age 12 years from 72.9% in 1979 to 63.7% in 2001. From the 2000 National Household Survey on Drug Abuse report, it can be seen that the average age at which drinking starts among those between 12 years and 20 years of age is 14 years. Furthermore, a person who starts drinking before the age of 15 years is about four times more likely to develop alcohol dependence—these rates increase with earlier ages of drinking onset. Thus, the most important factor that predicts progression into adulthood is an early age of onset of drinking problems, and the delay of drinking until adulthood reduces the risk of lifetime alcohol dependence. Nevertheless, not all cases of early problem drinking progress into adulthood. Only in approximately 20% to 30% of people who have early alcohol problems does this progress into adulthood. Children who drink alcohol frequently have prior behavioral problems, especially conduct disorder. Among adolescents, it appears that the symptoms of depression and anxiety often precede alcohol abuse.

Individuals who develop alcohol dependence after the age of 50 years tend to decrease their drinking as they get older. Importantly, however, the proportion of the elderly (i.e., older than age 65 years) who are dependent on alcohol continues to rise in the United States. Generally, the proportion of elderly women with at-risk drinking is 12%, compared with 10% for elderly men.

Ethnicity, Gender, Place of Residence, and Religion

Drinking patterns differ between men and women, as well as between ethnic and racial groups. Overall, whites have the highest alcohol consumption levels, followed by Hispanics and then African Americans. Despite a number of earlier references to epidemic drinking levels among Native Americans, this does vary tremendously between tribes. The trend toward reduced drinking with age is not uniform across ethnic groups. White men peak first (age 18 to 25 years), followed by Hispanic and African American men, with peak ages between 26 and 30 years. Interestingly, however, Hispanic men tend to maintain heavy drinking patterns acquired as adults even as they become elderly. The high levels of drinking persistence among Hispanic men are associated with elevated levels of partner abuse, and this subgroup may soon exert the heaviest burden of care on society for alcohol problems. Women are drinking more; nowadays, the proportion is approaching parity. Those who live in cities and suburbs, compared with those who reside in rural areas, have higher rates of alcohol dependence. Jews, Episcopalians, and Baptists living in rural areas exhibit low rates of alcohol dependence when compared with the general population.

Clinical Picture

Although there is no typical pattern that describes the progression of an individual from excessive drinking to alcohol dependence, and an exhaustive description that encompasses every heavy drinker is not possible, certain features appear to be dominant themes as the disease progresses. In the early phases of the disease process, the most obvious feature is excessive or binge drinking to the point of intoxication. Some alcohol-dependent individuals ascribe their desire to drink to be motivated by emotional factors such as dysthymic mood or negative affect and, sometimes, elation. In others, there is the description of what may be loosely termed as "craving" or a hard-to-suppress urge to drink. Contemporary research has, however, found it difficult to describe accurately what constitutes craving, and from the extensive literature that has developed on trying to reach an accepted definition, no consensus has emerged. Nevertheless, a large proportion of heavy drinkers are unable to provide a plausible explanation of what triggered the use of increasing amounts of alcohol. Increasingly, heavy drinking onset is not wholly precipitated by underlying emotional circumstances but out of a peer culture of drinking in school, in college, with friends, or with workmates. For some, there is a high level of exposure to drinking situations (e.g., working as a bartender), and the progression to heavier drinking patterns is not easily noticed. Increased *tolerance* to alcohol may drive a rise in consumption to maintain the same pharmacologic effect.

Once the bouts of drinking to *intoxication* become an embedded behavioral pattern, the likelihood that the individual will develop alcohol-related problems tends to increase. Typically, there are increasing days of sick leave taken from work, interpersonal relationships begin to break down, and driving while intoxicated not only leads to legal problems but also increases the risk of traumatic injury. Heavy drinking may become associated with "blackouts" with amnesia for events the night before, and "hangovers" on waking the next morning may become a common event. By this time, the chronic drinker's performance is generally impaired, he or she may appear to be more forgetful, and there is increasing neglect of comportment and attention to hygiene. Also, the chronic drinker may describe feelings of guilt, remorse, or disgust following drinking. These symptoms lead to concealment of drinking, with alcoholic beverages being hidden in the home, and drinking alone becomes a more frequent endeavor. An ingrained pattern of heavy drinking over many months can establish the physical features of alcohol-dependence syndrome, which become most marked with drinking cessation. That is, at this juncture, drinking cessation triggers symptoms of autonomic hyperactivity, which can include nervousness and tremulousness, and can develop into symptoms associated with greater neurologic impairment such as delirium tremens. "Relief drinking" may occur to avoid withdrawal symptoms that arise from temporary periods of abstinence.

On physical examination and laboratory testing, there are no pathognomonic features of alcoholism. There are, however, a range of signs and symptoms that should be sought in an established drinker or, if found, should increase the physician's suspicion that the patient may have an alcohol problem. It is important to remember that the alcohol-dependent individual can present in almost any medical setting.

Features Detectable by Physical Exam or Laboratory Tests

Skin and Muscle

Many skin conditions are exacerbated by heavy alcohol consumption. Exposure to sunshine leading to erythematous eruptions without blistering may be a sign of erythropoietic protoporphyria. Psoriasis vulgaris and acne rosacea (red nose) are also commonly found. Rarely, hepatic porphyrias can be triggered by alcohol and result in skin eruptions—porphyria cutanea tarda—which are characterized by bullous erosions, blistering, crusting, and scarred healing with hyperpigmentation or depigmentation, especially to the face, side of the neck, and back of the hands. Palmar erythema (red palms) may be seen, and with the onset of alcoholic liver disease, there may be spider nevi (angiomas of interlaced red blood vessels). Myopathy can be a rare complication of alcoholism.

Eyes

Arcus senilis may be present as a result of increased blood lipid levels in heavy drinkers. However, this sign is so ubiquitous as to be not of much diagnostic use. Rarely, prominent eye signs, such as ophthalmoplegia and nystagmus, which are features of Wernicke encephalopathy, can be manifested in individuals with chronic severe alcoholism. However, patients with this condition are unlikely to present in general practice.

Limbs

Tremulousness may be noticed as an early sign of alcohol withdrawal but is more likely to be associated with anxiety or a benign nonessential tremor. Sometimes, individuals with chronic alcoholism may present with peripheral neuropathy as a consequence of deficiencies of vitamin B_{12}, thiamin, or both. Asterixis or "liver flap" may be seen in individuals with established alcoholic liver disease.

Cardiovascular System

Excessive drinkers may present with hypertension. Although the etiology of most cases of hypertension is unknown, the possibility that heavy drinking may be involved should be considered. Arrhythmias are uncommon, but infrequently an individual may report having "butterflies in the chest" (i.e., bouts of atrial fibrillation) associated with heavy drinking episodes. When this occurs while on vacation, it is referred to as the *holiday heart syndrome*. Rare cardiac complications include cardiomyopathy.

Gastrointestinal System

Excessive drinking can bring about a range of gastrointestinal disorders. Enlarged salivary glands can occur. Also, heavy drinkers may describe episodes of reflux esophagitis with a burning or persistent raw feeling in the throat, and retching from vomiting can produce *Mallory-Weiss tears* to the esophagus and the vomiting of frank red blood. Rarely, long-standing esophagitis may predispose the individual to esophageal cancer. Generally, individuals with alcoholism have higher rates of oropharyngeal cancer than the general population. Stomach ulcers and gastritis are common; the patient may complain of dark stools, and intestinal malabsorption is possible. Diarrhea often signals the involvement of the colon; colonic polyps and rectal cancer are rare possibilities. The liver may be enlarged and easily palpated under the right costochondral margin, but it is usually nontender. Tenderness and pain in the upper abdominal cavity of an excessive drinker should lead to the suspicion of acute pancreatitis, typically with calcification.

Endocrine System

Heavy alcohol consumption can exacerbate hypoactivity of a number of endocrine organs, such as the thyroid, hyperthyroid, and pancreas, and should be considered as a complicating factor in individuals with these conditions who are not improving or who are treatment resistant.

Rheumatic and Immune System

With the onset of alcoholic liver disease, most alcoholics develop autoantibodies to smooth muscle, mitochondria, and nuclei, perhaps because of the cytosolic proteins modified by the metabolites of alcohol. Therefore, drinkers tend to experience a reduction in symptoms of autoimmune diseases such as systemic lupus erythematosus and rheumatoid arthritis. Heavy drinking may, however, precipitate attacks of gout, and less commonly there may be signs of osteoporosis and myopathy. Heavy drinkers are more susceptible to infections caused by an increase in the CD4:CD8 ratio; however, this would be difficult to distinguish from other conditions that may increase susceptibility to infections.

Erythropoiesis

Anemias are common and should be examined for clinically by inspecting the lower eyelids and the bed of the finger nails. Typically these are macrocytic; however, sideroblastic anemia also can occur. Microcytic anemia is typically associated with blood loss from ulcers or cancers. Thrombocytopenia can be a rare complication of alcoholism.

Mammary Glands

Chronically heavy-drinking women are at increased risk of breast cancer.

Central Nervous System

Impairment of cognitive function is a common complaint among chronic heavy drinkers. Of these, the specific deficit of Korsakoff syndrome needs to be tested for by the examination of short-term memory. Dementias caused by alcohol may complicate those of other etiologies, particularly those of the Alzheimer and multi-infarct type. Rare and complex neurologic disorders, such as central pontine myelinosis, also are associated with chronic heavy alcohol consumption.

Fetal Development

Alcohol and its metabolite acetaldehyde can have serious effects on the developing fetus. High levels of alcohol consumption in pregnant mothers can produce spontaneous abortion and *in utero* death. Infants born to mothers who drank heavily during pregnancy may suffer from fetal alcohol syndrome. Fetal alcohol syndrome can include severe mental retardation, small head, short stature, facial deformity (absent philtrum, flattened nasal bridge, and an epicanthal eye fold), syndactyly, and atrial septal defect.

Laboratory Tests

Laboratory tests may provide evidence that increases the physician's suspicion about the possibility that the patient may be a heavy drinker. Laboratory tests can also provide evidence to substantiate a history of heavy drinking. A complete blood count may lead to the finding of anemia, typically macrocytic, but it also could be microcytic or sideroblastic. Triglyceride levels are typically elevated. Abnormal liver function tests are common, particularly elevation of the enzyme, γ-glutamyl transferase (GGT). Bilirubin and uric acid levels also may be raised. Recently, measurement of percent carbohydrate-deficient transferrin (CDT) level, a carrier protein, was approved by the

Food and Drug Administration (FDA) as a marker of heavy drinking. Research evidence suggests that serial measurements of the combination of CDT and GGT are the best biochemical method in a particular individual to characterize heavy drinking behavior. Raised mean corpuscular volume (MCV) is a traditional measure of heavy drinking; however, its predictive power is low. Knowledge that heavy drinking may result in the derangement of multiple biochemical and hematologic measures has been used over the last two decades to develop the early detection of alcohol consumption (EDAC) score. The short version of the EDAC score compiles 13 tests—Na, Cl, K, bilirubin ratio, total protein, cholesterol, high-density lipoprotein, albumin, GGT, aspartate aminotransferase, MCV, white blood cell count, and monocytes. More specific biochemical markers of recent heavy alcohol consumption are under development.

Complications of Alcoholism

Acute Effects

The acute effects of alcohol depend on the time course of drinking. During the initial period of up to 30 minutes after ingesting even small amounts of alcohol (ascending curve), there is typically mood elevation, which is then followed by sedative and anxiolytic effects. Additionally, the blood alcohol concentration (BAC) reached is practically a direct function of the amount ingested.

Depending on the BAC reached, there are various consequences of intoxication. The acute consumption of large amounts of alcohol can lead to profound respiratory depression (especially if combined with tranquilizers), followed by coma and death. Rare acute complications of alcohol dependence include alcohol-induced psychotic disorder and Wernicke encephalopathy. *Alcohol-induced psychotic disorder* usually occurs in the presence of active drinking, but also has been described during withdrawal. It is characterized by the acute onset of visual and auditory hallucinations, and schizophreniform like delusions of a persecutory nature. A distinguishing feature between alcoholic hallucinosis and delirium tremens is that the former occurs in clear consciousness. Typically, alcohol-induced psychotic disorder lasts about 10 to 15 days. *Wernicke encephalopathy* is a life-threatening condition, and individuals with this disorder are typically managed in an intensive care unit, where fluid and electrolyte support and assisted mechanical ventilation, if needed, can be provided.

Chronic Effects

Perhaps the best-known chronic effect of heavy drinking is liver disease, which can manifest in two forms: *fatty liver* and *liver cirrhosis*. Although the former may progress to the latter, the relationship between the two conditions is not direct. Chronic alcoholism also tends to be associated with malabsorption and multiple vitamin B deficiencies, which typically present as *peripheral neuropathy*. A third disorder, *Korsakoff syndrome*, is also a chronic condition brought about by the deficiency of thiamin. Korsakoff syndrome is associated with damage to the mamillary bodies, and its most striking feature is short-term memory impairment. Because individuals with this disorder often confabulate to fill in memory gaps, diagnosis of this condition is often missed if memory is not specifically tested in the mental state examination.

Alcohol Withdrawal

Chronic heavy drinkers who abstain from alcohol for more than a few hours can experience *withdrawal* symptoms. These withdrawal symptoms can vary widely in intensity and typically start with tremulousness and signs of sympathetic overactivity such as palpitations and sweating. At its most extreme, alcohol withdrawal can produce the syndrome of *delirium tremens*, occurring about 24 to 48 hours after alcohol cessation, which is characterized by clouding of consciousness, phonemes (auditory and vivid visual hallucinations, typically of the persecutory type), and seizures. Rarely, individuals may experience seeing animals or people of small or diminished size, often in amusing guises; these are termed *Lilliputian hallucinations*. However, a more common and disturbing hallucination is that associated with the sensation of insects crawling over the skin (*tactile hallucinations*). The mortality rate from delirium tremens is approximately 5% to 15%. Typically, the signs and symptoms of alcohol withdrawal have a progressive nature from mild to severe. It is reasonable to expect that a chronic heavy drinker with confirmed abstinence for more than 72 hours with mild and nonprogressing withdrawal symptoms is unlikely to experience severe withdrawal symptoms from this episode a day or two later.

Comorbidity

Among addictive disorders, the highest association rates of alcoholism are with nicotine dependence. Alcoholism also occurs commonly with addiction to narcotics. For example, up to 89% of cocaine-dependent individuals are also dependent on alcohol. Prevalence estimates of alcohol misuse among cocaine-dependent individuals are twice as high as for opiates. Alcoholism is associated with greater severity of cocaine dependence, and increased alcohol misuse commonly follows the establishment of cocaine dependence. Misuse of other psychostimulants, sedatives (e.g., benzodiazepines, barbiturates, and marijuana), and hallucinogenic drugs also occurs commonly against a background of alcohol abuse or dependence.

An interesting feature of the comorbidity of alcoholism with other addictive disorders is that the association is greatest for those with the youngest age of onset of problem drinking. This raises the possibility that such individuals either may be particularly prone to inheriting a range of addictive or impulse dyscontrol disorders or may come from a familial or psychosocial background that encourages substance use, or both. Individuals with alcohol dependence also tend to have high rates of comorbidity with other psychiatric disorders. Of these, the more notable association appears to be with alcoholism and a variety of affective and anxiety-related disorders. For example, between 33% and 67% of individuals with alcohol dependence also have major depression, and up to 60% of people with bipolar disorder either abuse or are dependent on alcohol. Rates of alcohol abuse and dependence are high among those with anxiety or posttraumatic stress disorder. Antisocial personality disorder is common among those who develop problem drinking early in life, and tends to develop a few years before the problem drinking, leading to the proposition that antisocial personality disorder is the primary disorder in such individuals. Rates of alcohol abuse and dependence are also elevated among individuals with schizophreniform disorders. Although it is premature to posit an overarching theory that might explain the co-occurrence of alcoholism and other psychiatric disorders, it is tempting to speculate that these conditions might be related through dimensional constructs that affect impulse dyscontrol.

Treatment

The acute effects of alcohol are seldom treated as the symptoms tend to subside with time. Nevertheless, it is sometimes important to intervene medically, especially if there is a risk of profound respiratory depression. In this instance, flumazenil (a benzodiazepine antagonist) has been used to reverse alcohol-related respiratory suppression and coma. Typically, this treatment is administered on highly supervised medical units, where supportive therapy (which may include assisted mechanical ventilation) is available. Similarly, the treatment of Wernicke syndrome is a medical emergency requiring treatment on a highly supervised medical unit. The mainstay of treatment for Wernicke syndrome is intravenous hydration and thiamin. Magnesium sulfate is often a component of treatment to reduce the potential for seizures. The mortality rate from Wernicke encephalopathy may exceed 50%, even in specialized centers.

The chronic sequelae of alcohol dependence are typically managed in medical settings and are designed specifically to address the secondary disorder(s). For example, the treatment for alcohol-induced malabsorption leading to vitamin B deficiency disorders is, of course, to administer the appropriate vitamin supplements, usually for a period of several months. Of the other conditions, Korsakoff syndrome deserves special mention because it may be mostly reversible in some cases with appropriate treatment. It is important to administer thiamin at appropriate doses (100 mg/day) for at least 6 months, and in some cases, continued improvements have been seen with medication administration periods of up to 1 year or more.

The treatment of alcohol withdrawal depends on its severity. Individuals with mild withdrawal symptoms are typically treated with small doses of the long-acting benzodiazepine, chlordiazepoxide, for no more than a few days. Severe withdrawal syndromes, especially those complicated by neuropsychiatric disorders such as delirium tremens and seizures, require hospitalization. As a rough guide, individuals withdrawing from alcohol with clinical institute withdrawal assessment for alcohol scale–revised (CIWA-Ar) scores of less than 12 can often be managed as outpatients, but those above this threshold may require hospitalization; however, this decision should be based also on clinical condition, taking the particular characteristics of each individual into consideration.

The treatment of alcohol dependence *per se* usually starts with the individual's recognition that he or she needs treatment for the disorder. Unfortunately, because of the prevailing societal stigma of alcohol dependence, most people with alcohol dependence need to be confronted by a family member, friend, or health worker for them to present for treatment. New methods using a more empathetic approach, by highlighting the negative consequences of drinking to the patient and allowing the patient to move into advanced stages of readiness for change, show better success in getting individuals with alcohol dependence to seek treatment. Although some alcohol-dependent individuals with low levels of motivation and severely impaired lifestyles may require long-term rehabilitation, there is growing awareness that most people can be treated as outpatients. Irrespective of treatment setting, the modalities of available treatment are a variety of psychosocial treatments either alone or with the addition of pharmacotherapy.

Perhaps the best-known psychosocial intervention for individuals dependent on alcohol has been referral to Alcoholics Anonymous. This psychosocial treatment is, however, better described as 12-step facilitation. Basically, the treatment formalizes 12 steps through which the alcohol-dependent individual needs to progress to initiate recovery. The hallmark of treatment is that drinkers admit that they are powerless over alcohol, appraise their morals, admit the nature of their wrongs, make a list of everyone they have harmed, and make plans to make amends to those people. Cognitive–behavioral therapy also is a common treatment for alcohol dependence. The key to improvement is to teach the addicted individual cognitive and behavioral skills for changing the drinking behavior. Motivational enhancement therapy uses the addicted individual's own desire for change as the treatment vehicle. A landmark study comparing the relative effectiveness of 12-step facilitation, cognitive–behavioral therapy, and motivational enhancement therapy found them to be equally useful. Importantly, there is a growing and compelling literature on the use of brief interventions for the treatment of alcohol dependence. These have the advantage of being more easily delivered by nonspecialized staff in generic settings; however, some authorities have questioned their suitability for those with severe lifestyle impairment or a high chronicity of disease.

In the last decade, there has been growing interest in the use of pharmacotherapies for the treatment of alcohol dependence. Disulfiram (Antabuse) is perhaps the most widely used medication in the United States. Disulfiram works by inhibiting aldehyde dehydrogenase, thereby preventing the metabolism of the primary metabolite of alcohol: acetaldehyde; this leads to the production of a range of unpleasant side effects, such as nausea, vomiting, flushing, sympathetic overactivity, and palpitations, if drinking is initiated. However, disulfiram is effective only in those with a high level of motivation and a supportive partner to help ensure that it is taken—just the sort of alcohol-dependent individuals who are likely to abstain on their own. In 1995, the μ-opioid antagonist naltrexone was approved by the FDA for the treatment of alcohol dependence. Naltrexone presumably works at maintaining abstinence by reducing the craving for alcohol. Acamprosate is also used for the treatment of alcohol dependence. Other promising medications are in development for the treatment of alcohol dependence. For example, the serotonin-3 antagonist ondansetron (Zofran; 4 μg/kg) has shown promise in a double-blind, randomized clinical trial as a treatment for early onset alcoholism. Early onset alcoholics differ from those of late onset by having greater familial disease predisposition, serotonergic dysregulation, and a range of antisocial behaviors. The combination of ondansetron and naltrexone may be even more effective for the treatment of early onset alcoholism than either alone. Selective serotonin reuptake inhibitors may be effective as a treatment for late onset alcoholism. Finally, a recent double-blind trial showed that the anticonvulsant topiramate (Topamax; up to 300 mg/day) appears to be an effective treatment for alcoholism.

Despite the marked advances in alcoholism treatment, some individuals with alcohol dependence will go through several periods of alternating sobriety and relapse before attaining the ultimate goal of sustained sobriety. Therefore, treatment(s) that convert an individual's heavy drinking to nonpathologic levels may be a practical short-term goal. Although there is always the risk of relapse when alcohol-dependent individuals remain exposed to drinking, even at very low levels, there may be some advantages to a harm-reduction approach.

Conclusion

Increasingly new knowledge about the pathophysiology of alcoholism, and how a multitude of biologic, psychosocial, sociocultural, and environmental factors influence the alcoholism disease. The complexity of the potential sequelae of alcohol dependence means that a variety of physicians, and not only psychiatrists, as well as a range of treatment settings, are needed to provide a comprehensive level of care. Treatments for alcohol dependence are becoming even more effective, and developments in the neurosciences have promulgated important advances in the use of pharmacotherapies for the treatment of alcohol dependence.

Suggested Readings

Boehm SL II, Valenzuela CF, Harris RA. Alcohol: neurobiology. In: Lowinson JH, Ruiz P, Millman RB, et al., eds. *Substance abuse: a comprehensive textbook*, 4th ed. Philadelphia: Lippincott Williams & Wilkins; 2005:121–151.

DeWit DJ, Adlaf EM, Offord DR, et al. Age at first alcohol use: a risk factor for the development of alcohol disorders. *Am J Psychiatry.* 2000;157:745–750.

Johnson BA, Ait-Daoud N. Alcohol: clinical aspects. In: Lowinson JH, Ruiz P, Millman RB, et al., eds. *Substance abuse: a comprehensive textbook*, 4th ed. Philadelphia: Lippincott Williams & Wilkins; 2005:151–163.

Johnson BA, Ait-Daoud N. Neuropharmacological treatments for alcoholism: scientific basis and clinical findings. *Psychopharmacology.* 2000;149:327–344.

Johnson BA, Ruiz P, Galanter M, eds. *Handbook of clinical alcoholism treatment.* Baltimore: Lippincott Williams & Wilkins; 2003.

Kranzler HR, Pierucci-Lagha A, Feinn R, et al. Effects of ondansetron in early- versus late-onset alcoholics: a prospective, open-label study. *Alcohol Clin Exp Res.* 2003;27:1150–1155.

3

OPIATES

Opioid Receptors and Endogenous Opioid Peptides

In the 1940s and 1950s, a very active synthetic program was mounted by the pharmaceutical industry in an attempt to produce a nonaddictive analgesic. The work yielded a number of scientific findings, which gave rise to the hypothesis that opiate drugs must bind to highly specific sites or receptors on nerve cells in order to exert most of their effects. This hypothesis was based on the observation that many of the pharmacologic effects of these drugs exhibit considerable stereospecificity; that is, the levorotatory enantiomer is usually active, and the dextrorotatory form is essentially inactive. In 1973, evidence for the existence of stereospecific binding sites for opiates in animal brain was published, and it is now generally accepted that these binding sites are receptors that mediate various pharmacologic effects of the opiate drugs.

The important finding that specific receptors for opiate drugs exist led to the postulate that endogenous opiate-like ligands are likely to exist in the body. At least eight peptides with opioid activity have been found, including the endorphins, of which the most important is β-endorphin. Dynorphin is a very potent opioid peptide with Leu-enkephalin at its N-terminal. It is a very basic peptide; that is, it contains many basic amino acids, such as lysine and arginine, and is clearly not derived from β-lipotropin. Because these opioid peptides are thought to be the natural ligands of the opiate receptors, the latter have been renamed *opioid* receptors.

The techniques of molecular biology have permitted some order to be established among the many opioid peptides known. All the known opioid peptides are derived from three large precursor proteins—pro-opiomelanocortin (POMC), proenkephalin, and prodynorphin—each of which is encoded by a separate gene with known structure.

The discovery of POMC was of considerable importance for the entire field of biology. It was the first protein precursor found to give rise to several different and seemingly unrelated biologically active peptides. In addition to being the precursor of the endorphins, POMC gives rise to adrenocorticotropin (ACTH) and a family of melanocyte-stimulating hormones. The intermediate lobe of the pituitary is the major source of POMC, and β-endorphin is the major opioid peptide derived from this precursor. It exists mainly in the pituitary gland and the central nervous system (CNS). Proenkephalin has been cloned and sequenced from bovine and human tissues.

It contains one copy of Leu-enkephalin, four copies of Met-enkephalin, and two copies of C–terminal-extended Met-enkephalin peptides, a heptapeptide and an octapeptide. Prodynorphin, the last of the opioid peptide precursors to be characterized, has been isolated from various mammalian tissues, including brain and spinal cord, pituitary and adrenal glands, and reproductive organs. All of the opioid peptides derived from this protein, dynorphin A and B and α-neoendorphin and β-neoendorphin are C-terminal extensions of Leu-enkephalin.

There is considerable similarity between the three precursors and between their genes. They contain almost the same total number of amino acids. All have several opioid peptides contained largely in the C-terminal half of the molecule and framed by pairs of basic amino acids. They all possess a cysteine-rich N-terminal sequence preceded by similarly sized signal peptides. There is considerable amino acid sequence homology, which in the case of proenkephalin and prodynorphin exceeds 50%. The genes also exhibit similarity in the placement and size of their respective introns and exons. All this evidence has given rise to the hypothesis that the three genes developed from a common ancestor gene by gene duplication in the course of evolution.

All the opioid peptides produce a variety of pharmacologic effects when injected intraventricularly, including analgesia, respiratory depression, and a wide variety of behavioral changes. The peptides do not pass very efficiently through the blood–brain barrier, but a number of effects, particularly on memory and learning, have been reported for systemically administered opioid peptides. Presumably, only very tiny amounts of the peptides are required to penetrate into the CNS. The actions of the enkephalins tend to be short lived, probably as a result of their rapid destruction by peptidases. The longer-chain peptides tend to be more stable and produce effects of long duration. All the responses to endogenous opioids are readily reversed by opiate antagonists, such as naloxone and naltrexone.

Opioid Receptor Properties and Distribution

The discovery of the enkephalins led to the postulate of another receptor type with preference for these opioid pentapeptides. Enkephalins were much less effective than morphine in inhibiting electrically evoked contractions of the isolated guinea pig ileum, whereas the reverse was true in the isolated mouse vas deferens. The enkephalin-preferring receptor that seemed to predominate in the latter tissue was named delta (for *d*eferens).

Since then several additional types of receptors have been postulated, most notably a specific receptor for β-endorphin called epsilon and another receptor for the enkephalins, different from β receptors, called iota, because it seemed to predominate in intestines. Subtypes of receptors have also been suggested. The sigma receptor is not truly an opioid receptor, because actions mediated via this receptor are not reversed by the opiate antagonist naloxone, an operational definition of opioid receptors that is widely accepted.

The most recently discovered receptor is not really an opioid receptor, although it has very high amino acid homology with the opioid receptor family and especially with the κ receptor; it is called the opioid receptor like (ORL1) receptor. An endogenous peptide that appears to be the natural ligand for this receptor is called orphanin FQ (because ORL-1 had been for some time an "orphan" receptor in search of a ligand). The ligand has also been called nociceptin, because receptor activation alters nociception. The ORL-1 receptors do not bind opioid peptides or opiate drugs. This system is widely distributed in the brain and spinal cord. Its activation produces hyperalgesia in most instances, although analgesia and no effect on pain have also been reported.

Opioid Actions

Opioid drugs are defined and categorized in terms of their capacity to bind and activate opioid receptors. Those that bind and activate a receptor are *agonists* at that receptor. Those that bind but do not activate a receptor function as *antagonists* at that receptor. Opioids can differ greatly in their relative affinity for receptor types. They can also differ in their intrinsic activity in that they may bind very well to a receptor, but produce less than full receptor activation (a *partial agonist*), and under some circumstances, act as an antagonist at that same receptor.

Effects of opioids on pain and anticipation of pain and distress can be profound. At high enough doses, indifference to pain is sufficient to permit major surgery, but the profound respiratory depression that accompanies this level of opioid effect requires mechanical support of respiration. More commonly, opioids are used as analgesics in much lower doses. There appear to be significant differences among individuals in the way they feel when they take opioids. Postaddict volunteers usually experience an elevation of mood and increased sense of self-esteem (i.e., euphoria). Others given the same dose may complain of confusion and drowsiness, which they experience as unpleasant. Heroin addicts who do not have a high tolerance sometimes experience nausea and vomiting along with a sense of euphoria. When mu agonist opioids are self-administered intravenously (or, sometimes, when smoked) there is a sharp and rapid increase in brain opioid levels that produces a distinct, intense, and generally pleasurable sensation (a "flash" or "rush").

Included among the many other effects opioids produce through their CNS action are suppression of the cough reflex (which makes them useful antitussives) and effects on the neuroendocrine system. Most neuroendocrine effects, such as the inhibition of gonadotropin-releasing hormone—which results in decreased luteinizing hormone (LH) and follicle-stimulating hormone (FSH) and, ultimately, in decreased testosterone levels in males and disturbed menstrual function in females—are unwanted side effects. Opioid inhibition of corticotropin-releasing factor (CRF) results in decreased adrenocorticotropic hormone (ACTH) and decreased levels of cortisol.

μ-agonist opioids have effects on the gastrointestinal system, such as slowing the passage of food in the stomach, small intestine, and large intestine. Because of this action, opioid drugs are therapeutic agents in the treatment of diarrhea. Because little tolerance develops to this gut-slowing effect, patients with chronic pain given large doses of opioids are often constipated, as are heroin addicts if their supply is uninterrupted over long periods. Former addicts maintained on methadone also typically have problems with constipation. Mixed agonist–antagonist opioids and κ agonists have less-prominent constipating effects.

Some opioids, such as morphine, produce histamine release, which is associated with vasodilatation of skin vessels and itching. The nose scratching seen when addicts are quite intoxicated is probably related, in part, to this effect. However, pruritus is also seen with opioids that do not release histamine. The effects of most opioids on the cardiovascular system are not prominent except under special circumstances; one of these is hypovolemia, in which opioids can aggravate shock. In rare instances levo-alpha-acetylmethadol (LAAM) may produce prolongation of the QT interval and cardiac arrhythmias including torsades de pointes. Opioids also have effects on the bladder; they tend to increase sphincter tone and decrease the voiding reflexes; in this way, they can increase the likelihood of urinary retention.

Mechanisms of Opioid Action

Opioid peptides are thought to exert their actions at neuronal synapses as either neurotransmitters or neuromodulators. It is likely that the peptides act as neurotransmitters, that is, by altering (generally decreasing) the transsynaptic potential, when their receptors are localized presynaptically. On the other hand, evidence suggests that many opioid receptors are localized postsynaptically. In this case, the peptides modulate the release of a neurotransmitter.

It is now definitely established that all three major types of opioid receptors are coupled to G proteins. The early results were obtained in cell cultures, but more recent results show this to be true in the brain. The G proteins, in turn, can couple the receptors either to second messenger systems or directly to ion channels. It is thought that the slower effects of opioids may be exerted via inhibition of the enzyme adenylate cyclase, which synthesizes the second messenger, cyclic adenosine $3',5'$-monophosphate (cAMP). The level of cAMP affects the activity of an enzyme that is able to phosphorylate proteins (cAMP-activated protein kinase A). The phosphorylation of synaptic proteins would have relatively immediate effects. It is also possible that other proteins that act on gene expression can be phosphorylated, resulting in a downregulation or upregulation of gene transcription. This could be responsible for some of the very long-lasting changes produced by opiates.

It is a widely held view that many of the long-term effects of opiates are the result of somatic cell changes in gene expression. The signaling system that has been implicated in gene regulation is the mitogen-activated protein (MAP) kinase cascade. The phosphorylation of kinases in this pathway results in changes in gene expression in many situations. In 1995, it was shown that G protein–coupled receptors (GPCRs) were able to activate this pathway. This was quickly followed by the finding that opioid receptors are no exception. It has long been established that the phosphorylation of one or more receptor tyrosine residues is a prerequisite for the activation of the MAP kinase cascade. For some of the GPCRs it was demonstrated that this was accomplished by a cross-phosphorylation of tyrosine residues in a tyrosine kinase receptor, when the GPCR is activated. However, in the case of opioid receptors, tyrosine phosphorylation can, in fact, occur in the opioid receptor protein itself.

The rapid effects of opioids are most likely a result of direct action of activated opioid receptors on ion channels. It was established that the mu and delta opioid receptors open potassium channels, which results in reduction of calcium conductance. The activation of κ receptors was found to reduce calcium conductance by closing calcium channels. It was recently found that all three types of opioid receptors can act by both mechanisms; that is, they can open potassium channels or close calcium channels.

Pain and Its Modulation

Many early experiments involved attempts to demonstrate that nondrug-induced types of analgesia could be reversed by naloxone. If successful, this would suggest the involvement of endorphin release onto their receptors.

More direct evidence for the release of opioid peptides during analgesia has been obtained. Using indwelling intraventricular cannulae, it has been observed that a large increase in the amount of β-endorphin is released into the cerebrospinal fluid of patients with terminal cancer after analgesia caused by stimulation of electrodes implanted in the central gray region of the brain. There is also found an increased release of enkephalins during pain stimulation.

It is now widely accepted that all three of the major receptor types are involved in analgesia, but some evidence that they may be implicated in different kinds of pain is also becoming available. Thus, most reports suggest that supraspinal analgesia may be mediated via mu rather than delta or κ receptors. At the spinal level, analgesia against thermal pain stimuli seems to be mediated by both mu and delta mechanisms, whereas κ receptors seem to preferentially mediate analgesia against chemically induced visceral pain.

It is evident that much is yet to be learned regarding the mechanisms underlying analgesia and endogenous pain modulation. However, the evidence that suggests that the endogenous opioid system is involved in at least some of these mechanisms is quite impressive.

Drug Disposition

Conjugation with glucuronide is a major route of metabolism for several opioid agents. Glucuronidation of morphine involves its conversion to morphine-3-glucuronide, and to a lesser extent, morphine-6-glucuronide. Morphine-6-glucuronide is a more potent analgesic agent than morphine and may contribute significantly to the analgesic effects of morphine. Renal insufficiency can lead to a reduction in the clearance rate of morphine-6-glucuronide and the resultant high concentrations of this compound may have toxic effects.

The meperidine metabolite normeperidine may also accumulate to produce toxicity in patients with renal dysfunction. Normeperidine has no analgesic activity but can induce seizures and cause serious problems, such as twitching, tremors, and mental confusion. Problems can also arise when excessive amounts of meperidine (Demerol) are used, as in meperidine addiction.

In some instances, the drug administered is actually inactive, and only when metabolized does it readily attach to and activate opioid receptors (a prodrug). For example, heroin (diacetylmorphine) is not itself a potent mu agonist; but, because it is more lipid soluble than morphine, it can more rapidly enter the brain, where it is converted to 6-mono-acetyl-morphine and morphine. In the brain, heroin and morphine produce virtually identical effects because heroin acts primarily as morphine and 6-mono-acetyl-morphine. Very little heroin is detected in the urine of heroin addicts; what is excreted is morphine.

Codeine is also primarily a prodrug, and does not bind significantly to opioid receptors. However, in the body, a small percentage of codeine is converted to morphine, which then may produce its characteristic effects. Codeine is valuable clinically because it is well absorbed when given by mouth and is not deactivated by the liver as it is absorbed into the bloodstream. Individuals taking codeine for medical purposes usually have traces of morphine in their urine.

Drug Interactions

The biotransformation of several opioids is catalyzed by cytochrome P450 enzymes. Many compounds may selectively inhibit the activity of different isoforms of these enzymes. Some of these enzyme inhibitors may be substrates of specific enzymes; that is, their transformation is catalyzed by that enzyme, and they inhibit metabolism through competitive inhibition. Other compounds inhibit enzymes but are not substrates of these enzymes. These inhibitors may reduce enzyme activity by mechanisms such as noncompetitive inhibition.

The cytochrome enzyme CYP3A4 has been implicated as playing a major role in the metabolism of several opioids, including alfentanil, buprenorphine, fentanyl, LAAM, methadone, sufentanil, and tramadol. This enzyme mediates the dealkylation of buprenorphine, an action that is inhibited by the CYP3A4 inhibitor ketoconazole. The oxidative N-dealkylation of alfentanil, fentanyl, and sufentanil are all catalyzed by CYP3A4. Severe respiratory depression has occurred when fentanyl levels were markedly elevated after the administration of the CYP3A4 inhibitor, ritonavir (Norvir). Several agents, including troleandomycin (Tao), midazolam (Versed), ketoconazole (Nizoral), and nefazodone (Serzone) may inhibit CYP3A4 from catalyzing the biotransformation of alfentanil.

CYP3A4 plays a major role in the biotransformation of methadone into its main metabolite, EDDP. Inhibitors of CYP3A, including troleandomycin, ketoconazole, and fluvoxamine (Luvox), can readily block the formation of EDDP from methadone. Administration of ciprofloxacin, a CYP3A4 inhibitor, has produced marked respiratory depression when administered to a patient being treated with methadone. Plasma levels of methadone may be elevated by a number of CYP3A4 inhibitors, including fluconazole (Diflucan) and fluvoxamine. However, two inhibitors of CYP3A, ritonavir and nelfinavir (Viracept), paradoxically decrease methadone plasma concentrations via an unknown mechanism. The administration of substances that produce an induction of the CYP3A enzyme may produce a reduction in plasma methadone concentrations that, in turn, may lead to withdrawal in maintenance therapy patients. This can occur after the administration of the CYP3A inducer rifampin.

In addition to CYP3A4, the biotransformation of methadone may be metabolized by several other enzymes, including CYP2C9 and CYP2C19. The role played by the CYP2D6 enzyme in the metabolism of methadone remains unclear. Administration of either paroxetine (Paxil) or fluoxetine (Prozac), which are both inhibitors of CYP2D6, can produce elevations in the plasma concentrations of the active enantiomer (i.e., the R-enantiomer) of methadone.

The biotransformation of codeine is catalyzed by the CYP2D6 enzyme, which also catalyzes the transformation of hydrocodone into hydromorphone (Dilaudid) and oxycodone (OxyContin) into oxymorphone (Numorphan). Small subpopulations of individuals are poor metabolizers of these drugs as compared to most of the population who extensively metabolize these agents. Poor metabolizers of codeine will obtain less analgesia from codeine than will extensive metabolizers. A deficiency in the ability of individuals to metabolize codeine may result from polymorphisms of the CYP2D6 genes, which lead to altered enzyme activity. Between 4% and 10% of the white population are poor metabolizers of dextromethorphan.

Quinidine can inhibit the activity of CYP2D6 and the administration of this drug has the potential to reduce the analgesic potency of codeine and related compounds. Quinidine may inhibit the metabolism of tramadol, which is also dependent on CYP2D6 for its biotransformation into an active metabolite. The rate of biotransformation of tramadol, codeine, and related compounds metabolized by CYP2D6 may also be decreased by fluoxetine and paroxetine.

Other pharmacokinetic interactions may also have clinical importance. Propoxyphene (Darvon), which is structurally related to methadone, can inhibit the metabolism of carbamazepine (Tegretol). The metabolism of meperidine is increased by either phenytoin or phenobarbital treatment, resulting in increased normeperidine levels. Chronic carbamazepine treatment can lead to an increase in the rate at which tramadol is metabolized. Finally, the clearance of zidovudine (Retrovir) is reduced by both acute and chronic methadone administration. This action may result, in part, from the inhibition of the glucuronidation of zidovudine by methadone.

Certain opioid-related drug interactions do not involve the factors that regulate drug pharmacokinetics. Many CNS depressants, including barbiturates, benzodiazepines, propofol (Diprivan), and neuroleptics, may potentiate the sedative actions of opioids. The administration of either meperidine or tramadol to patients being treated with monoamine oxidase inhibitors (MAOIs), such as phenelzine (Nardil) or tranylcypromine (Parnate), can cause toxic reactions to occur. These reactions may result from alterations in cerebral serotonin levels and in the case of tramadol also norepinephrine levels. The administration of meperidine to a patient being treated with an MAOI may lead to hypertension, excitement, hyperreflexia, hyperthermia, and tachycardia. This reaction may progress to coma and sometimes death. The administration of tramadol may increase the risk of seizures in patients also being treated with tricyclic antidepressants, cyclobenzaprine (Flexeril), promethazine (Phenergan), selective serotonin-reuptake inhibitors, for example, fluoxetine, sertraline (Zoloft), paroxetine, and neuroleptic agents.

Opioid Addiction

Three major hypotheses have been put forth to account for continued opioid use: (a) after a period of opioid use (for whatever reason), people become physically dependent and continue use to avoid the distress of withdrawal; (b) people continue to use opioids because they like the effects (e.g., euphoria) produced; and (c) for some people opioids alleviate some pre-existing dysphoric or painful affective state (i.e., it is used for self-medication).

Although there is some comfort in the hypothesis that only a limited percentage of the population will experience opioid euphoria and, therefore, be vulnerable to opioid dependence, the proportion of the population that is vulnerable must be quite large. When heroin was widely available to U.S. Army personnel in Vietnam, 42% of enlisted men experimented with opioids and, of these, about half became physically dependent.

One of the most significant advances in understanding how opioids can lead to sustained drug-using behavior and relapse to opioid use after a period of withdrawal has been the recognition that both drug effects and drug withdrawal phenomena can become linked through learning to environmental cues and internal mood states. Because the concept of learned or conditioned craving tends to amplify and extend both the motivating effects of opioid withdrawal and their positive reinforcing actions, it is presented here not as a distinct hypothesis about continued opioid use, but as a process that should be considered whatever the initial or primary motives for use may have been.

There is little question that opioid withdrawal produces dysphoria and significant distress and that avoidance of opioid withdrawal can be a major motive for continuing opioid use. However, avoidance of withdrawal does not readily explain relapse once withdrawal phenomena have abated. Consequently, much current work focuses on how the acute effects of drugs come to have so much value for the individual that other values are subordinated to the goal of obtaining and using opioids, and on how emotions and environmental cues re-evoke the distress of withdrawal or the memory of opioid euphoria or opioid reduction of dysphoria.

Physical Dependence (Neuroadaptation) and Tolerance

Physical dependence is usually defined as an altered state of biology induced by a drug, such that when the drug is withdrawn (or displaced from its receptors by an antagonist), a complex set of biologic events (withdrawal or abstinence phenomena) ensue that are typical for that drug (or class of drugs) and that are distinct from a simple return to normal function. Physical dependence may develop within a single cell (e.g., a neuron in a culture), a complex of cells (e.g., the spinal cord), or the whole organism. Physical dependence can be observed with a number of pharmacologic classes that have psychoactive effects, including opioids, CNS depressants, and nicotine, as well as with drugs not ordinarily thought of as psychoactive agents.

The biologic changes responsible for opioid physical dependence begin as soon as opioid receptors are activated by opioid agonists. With prototypical μ-opioid agonists such as morphine, some degree of physical dependence can be induced in nontolerant human volunteers by single doses of opioids in the same dose range used for analgesia. The low degree of physical dependence induced in this way is of little clinical significance, and withdrawal symptoms are not typically seen when opioids are given briefly for acute pain. However, even this degree of physical dependence can easily be demonstrated by administering a specific antagonist such as naloxone. Subjects given up to 10 mg of naloxone 6 hours after a dose of morphine report nausea and other feelings of dysphoria and exhibit yawning, sweating, tearing, and rhinorrhea. Certainly, *tolerance* to opioids can develop quite rapidly in opioid users, and in experiments with volunteers the dose of morphine can be increased from ordinary clinical doses (e.g., 60 mg/day) to 500 mg/day over as short a period as 10 days.

Although the characteristics of the opioid withdrawal syndrome produced by a variety of available μ-opioid agonists are all qualitatively similar, they can differ considerably with respect to the time of onset of symptoms, peak intensity, time to peak intensity, and duration of signs and symptoms. The opioid withdrawal syndrome includes dysphoric mood, nausea, vomiting, muscle aches, tearing, rhinorrhea, pupil dilation, sweating, diarrhea, and insomnia. In general, the time course and intensity of the opioid withdrawal syndrome are related to how quickly the specific agonist is removed from its receptors. Drugs such as heroin, morphine, and hydromorphone have relatively short biologic half-lives (2 to 3 hours). When these drugs are stopped after a period of chronic use, the receptors are cleared relatively quickly. The onset of observable withdrawal is typically within 8 to 12 hours, and the acute syndrome reaches peak intensity within 48 hours and then begins to subside over a period of about 5 to 7 days. With drugs such as methadone or LAAM, which have half-lives after chronic administration ranging from 16 hours to more than 60 hours and are sequestered in body tissues, observable withdrawal may not develop until 36 to 48 hours or more after the last dose, peak intensity may not develop until the fourth to sixth day, and some signs may persist for more than 14 days. When naloxone is used to displace methadone from its receptors, the onset of withdrawal is within minutes and a brief (30 to 60 minutes) but severe syndrome develops. As the naloxone is excreted, the methadone that is still in the body again binds to the receptors and withdrawal subsides.

The phenomena of tolerance and physical dependence appear to be relatively receptor specific. Hence, induction of tolerance to a mu agonist such as morphine will induce some degree of tolerance to other mu agonists such as hydromorphone, levorphanol, and methadone but little cross-tolerance to drugs acting primarily at κ receptors. However, tolerance to mu agonists is generally accompanied by mu agonist physical dependence and therefore any effort to abruptly substitute a κ agonist with either no action or antagonistic actions at the mu receptor will generally be associated with varying degrees of withdrawal. Because clinically available opioids have somewhat different profiles of relative receptor affinity, some patients may respond better to one than to another and cross-tolerance is often incomplete. Yet the cross-tolerance between methadone and other mu agonists is such that patients maintained on oral methadone doses of 60 to 100 mg report little or no euphoria from doses of up to 25 mg of heroin.

Some available agents categorized as agonist–antagonists (such as butorphanol, nalbuphine, and pentazocine) appear to exert either weak agonist or antagonist actions at the mu receptor, but their actions at other receptors, such as κ, render them useful analgesics. However, if such an agent is administered to individuals dependent on a μ-agonist such as morphine or heroin, it may displace the more potent agonists and precipitate mu agonist withdrawal. In general, these agonist–antagonists have lower abuse potential than prototypical mu agonists, probably because their actions at κ receptors are such that, when the dose is increased, most individuals begin to experience dysphoria rather than greater euphoria.

Buprenorphine is best characterized as a partial mu agonist. Given to nontolerant and nondependent volunteers, it is generally identified as an opioid drug and produces elevation of mood and other effects typical of morphine like agents, and it is considered to have abuse potential. However, it appears to exhibit a different slope for its dose–effect curve so that increasing doses do not produce comparable increases in euphoria or mu agonist toxicity (i.e., respiratory depression). At low levels of mu agonist physical dependence, buprenorphine can substitute for morphine or heroin in suppressing mu agonist withdrawal. However, at very high levels of mu agonist physical dependence it may not substitute completely or may precipitate withdrawal. Another interesting characteristic of buprenorphine is the tenacity with which it binds to the mu receptor. One consequence of this characteristic is that unusually high doses of naloxone are required to reverse effects of overdoses or to precipitate withdrawal.

Opioid Physical Dependence and Addiction

Physical dependence and *addiction* are not (or should not be) interchangeable terms. When a patient with intractable pain becomes physically dependent, the situation should not evoke any sense of urgency about "getting the patient off narcotics." Ideally, in such a situation the issue is proper pain management, and withdrawal from opioids is undertaken only when there is some confidence that pain can be managed without opioid drugs.

Treatment of individuals who are dependent on illicit opioids may involve the use of either maintenance therapies or medically managed withdrawal. Maintenance therapy can consist of either methadone or buprenorphine. Many individuals who have been maintained on a maintenance agent elect (or are pressured) to withdraw from maintenance opioid therapy. The approach to withdrawal must take into account the current clinical situation of the patient (i.e., what specific opioid, for how long, at what dose, and for what reason), any associated medical or psychiatric problems, past experiences with withdrawal, the motives of the patient in seeking withdrawal, the available clinical resources, and the patient's social support network.

The objective of medically managed withdrawal is to make the syndrome more tolerable for the individual. In a hospital, oral methadone may be used; after a day or two of stabilization, the methadone is reduced by approximately 20% per day. Modest withdrawal typically begins about the third or fourth day and often persists for a number of days after the dose has been reduced to zero. Relapse to opioids after brief in-hospital detoxification is quite high.

Another agent still occasionally used to manage withdrawal is clonidine, which acts on noradrenergic neurons that become hyperactive during μ-opioid agonist withdrawal. Clonidine suppresses many of the autonomic signs and symptoms of withdrawal, although it does little to alleviate the muscle aches, back pain, insomnia, and craving for opioids. It is usually given orally, 0.1 to 0.3 mg every 6 hours up to a total of 2 mg in hospitalized patients, and 1.2 mg/day in outpatients. Side effects of sedation and marked hypotension and continued subjective withdrawal discomfort limit the use of this medication.

Buprenorphine appears to be a very useful agent for managing opioid withdrawal. In contrast to clonidine, buprenorphine does not tend to produce marked decreases in blood pressure. Patients transferred to buprenorphine experience little or no withdrawal and craving is generally suppressed. Buprenorphine can then be discontinued. During acute detoxification of opioid-dependent patients buprenorphine reduces subjective and physiologic withdrawal symptoms with an efficacy comparable or greater than that of clonidine.

Following successful withdrawal from opioids, the opioid antagonist naltrexone may be administered on a chronic basis to block the reinforcing effects of opioids during periods of relapse. It has been difficult to demonstrate the efficacy of naltrexone. Noncompliance is a major problem associated with the use of naltrexone. There is evidence that the chronic administration of an opioid antagonist such as naltrexone produces an upregulation of opioid receptors. Following discontinuation of naltrexone, there is increased sensitivity to opioid actions. In recently detoxified opioid addicts, this could result in an increased risk of overdosage if they experiment with opioids soon after naltrexone discontinuation.

Opioid Toxicity

When opioids are given orally under medical supervision, even prolonged periods of use appear to produce no major toxic effects on physiologic systems. However, in some individuals it is likely that prolonged exposure to opioids induces long-lasting adaptive changes that require continued administration of an opioid to maintain normal mood states and normal responses to stress. In contrast to the modest effects of medically supervised oral opioids, the toxic effects associated with unsupervised use of illicit, often contaminated, opioids by parenteral routes are severe and quite common. These toxic effects range from acute and sometimes fatal overdoses to a wide variety of infections associated with contaminated injection implements, to neurologic, muscular, pulmonary, and renal damage, the etiology of which is sometimes obscure. Opioid users are more likely than age-matched controls to die as a result of suicide or violence. Prior to the beginning of the human immunodeficiency deficiency virus (HIV) epidemic, mortality among illicit opioid users was two to three times higher than that of age- and gender-matched controls for older addicts, and 20-fold higher for younger addicts.

The characteristic signs of acute opioid toxicity include varying degrees of clouded consciousness (up to complete and unresponsive coma), severe respiratory depression, and markedly constricted (pinpoint) pupils. Often, there is pulmonary edema associated with the severe respiratory depression. Although blood pressure is reduced by such doses of opioids, severe hypotension and cardiovascular collapse do not generally occur unless hypoxia is severe and prolonged. In such situations, the pupils may be dilated.

The first response should be to re-establish adequate ventilation and to administer an opioid antagonist such as naloxone. This should be given intravenously, if possible. Doses of less than 0.5 mg of naloxone are sometimes adequate to reverse respiratory depression, and the response is typically seen within 1 or 2 minutes of initial intravenous administration. Generally, if there is no substantial response to 5 to 10 mg of naloxone, there is little likelihood that the coma and respiratory depression are solely caused by opioid overdose. One possible exception is in the case of buprenorphine. As noted above, buprenorphine appears to bind firmly to receptors, so that if an overdose does occur, it is likely to require in excess of 10 mg of naloxone to antagonize its effects. Mild degrees of pulmonary edema may clear when the respiratory rate is normalized. More severe pulmonary edema may require positive pressure ventilation.

Naloxone is a short-acting drug. If the opioid overdose is caused by an agent with a much longer half-life such as methadone, the patient may lapse back into coma when the naloxone is metabolized and the methadone still present reattaches to the receptors. In such instances, continued observation of the patient is called for. Alternatively, it may be possible to follow naloxone with a longer-acting antagonist such as naltrexone orally, recognizing that, unless used judiciously, naltrexone could precipitate severe withdrawal.

Suggested Readings

Inturrisi CE. Clinical pharmacology of opioids for pain. *Clin J Pain.* 2002;18:S3–S13.

Knapp CM, Ciraulo DA, Jaffe J. Opiates: clinical aspects. In: Lowinson JH, Ruiz P, Millman RB, et al., eds. *Substance abuse: a comprehensive textbook,* 4th ed. Philadelphia: Lippincott Williams & Wilkins; 2005:180–195.

Kreek MJ, Bart G, Lilly C, et al. Pharmacogenetics and human molecular genetics of opiate and cocaine addictions and their treatment. *Pharmacol Rev.* 2005;57:1–26.

Pasternak GW. The pharmacology of mu analgesics: from patients to genes. *Neuroscientist.* 2001;7:220–231.

Simon EJ. Opiates: neurobiology. In: JH Lowinson JH, P Ruiz P, RB Millman RB, et al., eds. *Substance abuse: a comprehensive textbook,* 4th ed. Philadelphia: Lippincott Williams & Wilkins; 2005:164–180.

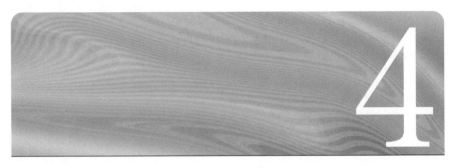

COCAINE

Neurobiologic Effects of Cocaine

Cocaine binds to the presynaptic transporter complexes inhibiting reuptake of dopamine (DA), noradrenaline, and serotonin, blocking the presynaptic reuptake of neurotransmitters and prolonging monoamine neurotransmission. The reinforcing properties of cocaine are believed to be associated with enhanced dopaminergic neurotransmission in mesocorticolimbic pathways. Hence there is a surplus of these neurotransmitters at the postsynaptic receptor sites. This surplus, in turn, activates responses along the sympathetic nervous system, producing such effects as vasoconstriction and acute increases in heart rate and blood pressure. DA neurons and DA release appear to demonstrate tolerance and diminished responses to chronic self-administration consistent with the notion of a functional DA deficit over time. By preventing DA reuptake, greater concentrations of DA remain in the synaptic cleft, with more DA available at the postsynaptic site for brain reinforcement, reward, or stimulation of specific salience-supporting receptors.

Clinical Pharmacology

Routes of Administration and Bioavailability

The principal routes of cocaine administration are oral, intranasal, intravenous, and inhalation. Oral absorption is the slowest, within 45 to 60 minutes. Although there is evidence that routes with quicker and higher peak absorption of cocaine lead to greater intoxication and addiction rates, any of the routes of administration can lead to absorption of large and toxic amounts of cocaine, especially once the onset of regular and addictive use is established. The absorption patterns parallel the behavioral and subjective effects of cocaine. Most controlled studies report close correlation between the plasma levels of cocaine and the physiologic and behavioral effects.

The purity of the preparations influences the rate and completeness of absorption of cocaine. In coca leaf chewing, the purity is 0.5%; it is higher for the cocaine hydrochloride form taken via the oral or intranasal route, with a wide range of 20% to 80%. The purity for intravenous preparations and the smoked form also varies, from 7% to 100% for the former, and from 40% to 100% for the latter.

Orally consumed cocaine has an area under the curve, or total amount absorbed, equal to that of the intranasal route, with bioavailability of 20% to 30%. The loss of cocaine after oral absorption is a result of the first-pass hepatic biotransformation, which metabolizes 70% to 80% of the dose. For oral absorption, the cocaine concentrations in the blood rise slowly such that at 10 to 15 minutes, levels are 30 to 50 ng/mL, with a peak of 160 ng/mL at about 60 minutes. The slow and more sloped peak blood level is thought to be responsible for the apparent low rate of addiction for the oral route.

After intranasal absorption, the loss of cocaine is a result of the poor penetration of the ionized form of cocaine (cocaine HCl) into biologic membranes, particularly the nasal mucosa; the vasoconstricting properties of cocaine limit its own passage into blood vessels. The onset of activity is within 3 to 5 minutes and the blood level peaks at 10 to 20 minutes, fading in 45 to 60 minutes. Because cocaine has a biologic half-life of 40 to 60 minutes, repeated self-administrations are necessary to maintain an effect.

After intravenous injection, the entire bolus of cocaine is delivered to the vessel chamber and has a bioavailability of 100%. The limiting factor for intravenous cocaine concentration is the original purity of the injected sample. The onset of activity is within 30 seconds, with a duration of action of 10 to 20 minutes. The venous system must still be traveled, with the sequence being from the peripheral veins back to the heart and subsequently through the pulmonary system for ejection by the left ventricle to the brain.

Cocaine inhalation became popular because it produces the quickest and highest peak blood levels to the brain without the risks of intravenous use. Freebase cocaine, whether in coca paste, freebase, or crack form, is much more volatile and lipid soluble than the leaf and powder forms. Because the freebase can be inhaled and thus delivered to the pulmonary bed, it is pumped by the heart directly into the brain. The bioavailability is low, at 6% to 32%, as a consequence of the pyrolysis that occurs on heating the cocaine for vaporization.

Metabolism and Excretion

Cocaine has a short half-life (<60 minutes), and is metabolized in the liver. Its primary metabolites are benzoylecgonine and ecgonine. Urine testing for cocaine detects benzoylecgonine, and detection of this metabolite may last for more than a week in cases of heavy, daily cocaine use. More typical acute use results in urinary detection for approximately 36 hours.

Acute Effects

Acute doses of cocaine produce a subjective feeling of increased alertness; electroencephalogram and electrocardiogram recordings show a general desynchronization of brain waves after cocaine administration. Such desynchronization, which indicates arousal, occurs in the part of the brain that is thought to be involved in the regulation of conscious awareness, attention, and sleep. Despite the feeling of arousal, individuals using cocaine do not gain any particular superior ability or greater knowledge. Their sense of omnipotence is only an illusion; they tend to misinterpret their enhanced confidence and lowered inhibitions as signs of enhanced physical or mental acuity.

DA inhibits secretion of prolactin. Hyperprolactinemia is the endocrine abnormality most often reported in clinical studies of cocaine abusers, with clear elevations in prolactin observed during abuse and withdrawal in animals.

Cocaine users report feeling more alert and more energetic. This reaction, in turn, produces a tremendous increase in self-confidence, self-image, and egocentricity; in some individuals this manifests as megalomania and feelings of omnipotence. Some groups, including athletes, salespeople, entertainers, musicians, and physicians, sometimes use cocaine to provide them with these effects, to enhance their energy, confidence, and "star image." But there are limits to the degree to which central nervous system (CNS) activity can be artificially stimulated. After chronic use, or following a prolonged binge, symptoms of depression, lack of motivation, sleeplessness, paranoia, irritability, and outright acute toxic psychosis may develop. States of severe transient panic accompanied by a terror of impending death can occur in persons with no pre-existing psychopathologic conditions, as can paranoid psychoses.

Chronic Effects

The tremendous attachment for cocaine and desire to repeat the pleasurable aspects of the cocaine experience and to counteract the depressive effects of the postcocaine crash can lead to compulsive chronic use of the drug. Such activity leads to a decrease or depletion in the neurotransmitter supply. The long-term results of such depletion include overt depression, dysphoria, hallucinatory experiences, and destructive antisocial behavior. More subtle changes in behavior include irritability, hypervigilance, psychomotor agitation, and impaired interpersonal relations. Cocaine is known to worsen the symptomatology of depression. Chronic cocaine use may lead to long-lasting and selective disruptions in serotonin pathways, which may be a neurochemical basis for mood changes that are commonly reported during cocaine withdrawal.

Use of cocaine can also produce a psychotic syndrome characterized by paranoia; impaired reality testing; anxiety; a stereotyped compulsive repetitive pattern of behavior; and vivid visual, auditory, and tactile hallucinations, such as the delusion that insects are crawling under the skin. Subjective and clinical data also show that cocaine can induce panic attacks.

Cocaine and Alcohol (Cocaethylene)

The combined use of cocaine and alcohol is common, with reports of 62% to 90% of cocaine abusers also being concurrent ethanol abusers. Cocaine users report that concurrent ethanol use prolongs the "high" and attenuates a number of the unpleasant physical and psychologic effects of cocaine. In the presence of cocaine and alcohol, the body creates cocaethylene, the ethyl ester of benzoylecgonine, which is similar to cocaine in neurochemical and pharmacologic properties and behavioral effects. Cocaethylene binds to the DA transporter, blocking DA uptake and increasing extracellular concentrations of DA in the nucleus accumbens, but unlike cocaine, it has little effect on the serotonin transporter. Although similar to cocaine and having effects on heart rate and reward, there are reports of increased lethality.

The longer half-life of cocaethylene (2 hours compared with 38 minutes for cocaine), and additive effect of cocaethylene on the DA transporter, and the 40-fold greater affinity for the serotonin transporter may explain the occurrence of lethal heart attacks and stroke (18-fold increase in the risk of sudden death compared to cocaine alone), the greater irritability, and the prolonged toxicity.

Epidemiology

Data from the 1990 National Household Survey on Drug Abuse (NHSDA) showed that the number of current cocaine users—people who had used the drug within the past 30 days—had decreased from 5.8 million in 1985 to 1.6 million in 1990. In 2001, rates were increasing again. An estimated 1.7 million Americans ages 12 years and older were current cocaine users and 406,000 were current crack users in 2001. The NHSDA also found that cocaine use increased among young adults age 18 to 25 years, from 1.4% in 2000 to 1.9% in 2001. Unlike other drugs of abuse, where rates are higher among youth and young adults, only 40% of cocaine users were age 12 to 25 years in 2001.

According to the U.S. Monitoring the Future annual survey, the peak lifetime use of cocaine decreased from 17.3% in 1985 to 5.9% in 1994 among high school seniors. However, it later increased and in 2001 was 8.2%. Crack use also decreased significantly among high school seniors between 1989 and 1990, but additional decreases have been difficult to demonstrate. The lifetime prevalence for crack use had a mild increase from 3.0% in 1994 to 3.7% in 2001. In 2003, 2.2% of 12th graders used crack in the last year and 0.9% used crack in the past month.

Cocaine-related emergency room visits in the United States declined 26% between 1988 and 1990. To a significant degree, the decline can be attributed to widespread public education about the dangers of cocaine. Despite this early decline, cocaine was the most frequently reported drug in emergency room visits in 2001. The Drug Abuse Warning Network (DAWN) reported a significant increase in emergency department mentions between 2000 and 2001, from 174,881 to 193,034 respectively. Cocaine is consistently among the top three drugs mentioned in mortality data from DAWN. Cocaine and cocaine in combination with alcohol were the most commonly mentioned drugs in suicide cases in 2001.

Clinical Effects: Acute Intoxication

Psychologic Effects

As a CNS stimulant, cocaine has many psychologic effects that are predictable and similar to those of other stimulants such as amphetamines and caffeine. Psychologic variations exist and are dependent on the user, environment, dose, and route of administration. Nonetheless, the intensity and duration of the acute manifestations correlate with the rate of increase and height of the peak blood level, and are subsequently reflected in brain concentrations. Crack smoking, which produces a faster rise and higher blood levels, results in earlier-onset and prominent clinical psychologic signs and symptoms. The dose and route of administration determine these pharmacokinetic parameters for cocaine absorption and distribution in the body. The acute psychologic effects begin when cocaine reaches the brain, which occurs within seconds by any route of administration.

The major psychologic functions affected by cocaine are mood; cognition; drive states such as hunger, sex, and thirst; and consciousness. An immediate and intense euphoria, analogous to a sexual orgasm, occurs and may last seconds or minutes. Other alterations arising from elevation in mood include giddiness, enhanced self-confidence, and a forceful boisterousness. The subsequent level of mood is milder euphoria mixed with anxiety, which can last for minutes, followed by a more protracted anxious state that persists for hours. During intoxication, a state virtually indistinguishable from hypomania or frank mania is typical. Thoughts race and the user speaks in a rapid, often pressured manner. The user is garrulous and grandiose with tangential and incoherent speech. Appetite is suppressed during the period of intoxication usually followed by a rebound increase in appetite as the cocaine is eliminated. In low doses, the libido is stimulated and sexual performance in men is reported to be enhanced by a prolonged erection and a heightened orgasm. The level of sensory awareness is altered and hypervigilance is typical. The user may develop ideas of reference and other mental alterations. Insomnia is common. With increasing doses, acts and decisions of poor judgment and indiscretions are more common. Motor activity is increased, as are driven atypical behaviors. Cocaine restlessness and fidgety behavior are accompanied by a driven state of perpetual motion.

Physiologic Effects

The acute physiologic effects result from sympathetic nervous discharge after cocaine releases norepinephrine, epinephrine, and DA. CNS stimulation lowers seizure threshold and causes other changes such as tremor, arousal, electrographic changes, emesis, and hyperpyrexia. Activation of the cardiovascular system results in tachycardia, hypertension, and diaphoresis. Peripheral nervous system stimulation results in urinary and bowel delay and retention, muscular contractions, and cutaneous flushing.

Clinical Effects: Tolerance and Dependence

Tolerance develops to some of the central effects of cocaine. Research indicates that tolerance is related to the reduction in the levels of DA and serotonin in the nucleus accumbens. Tolerance to the euphoria develops quickly and has been measured within 1 hour after a single intravenous dose, so that the dose must be escalated or the route and dose changed to experience the desired effects of equal intensity. Moreover, chronic cocaine users become tolerant to the rewarding effects of cocaine. A small degree of tolerance to effects on heart rate and blood pressure develops during the infusion of cocaine over the course of 4 hours; however, it is unlikely that significant tolerance to its cardiovascular actions is usually achieved. Tolerance does not seem to drive the use of cocaine. The adverse effects of, for example, anxiety, depression, financial expense, suicidal thinking, and disrupted lives increase as the euphoria decreases, so that tolerance would seem to be a rate-limiting factor at best.

Clinical Effects: Cocaine Withdrawal

Observations in humans and animal studies support the concept of a sometimes subtle but important cocaine abstinence state. The essential feature of cocaine withdrawal is the presence of a characteristic withdrawal syndrome that develops within a few hours to several days after the cessation of (or reduction in) cocaine use that has been heavy and prolonged. The withdrawal syndrome is characterized by the development of dysphoric mood accompanied by two or more of the following physiologic changes: fatigue, vivid and unpleasant dreams, insomnia or hypersomnia, increased appetite, and psychomotor retardation or agitation. Anhedonia and drug craving are often present, but are not part of the diagnostic criteria. These symptoms cause clinically significant distress or impairment.

Acute withdrawal symptoms ("a crash") are often seen after periods of repetitive high-dose use ("runs" or "binges"). These periods are characterized by intense and unpleasant feelings of lassitude and depression, generally requiring several days of rest and recuperation. Depressive symptoms with suicidal ideation or behavior can occur and are generally the most serious problems seen during "crashing" or other forms of cocaine withdrawal.

A substantial number of individuals with cocaine dependence have few or no clinically evident withdrawal symptoms on cessation of use, and in general, cocaine withdrawal is neither acutely life-threatening nor problematic in a secure, locked environment, but relapse is easily provoked by a host of conditioned cues.

Medical Complications of Cocaine Abuse

Cardiovascular System

Cocaine produces a number of cardiovascular effects that may lead to the development of different forms of arrhythmia. Tachycardia often occurs within minutes of cocaine ingestion. Other forms of arrhythmia associated with cocaine use include sinus bradycardia, ventricular premature depolarization, ventricular tachycardia degenerating to defibrillation, and asystole. Cocaine is known to elevate blood pressure through adrenergic stimulation. The pressor effects of cocaine continue to rise as dosage increases. The sudden increase in blood pressure may cause spontaneous bleeding in people with normal blood pressure and may underlie many incidents of cerebrovascular accidents associated with cocaine use.

Evidence suggests that cocaine can induce spasms in a number of vascular systems, including the coronary arteries. These spasms can produce myocardial infarction even in a person whose endothelium is otherwise intact. The pathologic changes in the vasculature, regardless of the route of cocaine self-administration, that place individuals at high risk for a cardiovascular or cerebrovascular accident appear to include arteriolar thickening, increased perivascular deposits of collagen and glycoprotein, and inflammation.

Most of the case reports of cocaine-related cardiovascular toxicity involve myocardial infarctions, which may occur regardless of dosage level or route of administration. Cocaine increases myocardial oxygen consumption, but at the same time it interferes with the ability of the coronary circulation to adjust to this increased demand by decreasing its resistance to blood flow.

Respiratory System

Smoking crack can induce severe chest pain or dyspnea. One explanation for this effect may be that cocaine significantly reduces the ability of the lungs to diffuse carbon monoxide. Often it is this symptom of chest pain that drives patients to seek medical attention.

Other respiratory effects of cocaine smoking include lung damage, pneumonia, pulmonary edema, cough, sputum production, fever, hemoptysis, pulmonary barotraumas, pneumomediastinum, pneumothorax, pneumopericardium, and diffuse alveolar hemorrhage. Cocaine inhalation can cause or contribute to asthma. Respiratory failure, resulting from cocaine-induced inhibition of medullary centers in the brain, may lead to sudden death. Chronic cocaine inhalation can cause progressive destruction of the hard palate, soft palate, septum, nasal cartilage, and can even progress to midfacial osteomyelitis.

Neurotoxicity

The spectrum of neuropathologic changes encountered in the brains of cocaine abusers is broad, but the major findings consist of ischemic and hemorrhagic stroke, subarachnoid and intracerebral hemorrhages and cerebral ischemia. Especially persons with underlying arteriovenous malformation or aneurysm are at risk for such events. In addition to pharmacologically induced vasospasm, vasculitis, impaired hemostasis and platelet function, and decreased cerebral blood flow appear to play a role.

Cocaine is an epileptogenic agent that can provoke generalized seizures, even after a single dose. With repeated administration, the ability of cocaine to produce clonic convulsions increases. This phenomenon, known as kindling, may result from sensitization of receptors in the brain. Because seizure disorders can be unmasked or induced by the kindling effect of cocaine on the brain, proper medical evaluation of patients must rule out epilepsy.

CNS stimulants such as cocaine can also cause tics, persistent mechanical repetition of speech or movement, ataxia, and disturbed gait, which may disappear after drug use is stopped.

Impact on Sexuality

Many users claim that cocaine is an aphrodisiac. The feeling of sexual excitement that sometimes accompanies cocaine use may be the result of its impact on the DA system and may produce spontaneous orgasm. Nonetheless, chronic cocaine abuse causes derangements in reproductive function including impotence and gynecomastia. These symptoms may persist for long periods, even after use of cocaine has stopped. Men who abuse cocaine chronically and in high doses may have difficulty maintaining an erection and ejaculating. Many men report experiencing periods when they completely lose interest in sex. In women, cocaine abuse has adverse effects on reproductive function, including derangements in the menstrual cycle function, galactorrhea, amenorrhea, and infertility. Some women who use cocaine report having greater difficulty achieving orgasm.

Other Adverse Effects

Chronic cocaine abuse may induce persistent hyperprolactinemia, apparently because it disrupts the ability of DA to inhibit prolactin secretion. This effect may continue for long periods even after a person has stopped using cocaine. As a result of the effects of the drug on the primary eating drive, many individuals who use cocaine compulsively lose their appetites and can experience significant weight loss. Cocaine also produces hyperpyrexia, or extremely elevated body temperatures, which can contribute to the development of seizures, life-threatening cardiac arrhythmias, and death. This effect results from hypermetabolism combined with severe peripheral vasoconstriction and the impact of cocaine on the ability of the thalamus to regulate body heat.

Different routes of cocaine administration can produce different adverse effects. Intranasal use can lead to sinusitis, loss of the sense of smell, atrophy of the nasal mucosa, nosebleeds, perforation of the nasal septum, problems with swallowing, and hoarseness. Ingested cocaine can cause severe bowel ischemia or gangrene as a consequence of vasoconstriction and reduced blood flow. Persons who inject cocaine have puncture marks and "tracks," most commonly on their forearms, as seen in those with opioid dependence. Human immunodeficiency virus (HIV) infection is associated with cocaine dependence as a result of the frequent intravenous injections and the increase in promiscuous sexual behavior. HIV seropositivity is associated with crack smoking without intravenous use.

Other sexually transmitted diseases, hepatitis, tuberculosis, and other lung infections are also seen in cocaine abusers. Intravenous use is associated with diseases introduced by dirty needles contaminated with the blood of previous users, as well as with extra substances in the drug. The most common severe complications from intravenous cocaine use are bacterial or viral endocarditis, hepatitis, and acquired immune deficiency syndrome (AIDS). Other conditions arising from parenteral cocaine use include cellulitis, cerebritis, wound abscess, sepsis, arterial thrombosis, renal infarction, and thrombophlebitis.

Cocaine and Pregnancy

Placental abruption, or premature separation of a normally implanted placenta, occurs in approximately 1% of pregnancies in women who use cocaine, making the drug a significant cause of maternal morbidity, as well as of fetal mortality. Women who use cocaine during pregnancy have a rate of spontaneous abortion higher than that of heroin users.

Cocaine may produce toxic effects on the fetus at concentrations that are apparently nontoxic to the mother. The drug decreases blood flow to the uterus, increases uterine vascular resistance, and reduces fetal oxygen levels. The vasoconstriction, tachycardia, and increased blood pressure associated with cocaine use increase the risk of intermittent intrauterine hypoxia, preterm or precipitous labor, and placental abruption. Cocaine has a significant effect on the ability of fetal hearts to produce action potentials of normal rising velocity, amplitude, and duration. Cocaine can cause fetal cerebral infarction, growth retardation, and fetal death.

Cocaine and Other Psychiatric Disorders

Overall rates for other psychiatric disorders in cocaine abusers are approximately 50% for current, and 75% to 85% for lifetime diagnoses. Such high rates of comorbidity may be related to the poor outcomes reported for some studies of cocaine treatment. Some investigators have reported comorbidity of up to 25% for bipolar-spectrum illnesses (mania, hypomania, cyclothymia) in cocaine-dependent patients. Lifetime major depression is diagnosed in approximately 50% of patients, whereas dysthymia is diagnosed in another 25% to 50%. Rates of antisocial personality disorder are high in some studies of cocaine dependent patients (as high as 40 to 50%), and it is not uncommon to find a lifetime history of an eating disorder in persons with cocaine use. Rates for alcoholism are also quite high, with as many as 60% having clear lifetime diagnoses. marijuana use is common and may be related to cocaine pharmacokinetics.

Treatment of Cocaine Addiction
Diagnosis

The first step in treatment is to diagnose the patient's condition accurately. A diagnosis of cocaine abuse or dependence should be made based on DSM-IV-TR criteria. Other less common cocaine-related diagnoses include cocaine withdrawal, cocaine delusional disorder, and cocaine delirium. A diagnosis of cocaine withdrawal can be made if the patient has stopped or reduced heavy use of the drug after a prolonged period (several days or longer) and experiences dysphoric mood (depression, irritability, anxiety) and fatigue, sleep disturbance, or psychomotor agitation. Cocaine delirium is marked by disorganized thinking, sensory misperceptions, and disorientation within 24 hours after drug use. Typically, patients experience tactile or olfactory hallucinations, and affect is often labile. The essential feature of cocaine delusional disorder involves the presence of persecutory delusions developing shortly after the use of cocaine.

Inpatient versus Outpatient Care

If circumstances permit, outpatient treatment is the preferred modality for delivery of care for several reasons. Many cocaine abusers can be treated as outpatients, because use of the drug usually can be stopped abruptly without medical risk or significant discomfort. The goal of treatment is to return the patient to a normal life; by definition there can be no "normal" life inside the hospital. The cost of out-patient treatment is lower, and many patients are more willing to accept help on an outpatient basis because it carries less of a social stigma and is less disruptive to daily life. However, inpatient or residential treatment provides an ideal transition from drug use and dependency to abstinence and daily meetings. When drug use is severe, or if outpatient care is not possible or has failed in the past, hospitalization is indicated.

Treatment Strategies

The physician should take a complete family, medical, and forensic history, as well as a history of all drug use. The patient should undergo a thorough physical and dental examination. Chest radiographs and electrocardiograms may supply useful informa-tion and may help to reassure patients about their state of health. Immediately follow-ing the physical examination, blood and/or supervised urine samples should be collected and sent for analysis.

Medical Treatment of Withdrawal and Cocaine-Related Emergencies

As a rule, symptoms of cocaine withdrawal are not medically dangerous. Detoxification from cocaine requires no treatment other than abstinence. However, many patients find the symptoms of withdrawal intensely dysphoric. Any medical treatment that helps relieve withdrawal symptoms therefore improves the initial prognosis. However, suc-cessful amelioration of withdrawal appears to be of limited long-term clinical signifi-cance. More recently, researchers have focused the development of treatments on the direct prevention of further drug use as measured by urinalysis or have tried to reduce the likelihood of relapse.

The choice of treatment for cocaine toxicity depends on the clinical signs and symptoms. Supportive therapy is the rule. Treating hyperthermia with vigorous body cooling may be a positive first step. Cardiac and neurologic status should be monitored closely, with medical strategies directed at providing symptom relief. Hospitalization with respiratory assistance and a life support system may be necessary in cases of severe cocaine overdose reaction. Treatment of overdose is often complicated by the presence of sedative–hypnotics, opiates, or alcohol, drugs that are frequently taken to mitigate the unpleasant effects of excessive cocaine use.

Typically, cocaine psychosis lasts for 3 to 5 days following cessation of use; if it persists for a longer period, or if the patient becomes increasingly difficult to manage, a re-evaluation of the diagnosis is indicated and an antipsychotic medication may be tried.

Preventing Relapse

Despite progress in treatment for cocaine use, the risk of relapse is extremely high. Persistence of cocaine abstinence may be manifested in persistent dysphoria and cocaine self-administration. It is not uncommon for such persistent dysphoria, anxiety, or panic symptoms to persist after discontinuation of cocaine and thus constitute a feature of the prolonged abstinence phase.

Relapse prevention strategies developed according to a social learning theory model have been adapted to chemical dependency treatment. Some of these techniques are helping the patient to recognize the warning signs of relapse; combating the powerful memories of euphoria; reinforcing the negative aspects of drugs; overcoming the desire to attempt to regain control over drug use; avoiding the people, places, and things that may trigger drug urges; preventing occasional "slips" from developing into full-blown binges; learning other ways to cope with dysphoric feelings that in the past may have led to drug use; and developing an array of pleasurable and rewarding alternatives to drugs.

The mainstay of treatment for cocaine dependence remains behavioral. In treating physicians and celebrities addicted to cocaine, persistent abstinence can be achieved by contingent drug test–related contracting with swift consequences related to abstinence violation. For others, opposite reinforcement paradigms with monetary reward for abstinence have been successful. Community payment for abstinence or the "reinforcement approach" has shown more efficacy than traditional counseling or pharmacotherapies. Payment for abstinence by focusing on drug-free and cocaine-free urines rather than a more amorphous outcome can succeed where standard drug abuse counseling fails in retaining cocaine-dependent individuals in outpatient treatment. Considering the widespread use of incentives in society, the systematic use of incentives to foster cocaine abstinence may be warranted. Community reinforcement, payment for abstinence, and relapse prevention are the three major types of cocaine treatment programs in widespread use in the United States.

Medications and the Treatment of Cocaine Abuse/Dependence

Numerous medications have been tested for possible efficacy in the treatment of cocaine abuse or dependence. In general, the overwhelming majority of these have not been shown to be consistently effective, although there continues to be interest in some which may yet be found useful under certain circumstances (e.g., when linked to voucher incentives or other behavioral treatments to enhance compliance), or for certain populations (e.g., patients with higher levels of cocaine dependence). A partial listing of agents tested includes amantadine, baclofen, bromocriptine, bupropion, carbamazepine, desipramine, divalproex, doxepin, fluoxetine, lithium, mazindol, methylphenidate, modafinil, olanzapine, ondansetron, propranolol, risperidone, ritanserin, trazadone, selegline, and vigabatrin. Notably, one agent, disulfiram, has been shown in several clinical trials to have possible efficacy. Initial studies of disulfiram were based on the high rate of comorbid alcohol use found in patients with cocaine use disorders. Now, it appears that disulfiram may have efficacy for cocaine use even in patients without concurrent alcohol use. However, it is not approved as a treatment for cocaine use disorders. Finally, immunotherapies for cocaine abuse/dependence (a cocaine vaccine) are under active investigation, and may provide an alternative mechanism for treating patients with cocaine use.

Conclusion

Cocaine dependence remains an intractable public health problem that contributes to many disturbing social crises, including violent crime, unsafe streets, urban decay, accidents, unnecessary medical costs, the spread of infectious disease, failures in school and work performance, and neonatal drug exposure. Clinicians should realize that the experience of recent years has proved that effective education prevents drug abuse and results in abstinence. A wide range of efforts based in schools, the community, the workplace, religious groups, and the family aimed at reducing drug use has resulted in a dramatic reduction of drug use. Physicians should play a significant role in reducing cocaine use by never failing to consider the possibility of substance abuse in their patients and by inoculating their patients, especially their younger ones, with accurate information about this dangerous and deadly drug. Effective treatment interventions at present involve use of cognitive–behavioral therapies, with 12-step involvement an often valuable component of comprehensive treatment for many patients. The hope is that continued study of medications for cocaine use disorders will soon lead to an effective pharmacologic intervention similar to medications used to treat alcohol, nicotine, and opioid use disorders.

Suggested Readings

Benzaquen BS, Cohen V, Eisenberg MJ. Effects of cocaine on the coronary arteries. *Am Heart J.* 2001; 142(3):402–410.

Gold MS, Jacobs WS.: Cocaine and crack: clinical aspects. In: Lowinson JH, Ruiz P, Millman RB, et al., eds. *Substance abuse: a comprehensive textbook*, 4th ed. Philadelphia: Lippincott Williams & Wilkins; 2005:218–251.

Lima MS, Reisser AA, Soares BG, et al. Antidepressants for cocaine dependence. *Cochrane Database Syst.* 2001;(4):CD002950.

Repetto M, Gold MS. Cocaine and crack: neurobiology. In: Lowinson JH, Ruiz P, Millman RB, et al., eds. *Substance abuse: a comprehensive textbook*, 4th ed. Philadelphia: Lippincott Williams & Wilkins; 2005:195–218.

Simpson DD, Joe GW, Broome KM. A national 5-year follow-up of treatment outcomes for cocaine dependence. *Arch Gen Psychiatry.* 2002;59(6):538–544.

Soares BG, Lima MS, Reisser AA, et al. Dopamine agonists for cocaine dependence. *Cochrane Database Syst.* 2001;(4):CD003352.

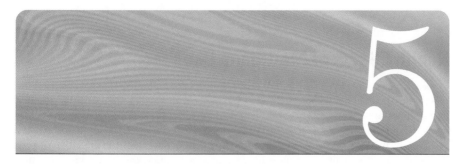

MARIJUANA

Cannabis, along with opium, is one of the oldest drugs in pharmaceutical use in the world. Cannabis use dates back more than 12,000 years. The cannabis plant was introduced to the New World for nonpharmacologic purposes. The ability of cannabis to survive and produce large amounts of fiber during the short growing season made hemp a valued commodity. The warm, temperate, and subtropical climates of the southern and southwestern United States produced a plant with less fiber and more psychoactive potency than that of the northern and midwestern areas. Once the pharmacologic properties of cannabis were realized, marijuana was included in the U.S. Pharmacopoeia in 1850, and in the U.S. Dispensary in 1851. Cannabis tinctures were recommended for a variety of maladies, including gout, rheumatism, depression, and convulsions, and as treatment for constipation and malaria.

Advances into the pharmacology of the cannabinoids have been made in large part as a result of the cloning of receptors and the development of specific antagonists for those receptors. Many critical questions remain regarding the role of the endo-cannabinoid system in human physiology and pathophysiology. Much controversy surrounds the use of tetrahydrocannabinol (THC) or another cannabinoid analogue in a variety of disease states. As was evident from the ancient sources, cannabinoids appear to have a variety of potentially useful therapeutic effects, but are not devoid of undesirable side effects. If novel non-CB_1, non-CB_2 cannabinoid receptors were to be found, it certainly will become a therapeutic target it certainly will become a therapeutic target. In addition, the increasing knowledge of the role of the endocannabinoid system in tonic regulation of analgesia, cognition, food intake, and cardiovascular tone indicates that possible analogues of the endocannabinoids, or modulators of endocannabinoid pathways, may become targets for drug development. The endo-cannabinoids and cannabinoid receptors are highly conserved phylogenically. For today's researcher remains the task of determining the reasons for the preservation of the cannabinoid system through both invertebrate and vertebrate evolution, and the roles such receptors, known and yet to be found, play in diseases, including addictive behaviors. The goal of novel therapeutic interventions is to decrease the potential for tolerance to and dependence on the cannabinoid drugs.

The use of marijuana reached a high point in the late 1970s and early 1980s, declined until the early 1990s, then began to rise slightly. In a 1978 National Institute on Drug Abuse (NIDA) survey, 37% of high school seniors said that they had smoked marijuana in the past 30 days. In 1989, that number fell to 17%, but by 2001, it had risen again to 22%.

Health Effects of Marijuana Use

In recent years, the psychologic and physical effects of long-term use have caused the most concern. Studies are often conflicting and permit various views of the possible harmfulness of marijuana. This complicates the task of presenting an objective statement about the issue.

One of the first questions asked about any drug is whether it is addictive or produces dependence. This question is hard to answer because the terms *addiction* and *dependence* have no agreed-to definitions. Two recognized signs of addiction are tolerance and withdrawal symptoms; these are rarely a serious problem for marijuana users. In the early stages, users actually become more sensitive to the desired effects. After continued heavy use, some tolerance to both physiologic and psychologic effects develops, although it seems to vary considerably among individuals. Almost no one reports an urgent need to increase the dose to recapture the original sensation. What is called *behavioral tolerance* may be partly a matter of learning to compensate for the effects of high doses, and may explain why farm workers in some Third World countries are able to do heavy physical labor while smoking a great deal of marijuana.

A mild withdrawal reaction also occurs in animal experiments and possibly in some human beings who take high doses for a long time. The rarely reported mild symptoms are anxiety, insomnia, tremors, and chills, lasting for a day or two. It is unclear how common this reaction is.

In a more important sense, dependence means an unhealthy and often unwanted preoccupation with a drug to the exclusion of most other things. People suffering from drug dependence find that they are constantly thinking about the drug, or intoxicated, or recovering from its effects. The habit impairs their mental and physical health and hurts their work, family life, and friendships. They often know that they are using too much and repeatedly make unsuccessful attempts to cut down or stop. These problems seem to afflict proportionately fewer marijuana smokers than users of alcohol, tobacco, heroin, or cocaine.

It is often difficult to distinguish between drug use as a cause of problems and drug use as an effect; this is especially true in the case of marijuana. Most people who develop a dependency on marijuana would also be likely to develop other dependencies because of anxiety, depression, or feelings of inadequacy. The original condition is likely to matter more than the attempt to relieve it by means of the drug. The troubled teenager who smokes cannabis throughout the school day certainly has a problem, and excessive use of marijuana may be one of its symptoms.

The idea has persisted that in the long run smoking marijuana causes some sort of mental or emotional deterioration. In three major studies conducted in Jamaica, Costa Rica, and Greece, researchers compared heavy long-term cannabis users with nonusers and found no evidence of intellectual or neurologic damage, no changes in personality, and no loss of the will to work or participate in society. The Costa Rican study showed no difference between heavy users (seven or more marijuana cigarettes a day) and lighter users (six or fewer cigarettes a day). Experiments in the United States show no effects of fairly heavy marijuana use on learning, perception, or motivation over periods as long as 1 year.

On the other side are clinical reports of a personality change called the *amotivational syndrome*. Its symptoms are said to be passivity, aimlessness, apathy, uncommunicativeness, and lack of ambition. Some proposed explanations are hormone changes, brain damage, sedation, and depression. Because the amotivational syndrome does not seem to occur in Greek or Caribbean farm laborers, some writers suggest that it affects only skilled and educated people who need to do more complex thinking. However, there is no credible evidence that what is meant by this syndrome is related to any inherent properties of the drug rather than to different sociocultural adaptations on the part of the users.

The problem of distinguishing causes from symptoms is particularly acute here. Heavy drug users in our society are often bored, depressed, and listless, or alienated, cynical, and rebellious. Sometimes the drugs cause these states of mind, and sometimes they result from personality characteristics that lead to drug abuse. Drug abuse can be an excuse for failure, or a form of self-medication. Because of these complications and the absence of confirmation from controlled studies, the existence of an amotivational syndrome caused by cannabis use has to be regarded as unproved.

Much attention has also been devoted to the idea that marijuana smoking leads to the use of opiates and other illicit drugs—the steppingstone hypothesis, now commonly referred to as the gateway hypothesis, which was rejected after extensive study by the Institute of Medicine and the Canadian Senate. In this country, almost everyone who uses any other illicit drug has smoked marijuana first, just as almost everyone who smokes marijuana drank alcohol first. Anyone who uses any given drug is more likely to be interested in others, for some of the same reasons. People who use illicit drugs, in particular, are somewhat more likely to find themselves in company where other illicit drugs are available. None of this proves that using one drug leads to or causes the use of another. Most marijuana smokers do not use heroin or cocaine, just as most alcohol drinkers do not use marijuana. The metaphor of steppingstones suggests that if no one smoked marijuana it would be more difficult for anyone to develop an interest in opiates or cocaine. There is no convincing evidence for or against this. What is clear is that at many times and places marijuana has been used without these drugs, and that these drugs have been used without marijuana.

Only the unsophisticated continue to believe that cannabis leads to violence and crime. Indeed, instead of inciting criminal behavior, cannabis may tend to suppress it. The intoxication induces a mild lethargy that is not conducive to any physical activity, let alone the commission of crimes. The release of inhibitions results in fantasy and verbal (rather than behavioral) expression. During the "high", marijuana users may say and think things they would not ordinarily say and think, but they generally do not do things that are foreign to their nature. If they are not already criminals, they will not commit crimes under the influence of the drug.

Does marijuana induce sexual debauchery? This popular impression may owe its origin partly to writers' fantasies and partly to the fact that users in the Middle East once laced the drug with what they thought were aphrodisiacs. In actuality, there is little evidence that cannabis stimulates sexual desire or power. On the other hand, there are those who contend, with equally little substantiation, that marijuana weakens sexual desire. Many marijuana users report that the high enhances the enjoyment of sexual intercourse, and it has been an aid to tantric sexual meditation in India and Tibet since ancient times. This appears to be true in the same sense that the enjoyment of art and music is apparently enhanced. It is questionable, however, whether the intoxication breaks down barriers to sexual activity that are not already broken.

In the LaGuardia study in New York City, an examination of chronic users who had averaged about seven marijuana cigarettes a day (a comparatively high dosage) over a long period (the mean was 8 years) showed that they had suffered no demonstrable mental or physical decline as a result of their use of the drug.

A common assertion made about cannabis is that it may lead to psychosis. The literature on this subject is vast, and it divides into all shades of opinion. Our own clinical experience and that of others suggests that cannabis may precipitate exacerbations in the psychotic processes of some patients with schizophrenia at a time when their illnesses are otherwise reasonably well controlled with antipsychotic drugs. In these patients, it is often difficult to determine whether the use of cannabis is simply a precipitant of the psychosis or whether it is an attempt to treat symptomatically the earliest perceptions of decompensation; needless to say, the two possibilities are not mutually exclusive. There is little support for the idea that cannabis contributes to the etiology of schizophrenia. And in one recently reported case, a 19-year-old woman with schizophrenia was more successfully treated with cannabidiol (one of the cannabinoids in marijuana) than she had been with haloperidol (Haldol).

A recent study from Sweden on schizophrenia is most suspect. The authors examined Swedish conscripts from 1969. This investigation seems to be an attempt to rehabilitate a study of the same cohort published in 1987, which had been thoroughly criticized. In the current study, the authors claim that based on their data, up to 13% of schizophrenia incidence could be attributable to cannabis. This is an unsubstantiated allegation, given that only 1.4% of the conscripts who ever smoked cannabis wound up schizophrenic. Men of such age are at the critical time in development of the disorder. All the eventual schizophrenics in the earlier study were recognized to have some psychiatric issue before they entered the service!

Another recent study examined a cohort of young New Zealanders for cannabis use versus development of adult psychosis. In this brief article, "controls" smoked cannabis zero to two times, whereas "cannabis users" took the drug "three times or more" by age 15 years and continued at some unspecified rate of intake by age 18 years. Supposedly, smoking cannabis increased the incidence of psychosis in adults, and it was more likely the earlier they began. If cannabis were truly etiologic in the development of psychosis, it would be reasonable to expect some dose–response effect. That is not evident here in any respect.

Interestingly, cannabis may ameliorate certain symptoms of psychosis, including activation symptoms and subjective complaints of depression, anxiety, insomnia, and pain. It is noteworthy that levels of anandamide are elevated in the brains of individuals with schizophrenia.

Although there is little evidence for the existence of a cannabis psychosis, it seems clear that the drug may precipitate in susceptible people one of several types of mental dysfunction. The most serious and disturbing of these is the toxic psychosis. This is an acute state that resembles the delirium of a high fever. It is caused by the presence in the brain of toxic substances that interfere with a variety of cerebral functions. Generally speaking, as the toxins disappear, so do the symptoms of toxic psychosis. This type of reaction may be caused by any number of substances taken either as intended or as inadvertent overdoses. The syndrome often includes clouding of consciousness, restlessness, confusion, bewilderment, disorientation, dream-like thinking, apprehension, fear, illusions, and hallucinations. It generally requires a rather large ingested dose of cannabis to induce a toxic psychosis. Such a reaction is apparently much less likely to occur when cannabis is smoked, perhaps because not enough of the active substances can be absorbed sufficiently rapidly, or possibly because the process of smoking modifies in some yet unknown way those cannabinoids that are most likely to precipitate this syndrome.

Some marijuana users suffer what are usually short-lived, acute, anxiety states, sometimes with and sometimes without accompanying paranoid thoughts. The anxiety may reach such proportions as properly to be called panic. Such panic reactions, although uncommon, probably constitute the most frequent adverse reaction to the moderate use of smoked marijuana. During this reaction, the sufferer may believe that the various distortions of bodily perceptions mean that the sufferer is dying or is undergoing some great physical catastrophe, and similarly the individual may interpret the psychologic distortions induced by the drug as an indication of the sufferer's loss of sanity. Panic states may, albeit rarely, be so severe as to incapacitate, usually for a relatively short period of time. The anxiety that characterizes the acute panic reaction resembles an attenuated version of the frightening parts of an lysergic acid diethylamide (LSD) or other psychedelic experience—the so-called bad trip. Some proponents of the use of LSD in psychotherapy assert that the induced altered state of consciousness involves a lifting of repression. Although the occurrence of a global undermining of repression is questionable, many effects of LSD do suggest important alterations in ego defenses. These alterations presumably make new percepts and insights available to the ego; some, particularly those most directly derived from primary process, may be quite threatening, especially if there is no comfortable and supportive setting to facilitate the integration of the new awareness into the ego organization. Thus, psychedelic experiences may be accompanied by a great deal of anxiety, particularly when the drugs are taken under poor conditions of set and setting; to a much lesser extent, the same can be said of cannabis.

These reactions are self-limiting, and simple reassurance is the best method of treatment. Perhaps the main danger to the user is that the user will be diagnosed as having a toxic psychosis. Users with this kind of reaction may be quite distressed, but they are not psychotic. The *sine qua non* of sanity, the ability to test reality, remains intact, and the panicked user is invariably able to relate the discomfort to the drug. There is no disorientation, nor are there true hallucinations. Sometimes this panic reaction is accompanied by paranoid ideation. The user may, for example, believe that the others in the room, especially if they are not well known, have some hostile intentions, or that someone is going to inform on the user, often to the police, for smoking marijuana. Generally speaking, these paranoid ideas are not strongly held, and simple reassurance dispels them. Anxiety reactions and paranoid thoughts are much more likely in someone who is taking the drug for the first time or in an unpleasant or unfamiliar setting, than in an experienced user who is comfortable with the surroundings and companions; the reaction is very rare where marijuana is a casually accepted part of the social scene. The likelihood varies directly with the dose and inversely with the user's experience; thus, the most vulnerable person is the inexperienced user who inadvertently (often precisely because the inexperienced user lacks familiarity with the drug) takes a large dose that produces perceptual and somatic changes for which the user is unprepared.

One rather rare reaction to cannabis is the flashback, or spontaneous recurrence of drug symptoms while not intoxicated. Although several reports suggest that this may occur in marijuana users even without prior use of any other drug, in general, it seems to arise only in those who have used more powerful hallucinogenic or psychedelic drugs. There are also some people who have flashback experiences of psychedelic drug trips while smoking marijuana; this is sometimes regarded as an extreme version of a more general heightening of the marijuana high that occurs after the use of hallucinogens. Many people find flashbacks enjoyable, but to others they are distressing. They usually fade with the passage of time. It is possible that flashbacks are attempts to deal with primary process derivatives and other unconscious material that has breached the ego defenses during the psychedelic or cannabis experience.

Rarely, but especially among new users of marijuana, there occurs an acute depressive reaction. It is generally rather mild and transient but may sometimes require psychiatric intervention. This type of reaction is most likely to occur in a user who has some degree of underlying depression; it is as though the drug allows the depression to be felt and experienced as such. Again, set and setting play an important part. Cannabis has been of benefit in mood stabilization in case reports from patients with bipolar disease.

Most recent research on the health hazards of marijuana concerns its long-term effects on the body. The main physiologic effects of cannabis are increased appetite, a faster heartbeat, and slight reddening of the conjunctiva. Although the increased heart rate could be a problem for people with cardiovascular disease, dangerous physical reactions to marijuana are almost unknown. No human is known to have died of an overdose. By extrapolation from animal experiments, the ratio of lethal to effective (intoxicating) dose is estimated to be about 20,000:1.

Studies have examined the brain, the immune system, the reproductive system, and the lungs. Suggestions of long-term damage come almost exclusively from animal experiments and other laboratory work. Observations of marijuana users and the Caribbean, Greek, and other studies reveal little disease or organic pathology associated with the drug.

For example, there are several reports of damaged brain cells and changes in brain-wave readings in monkeys smoking marijuana, but neurologic and neuropsychologic tests in Greece, Jamaica, and Costa Rica found no evidence of functional brain damage. A recent study of enrolled patients in the Compassionate Use Investigational New Drug Program in the United States also demonstrated no significant electroencephalograph (EEG) or P300 changes. Damage to white blood cells has also been observed in the laboratory, but again, its practical importance is unclear. Whatever temporary changes marijuana may produce in the immune system, they have not been found to increase the danger of infectious disease or cancer. If there were significant damage, we might expect to find a higher rate of these diseases among young people beginning in the 1960s, when marijuana first became popular. There is no evidence of that. Recent studies in human immunodeficiency virus (HIV) and in the Missoula Chronic Use Study also failed to demonstrate deleterious effects on white blood cell or CD4 counts.

The effects of marijuana on the reproductive system are a more complicated issue. In men, a single dose of THC lowers sperm count and the level of testosterone and other hormones. Tolerance to this effect apparently develops; in the Costa Rican study, marijuana smokers and controls had the same testosterone levels. Although the smokers in that study began using marijuana at an average age of 15 years, it had not affected their masculine development. There is no evidence that the changes in sperm count and testosterone produced by marijuana affect sexual performance or fertility.

In animal experiments, THC has also been reported to lower levels of female hormones and to disturb the menstrual cycle. When monkeys, rats, and mice are exposed during pregnancy to amounts of THC equivalent to a heavy human smoker's dose, stillbirths and decreased birth weight are sometimes reported in their offspring. There are also reports of low birth weight, prematurity, and even a condition resembling the fetal alcohol syndrome in some children of women who smoke marijuana heavily during pregnancy. The significance of these reports is unclear because controls are lacking and other circumstances make it hard to attribute causes. No endocrine changes were observed in the Missoula Chronic Use Study. To be safe, pregnant and nursing women should follow the standard conservative recommendation to avoid all drugs, including cannabis, that are not absolutely necessary. Nonetheless, evidence from a well-controlled study of cannabis-only smokers in Jamaica is supportive of a low risk to their children.

A well-confirmed danger of long-term, heavy marijuana use is its effect on the lungs. Smoking narrows and inflames air passages and reduces breathing capacity; damage to bronchial cells has been observed in hashish smokers. The possible side effects include bronchitis, emphysema, and lung cancer. Interestingly, one study failed to demonstrate emphysematous degeneration in cannabis smokers over time. Marijuana smoke contains the same carcinogens as tobacco smoke, usually in somewhat higher concentrations, at least in cannabis supplied by the NIDA. THC may actually interfere with a key biochemical step in carcinogenesis. Marijuana is also inhaled more deeply and held in the lungs longer, which increases the danger. On the other hand, almost no one smokes 20 marijuana cigarettes a day. Marijuana of higher potency may reduce the danger of respiratory damage, because less smoking is required for the desired effect. There is now some experimental evidence demonstrating that high-potency THC cigarettes are smoked less vigorously than those of low potency; the user takes smaller and shorter puffs, inhaling less with each puff. Vaporization technology may also reduce risks.

It is appropriate to consider psychotherapy for the frequent adolescent users of marijuana. The picture that emerges is *one of a troubled adolescent who is interpersonally alienated, emotionally withdrawn, and manifestly unhappy, and who expresses his or her maladjustment through undercontrolled, overtly antisocial behavior.* Such users are described as being *overreactive to minor frustrations, likely to think and associate to ideas in unusual ways, having brittle ego-defense systems, self-defeating, concerned about the adequacy of their bodily functioning, concerned about their adequacy as persons, prone to project their feelings and motives onto others, feeling cheated and victimized by life, and having fluctuating moods.*

Obviously, psychotherapy is not inappropriate for individuals who exemplify this description. But it should be emphasized that this is not psychotherapy for marijuana abuse; it is therapy for the underlying psychopathology, one of whose symptoms is the abuse of cannabis. It is no more appropriate to see marijuana as the cause of the problem here than it is to see repetitive hand washing as the cause of obsessive–compulsive disorder. The individual may be brought to psychiatric attention because of the hand washing, but the therapy will address the underlying disorder. Becoming attached to cannabis is not so much a function of any inherent psychopharmacologic property of the drug as it is emotionally driven by the underlying psychopathology. Success in curtailing cannabis use requires dealing with that pathology.

Medicinal Uses of Cannabis

Cannabis usage as a medicament is ancient, and it has included indications for headache, other types of pain, obstetric and gynecologic conditions, and psychiatric disorders.

The history of cannabis as a Western medicine begins in 1839. In the 19th century the drug was widely prescribed in the Western world for various ailments and discomforts, such as coughing, fatigue, rheumatism, asthma, delirium tremens, migraine headache, and painful menstruation. Although its use was already declining somewhat because of the introduction of synthetic hypnotics and analgesics, it remained in the U.S. Pharmacopoeia until 1941. The difficulties imposed on its use by the Marijuana Tax Act of 1937, as well as quality-control issues with uncertain supplies, completed its medical demise, and, from that time on, physicians allowed themselves to become ignorant about the drug.

The greatest advantage of cannabis as a medicine is its unusual safety. The ratio of lethal dose to effective dose is estimated on the basis of extrapolation from animal data to be about 20,000:1. Huge doses have been given to dogs without causing death, and there is no reliable evidence of death caused by cannabis in a human. Cannabis also has the advantage of not disturbing any physiologic functions or damaging any body organs when it is used in therapeutic doses. It produces little physical dependence or tolerance; there has never been any evidence that medical use of cannabis has led to habitual use as an intoxicant.

There are many anecdotal reports of marijuana smokers using the drug to reduce postsurgery pain, headache, migraine, menstrual cramps, phantom limbs, and other kinds of pain. It is the case that cannabis acts by mechanisms different from those of other analgesics through the endocannabinoid pain mechanisms, and that cannabis may be more effective than opiates in neuropathic pain states. Again, some new synthetic derivatives might prove useful as an analgesic, but this is not an immediate prospect.

Because of reports that some people use less alcohol when they smoke marijuana, cannabis has been proposed as an adjunct to alcoholism treatment, but so far it has not been found useful. Most alcoholics neither want to substitute marijuana nor find it particularly helpful. But there might be some hope for use of marijuana in combination with disulfiram (Antabuse). Certainly a cannabis habit would be preferable to an alcohol habit for anyone who could not avoid dependence on a drug but who was able to substitute one drug for another.

Approximately 20% of patients with epilepsy do not get much relief from conventional anticonvulsant medications. Cannabis has been explored as an alternative, at least since a case was reported in which marijuana smoking, together with the standard anticonvulsants phenobarbital and diphenylhydantoin (Dilantin), was apparently necessary to control seizures in a young man with epilepsy. Recent reports support the role of THC endocannabinoids in modulation of seizure threshold. Cannabidiol also demonstrates anticonvulsant properties.

Marijuana also reduces muscle spasm and tremors in some people who suffer from spastic disorders, including multiple sclerosis, cerebral palsy, and various causes of hemiplegia and quadriplegia, such as spinal cord injury or disease. Anecdotal reports of the use of cannabis for the relief of asthma abound. The antiasthmatic drugs that are available all have drawbacks—either limited effectiveness or side effects. Because marijuana dilates the bronchi and reverses bronchial spasm, cannabis derivatives have been tested as antiasthmatic drugs. Smoking marijuana would probably not be a good way to treat asthma because of chronic irritation of the bronchial tract by tars and other substances in marijuana smoke, so recent research has sought a better means of administration. THC in the form of an aerosol spray has been investigated extensively. Other cannabinoids, such as cannabinol and cannabidiol, may be preferable to THC for this purpose. An interesting finding for future research is that cannabinoids may affect the bronchi by means of a mechanism different from that of the familiar antiasthmatic drugs. A promising new medical use for cannabis is treatment of glaucoma, the second leading cause of blindness in the United States. About a million Americans suffer from the form of glaucoma (wide angle) treatable with cannabis. Marijuana causes a dose-related, clinically significant drop in intraocular pressure that lasts several hours in both normal subjects and in those with the abnormally high ocular tension produced by glaucoma. Oral or intravenous THC has the same effect, which seems to be specific to cannabis derivatives rather than simply a result of sedation. Cannabis does not cure the disease, but it can retard the progressive loss of sight when conventional medication fails and surgery is too dangerous. A recent comprehensive review supports the use of cannabinoids as antioxidant protective agents in the development of vascular retinopathy of glaucoma, a process independent of intraocular pressure.

Cannabis derivatives have several minor or speculative uses in the treatment of cancer, and one major use. As appetite stimulants, marijuana and THC may help to slow weight loss in patients with cancer, as they have in patients with AIDS. THC has also retarded the growth of tumor cells in some animal studies, but results are inconclusive, and another cannabis derivative, cannabidiol, seems to increase tumor growth. Possibly cannabinoids in combination with other drugs will turn out to have some use in preventing tumor growth. THC may promote apoptosis (programmed cell death) in some malignant cells. Limonene, a monoterpenoid component of cannabis resin, has similar activity on breast tumor cells. But the most promising use of cannabis in cancer treatment is the prevention of nausea and vomiting in patients undergoing chemotherapy. About half of patients treated with anticancer drugs suffer from severe nausea and vomiting. In 25% to 30% of these cases, the commonly used antiemetics do not work. The nausea and vomiting are not only unpleasant, but are a threat to the effectiveness of the therapy. Retching can cause tears of the esophagus and rib fractures, prevent adequate nutrition, and lead to fluid loss.

The antiemetics most commonly used in chemotherapy are prochlorperazine (Compazine) and the newer ondansetron (Zofran) and granisetron (Kytril). The suggestion that cannabis might be useful arose in the early 1970s when some young patients receiving cancer chemotherapy found that marijuana smoking, which was, of course, illegal, reduced their nausea and vomiting. In one study of 56 patients who got no relief from standard antiemetic agents, 78% became symptom free when they smoked marijuana. Previously unpublished state studies of smoked cannabis have demonstrated 70% to 100% relief of vomiting in some 748 chemotherapy patients.

Several of the most urgent medical uses of cannabis are for the treatment of the nausea and weight loss suffered by many patients with AIDS. The nausea is often a symptom of the disease itself and a side effect of some of the medicines, particularly azidothymidine (zidovudine or AZT). For many AIDS patients the most distressing and threatening symptom is cachexia. Marijuana will retard weight loss in most patients and even helps some regain weight.

Under federal and most state statutes, marijuana is listed as a Schedule I drug: high potential for abuse, no currently accepted medical use, and lacking in accepted safety for use under medical supervision. It cannot ordinarily be prescribed and may be used only under research conditions. Cannabis was recently legalized for medical use in Canada and Holland, and liberalization of laws is proceeding in the United Kingdom and elsewhere in Western Europe.

Most recent research is tentative, and initial enthusiasm for drugs is often disappointed after further investigation. But it is not as though cannabis were an entirely new agent with unknown properties. Studies done during the past 10 years confirm a centuries-old promise. With the relaxation of restrictions on research and the further chemical manipulation of cannabis derivatives, this promise will eventually be realized. The weight of past and contemporary evidence will probably prove cannabis to be valuable in a number of ways as a medicine.

Suggested Readings

Arsenault L, Cannon M, Poulton R, et al. Cannabis use in adolescence and risk for adult psychosis: longitudinal prospective study. *BMJ.* 2002;325:1212–1213.

Grinspoon L, Bakalar JB, Russo E.: Marijuana: clinical aspects. In: Lowinson JH, Ruiz P, Millman RB, et al., eds. *Substance abuse: a comprehensive textbook,* 4th ed. Philadelphia: Lippincott Williams & Wilkins; 2005:263–276.

Grotenhermen F, Russo EB. *Cannabis and cannabinoids: pharmacology, toxicology and therapeutic potential.* Binghamton, N.Y.: Haworth Press; 2002.

Russo EB, Mathre ML, Byrne A, et al. Chronic cannabis use in the Compassionate Investigational New Drug Program: an examination of benefits and adverse effects of legal clinical cannabis. *J Cannabis Ther.* 2002;2(1):3–57.

Smith NT. A review of the published literature into cannabis withdrawal symptoms in human users. *Addiction.* 2002;97(6):621–632.

Welch SP. The neurobiology of marijuana. In: Lowinson JH, Ruiz P, Millman RB, et al., eds. *Substance abuse: a comprehensive textbook,* 4th ed. Philadelphia: Lippincott Williams & Wilkins; 2005:252–263.

6

AMPHETAMINES AND OTHER STIMULANTS

Pharmacology

Central Effects

The amphetamines are indirect catecholamine agonists and administration results in the release of newly synthesized norepinephrine and dopamine. Several lines of evidence indicate that amphetamine acts on newly synthesized, versus stored, pools of catecholamines, by reversing the transporter, thereby reversing the transport of cytosolic neurotransmitter. In addition, high doses of amphetamines release 5-hydroxytryptamine and may affect serotonergic receptors. High doses of amphetamines will also decrease tyrosine hydroxylase (TH) activity, and in much the same way that amphetamine affects TH activity, amphetamine also results in a decrease of tryptophan hydroxylase activity following acute administration. These synthesis-sensitive mechanisms are in contrast to other types of stimulants, such as methylphenidate and cocaine, which act through storage pools (but not on newly synthesized pools) of catecholamines.

The systemic administration of amphetamines generally results in a dose-dependent depression of the firing rate of catecholaminergic neurons, and noradrenergic neurons in the locus ceruleus. This suppression of firing rate is caused by somatodendritic autoregulation. In contrast to the inhibitory effects of amphetamine on dopaminergic neurons in the substantia nigra, the effects of amphetamine in the neostriatum are biphasic. Low doses of amphetamine inhibit the firing rate of spontaneously active neostriatal neurons, whereas at higher doses there is an excitation of the firing rate. In the caudate putamen, administration of d-amphetamine results in a transient increase in the firing rate of dopaminergic neurons within the first 10 minutes and then a profound inhibition of the firing rate of these neurons.

Behavioral Effects

Locomotion

Low acute doses of amphetamine result in increased locomotor activity, running, and forward motion associated with exploratory behaviors. Several lines of evidence indicate that this increase in locomotor activity is mediated by the mesolimbic dopaminergic system. The effects of chronic stimulant (amphetamine and cocaine) administration on behavior and dopaminergic neurotransmission depend on the route and temporal pattern of administration. Daily intermittent injections induce enhanced locomotion and stereotypies, whereas the continuous infusion of an equivalent daily dose of cocaine induces tolerance to the behavioral effects of cocaine. These behavioral effects are associated with alterations in dopaminergic neurotransmission.

Although research indicates that the locomotor properties are mediated by the mesolimbic dopamine system, several lines of evidence indicate that the serotonergic system plays an inhibitory modulating role on the effects of amphetamine. In addition, several reports indicate that endogenous opiate systems are important in the regulation of amphetamine-induced locomotion and dopamine release.

Stereotypies

ACUTE EFFECTS

High doses of amphetamines result in stereotyped behaviors that are representative for the respective species. These behaviors are continually repetitive acts that serve no apparent purpose. For example, the stereotyped behavior elicited in the rat generally consists of sniffing, licking, biting, or gnawing. The pattern of these would seem to indicate that an intact caudate putamen is necessary for the development of the intense gnawing/biting portion of the stereotypy.

CHRONIC EFFECTS

The effects of chronic amphetamine and cocaine administration depend, in part, on the dosing regimen used. Use of a daily, intermittent dosing regimen results in sensitization (i.e., an augmentation of the effects of amphetamine). Daily injections of amphetamine result in the pre-empting of locomotor stimulation by periods of intense, focused stereotypies. As the duration of amphetamine administration lengthens, tolerance to the dopamine effects of amphetamine develops and various "end-stage" behaviors appear; these behaviors are characterized by limb flicks, abortive grooming, increased startle responses to existent and nonexistent stimuli, and abnormal dystonic postures. In other words, animals progress from an initial stage in which they exhibit "exploratory, investigative," and repetitive movements to a stage characterized by intense stereotypies interspersed with bizarre behavior. This behavior is unrelated to environmental cues and may consist of bits and pieces of earlier patterns and sequences of behavior that at one time served a purpose.

SOCIAL BEHAVIOR

Results from preclinical studies suggest increasing behavioral disintegration and social isolation during chronic amphetamine administration. The behavioral repertoire becomes increasingly restricted, and the animal becomes increasingly responsive to existent and nonexistent stimuli. In other words, the animal is increasingly losing contact with reality. Even months after withdrawal, a single moderate dose of amphetamine can reintroduce the original repertoire of intense bizarre behaviors that originally may have taken months to develop.

Chronic amphetamine administration is associated with decreased dopamine stores and TH activity. In addition to the effects on dopaminergic functioning, a profound depletion of serotonin and tryptophan hydroxylase activity has also been reported, although it seems that this effect is more specific to methylamphetamine than to *d*- or *l*-amphetamine.

AGGRESSION

The effects of amphetamine on aggressive behavior are complex and poorly understood. However, in general, the effects seem to depend on the dose, the environment, and the individual. Amphetamine use has been associated with the potential for sudden violent outbursts for quite a while; indeed, a common street warning of the 1960s and 1970s was "speed kills."

Several murders and other violent offenses have been attributed to amphetamine intoxication. Experimental research in humans indicates that acute doses of amphetamine can increase aggressiveness in humans. Humans exposed to a competitive task could deliver blasts of white noise or take money from a competitor. The results indicated that 5-mg and 10-mg doses increased the frequency of noise deliveries and the taking away of money, suggesting an increase in aggressive behavior. In contrast to these results, caffeine reduced the frequency of such aggressive behavior, indicating that the effects are specific to amphetamine.

In spite of this evidence indicating that amphetamine increases aggressive behavior, other evidence indicates that amphetamine can decrease aggressive behavior. Amphetamine treatment is used to treat aggression in children diagnosed with hyperkinesis and/or attention-deficit–hyperactivity disorder (ADHD). This effect has been repeatedly confirmed in controlled, double-blind studies. Not all surveys of prison populations and juvenile delinquents report finding a relation between aggression or hostility and amphetamine abuse.

ANOREXIA

Amphetamines are potent anorectics. The evidence indicates that this effect of the amphetamines is mediated by dopaminergic neurotransmission. Although research indicates that the amphetamines probably work through a dopaminergic mechanism, several lines of evidence indicate that structurally related compounds such as fenfluramine seem to act via a serotonergic mechanism.

Elimination and Pharmacokinetics

Renal Excretion

Amphetamine is a basic (pK_a 9.90), highly lipid-soluble drug, and a primary mode of elimination is excretion of the unchanged drug in the urine. Renal excretion is strongly determined by the pH of the urine; with acidic urine (e.g., pH 5), approximately 99% of a dose of amphetamine is ionized by glomerular filtration, and only the remaining nonionized portion of the drug is reabsorbed into the circulatory system. Hence, a treatment of amphetamine overdose is to acidify the urine.

Metabolism

There are several metabolic pathways for the biotransformation of the amphetamines. One pathway is aromatic hydroxylation. p-Hydroxyamphetamine, a major metabolite of this metabolic pathway, is also extremely biologically active. A second metabolic pathway is β-hydroxylation. This process is carried out by the enzyme dopamine β-hydroxylase, which converts dopamine to norepinephrine, and it is apparently restricted to the primary amines. Finally, by far the most important metabolic pathways for the amphetamines are those involving oxidation of the nitrogen and its carbons (i.e., N-dealkylation and deamination). Both reactions result in a primary amine and a carbonyl function. Deamination results in the excretion of the corresponding ketone, secondary alcohol, or benzoic acid, although the major metabolite excreted is benzoic acid.

After chronic administration of amphetamines, the tissue and brain contents of p-hydroxyamphetamine and p-hydroxynorephedrine are not significantly different from those of saline-treated control subjects, indicating that the rate of removal of amphetamine is not affected by chronic administration.

These results indicate that the metabolism of amphetamine is different from that of most other drugs. Chronic amphetamine administration does not seem to result in enzyme induction as indicated by the lack of an increase in the rate of removal, or the production of hydroxylated metabolites. However, during chronic administration, amphetamine and p-hydroxyephedrine may accumulate in a pool that could eventually disrupt cellular functioning. Finally, the brain and heart levels of amphetamine in chronically treated animals are significantly higher than those in control animals, and this difference may in part account for the sensitization often produced by chronic amphetamine administration.

Toxicity

Central Toxicities

The classical view of amphetamine neurotoxicity centers on necrotic cell death induced by free radical formation (reactive oxygen and nitrogen species). Briefly, amphetamine enters dopaminergic or serotonergic neurons via the respective transporter, and displaces vesicular and cytosolic neurotransmitter. Dopamine is metabolized by monoamine oxidase (MAO) into dihydroxyphenylacetic acid (DOPAC) and hydrogen peroxide (H_2O_2), or dopamine can be oxidized by molecular O_2 via autooxidative processes. Alternatively, the stimulation of N-methyl-D-aspartic acid (NMDA) receptors (via accumulation of synaptic glutamate levels) results in Ca^{2+} influx into the neuron, where Ca^{2+}–calmodulin binding activates neuronal nitric oxide synthase (nNOS). nNOS produces nitric oxide (NO) and hence the reactive nitrogen species peroxynitrite. Cell necrosis occurs as a direct result of the production of these reactive oxygen and nitrogen species. However, research also suggests that other mechanisms may be involved in the neurotoxicity of amphetamine. For example, amphetamine may exert a neurotoxic effect by the induction of apoptosis. Amphetamine is a highly lipophilic compound that can pass the neuronal membrane. Amphetamine can then, either directly or indirectly, interfere with mitochondrial function.

Changes in cerebral vasculature have also been reported following chronic amphetamine administration. High-dose amphetamines, both experimentally and clinically, induce hypertensive episodes associated with cerebral hemorrhage. Indeed, several cases of death have been attributed to hemorrhages induced by chronic amphetamine use.

Peripheral Toxicities

The cardiovascular effects of amphetamine are prominent. Amphetamine raises both systolic and diastolic blood pressure, and heart rate is reflexively slowed. Tachycardia and cardiac arrhythmias are not uncommon following high doses of amphetamines.

The amphetamines also result in peripheral hyperthermia via activation of the sympathoadrenal system. However, the amphetamines produce hypothermia centrally, and this seems to be mediated by the activity of the anterior hypothalamus.

Medical Uses of Amphetamines

In the late 1960s, at the height of the amphetamine-abuse epidemic in the United States, there were approximately 31 million prescriptions for anorectic stimulant drugs, yet enough was legally manufactured for 8 billion pills. This lax legal and social attitude of prescription-and-supply regulation was followed in most industrial nations by very strict control. From 1969 to 1971, the US government (a) markedly reduced the production of amphetamines by 80%, (b) alerted physicians to their dependence-producing effects, and (c) through the Food and Drug Administration (FDA) rescheduled amphetamines to Schedule II. The pendulum has swung back to the point that potentially important clinical uses are being avoided by physicians.

Stimulant Treatment of Attention-Deficit–Hyperactivity Disorder

The treatment of first choice for ADHD involves the use of psychostimulants, primarily methylphenidate (Ritalin), dextroamphetamine (Dexedrine), or pemoline (Cylert). Methylphenidate, the most common treatment, is a piperidine derivative structurally related to amphetamine and is a milder central nervous system stimulant than amphetamine. Numerous studies indicate that methylphenidate is highly effective in increasing attentiveness, reducing hyperactivity and destructive behavior, and improving classroom behavior and academic performance. The improvements in behavior and academic performance seem to persist as long as the drug is taken, with the behavior problems returning upon cessation of methylphenidate. Dextroamphetamine and pemoline are second-line stimulants used for those individuals who may not respond to methylphenidate. These drugs are reported to be as effective as methylphenidate in the treatment of ADHD. Several reports suggest that stimulants are also efficacious treatments for adult attention-deficit disorder.

Side Effects in the Use of Stimulants to Treat ADHD

There is clear evidence of temporary retardation in growth in weight and a suggestion of temporary slowing of stature growth related to drug dose and absence of drug holidays during the prepubertal period. To allow for growth rebound, the importance of drug holidays is evident in children requiring higher doses and manifesting drug plateaus. ADHD is associated with a variety of comorbid conditions, one of which is later substance abuse. However, treatment of ADHD significantly decreases the risk of later developing a substance abuse disorder.

Use of Stimulants as Anorectics

The effectiveness of stimulants as anorectics is well documented. The problem with the use of anorectics, besides their abuse potential, is that only a small percentage of patients maintain weight loss after cessation of anorectics. Where possible, stimulants with lower abuse potential should be used. With any clinical use of psychostimulants, careful history taking of previous drug misuse is warranted. Previous abusers of other stimulants should be excluded from treatment even when medically warranted.

Stimulant Treatment of Depression

In Europe, some countries have prohibited any use of stimulants. In 1968, an English report concluded that, with regard to the previous clinical use for depression, "amphetamines . . . have no place in the treatment of depression." On balance, there is no evidence to justify the use of stimulants as a first-line or routine treatment for the usual patient with depression. In patients with endogenous depression, stimulants may be useful to potentiate other antidepressant medications when used judiciously by experienced clinicians. Augmentation with stimulants may be effective in treatment-failure depressions.

Abuse

Amphetamines have been abused almost since their introduction. For example, benzedrine inhalers were abused by a wide segment of the population (e.g., athletes, professionals, and students) during the 1930s to overcome fatigue and increase alertness. Amphetamines were routinely available during World War II and the Vietnam War to keep soldiers alert during combat conditions. Amphetamine epidemics have been reported in Japan, Sweden, and the United States. These epidemics are generally associated with increasing levels of violence and the development of a "speed culture." These epidemics often start by introducing segments of the population to amphetamines for medical purposes, with a subsequent diversion of licit amphetamines to illicit markets.

In an individual, the development of stimulant abuse follows a developmental pattern that has been qualitatively described. This profile describes the behavioral pathologies that emerge during the active abuse and withdrawal phases.

Initiation Phase

During the initial, single-dose phase, the acute reinforcing actions of amphetamine are determined by the pharmacologic effects (i.e., release of dopamine) and the resulting euphoria, increase in energy, and enhancement of vocational and social interactions that occur following consumption. The individual may initially increase the number of settings and occasions on which the drug is used (e.g., for studying, at parties). During this phase, conditioning occurs: settings in which the drug is consumed become associated with the euphoriant and energizing effects of the drug, and this is especially true for individuals using rapid routes of administration (such as intravenous or smoking).

The initiation phase is primarily concerned with classical conditioning of drug cue or reinforcement properties. During this phase, both anticipatory acts and the stimulus properties of the drug are gradually linked in classically and operantly conditioned sequences. Anticipatory acts may include drug-seeking behaviors. Drug stimulus properties include not only the reinforcing efficacy of the drug but also the cascade of other discriminative or internally appreciated drug cues (e.g., subjective effects) associated with the consumption of the drug.

Consolidation Phase

With prolonged, intermittent consumption, the user discovers that higher doses produce greater effects; the individual starts to consume higher doses regularly, if the resources are available. Indeed, before the development of tolerance, the euphoriant effects of stimulants are proportional to amphetamine plasma levels. However, as stimulant use continues, tolerance to the euphoriant effects develops, and the individual starts to escalate the frequency and dose in an attempt to chase the "flash" or "rush" of amphetamine administration. During the high-dose transition phase, the individual resorts to rapid routes of administration, such as smoking or intravenous administration. In spite of any tolerance that may have developed, these routes of administration result in a rapid rise in plasma amphetamine levels, which produces an intense euphoria.

The individual may start binging during this period. A binge is characterized by the repeated readministration of the drug, resulting in frequent mood swings. Binges typically last 12 to 18 hours, but may last as long as 2, 3, or even 7 days. Such binges are facilitated by acute tolerance; the effects of the drug diminish rapidly. Acute tolerance, coupled with the memory of the preceding "flash," produces the desire to reinstate the drug effect; this is accomplished by the repeated consumption of the drug. These euphoric states result in strong memories of the drug effects and in the conditioning of previously neutral stimuli to the drug effects. During this period, the pattern of acquisition and intake becomes stereotyped and restricted; the individual's behavior focuses on the purchase and consumption of amphetamine, and the number of settings in which amphetamine is consumed becomes progressively restricted.

Withdrawal Phase

At the end of a binge, the individual enters the "crash" phase, which is characterized by initial depression, agitation, anxiety, anergia, and high drug craving. In the middle period of the crash phase, drug craving is replaced by fatigue, depression, loss of desire for the drug, and insomnia accompanied by an intense desire for sleep. During this time, the individual may use alcohol, benzodiazepines, or opiates to induce the desired sleep. During the late period of the crash phase, hypersomnolence is followed by awakening in a hyperphagic state.

Following the crash period, if individuals remain abstinent, they enter an intermediate withdrawal phase with effects that are generally opposite those of the drug: loss of physical and mental energy necessary to most naturally occurring incentive behaviors. Individuals experience fatigue, decreased mental energy, limited interest in the environment, and anhedonia. These symptoms gradually increase in intensity during the 12 to 96 hours following the crash phase.

During late withdrawal, or the extinction phase, brief periods of drug craving can occur. The individual may experience conditioned combinations of stimulus properties of both the drug and withdrawal "hunger" effects in the form of "urges" or "cravings." These episodes of craving are triggered by conditioned stimuli (circumstances and objects) that were previously associated with the drug effects. If the individual experiences these cues without the associated drug effects, then the ability of these cues to elicit drug craving will diminish over time, and the individual will experience less-intense drug cravings, which should lessen the probability of relapse.

Amphetamine Psychosis

During the phase of chronic, high-dose consumption of amphetamines, the individual may develop "amphetamine psychosis." The stimulant psychosis is more prevalent with amphetamine than with cocaine, probably because of the difficulty in sustaining high chronic levels of cocaine. This psychosis has several profiles. First, and most commonly, the individual develops paranoid ideation. This paranoia usually is accompanied by ideas of reference and an extremely well-formed delusional structure. In the beginning there is an exploratory, pleasurable, vague suspiciousness in which the individual continually wants to look beneath the surface of things (i.e., from the original term *subspicio*), and the individual watches others intensely. Later there is a phase reversal in which the person feels that others are watching and following him or her. As consumption continues, the individual may overreact to stimuli in the peripheral field of vision and may start to hallucinate. During the later stages of psychosis development, the individual may lose all insight and develop extremely well-structured delusions of persecution.

Another prominent aspect of amphetamine psychosis is the development of stereotyped behavior patterns that typically consist of activities that the individual normally engaged in and enjoyed doing. Many psychotic and prepsychotic individuals engage in the repetitive disassembling and reassembling of radios, engines, and various gadgets. Although individuals engaged in such activities are aware that the behavior is meaningless and serves no purpose, they report being unable to stop and become irritable and anxious if forced to stop. Furthermore, during engagement in the activity, the individuals report feeling an exploratory pleasure; they do not feel anxious.

Treatment of Amphetamine Abuse

An enormous research effort is based on the assumption that an understanding of the rate-limiting mechanisms underlying stimulant reinforcement, residual withdrawal states, and toxic consequences would lead to effective treatment regimens. Although a great deal has been learned about the neurobiologic mechanisms underlying these aspects of high-dose stimulant use, the development of rational treatment strategies has lagged.

Pharmacotherapy

No specific medication has gained widespread acceptance as having broad clinical effectiveness in the treatment of stimulant dependence. Nevertheless, medications are useful in managing particular manifestations of dependence in selected patients. Potential indications for pharmacotherapy include treatment of comorbid psychiatric disorders, management of stimulant withdrawal and other drug-induced mental disorders, treatment of concurrent substance use disorders (e.g., alcohol dependence), and facilitation of initial abstinence.

Behavioral Therapy

Extinction

During the active abuse phase, the pharmacologic effects of amphetamine consumption (e.g., euphoria and behavioral activation) become associated with various environmental stimuli via the process of classical conditioning. During the withdrawal phase, exposure to these same stimuli can elicit drug craving and urges. These cravings and urges are conditioned responses that extinguish slowly and that are not systematically affected by detoxification or the simple passage of time (i.e., forgetting). Hence, one behavioral treatment is to accelerate the extinction of these conditioned responses by exposing the individual, in a laboratory or clinical setting, to drug-related stimuli in the absence of any drug effects. Over repeated exposures, the cravings and urges diminish. This type of treatment is used with some success in the treatment of cocaine and opiate abusers.

Another behavioral therapy approach is contingency contracting. In this treatment, the abuser signs a "contract" stating that the abuser will perform certain behaviors; under the terms of some contracts, failure to perform these behaviors results in aversive consequences (e.g., the abuser's money being sent to the abuser's most disliked charity, the loss of a license to practice a profession); conversely, the fulfillment of the conditions of the contract may result in positive consequences (e.g., receiving money). Some behavioral contracts incorporate both positive and negative consequences. Contingency contracts are commonly used in urine-monitoring programs. In this treatment procedure, the individual agrees to participate in a urine-monitoring program, and failure to provide either a drug-free urine or a scheduled urine sample results in an aversive consequence; this aversive consequence is obtained from the abuser's own statements. It is important that any positive or negative consequences be derived from the abuser's own statements; otherwise, they will not be optimally effective.

Conclusion

The consumption of amphetamines for nonmedical reasons probably occurs because of their euphoriant and psychomotor-stimulating properties. Chronic consumption of amphetamine results in the development of stereotyped behavior, paranoia, and possibly aggression. During the protracted withdrawal phase from amphetamine, individuals experience anhedonia and anergia. This may be the result of long-lasting, and possibly permanent, changes in the neurobiologic substrates that mediate reward. In addition to these effects, acute and chronic consumption of amphetamine can be highly toxic. Deaths from amphetamine overdose are not uncommon and are caused by hyperpyrexia, cardiac failure, convulsions, and cerebral hemorrhage.

Suggested Readings

Baker A, Lee NK. A review of psychosocial interventions for amphetamine use. *Drug Alcohol Rev.* 2003;22:323–335.

Davidson C, Gow AJ, Lee TH, et al. Methamphetamine neurotoxicity: necrotic and apoptotic mechanisms and relevance to human abuse and treatment. *Brain Res Brain Res Rev.* 2001;36:1–22.

King GR, Ellinwood EH. Amphetamines and other stimulants. In: Lowinson JH, Ruiz P, Millman RB, et al., eds. *Substance abuse: a comprehensive textbook*, 4th ed. Philadelphia: Lippincott Williams & Wilkins; 2005:277–302.

Srisurapanont M, Jarusuraisin N, Kittirattanapaiboon P. Treatment of amphetamine dependence and abuse. *Cochrane Database Syst Rev.* 2001;(4):CD003022.

Willens TE, Spencer TJ, Biederman J. A review of the pharmacotherapy of adults with attention-deficit/hyperactivity disorder. *J Atten Disord.* 2002;5:189–202.

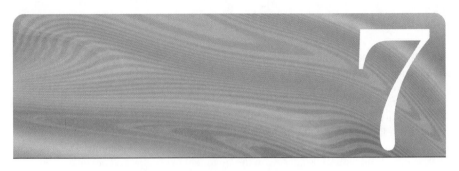

SEDATIVE–HYPNOTICS

This chapter focuses on the benzodiazepines and newer sedative–hypnotics because they have largely replaced the short-acting barbiturates and older non-barbiturate hypnotics in medical therapeutics. Abuse of older sedative–hypnotics has been greatly curtailed by controls on their availability, by the availability of new medications, and by changes in physician prescribing practices.

Some tricyclic antidepressants, such as amitriptyline, have sedation as a prominent side effect. Although not usually classified as sedative–hypnotics, they have properties that are sometimes used therapeutically as an alternative to classical sedative–hypnotics for treatment of insomnia.

Anticholinergics, commonly used to counteract the side effects of neuroleptic medication, can have sedative effects and some patients with schizophrenia take them in doses larger than prescribed. They are not widely abused, but are included here because alcoholics and other sedative–hypnotic abusers sometimes seek them for their sedative–hypnotic effects.

Sodium oxybate (also known as γ-hydroxybutyrate or GHB) is a sedative– hypnotic and a common drug of abuse. Sodium oxybate is now marketed for treatment of cataplexy associated with narcolepsy under the trade name Xyrem.

Although the use of sedative–hypnotics is ubiquitous in American society, mainstream society is ambivalent about the appropriate role of sedative–hypnotics. As a consequence, laws relating to sedative–hypnotics are complex, bewildering, and inconsistent. Alcohol is socially sanctioned as an intoxicant; marijuana—although still the focus of vigorous criminal prosecution and crop eradication in some states—is grudgingly tolerated; and medical prescription of sedative–hypnotics is increasingly subjected to controls (e.g., benzodiazepines have been put on triplicate prescription in New York, and because of its abuse, methaqualone has been removed from the American market). Sedative–hypnotic abuse is often attributed to physicians' overprescribing. What constitutes overprescribing, however, is a complex judgment that is molded by beliefs about the cause and appropriate treatment of anxiety and insomnia.

Opposition to treating anxiety with tranquilizers also comes from psychotherapists. Psychotherapists with a psychodynamic orientation view anxiety as a secondary symptom of an underlying psychopathology. Psychotherapeutic treatment is directed toward understanding and resolving the underlying reasons for anxiety. All mood-altering prescription medications are viewed as risky for a drug addict because the medication may trigger a return to drug-seeking behavior, particularly among recovering addicts who previously abused prescription medications.

Physicians are often faulted for "giving in" to their patients' request (or demand) for sedative–hypnotics. Clinically experienced physicians know, however, that trying to talk some patients out of taking sedative–hypnotics is futile, even when the distress is because of family discord, grief, an intolerable life situation, or an acute loss. When a physician refuses a patient's request for sedative–hypnotic medication, the patient generally concludes that the physician does not understand the severity of the patient's distress and consults another physician.

Benzodiazepines

Benzodiazepine use and abuse continues to generate professional controversy, legislative hearings, and articles in the lay press. Legislative concern about benzodiazepines generally involves the contribution of benzodiazepines to the cost of medical care or to benzodiazepine abuse and dependence.

The term *misuse* is commonly applied to prescription sedative–hypnotics. When medications are taken in higher doses or more frequently than prescribed, or taken by someone other than the person for whom the medication was prescribed, or taken for reasons other than what would normally be considered medical use, the behavior is generally considered misuse of the medication.

The criteria for abuse and dependence apply as uniformly as possible across classes of drugs, and the criteria do not distinguish the source of the medication or the intended purpose for which it was taken. Furthermore, when most people, including physicians, speak of drug *dependence*, they are referring to *physical dependence*. A diagnosis of substance dependence is only made when a patient has dysfunctional behaviors that are a result of the drug use.

In a regulatory context, "benzodiazepine abuse" can mean many things: self-administration of a benzodiazepine to produce intoxication or long-term prescription of benzodiazepines at therapeutic doses to patients who subsequently develop physical dependence on the benzodiazepines; or patients escalating their dose of benzodiazepines beyond that prescribed by their physicians; or use of a benzodiazepine by heroin or cocaine addicts to self-medicate symptoms of heroin withdrawal or cocaine toxicity; or intentional benzodiazepine overdose in a suicide or suicide attempt.

Epidemiology of Benzodiazepine Abuse

The incidence and prevalence of benzodiazepine abuse depend on how abuse is defined. If any nonmedical use of a benzodiazepine is defined as abuse, then benzodiazepine abuse is common.

Given the frequency with which benzodiazepines are prescribed, the rates of their abuse, even those such as alprazolam that are widely prescribed, is remarkably low. The abuse of benzodiazepines and other sedative–hypnotics is, however, a significant problem among some subgroups of patients, such as those on methadone maintenance. Benzodiazepine abuse, particularly flunitrazepam abuse, is associated with death of patients treated with buprenorphine (Buprenex).

Benzodiazepines are generally not primary drugs of abuse; that is, they are rarely taken by themselves to produce intoxication. Most people who take benzodiazepines do so for anxiolysis or sleep induction. After chronic use, they may also be taking them to ameliorate benzodiazepine withdrawal symptoms. Some alcohol and sedative–hypnotic abusers find the subjective effects of benzodiazepines desirable, but even among this population, benzodiazepines are rarely used alone to produce intoxication.

Benzodiazepines are commonly self-administered by drug addicts, sometimes to ameliorate withdrawal from heroin, alcohol, or other drugs or to attenuate the side effects of cocaine or methamphetamine intoxication. Addicts may also combine benzodiazepines with heroin, marijuana, or alcohol to enhance their effects.

Flunitrazepam is an effective hypnotic marketed in many countries for treatment of insomnia. Although not marketed in the United States or Canada, 1- and 2-mg tablets of flunitrazepam are available by prescription in Mexico, in Central and South America, and in many countries in Europe, Asia, and Africa. Until 1996, small quantities of flunitrazepam could be brought legally into the United States, but flunitrazepam is now subject to confiscation by U.S. Customs. Flunitrazepam abuse is most visible in Florida and Texas, although sporadic reports from drug abuse treatment clinics and police seizures of flunitrazepam in other areas suggest a broader distribution. Street names of flunitrazepam vary by region. In Florida, flunitrazepam is most often referred to as "roSHAY" or "roofies"; in Texas, it is often called "Roche." In the street-drug marketplace, deception is common, and many different kinds of tablets are being sold under these street names.

The popular media have given flunitrazepam abuse considerable attention in the United States. Newspapers and television coverage have focused on its use for "date rape." Although the publicity is framed to warn women that men may slip flunitrazepam into their drinks, another potential result of the publicity is to instruct unscrupulous men in its use.

A study of "Roche" abuse along the Texas–Mexico border from Brownsville to Laredo found that flunitrazepam abuse was only one of many benzodiazepines being abused. Although users in the area prefer white tablets imprinted with Roche and the number 2, many were not specifically seeking Rohypnol. From users' descriptions of the tablets and from police seizures of tablets at schools, it appears that many users are taking Rivotril (the trade name for clonazepam marketed in Mexico), Lexotán (the trade name for bromazepam, another benzodiazepine–hypnotic marketed in Mexico), and Valium (the trade name for diazepam), which is different in appearance from the Valium marketed in the United States.

Medical Uses of Benzodiazepines

Benzodiazepines have many important medical uses. Treatment of anxiety disorders, short-term treatment of insomnia, treatment of seizure disorders, and preoperative sedation and anesthesia are the most common uses. From an addiction medicine perspective, it is easy to lose sight of their medical utility because addiction medicine specialists treat patients who often misuse or abuse benzodiazepines or patients who have developed a dependence on them.

Benzodiazepines are still among the most widely prescribed medications, although there has been a steady decline in their prescription worldwide because new medications have been introduced for the same purposes and because there is concern about their overuse, misuse, and abuse. Benzodiazepines have been subject to increasing control and, in New York, have been placed on triplicate status. Benzodiazepines have a significant advantage over the previously available sedative–hypnotics. The short-acting and intermediate-acting barbiturates meprobamate and ethchlorvynol are lethal if taken in excess of ten times a single therapeutic dose. Benzodiazepines, on the other hand, are virtually nonlethal unless combined with alcohol or other drugs. Because children may accidentally overdose on prescription medications and because adults who overdose in suicide attempts often take everything in the family medicine cabinet, it is of significant public health benefit to have nonlethal medications in the family medicine cabinet.

Some patients with debilitating anxiety symptoms derive great benefit from benzodiazepine treatment, even from long-term treatment, and tolerance to the therapeutic effects and physical dependence do not inevitably occur.

Adverse Effects of Benzodiazepines

Separate from issues of addiction and dependence, the prescription of benzodiazepines can be associated with adverse effects that may bring patients to the attention of addiction specialists. Alprazolam (Xanax) is noteworthy because it is prescribed for treatment of panic attacks and depression in relatively high doses (4 to 10 mg/day) for extended periods of time. Initial clinical trials suggested few side effects or adverse events. With accumulated clinical experience, there have been case reports of alprazolam-released hostility, rebound insomnia, major depression, amnesia, and aggressive and violent behavior. Physical dependence can result when higher-than-usual therapeutic doses are used daily for about a month and when usual therapeutic doses are used for several months.

The prescription of psychotropic medications is malevolent only when medication robs a patient of the opportunity to develop a more satisfactory nonpharmacologic solution or when the patient develops drug dependence or other adverse effects that compound the patient's difficulties.

Liking of Drug by Addicts

Current and former drug abusers may have different subjective responses to psychoactive drugs than do nondrug abusers. The different response may have a biologic component, because altered response to benzodiazepines has been observed in children of alcoholics. The extent to which altered drug effects are learned, are the result of some genetically determined biochemical or receptor site differences, or are caused by perturbations of metabolism or receptor site function induced by long-term exposure to drugs is not well delineated. Whatever the cause, some drugs have desirable or reinforcing effects in people with current or past histories of alcohol and other drug abuse that are not present in nondrug abusers. Most nondrug abuser or nonanxious people do not like the effects of benzodiazepines and prefer a placebo. Studies in former drug abusers generally show that benzodiazepines are reinforcing, but less so than short-acting barbiturates. Of the benzodiazepines, addicts generally prefer diazepam or alprazolam to other benzodiazepines. Outside the laboratory setting, the benzodiazepine actually used by addicts is determined both by preference and accessibility.

Other Sedative–Hypnotics

When the short-acting sedative–hypnotics such as secobarbital (Seconal) and pentobarbital (Nembutal) were commonly prescribed, they were often taken orally or by injection to produce intoxication. Intoxication with sedative–hypnotics is qualitatively similar to intoxication with alcohol. The desired effect is a state of *disinhibition* in which mood is elevated; self-criticism, anxiety, and guilt are reduced; and energy and self-confidence are increased. During intoxication, the mood is often labile and may shift rapidly from euphoria to sadness. The user does not always obtain the desired effects and, while intoxicated, may be irritable, hypochondriacal, anxious, and angry to the point of rage. Pre-existing personality, expectations, and circumstances under which the drug is used all interact. Users' perception that a drug effect is pleasurable is partly learned and partly the pharmacology of the drug.

A person intoxicated on sedative–hypnotics commonly has an unsteady gait, slurred speech, sustained horizontal nystagmus, and poor judgment. Intoxication with sedative–hypnotics may produce an amnesia for events that occur while intoxicated that is similar to alcoholic blackouts. Amnesia appears particularly likely to occur with benzodiazepine intoxication.

Sedative–Hypnotic Withdrawal

The sedative–hypnotic withdrawal syndrome is a spectrum of signs and symptoms that occur after stopping or markedly reducing the daily intake of a sedative–hypnotic. Signs and symptoms do not always follow a specific sequence. Common signs and symptoms include anxiety, tremors, nightmares, insomnia, anorexia, nausea, vomiting, postural hypotension, seizures, delirium, and hyperpyrexia. The withdrawal syndrome is similar for all sedative–hypnotics, but the severity and time course depend on the particular sedative–hypnotic. With short-acting medications, such as pentobarbital, secobarbital, meprobamate, and methaqualone, withdrawal symptoms typically begin 12 to 24 hours after the last dose and peak in intensity between 24 and 72 hours after the last dose. If the patient has liver disease or is over the age of 65, symptoms may develop more slowly. With long-acting medications such as phenobarbital, diazepam, and chlordiazepoxide (Librium), the withdrawal syndrome usually begins 24 to 48 hours after the last dose and peaks on the fifth to eighth day.

During untreated sedative–hypnotic withdrawal, the electroencephalogram may show bursts of high-voltage, slow-frequency activity that precede clinical seizure activity. The withdrawal delirium may include disorientation as to time, place, and situation, and auditory and visual hallucinations. The delirium generally follows a period of insomnia. Some patients may have only delirium, others only seizures, and some may have both delirium and seizures.

With the exception of buspirone (BuSpar), which apparently does not have a withdrawal syndrome, the other sedative–hypnotics can produce clinically significant withdrawal signs and symptoms when taken at two or more times the maximum therapeutic range for more than 1 month.

Low-Dose Benzodiazepine Withdrawal Syndromes

Many patients who have taken benzodiazepines in therapeutic doses for months to years can abruptly discontinue the drug without developing withdrawal symptoms. The symptoms for which the benzodiazepine was being taken often return or intensify. The return of symptoms is called *symptom re-emergence* (or *recrudescence*). Patients' symptoms of anxiety, insomnia, or muscle tension abate during benzodiazepine treatment. When the benzodiazepine is stopped, symptoms return to the same level as before benzodiazepine therapy. The reason for making a distinction between symptom rebound and symptom recurrence is that symptom recurrence suggests persistence of the original symptoms, whereas symptom rebound suggests a transient withdrawal syndrome.

Other patients chronically taking similar amounts of a benzodiazepine in therapeutic doses develop symptoms ranging from mild to severe when the benzodiazepine is stopped or when the dosage is substantially reduced. Characteristically, patients tolerate a gradual tapering of the benzodiazepine until they are at 10% to 20% of their peak dose. Further reduction in benzodiazepine dose causes patients to become increasingly symptomatic. In addiction medicine literature, the low-dose benzodiazepine withdrawal syndrome may be called therapeutic-dose withdrawal, normal-dose withdrawal, or benzodiazepine discontinuation syndrome.

Many patients experience a transient increase in symptoms for 1 to 2 weeks after benzodiazepine withdrawal. The symptoms are an intensified return of the symptoms for which the benzodiazepine was prescribed. The transient form of symptom intensification is called *symptom rebound*. The term comes from sleep research in which "rebound insomnia" is commonly observed following sedative–hypnotic use. Symptom rebound lasts a few days to weeks following discontinuation of the benzodiazepine. Symptom rebound is the most common withdrawal consequence of prolonged benzodiazepine use.

A few patients experience a severe, protracted withdrawal syndrome that includes symptoms (e.g., paresthesias and psychosis) that were not present before. It is this latter withdrawal syndrome that has generated much of the concern about the long-term *safety* of the benzodiazepines when taken daily for months to years.

Protracted Benzodiazepine Withdrawal Syndrome

In some patients, protracted benzodiazepine withdrawal consists of relatively mild withdrawal symptoms such as mild to moderate anxiety, mood instability, and sleep disturbance. In others, however, the protracted withdrawal syndrome consists of increased sensitivity to light and sound, psychosis, and severe insomnia. The symptoms can be severe and disabling and last many months.

There is considerable controversy surrounding even the existence of this syndrome. The notion of a protracted withdrawal syndrome evolves primarily from the addiction medicine literature. Many symptoms are nonspecific and often mimic an obsessive–compulsive disorder with psychotic features. As a practical matter, it is often difficult in the clinical setting to separate symptom re-emergence from protracted withdrawal. New symptoms such as paresthesias and increased sensitivity to sound, light, and touch are particularly suggestive of low-dose withdrawal.

The waxing and waning of symptom intensity from day-to-day is characteristic of the low-dose protracted benzodiazepine withdrawal syndrome. Patients are sometimes asymptomatic for several days; then, without apparent reason, they become acutely anxious. Often there are concomitant physiologic signs, for example, dilated pupils, increased resting heart rate, and increased blood pressure. The intense waxing and waning of symptoms is important in distinguishing low-dose withdrawal symptoms from symptom re-emergence.

Risk Factors for Low-Dose Withdrawal

Some drugs or medications may facilitate neuroadaptation by increasing the affinity of benzodiazepines for their receptors. Phenobarbital, for example, increases the affinity of diazepam to benzodiazepine receptors, and prior treatment with phenobarbital has been found to increase the intensity of chlordiazepoxide (45 mg/day) withdrawal symptoms. Patients at increased risk for development of the low-dose withdrawal syndrome are those with a family or personal history of alcoholism, those who use alcohol daily, and those who concomitantly use other sedatives.

Pharmacologic Treatment of Withdrawal

The strategies for treating physical dependence on sedative–hypnotics involve gradual reduction of a sedative–hypnotic or substitution of an anticonvulsant medication that allows the physiologic readjustment to occur gradually. There are three basic strategies: (a) use gradually decreasing doses of the sedative–hypnotic; (b) substitute long-acting barbiturate for the sedative–hypnotic of abuse and gradually withdraw the long-acting sedative–hypnotic; and (c) substitute an anticonvulsant such as carbamazepine (Tegretol) or valproate (Depakene).

Abrupt discontinuation of a sedative–hypnotic in a patient who is physically dependent on it is not acceptable medical practice. Unlike opiate withdrawal, whose withdrawal symptoms are unpleasant but not life threatening in an otherwise healthy patient, abrupt withdrawal of sedative–hypnotics can be fatal.

Withdrawal of the Drug of Dependence

The classical treatment of a sedative–hypnotic patient is a gradual withdrawal of the drug of dependence. Although the method is sound from a pharmacologic point of view, it has some disadvantages. When the drug of dependence is a short-acting hypnotic, such as a short-acting barbiturate, patients may become intoxicated and disinhibited, resulting in behavior problems. Giving an addict their drug of abuse, even in a therapeutic context, is problematic.

A gradual taper of the drug of dependence is more often used in the context of therapeutic discontinuation of patients from long-acting sedative–hypnotics. With long-term benzodiazepine therapy, for example, physical dependence can develop in patients who do not have a substance abuse disorder. In this situation, gradual taper of the drug of dependence can be an appropriate therapeutic strategy.

Substitution of Phenobarbital

Phenobarbital substitution has a number of advantages over withdrawal from the drug of dependence. First, phenobarbital is long acting, and small changes in blood levels of phenobarbital occur between doses, allowing the safe use of smaller daily doses. Second, phenobarbital is safer than the shorter-acting barbiturates, because the lethal dose of phenobarbital is many times higher than the toxic dose and the signs of toxicity (e.g., sustained nystagmus, slurred speech, and ataxia) are easy to observe. Third, phenobarbital intoxication does not usually produce disinhibition, so most patients view it as a medication, not as a drug of abuse. Finally, the phenobarbital technique can be applied to a broad range of sedative–hypnotics and with patients who abuse a mixture of alcohol and/or sedative–hypnotics.

The disadvantages to phenobarbital substitution are that the calculations for making the conversion between the drug or drugs of abuse are tedious, and 1% to 5% of patients treated with phenobarbital develop a rash.

STABILIZATION PHASE

The substitution dose of phenobarbital is calculated by substituting 30 mg of phenobarbital for each hypnotic dose of the drug of abuse. Phenobarbital withdrawal conversion equivalence is not the same as therapeutic dose equivalency. The phenobarbital withdrawal equivalence is the amount of phenobarbital that can be substituted to prevent emergence of serious sedative–hypnotic withdrawal signs and symptoms.

For sedative–hypnotics that are not marketed as sleeping pills, the upper recommended therapeutic single dose is considered equivalent to the hypnotic dose. For medications marketed primarily for treatment of insomnia, the lower recommended dose is considered a "hypnotic dose." The conversion is, at best, a clinical approximation, and published tables sometimes show different withdrawal equivalent values for phenobarbital. Phenobarbital equivalents do, however, provide a clinically appropriate starting dose of phenobarbital that will usually prevent the emergence of medically serious withdrawal symptoms. Because phenobarbital has a long half-life, blood levels of phenobarbital will continue to increase even with a fixed daily dose. The key to successful clinical use of phenobarbital is careful monitoring of the patient before each dose. If signs of sedative–hypnotic intoxication occur (e.g., slurred speech, sustained nystagmus), the dose is adjusted downward; if symptoms of withdrawal occur (e.g., intense nightmares, muscle twitching, psychosis), the dose is increased.

Regardless of the computed dose, the maximum starting daily dose of phenobarbital should not exceed 500 mg per day.

If, on initial evaluation, the patient is in acute sedative–hypnotic withdrawal and has had a withdrawal seizure, the initial dose of phenobarbital is administered by injection. If nystagmus, slurred speech, or ataxia develop 1 to 2 hours after the intramuscular dose, the patient is in no immediate danger from sedative–hypnotic withdrawal. Patients are maintained on the initial calculated schedule of phenobarbital for 2 days. Patients who have neither signs of sedative–hypnotic withdrawal nor signs of phenobarbital intoxication are ready to begin phenobarbital withdrawal.

WITHDRAWAL PHASE

For inpatients the daily phenobarbital dose is decreased 30 mg per day unless the patient develops signs or symptoms of phenobarbital toxicity or sedative–hypnotic withdrawal. (Outpatient withdrawal generally proceeds more slowly.) If signs of phenobarbital toxicity appear, the daily phenobarbital dose is decreased by 50%, and the 30-mg-per-day withdrawal is continued from the reduced phenobarbital dose. If the patient has objective signs of sedative–hypnotic withdrawal, the daily phenobarbital dose is increased 50%, and the patient is restabilized before continuing the withdrawal.

Substitution of an Anticonvulsant

Protocols using carbamazepine or valproic acid (Depakote, Depakene) have been used clinically for treatment of sedative–hypnotic withdrawal. Both medications enhance γ-aminobutyric acid (GABA) function. Both are effective in suppressing benzodiazepine withdrawal symptoms. Neither carbamazepine nor valproic acid produces effects that sedative–hypnotic abusers find desirable.

The use of valproate as a withdrawal protocol was suggested in 1989, and there are clinical case reports of its use in benzodiazepine withdrawal. Valproic acid in a dosage up to about 1,200 mg per day is useful both in acute withdrawal and in treatment of persistent symptoms following withdrawal.

Carbamazepine is reported to be useful in benzodiazepine withdrawal and in alcohol withdrawal. It is also useful in treating benzodiazepine withdrawal in benzodiazepine-dependent, methadone-maintained patients. Both carbamazepine and phenobarbital can increase the metabolism of methadone and require that the dose of methadone be adjusted. In patients with seizure disorders, valproic acid appears to be better tolerated than carbamazepine.

Zolpidem

Zolpidem (Ambien) is an imidazopyridine hypnotic, chemically unrelated to the benzodiazepines. Although zolpidem is not chemically a benzodiazepine, its pharmacologic profile is similar to a benzodiazepine, and it binds to a subunit of the same GABA-benzodiazepine (GABA-BZ) receptor as the benzodiazepines. Its sedative effects are reversed by the benzodiazepine antagonist flumazenil. Zolpidem is rapidly absorbed and has a short half-life ($T_{1/2}$ = 2.2 hours). Its sedative effects are additive with alcohol. Like triazolam, zolpidem decreases brain metabolism of glucose.

Zaleplon

Zaleplon (Sonata) is a pyrazolopyrimidine that the Food and Drug Administration (FDA) approved for marketing in the United States in 1999. Like zolpidem, it is chemically unrelated to the benzodiazepines and binds to the ω-1-receptor, which is a subunit of the GABA-BZ receptor. Studies in baboons and healthy volunteers with a history of drug abuse suggest abuse potential similar to triazolam.

Buspirone

Buspirone is an anxiolytic that is not chemically or pharmacologically related to the benzodiazepines, barbiturates, or other sedative–hypnotics. Buspirone is not cross-tolerant with classical sedative–hypnotics and will not prevent acute benzodiazepine withdrawal signs and symptoms even when the buspirone is begun 4 weeks before benzodiazepine withdrawal is initiated. From the neuropharmacology of benzodiazepine withdrawal, buspirone appears to have clinical utility in benzodiazepine discontinuation.

The anxiolytic effects of buspirone take days to weeks to develop. Buspirone has been proposed as an alternative to benzodiazepines in postdetoxification treatment of anxiety in patients who are alcohol or sedative–hypnotic dependent.

Anticholinergics

Trihexyphenidyl (Artane) and benztropine (Cogentin) are commonly used to ameliorate neuroleptic-induced extrapyramidal symptoms. In a case series ($n = 214$) from a hospital in Israel, evidence for abuse of trihexyphenidyl was found in 6.5% of admissions for schizophrenia. Although anticholinergics in low doses can have sedative–hypnotic effects, a case report suggests that patients may abuse high doses of trihexyphenidyl for nonspecific stimulant or euphoric effects. Long-term abuse of trihexyphenidyl has been reported to produce impairment of memory and cognitive function, which clears after withdrawal of the medication. The frequency of benztropine abuse in the severely mentally disturbed population has been reported to be as high as 30%, and treatment of benztropine abuse can require hospitalization.

Conclusion

The benzodiazepines remain valuable medications and their general safety in terms of overdose lethality remains unchallenged. Most of the controversy or difficulty with benzodiazepines revolves around (a) the neuroadaptive changes that may occur with chronic use; (b) their prescription to addicts in recovery and their use by addicts to self-medicate drug toxicity from cocaine and methamphetamine; (c) their use by opioid addicts to boost methadone or buprenorphine effects; and (d) their nonmedical use as incapacitating agents for robbery or date-rape. Physical dependence may occur in the context of chronic therapeutic benzodiazepine use.

Some of the conditions for which benzodiazepines have been chronically prescribed— treatment of generalized anxiety disorder, pain attacks, and insomnia—have been supplanted by the selective serotonin reuptake inhibitors and newer hypnotics. Therapeutic use of benzodiazepines in treatment of psychiatric disorders is still evolving and beyond the scope of this chapter, which focuses on diagnosis and treatment of benzodiazepine abuse and dependence.

Suggested Readings

Buhrich N, Weller A, Kevans P. Misuse of anticholinergic drugs by people with serious mental illness. *Psychiatr Serv.* 2000;51(7):928–929.

Piercey MF, Hoffmann WE, Cooper M. The hypnotics triazolam and zolpidem have identical metabolic effects throughout the brain: implications for benzodiazepine receptor subtypes. *Brain Res.* 1991;554(1–2):244–252.

Rickels K, Case WG, Schweizer, et al. Benzodiazepine dependence: management of discontinuation. *Psychopharmacol Bull.* 1990;26(1):63–68.

Rush CR, Frey JM, Griffiths RR. Zaleplon and triazolam in humans: acute behavioral effects and abuse potential. *Psychopharmacology (Berl).* 1999;145(1):39–51.

Sellers EM, Ciraulo DA, DuPont RL, et al. Alprazolam and benzodiazepine dependence. *J Clin Psychiatry.* 1993;54(Suppl 10):64–75.

Wesson DR, Smith DE, Ling W, et al. Sedative–hypnotics. In: Lowinson JH, Ruiz P, Millman RB, et al., eds. *Substance abuse: a comprehensive textbook,* 4th ed. Philadelphia: Lippincott Williams & Wilkins; 2005:302–313.

8

HALLUCINOGENS

Data indicate that the use of hallucinogens is on the rise, especially among adolescents. The trend of decreased use of the hallucinogens in the United States, from the mid-1970s through the 1980s has begun to reverse. Moreover, in recent years the Internet has become a widely used source of information on hallucinogens, and a vehicle for obtaining the drugs. Although during the 1980s little research was conducted wherein humans were administered hallucinogens, over the last few years there has been a resurgence of clinical studies carried out under highly controlled conditions. The results obtained from controlled clinical studies should provide important information, in contrast to some of the clinical data that previously have come from anecdotal information. This resurgence in clinical research has taken place at the same time that there have been major advances regarding the possible mechanisms of action of the hallucinogens. Although in the past decade there had been an ever-widening discrepancy between our limited knowledge of the clinical pharmacology of the hallucinogens and information on their mechanisms of action obtained from preclinical studies, we now may be reaching a point where we can begin to develop a unified conceptual framework regarding the fundamental mechanisms underlying their pharmacologic effects in humans.

Historical Perspective

In the early 1960s, Timothy Leary, then a young psychology instructor at Harvard, began experimenting with hallucinogens, particularly lysergic acid diethylamide (LSD). He claimed that it provided instant happiness, enhanced creativity in art and music, facilitated problem-solving ability, increased self-awareness, and might be useful as an adjunct to psychotherapy. Leary popularized this on college campuses, coining the phrase "turn on, tune in, drop out." When he was not reappointed to the faculty at Harvard, he became a highly publicized self-proclaimed martyr to his cause, and his followers began to proselytize for LSD. Leary's advocates organized their lifestyle around LSD and developed a subculture of fellow LSD users who shared this common interest. They would never give it to anyone without their knowledge, and they would not use other classes of drugs. For example, they would not smoke tobacco, use amphetamine or amphetamine-like psychostimulants or barbiturates, or even drink alcohol. Thus, very little polydrug abuse occurred among these LSD users. In contrast to later patterns of hallucinogen use, the early users of LSD were older; a study published in 1968 revealed that the average age of persons using and in difficulty from LSD was 21 years. At that time the quality of street LSD was equivalent to that made by legitimate chemists at Sandoz Laboratories, the original manufacturer of the drug.

Subcultures experimenting with LSD began to emerge in many East and West Coast cities. Other hallucinogenic compounds, such as mescaline and psilocybin, began to be taken as well, although LSD remained the most widely used hallucinogen because it was the most readily available on the street. Later, younger individuals began to experiment with LSD, and its use began to increase in all socioeconomic groups, particularly among middle-class and affluent youth. About this time, various adverse reactions began to be recorded. The populace reacted with anxiety and fear, worrying that many of the young would soon become acidheads.

Eventually, many LSD users became involved in polydrug abuse, using other drugs besides hallucinogens. In the search for new drugs with different and improved characteristics, such as more or less euphoria, hallucinogenic activity or stimulant properties, and a longer or shorter duration of action, literally hundreds of so-called designer drugs were synthesized, for example, dimethoxy-methylamphetamine (DOM), methylene-dioxymethamphetamine (ecstasy or MDMA), dimethyltryptamine (DMT).

Concern about drug abuse rose until it finally was perceived as one of the nation's most pressing problems, along with the economy and the war in Vietnam. The nation geared up to declare war on drug abuse, and the national drug abuse effort expanded from a relatively small research-oriented program under the National Institute of Mental Health (NIMH) to the then newly created National Institute on Drug Abuse (NIDA) and the National Institute on Alcohol Abuse and Alcoholism (NIAAA).

By the mid-1960s more than a thousand articles on LSD had appeared in the medical literature. Sandoz Laboratories stopped distributing the drug in late 1966 because of the reported adverse reactions and the resulting public outcry. At that time, all of the existing supplies of LSD were turned over to the government, which was to make the drug available for legitimate and highly controlled research; however, research on humans essentially was discontinued. Although some of the hallucinogens originally were developed and studied for use in chemical warfare, the results of these experiments remain classified. Today, LSD, along with heroin and marijuana, remains classified as a Schedule I drug. Legally, LSD is regarded as having no currently accepted medical use in the United States, a high potential for abuse, and to be unsafe even when administered by a physician. The therapeutic potential of LSD as an adjunct to psychotherapy, in the management of the dying patient, and in the treatment of alcoholism and neuropsychiatric illness such as obsessive–compulsive disorder remains unresolved. Nevertheless, black market LSD remains widely available on the street.

Definitions and Terminology

The term *hallucinogen* means "producer of hallucinations." Many drugs, when taken in sufficient quantity, are psychoactive and can cause auditory and/or visual hallucinations. Such hallucinations may be present as part of a delirium, accompanied by disturbances in judgment, orientation, intellect, memory, emotion, and level of consciousness (e.g., organic brain syndrome). Delirium also may result from drug withdrawal (e.g., sedative–hypnotic withdrawal or delirium tremens in alcohol withdrawal). Hallucinogen, however, generally refers to compounds that alter consciousness without producing delirium, sedation, excessive stimulation, or intellectual or memory impairment as prominent effects. True LSD-induced hallucinations are rare; what are commonly seen are illusory phenomena. An illusion is a perceptual distortion of an actual stimulus in the environment: to see someone's face seeming to be melting is an illusion, whereas to see a melting face when no face is present is a hallucination.

There are a variety of widely accepted synonyms for the hallucinogens, including the term *psychedelic*. Unfortunately, those who use the term psychedelic are criticized as being "prodrug," much as those who use the term hallucinogen are accused of being "antidrug." Other suggested names include phantastica, psychotaraxic, psycholeptic, and psychotomystic. The term *psychotomimetic*, meaning "a producer of psychosis," also has been widely used.

Epidemiology

The epidemiologic data on the use of hallucinogens centers on the use of LSD in the United States. Both the use of LSD and its availability decreased from the mid-1970s through the 1980s. These downward trends appear to be reversing beginning in the 1990s. In 1992, there was an increase in prevalence in the use of LSD by school-age children and young adults, but there are indications that since that time increases have continued only in high school students. There are ethnic differences in the use of hallucinogens; in the 12th grade whites have a higher usage of LSD and hallucinogens than either African Americans or Hispanics. Other studies have shown even higher rates of hallucinogen usage. For example, a random survey of Tulane University undergraduates in 1990 indicated that the number of students reporting having tried LSD was more than 17%.

Hallucinogens appear to be readily available on the street. In 1994, more than 24% of 18-year-olds said that they were "exposed" (friends using drug or around people using drug) to LSD, whereas 14% said that they were "exposed" to other hallucinogens. There also have been changes in attitudes toward their use. Among high school students there has been a decrease in the proportions disapproving of LSD use and associating risk with its use; in contrast, older groups are more likely to perceive LSD as dangerous. These changes in attitude are likely linked to the increase in use in those age groups.

Chemical Classification

The commonly abused hallucinogenic substances can be classified according to their chemical structure. All of these drugs are organic compounds and some occur naturally.

Indolealkylamines

All the indole-type hallucinogens have structural similarities to the neurotransmitter serotonin (5-hydroxytryptamine, 5-HT), suggesting that their mechanism of action could involve the alteration of serotonergic neurotransmission.

Lysergic Acid Derivatives

Lysergic acid is one of the constituents of the ergot fungus that grows on rye. It has inadvertently been baked into bread, with profound mental changes occurring in those who consumed it. Because the presence of the diethylamide group is a prerequisite for hallucinogenic activity, it is not clear whether these reported epidemics actually were caused by ergot in the bread, or by some other related substances or (psychologic) phenomena. LSD was first synthesized by Hofmann in 1938, and it was called LSD-25 because it was the 25th compound made in this series of experiments on ergot derivatives. In 1943, Hofmann accidentally ingested some of the compound, and soon had the first LSD trip, a famous bicycle ride home from his laboratory. The seeds of the morning glory (*Ipomoea*) contain lysergic acid derivatives, particularly lysergic acid amide. Commercial packages of seeds often have been treated with insecticides, fungicides, and other toxic chemicals.

Substituted Tryptamines

Psilocybin and psilocin occur naturally in a variety of mushrooms that have hallucinogenic properties. The most publicized is the Mexican or "magic" mushroom, *Psilocybe mexicana*, which contains both psilocybin and psilocin, as do some of the other *Psilocybe* and *Conocybe* species. DMT, although found in the psychoactive ayahuasca, is usually produced synthetically.

Substituted Phenethylamines

The substituted phenethylamine-type hallucinogens are structurally related to the catecholamine neurotransmitters dopamine, norepinephrine, and epinephrine.

Mescaline

Mescaline is a naturally occurring hallucinogen present in the peyote cactus (*Lophophora williamsii* or *Anhalonium lewinii*), which is found in the southwestern United States and northern Mexico. Peyote was used by the Indians in these areas in highly structured tribal religious rituals.

Phenylisopropylamines

The phenylisopropylamine hallucinogens DOM (or STP, from "serenity, tranquility, and peace"), MDA (or "Eve"), and MDMA (or ecstasy) are synthetic compounds and are structurally similar to mescaline as well as the psychostimulant amphetamine. They have inaccurately been called "psychotomimetic amphetamines" and sometimes are referred to as "stimulant-hallucinogens." It should be pointed out that literally hundreds of analogues of the aforementioned compounds, the so-called designer drugs, have been synthesized and sometimes are found on the street.

Acute Psychologic Effects

The overall psychologic effects of many of the hallucinogens are quite similar; however, the rate of onset, duration of action, and absolute intensity of the effects differ among the drugs. Moreover, the various hallucinogens vary widely in potency and the slope of the dose–response curve. Thus, some of the apparent qualitative differences among hallucinogens may be partly a result of the amount of drug ingested relative to its specific dose–response characteristics.

LSD is one of the most potent hallucinogens known, with behavioral effects occurring in some individuals after doses as low as 20 μg. In the past, typical street doses ranged from 50 to 300 μg ; however, some anecdotal evidence indicates that today's street LSD is less potent. The reported street dose is often highly inaccurate.

Because of its high potency, LSD can be applied to paper blotters or the backs of postage stamps. The absorption of LSD from the gastrointestinal tract occurs rapidly, with drug diffusion to all tissues, including the brain. The onset of psychologic and behavioral effects occurs approximately 60 minutes after oral administration and peaks 2 to 4 hours after administration, with a gradual return to the predrug state in 10 to 12 hours.

The first 4 hours after LSD ingestion are sometimes called a "trip." The effects of LSD are dramatic, and can be divided into somatic (dizziness, paresthesias, weakness, and tremor), perceptual (altered visual sense and changes in hearing), and psychic (changes in mood, dream-like feelings, altered time sense, and depersonalization). Somatic symptoms usually occur first. Later, visual alterations are marked and sounds are intensified. Visual distortions and illusory phenomena occur, but true hallucinations are rare. Dream-like imagery may develop when the eyes are closed, and afterimages are prolonged. Sensory input becomes mixed together, and synesthesia ("seeing" smells, "hearing" colors) is commonly reported. Touch is magnified and time is markedly distorted. Feelings of attainment of true insight are common, as is the experience of delusional ideation. Separating one object from another and self from environment becomes difficult, and depersonalization can develop. Emotions become intensified, and extreme and rapid affective lability may be observed. Several emotional feelings may occur at the same time. Performance on tests involving attention, concentration, and motivation is impaired. Several hours later, subjects sometimes feel that the drug is no longer active, but later they recognize that at that time they had paranoid thoughts and ideas of reference. This is a regular, but little publicized, aftereffect that finally dissipates 10 to 12 hours after the dose. From 12 to 24 hours after the trip there may be some slight letdown or a feeling of fatigue. There is no immediate craving to take more drug to relieve this boredom; one trip usually produces "satiation" for some time. Memory for the events that occurred during the trip is quite clear.

DMT produces effects that are similar to those produced by LSD, but DMT is inactive after oral administration and must be injected, sniffed, or smoked. It has a rapid onset, almost immediately after intravenous administration, and a short duration of action, about 30 minutes. Because of its short duration of action, DMT was once known as the "businessman's LSD" (i.e., one could have a psychedelic experience during the lunch hour and be back at work in the afternoon). However, the sudden and rapid onset of a period of altered perceptions that soon terminates is disconcerting to some. DMT has never been a widely, steadily available or popular drug on the streets. The effects of ayahuasca, a psychoactive beverage that contains DMT, last about 4 hours.

In contrast to DMT, the effects of DOM have a very slow onset, but the effects have been reported to last more than 24 hours. Mescaline is approximately two to three orders of magnitude less potent than LSD, and its effects last about 6 to 10 hours, whereas the effects of psilocybin last about 2 hours.

Autonomic and Other Effects

The hallucinogens also possess significant autonomic activity. LSD produces marked pupillary dilation, hyperreflexia, increases in blood pressure and body temperature, tremor, piloerection, and tachycardia. Some autonomic effects of hallucinogens are variable and might be partly a result of the anxiety state of the user. DMT and ayahuasca also increase heart rate, pupil diameter, and body temperature. LSD also can cause nausea, and nausea and vomiting are especially noteworthy after the ingestion of mescaline or peyote. The hallucinogens also alter neuroendocrine function. For example, in humans, DMT elevates plasma levels of cortisol, adrenocorticotropic hormone (ACTH), and prolactin. Similarly, LSD and the hallucinogen 1-(2,5-dimethoxy-4-iodophenyl)-2-aminopropane (DOI) increase plasma glucocorticoids in the rat.

Effects of Chronic Use

A high degree of tolerance develops to the behavioral effects of LSD after repeated administration. Such behavioral tolerance develops rapidly, after only several days of daily administration, and tolerance is also lost rapidly after the individual stops taking the drug for several days. Because of this rapid development of tolerance, LSD users usually limit themselves to taking the drug once or twice weekly. Cross-tolerance develops between LSD and other hallucinogens, such as mescaline and psilocybin, suggesting a similar mechanism of action. However, cross-tolerance does not develop to other classes of psychotropic agents that are thought to have different underlying mechanisms of action, such as amphetamines, phencyclidine, and marijuana. Little tolerance develops to the various autonomic effects produced by the hallucinogens. There is no withdrawal syndrome after the cessation of the chronic administration of the hallucinogens.

Mechanisms of Action

The exact mechanisms of action of LSD and other hallucinogens still remain unclear. LSD affects the electrical activity of neurons in the locus ceruleus and certain cortical regions, and at a system level, these effects could change how the brain handles sensory information, as well as alter cognitive and perceptual processing. Although hallucinogenic drugs interact with several neurotransmitter systems, their ability to alter neurotransmission mediated by the neurotransmitter serotonin appears to be of critical importance. It is important to note that an ever-increasing number of serotonin receptors have been identified, and the terminology for these serotonin receptor families and subtypes is in a state of flux. Some of the receptors have been renamed or reclassified, and caution must be used in comparing results and conclusions drawn from older studies with the nomenclature currently used.

Early on it was noted that many hallucinogens, including LSD, were structurally similar to serotonin. However, it was found that brom-LSD, an LSD analogue that does not produce hallucinations, also has serotonergic antagonist activity. Thus, the hallucinogenic activity of LSD could not be explained solely by its direct serotonergic antagonist activity.

In 1961, to provide direct evidence was found that LSD acted on serotonergic systems within the central nervous system. It was found that LSD increases the levels of serotonin in rat brain, but decreases the levels of serotonin metabolites, whereas the nonhallucinogenic analogue brom-LSD failed to have the same effects. That brom-LSD does not produce hallucinatory phenomena suggests that the hallucinogenic effects of LSD might be caused by LSD-induced decreases in serotonin turnover (synthesis and release) in the brain.

LSD inhibits the firing of serotonergic neurons in the dorsal raphe nucleus, most likely by interacting with presynaptic autoreceptors (5-HT_{1A} receptors). Other indole-type hallucinogens, such as psilocin and DMT, also produce this effect. A decrease in firing rate of serotonergic neurons would account for LSD increasing the levels of serotonin, but decreasing the levels of serotonin metabolites. However, strong evidence refutes a direct linkage between the presynaptic effects of LSD and its hallucinogenic activity: (a) phenethylamine hallucinogens, such as mescaline, do not have the same inhibitory effects on the firing of serotonergic neurons; (b) there is no correlation between the activity of drugs at presynaptic 5-HT_{1A} receptors and their hallucinogenic activity; and (c) tolerance does not develop to the effects of the hallucinogens on neuronal firing, but behavioral tolerance rapidly develops after the repeated administration of hallucinogens. These findings suggest that interactions with presynaptic 5-HT_{1A} receptors cannot be the sole mechanism of action of the hallucinogens, and other factors must be involved.

Both indole-type and phenethylamine-type hallucinogens bind to the serotonin 5-HT_{2A} receptor subtype (formerly called the 5-HT_2 receptor), where they act as agonists or partial agonists. This receptor subtype is found in high concentrations in cortical and limbic regions, and these receptor interactions appear to underlie the mechanism of action of the hallucinogens.

Even though the interaction of hallucinogens with 5-HT_{2A} receptors appears to be critical, other serotonergic receptor subtypes also might be involved. For example, interactions with the closely related 5-HT_{2C} receptors (formerly called 5-HT_{1C} receptors) might contribute to the psychoactive effects. Although apparently not critical for hallucinogenic activity, interactions with presynaptic 5-HT_{1A} receptors might contribute to the effects of some hallucinogens. The differential interactions of the various hallucinogens with numerous sites and systems might underlie the qualitative differences between the drugs. However, the commonality of interactions with 5-HT_{2A} receptors suggests that drugs that possess 5-HT_{2A} receptor antagonist activity might be useful in blocking the behavioral effects of the hallucinogens in humans.

Adverse Reactions

Acute Adverse Reactions

A person's reaction to the effects of a drug may be felt to be either a pleasant or an unpleasant experience; a perceptual distortion or illusion may cause intense anxiety in one person and be a pleasant and amusing interlude in another. Individuals who place a premium on self-control, advance planning, and impulse restriction may do particularly poorly on LSD. Traumatic and stressful external events can precipitate an adverse reaction. Prediction of who will have an acute (or other) adverse reaction is unreliable, and the occurrence of multiple previous pleasurable LSD experiences renders no immunity from an adverse reaction. Adverse reactions have occurred after doses of LSD as low as 40 μg, and no adverse effects have been observed in some individuals after ingesting 2,000 μg, although in general the hallucinogenic effects are dose dependent. Thus, acute adverse behavioral reactions generally are a function of personal predisposition, setting, and circumstance. Because of the perceptual distortions (and subsequent deficits in judgment), there is always the risk that self-destructive behavior will occur. Some of the adverse reactions that occur after ingesting hallucinogens can be caused by other contaminants in the product, such as strychnine, phencyclidine, or amphetamine. Once commonly reported by medical facilities, acute adverse LSD reactions are rarely seen today, yet the drug remains in use. Moreover, the paucity of users seeking emergency medical treatment may reflect increased knowledge of how to deal with such situations on the part of the "drug-using community," as well as a decrease in the doses of LSD currently used compared to those used in the past.

Acute anxiety or panic reactions, the so-called bad trip, are the most commonly reported acute adverse reactions. They usually wear off before medical intervention is sought; most LSD is metabolized and excreted within 24 hours, and acute panic reactions usually subside within this timeframe. Depression with suicidal ideation can occur several days after LSD use.

Paranoid ideation, hallucinations, and a confusional state (organic brain syndrome) are other commonly reported acute adverse reactions. Initially it was thought that LSD could replicate the signs and symptoms of schizophrenia in some subjects, and the induction of such a model psychosis could be used to study and potentially find a cure for this major psychiatric illness. These hopes did not materialize, as major differences have been found between hallucinogen-induced psychosis and the schizophrenic state. More recently, using single-photon emission computed tomography (SPECT), it was found that the administration of mescaline to controls produced a *hyperfrontal* pattern, whereas *hypofrontality* has been observed in subjects with schizophrenia. However, positron emission tomography shows that psilocybin produces changes in glucose metabolism similar to those in patients with acute schizophrenia.

In terms of adverse physiologic effects, LSD has a very high therapeutic index. An elephant was killed after the experimental administration of a massive dose relative to brain weight, 0.15 mg/kg, or approximately 300,000 μg of LSD. The lethal dose in humans has not been determined, and fatalities that have been reported usually are secondary to perceptual distortions with resultant accidental death (e.g., "flying" off a roof, merging with an oncoming automobile on the freeway).

Treatment of Acute Adverse Reactions

Treatment of the acute adverse reactions to hallucinogens first must be directed toward preventing the patient from physically harming self or others. Anxiety can be handled by means of interpersonal support and reassurance. Psychotherapeutic intervention consists of reassurance, placing the patient in a quiet room, and avoidance of physical intrusion until the patient begins to calm down. The use of a benzodiazepine, such as lorazepam (Ativan), also can be effective. The oral route can be used for administering such medication in mildly agitated patients; however, it can be difficult to convince severely agitated or paranoid patients to swallow a pill, in which case parenteral administration might be necessary. Severely agitated patients who fail to respond to a benzodiazepine may be given a neuroleptic agent. Caution must be used in administering neuroleptics because they can lower the seizure threshold and elicit seizures, especially if the hallucinogen has been cut with an agent that has convulsant activity, such as strychnine. Phenothiazines, such as chlorpromazine (Thorazine), given orally or intramuscularly can end an LSD trip and are effective in treating LSD-induced psychosis. Because anticholinergic crises can develop with chlorpromazine in combination with other drugs with anticholinergic activity, such as phencyclidine (PCP) and DOM, haloperidol (Haldol) is a safer drug to use when the true nature of the drug ingested is unknown. It has been suggested that a combination of intramuscular haloperidol and lorazepam is particularly effective in treating acute adverse reactions. Theoretically, selective 5-HT_{2A} antagonists should block the effects of hallucinogens; however, other drugs with significant 5-HT_{2A} antagonist activity, for example, clozapine (Clozaril), olanzapine (Zyprexa), and risperidone (Risperdal), also might be effective. It should be noted that there is some indication that risperidone might exacerbate flashbacks.

Drug Interactions

Drugs interactions involving the hallucinogens do not appear to be an important source of adverse reactions. There are reports that the effects of LSD are reduced after the chronic administration of monoamine oxidase inhibitors or selective serotonin reuptake inhibitor antidepressants such as fluoxetine (Prozac), whereas the effects of LSD are increased after the chronic administration of lithium or tricyclic antidepressants.

Long-Term Adverse Effects

Chronic adverse reactions include psychoses, depressive reactions, acting out, paranoid states, and flashbacks. The use of LSD has been found to coincide with the onset of depression, suggesting a possible role in the etiology of some depression. Flashbacks are a well-publicized adverse reaction. They now have been renamed "hallucinogen-persisting perception disorder," and have specific diagnostic criteria. Only a small proportion of LSD and other hallucinogenic users experience flashbacks. They can occur spontaneously a number of weeks or months after the original drug experience, appear not to be dose related, and can develop after a single exposure to the drug. During a flashback, the original drug experience is re-created complete with perceptual and reality distortion. Even a previously pleasant drug experience may be accompanied by anxiety when the people realize that they have no control over its recurrence. In time, flashbacks decrease in intensity, frequency, and duration (although initially they usually last only a few seconds), whether treated or not. Flashbacks may or may not be precipitated by stressors or the subsequent use of other psychoactive drugs, such as psilocybin or marijuana. The administration of selective serotonin reuptake inhibitor antidepressants and risperidone is reported to initiate or exacerbate flashbacks in individuals with a history of LSD use. Flashbacks usually can be handled with psychotherapy. An anxiolytic or neuroleptic may be indicated, but probably is as much for the reassurance of the therapist as for the patient. The exact mechanism underlying this phenomenon remains obscure. Individuals with flashbacks have a high lifetime incidence of affective disorder when compared to substance abusers who do not abuse LSD. LSD users have long-term changes in visual function. For example, a visual disturbance consisting of prolonged afterimages (palinopsia) has been found in individuals several years after the last reported use of LSD. Such changes in visual function might underlie flashbacks.

Psychosis can develop and persist after hallucinogen use, but it remains unclear whether hallucinogen use can "cause" long-term psychosis, or if it has a role in precipitating the onset of illness. For example, hallucinogens may have a variety of effects in a person who is genetically predisposed to schizophrenia: (a) they may cause the psychosis to manifest at an earlier age; (b) they may produce a psychosis that would have remained dormant if drugs had not been used; or (c) they may cause relapse in a person who has previously suffered a psychotic disorder.

There are few if any long-term neuropsychologic deficits attributable to hallucinogen use. Chronic personality changes with a shift in attitudes and evidence of magical thinking can occur after the use of hallucinogens. There is always the risk that such thinking can lead to destructive behavior, in acute as well as chronic reactions. The effects of the chronic use of LSD must be differentiated from the effects of personality disorders, particularly in those who use a variety of drugs in polydrug abuse patterns. In some individuals with well-integrated personalities and with no previous psychiatric history, chronic personality changes have resulted from repeated LSD use. Personality changes that result from LSD use can occur after a single experience, unlike other classes of drugs (PCP, perhaps, excepted). In addition, the hallucinogenic drugs interact in a variety of nonspecific ways with the personality. The suggestibility that may come from many experiences with LSD may be reinforced by the social values of a particular subculture in which the drug is used. Treatment of chronic hallucinogen abuse can include psychotherapy on a long-term basis to determine what needs are being fulfilled by the use of the drug for this particular person. Twelve-step meetings also might be crucial for reinforcement of the decision to remain abstinent. There is no generally accepted evidence of brain cell damage, chromosomal abnormalities, or teratogenic effects after the use of the indole-type hallucinogens and mescaline.

Suggested Readings

Nelson DL. 5-HT5 receptors. *Curr Drug Targets CNS Neurol Disord.* 2004;3:53–58.

Nichols DE. Hallucinogens. *Pharmacol Ther.* 2004;101:131–181.

Passie T, Seifert J, Schneider U, et al. The pharmacology of psilocybin. *Addict Biol.* 2002;7: 357–364.

Pechnick RN, Ungerleider JT. Hallucinogens. In: Lowinson JH, Ruiz P, Millman RB, et al., eds. *Substance abuse: a comprehensive textbook,* 4th ed. Philadelphia: Lippincott Williams & Wilkins; 2005:313–323.

Weinstein H. Hallucinogen actions on 5-HT receptors reveal distinct mechanisms of activation and signaling by G protein-coupled receptors. *AAPS.* 2006;7:E871–E884.

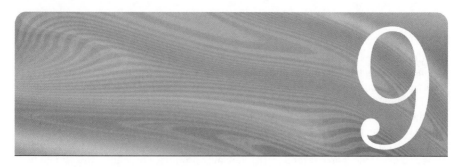

PHENCYCLIDINE

Phencyclidine—1-1(phenylcyclohexyl) piperidine; PCP; "angel dust"—was developed by Parke-Davis under the trade name Sernyl during the 1950s in a research program targeting general anesthetics. It and the related compounds cyclohexamine and ketamine are classified as "dissociative anesthetics." Despite its physiologic advantages over traditional anesthetics, PCP was removed from the market in 1965 and officially limited thereafter to veterinary applications. Up to half of patients subjected to PCP anesthesia developed severe intraoperative reactions, including agitation and hallucinations. Many of these patients went on to develop psychotic reactions, which persisted beyond emergence from anesthesia, and in some cases persisted for an additional 12 to 240 hours.

PCP is often adulterated and misrepresented on the street as tetrahydrocannabinol (THC), LSD, mescaline, psilocybin, amphetamine, or cocaine. Because of the high frequency with which it is used in combination with other drugs, the user may not be aware of having ingested PCP. To add to the confusion, the street names for PCP vary considerably: angel dust, dust, crystal, cyclones, embalming fluid, wet, killer weed, mintweed, PeaCe Pill, goon, surfer, Illy, crazy Eddie, Purple Rain, and Milk. PCP was originally ingested orally, but because the risk of overdose is greater with the oral form of the drug, it is now more commonly smoked or snorted, allowing the user more control of dosage. It has also been injected.

Initial use is usually in a smoking form (about 1 to 100 mg of PCP per joint) in conjunction with marijuana, tobacco, or parsley. Chronic users may take from 100 mg to 1 g within a single 24-hour period. The effects last between 4 and 6 hours with a longer "coming down" period. It is most often used as a social drug, with other users. PCP is used by people from all socioeconomic backgrounds, with and without formal premorbid psychopathology. For those who become chronic users, PCP is generally a primary drug of choice. Studies of chronic users show persistent cognitive and memory problems, speech difficulties, mood disorders, loss of purposive activities, and weight loss, lasting a year or more after last use. Late-stage chronic use is associated with paranoia and violent behavior with auditory hallucinations.

Neurobiology

Identification and Characterization of the PCP Receptor

The central nervous effects of PCP are initiated by binding of the drug to high-affinity PCP receptors whose existence in rat brain membranes was demonstrated in 1979. PCP receptors are highly selective for drugs that elicit PCP-like effects on behavior, including PCP and related arylcyclohexylamines, the F-opioids, the dioxolanes (a class of dissociative anesthetics), and MK-801 (dizocilpine). Several classes of drugs not chemically derived from PCP, including the F-opiates, the dioxolane derivatives dexoxadrol and etoxadrol, and the anticonvulsant MK-801, are active in the [^{3}H]PCP binding assay and exhibit PCP-like behavioral activity. All these drugs mimic PCP in conditioned and unconditioned behavioral assays and generalize to PCP in the highly selective rat two-lever drug discriminative stimulus test. The relative potencies of these drugs in eliciting PCP-like behaviors are proportional to their potencies in competing for radioligand binding to the PCP receptor. More than 100 such derivatives have been so characterized. Drugs that exhibit PCP-like behavioral effects also block N-methyl-D-aspartate (NMDA)-activated channels in electrophysiologic assays. The rank order of potency of such drugs as channel blockers parallels their behavioral potencies and their potencies in binding to the PCP receptor. By contrast, a wide range of neurotransmitters, known agonists, and antagonists of other receptors (including the classical opiates and the psychotomimetic drugs LSD, THC, cocaine, and mescaline) are inactive in the PCP-binding assay and fail to elicit PCP-like behaviors or channel-blocking activity.

PCP–NMDA Receptor Interactions

Following the demonstration of PCP receptors, the next major advance in determining the molecular mechanism of PCP occurred in the early 1980s, with the demonstration that PCP receptor ligands potently inhibit neurotransmission mediated at NMDA-type glutamate receptors. NMDA receptors are one of several receptor types for the excitatory amino acid neurotransmitter glutamate. As opposed to other glutamate receptors, NMDA channels are permeable to Ca^{2+} along with Na^{+}. Following NMDA receptor activation, NMDA-mediated Ca^{2+} flux may lead to stimulation of calmodulin-dependent kinases and activation of postsynaptic second messenger pathways. A unique functional property of the NMDA channel is that it is blocked in a voltage-dependent manner by the endogenous Mg^{2+} ion. The dual voltage and ligand dependence of NMDA receptors permits them to function in a Hebbian manner to integrate information from multiple input streams. One stream is represented as a modulation of presynaptic glutamate release; additional streams are reflected in modulation of resting membrane potential on the postsynaptic NMDA-bearing dendrites. Ca^{2+} flowing through open, unblocked NMDA channels may serve as the trigger for long-term potentiation, which, in turn, may represent the neurophysiologic substrate underlying learning and memory formation. In rodents, PCP and other NMDA antagonists lead to profound memory disturbances that are linked to inhibition of hippocampal long-term potentiation. Profound amnesia is also characteristic of both PCP psychosis and ketamine anesthesia.

Glycine Sensitivity of NMDA Receptor Activation

As opposed to most receptors, which require the presence of only a single neurotransmitter, NMDA receptors possess two distinct agonist-binding sites, one for glutamate and other excitatory amino acids, and a second for glycine. Binding of both glycine and glutamate are required for NMDA receptor activation to occur, and, *in vitro*, total removal of glycine from the incubation medium prevents NMDA receptor activation by glutamate. From a technical viewpoint, therefore, glutamate and glycine should be considered co-agonists at the NMDA receptor complex. However, the functional roles played by glutamate and glycine *in vivo* appear quite different. Thus, glutamate is released from presynaptic nerve endings in a pulsatile fashion and rapidly deactivated following release, as is the case for most classical neurotransmitters. In contrast, glycine in forebrain does not appear to be concentrated in presynaptic nerve endings nor released in response to electrical stimulation. Moreover, endogenous glycine levels are typically at or above the K_d (dissociation constant) of the NMDA-associated glycine site for these agents, indicating that activity-stimulated release of glycine is not required for neurotransmission. It has even been suggested that the glycine site may be saturated under normal brain conditions, and thus physiologically irrelevant, although this appears not to be the case. Instead, glycine appears to set the tonic level of NMDA excitability, determining the degree to which presynaptic glutamate release leads to postsynaptic excitation. Postsynaptic excitation, however, is triggered by presynaptic glutamate release. Therefore, glycine functions more similarly to a neuromodulator than a classical neurotransmitter. In addition to glycine, the NMDA-associated glycine site shows high affinity for D-serine, which may also serve as an endogenous NMDA agonist.

Use-Dependent Blockade

Because PCP mediates its effects at a binding site located within the NMDA channel, access of PCP to its site of action is affected by the degree of NMDA receptor activation. Opening of the NMDA channel facilitates access of PCP to its receptor, accelerating the rate at which PCP-induced blockade of NMDA receptor-mediated neurotransmission is observed. Thus, *in vitro*, NMDA currents show marked use dependence, with greater use being associated with more rapid blockade over the course of seconds to minutes. However, the phenomenon of use dependence appears to be true only over the course of minutes. When incubations are continued for several hours, significant PCP receptor occupancy is observed even in the absence of NMDA activation. The slow onset of closed channel blockade is most likely a result of the ability of PCP receptor ligands, all of which are highly lipophilic, to reach the NMDA channel by diffusion through the lipid bilayer.

Neurotoxicity

In the range of concentrations most associated with behavioral hyperactivity, PCP does not appear to cause significant long-lasting brain toxicity. At doses significantly above those used for behavioral studies (e.g., 5 to 50 mg/kg), however, PCP induces neuronal vacuolization, particularly in neurons in posterior cingulate/retrosplenial cortex. Similar vacuolization is observed following of administration of MK-801 and ketamine, indicating that the effect is probably NMDA receptor mediated. The effect is initially observed in layers III and IV of the cortex. At lower doses (e.g., 5 mg/kg), the effect is transient, reaching peak levels approximately 12 hours after PCP or MK-801 administration and then resolving over 12 to 18 hours. Extremely large doses of drug, however, may lead to neuronal necrosis, which is apparent even 48 hours after drug administration. Although posterior cingulate/retrosplenial cortex appears most susceptible to the effects of PCP, other hippocampus and limbic brain regions may be affected at higher doses. Along with vacuolization, administration of high-dose PCP leads to elevation of glucose uptake, expression of heat shock protein, and glial fibrillary acidic protein in the affected regions. Vacuolization can be inhibited by prior administration of antipsychotic, anticholinergic, or γ-aminobutyric acid (GABA)-ergic agents, and is potentiated by administration of pilocarpine.

Behavioral Pharmacology

The behavioral effects of PCP in animals depend on the species. In rodents, PCP induces a characteristic syndrome of hyperactivity and stereotypies. These effects respond partially to treatment with neuroleptics, and may also be reversed by agents such as glycine that augment NMDA receptor-mediated neurotransmission. Because the serum half-life of PCP is shorter and the volume of distribution is larger, rodents typically require doses of PCP higher than those used clinically than in humans. Sensitization to the behavioral effects of PCP may occur following daily administration. In rodents, PCP may also inhibit social behavior. The effects of PCP on social behaviors are poorly reversed by typical or atypical antipsychotic agents.

PCP-induced hyperactivity in rodents is mediated at least in part by disruption of NMDA-mediated interaction with ascending midbrain dopamine systems. PCP-induced hyperactivity appears to be reflective of increased dopaminergic neurotransmission within nucleus accumbens, because this effect can be selectively inhibited by accumbens lesions. Other components of the PCP-induced behavioral syndrome (e.g., alterations in social behavior, stereotypies) persist even following accumbens lesion, however, suggesting that those behaviors may be mediated by other brain regions. In addition to being present in dopaminergic terminal fields, NMDA receptors are also present in substantia nigra (A9) and ventral tegmental area (A10). Glutamatergic innervation of substantia nigra from prefrontal cortex is a major determinant of dopaminergic activity levels and NMDA receptors appear to be the primary mediators of glutamate-induced stimulation of midbrain dopaminergic neurons. To the extent that NMDA receptors stimulate A9 and A10 neurons, PCP would, paradoxically, be expected to decrease dopaminergic outflow in striatum and accumbens. However, it has been found that direct application of PCP to A10 does not inhibit dopamine cell firing or alter dopamine release in accumbens, although it does prevent NMDA-induced neuronal activation. Thus, the predominant behavioral effects of PCP in rodents appear to be a result of its interactions within dopamine terminal fields, rather than within dopaminergic midbrain nuclei.

In monkeys, doses of approximately 0.5 mg/kg PCP produce a tranquilization in which animals appear awake but unresponsive to the environment. At doses of 1.0 mg/kg, PCP induces a cataleptoid state in which animals show waxy flexibility and rigidity closely resembling catatonic schizophrenia. Doses of 2.5 mg/kg lead to stupor, 5.0 mg/kg to surgical anesthesia, and 15 mg/kg to convulsive seizures.

In both rats and monkeys, PCP administration also leads to profound disruption in learning and memory. In rodents, noncompetitive NMDA antagonists lead to disruptions in spatial delayed alteration performance, which can be reversed by dopamine (D2) receptor antagonists. Thus, in cortex, as in striatum, the effects of NMDA antagonists may, in part, reflect secondary dysregulation of dopaminergic neurotransmission. In monkeys, NMDA antagonists lead to impairments in learning and working memory performance that are not reproduced by amphetamines, indicating that the effect cannot be wholly attributed to increased dopaminergic neurotransmission. However, NMDA antagonists do lead to potentiation of the disruptive effects of amphetamines on learning in monkeys, indicating that interactions between the NMDA and dopamine systems may nevertheless be important.

Anatomic Localization

The anatomic localization of the PCP receptor in the rat brain has been determined by receptor autoradiography. High densities of PCP receptors are found in anterior forebrain areas, including neocortex and olfactory structures. The highest selective localization is observed in the dentate gyrus and the CA1 and CA2 subfields of the hippocampus. Within the spinal cord, sites are localized primarily to laminae I and II in cervical and thoracic spinal segments. In lamina I the density of sites decreases along a rostral to caudal gradient. Autoradiographic evidence indicates that PCP receptors are located postsynaptically rather than presynaptically in the perforant path-dentate granule cell system of the adult rat. A phylogenetic study indicates that PCP receptors are old from an evolutionary standpoint, occurring in the neural tissue of a large number of animal species, including monkey, guinea pig, chicken, turtle, frog, goldfish, shark, planarian, and sea anemone, although their pharmacology in invertebrates is not congruent with that found in vertebrates.

Molecular Characterization of the PCP Receptor

On a molecular level, the NMDA receptor complex is hetero-oligomeric in structure, consisting of combinations of NMDAR1 and NMDAR2 subunits. NMDAR1 is the key subunit in the formation of the receptor complex. All functional NMDA receptor complexes contain a type 1 (NR1) subunit; complexes may also contain variable numbers of modulatory subunits (NR2A-D). The sensitivity of NMDA receptors to modulatory effects of glycine is conferred by residues within the NR1 subunit itself. Thus, in general, all functional NMDA receptor complexes should be sensitive to glycine. Eight variants of NMDAR1 (NMDAR1a to h) have been identified, which reflect alternative messenger ribonucleic acid (mRNA) splicing. These clones have distinct sensitivities to agonists, antagonists, Zn^{2+}, and polyamines. Polyamines are also conferred by regulatory (NR2) subunits that are differentially expressed across brain regions. NMDA receptors are primarily postsynaptic in localization and occur on both projection and interneurons. In some brain regions, however, especially in target areas of the mesolimbic/mesocortical system, NMDA receptors may also be localized presynaptically and thus may regulate release of dopamine from presynaptic terminals. It has been suggested that such receptors consist solely of NR1 subunits and thus may have a different pharmacologic profile from postsynaptic receptors.

Psychopharmacology

Pharmacokinetics

In practical terms, PCP must be considered an extremely potent compound among drugs of abuse. It is extremely lipid soluble and can reach significant brain levels upon administration via any one of several routes, including oral, inhalation, smoking, and topical. A typical street dose is about 5 mg (one pill, joint, or line). Based on the pharmacokinetics of PCP, such a dose would result in a serum PCP concentration between 0.01 and 0.1 μmol/L. Marked psychotic reactions have been observed associated with undetectably low serum concentrations (<0.02 μmol/L), whereas concentrations of >0.4 μmol/L induce gross impairment of consciousness. Abusers characteristically titrate their dose in an effort to maximize the "high" while avoiding unconsciousness. Failures of judgment or variations in purity of supplies often result in inadvertent overdose, which may lead to severe medical complications. Serum concentrations above 1.0 μmol/L are strongly associated with coma, seizures, respiratory arrest, and death. The highest recorded serum and cerebrospinal fluid concentrations are in the range of 1.0 to 2.0 μmol/L.

PCP manifests a volume of distribution of 6.2 L/kg. Its lipophilicity facilitates accumulation in fatty body tissues, including the brain. Mobilization of adipose stores, as with exercise, may release sequestered PCP, leading to *flashbacks*.

Metabolism is primarily hepatic, with renal secretion of hydroxylase metabolites. The pK_a of 8.5 implies that PCP is largely ionized while in the stomach or the urinary tract. In passing through the pyloric valve, PCP enters a nonacidic environment in the small intestine in which it becomes largely nonionized and readily absorbed across the mucosal membrane, whereupon enterohepatic recalculation can account for the fluctuating clinical course so often observed in intoxication.

Chemistry

A phenylcyclohexylamine, PCP is easily synthesized from the starting materials piperazine, cyclohexanone, and potassium cyanide. The synthesis proceeds through the intermediate 1-piperidinocyclohexanecarbonitrile (PC), which is reacted with phenylmagnesium bromide to form PCP. The simplicity of this reaction, which enables PCP to be synthesized with almost no training or equipment, suggests that a resurgence of PCP abuse may follow successful efforts to eliminate from the marketplace drugs of abuse derived from natural products. During the 1970s, analytic surveys of street samples revealed that a large portion of drugs marketed as THC, mescaline, and LSD were actually PCP. Another consequence of the ease of synthesis is the contamination of significant percentages of analyzed street samples of PCP by dangerously high amounts of residual PC. In physiologic saline, PC decomposes to hydrocyanic acid. When PC-contaminated PCP is smoked, approximately 58% of the PC breaks down to cyanide and organic by-products. Although devoid of PCP-like pharmacologic activity, PC is more acutely toxic and may be implicated in some PCP-related fatalities.

Psychotomimetic Effects

In normal volunteers, single, small, intravenous subanesthetic doses (0.05 to 0.1 mg/kg) of PCP acutely induced a psychotic state in which subjects became withdrawn, autistic, negativistic, and unable to maintain a cognitive set, and manifested concrete, impoverished, idiosyncratic, and bizarre responses to proverbs and projective testing. Some subjects showed catatonic posturing. These schizophrenia-like alterations in brain functioning went beyond the symptom level; thus, in formal studies of neuropsychologic function, PCP induced a spectrum of specific disturbances in attention, perception, and symbolic thinking strikingly similar to those seen in schizophrenia. The most severe impairment caused by PCP was observed in tests requiring selective attention and paired-association learning. An important clinical correlate of this data is that any person under the influence of even a small dose of PCP or a similar drug will have profound alterations of higher emotional functions affecting judgment and cognition, even in the absence of gross neurologic findings.

In recompensated schizophrenic subjects, single low doses of PCP caused rekindling of presenting symptomatology lasting as long as 6 weeks, without evocation of any symptoms or signs not typical of the schizophrenic illness. An important clinical correlate of this data is that people with schizophrenia or preschizophrenia abusing a PCP-type drug run an extremely high risk of severe psychiatric morbidity.

The epidemic of PCP abuse during the 1970s yielded considerable data on psychotomimetic effects in other than experimental subjects. This literature cannot be used directly to ascertain risks because no firm evidence is available of what percentage of PCP users sought or were brought to medical attention. However, it is striking that in retrospective studies of patients hospitalized for complications of PCP use, PCP-intoxicated patients could not be distinguished from patients with schizophrenia based on presenting symptomatology.

Reinforcing Effects

Self-Administration

A series of studies established that monkeys avidly self-administer large doses of PCP intravenously and orally. In such studies the finding that the monkeys, given unlimited access to PCP, maintained nearly continuous intoxication distinguished abuse patterns of PCP from those of classical stimulants. In this respect the reinforcing properties of PCP resemble those of opiates and central nervous system (CNS) depressants more than they resemble those of stimulants. Furthermore, as distinct from findings on opiate self-administration, monkeys self-administered doses of PCP high enough to cause marked behavioral effects. Given the similarities between behavioral effects of PCP in monkeys and humans, this research validates the clinical impression of avid human self-administration of PCP. PCP-like drugs stimulate brain reward areas, lowering the threshold for intracranial self-stimulation.

Tolerance

In rats and monkeys, repeated administration of PCP on a daily or more frequent schedule leads to two-fold to fourfold rightward shifts in dose–response curves. The major determinant of this moderate tolerance appears to be biodispositional. Unlike the modest degree of tolerance observed upon intermittent dosing, it appears that much greater degrees of tolerance are induced by continuous self-administration. In humans, there is a paucity of scientific data on PCP tolerance, but tolerance has been observed in burn patients given repeated doses of ketamine for analgesia.

Dependence

After unlimited-access self-administration of PCP for 1 month or longer, severe signs of withdrawal reaction were observed in monkeys when the drug was discontinued. These included vocalizations, bruxism, oculomotor hyperactivity, diarrhea, piloerection, somnolence, tremor, and seizures. Similarly severe reactions might be expected following binging on PCP by human abusers.

Clinical Toxicology

The range of clinical effects of PCP can be correlated with dose and serum PCP concentration. The variety of effects of PCP are a result of its interaction with a variety of molecular target sites. The highest-affinity target site is the CNS PCP/NMDA receptor, which would be the only system affected significantly at very low PCP doses. Serum PCP levels up to about 0.1 μmol/L would correspond with a clinical state manifesting psychotomimetic symptoms without overt physiologic disturbances of vital functions. Serum levels just higher than 0.1 μmol/L correspond to dissociative anesthesia. At still higher doses, as additional receptor sites are occupied, acute brain syndrome accompanied by prominent neurologic and cardiovascular complications ensues. Serum levels of 1.0 μmol/L and above are associated with coma and lethal complications. The PCP-induced organic mental syndrome and coma result from the summation of actions of PCP noncompetitively inhibiting the PCP/NMDA receptor, blocking the reuptake sites for catecholamines and indolamines, and blocking sodium and potassium channels and nicotinic and muscarinic cholinergic receptors. Because it is not currently feasible to design and administer treatments specifically targeting each of the molecular sites at which PCP exerts its toxic effects, treatment must address each symptom cluster and organ system.

Measures to Reduce Systemic PCP Levels

Trapping of ionized PCP in the stomach has led to the suggestion of continuous nasogastric suction for PCP intoxication. However, such a strategy can be needlessly intrusive and can lead to complications such as electrolyte imbalances. The same principle can be more safely implemented by administration of activated charcoal, which binds PCP and diminishes the toxic effects of PCP in animals.

Trapping of ionized PCP in urine has led to the suggestion of urinary acidification as an aid to drug elimination. Current thinking is this strategy is ineffective and potentially dangerous, for several reasons: only a small portion of PCP is excreted in urine; metabolic acidosis itself carries significant risks; and acidic urine would increase the risk of renal failure secondary to rhabdomyolysis. Finally, the extremely large volume of distribution of PCP implies that neither hemodialysis nor hemoperfusion significantly promotes drug clearance.

At present no drug functions as a "PCP antagonist." No drug will work for PCP as naloxone (Narcan) works for heroin because any compound binding to the PCP receptor, which is located within the ion channel of the NMDA receptor, would block NMDA receptor-mediated ion fluxes as does PCP itself. Recent progress in elucidation of NMDA receptor mechanisms suggests concepts that could lead to pharmacologic strategies promoting NMDA receptor activation, such as administration of glycine or polyamines (or derivatives or precursors of such substances). Increasing channel open time would promote dissociation of PCP from its binding sites. There is evidence that oral glycine in massive doses can antagonize PCP-induced behaviors in the mouse. However, no clinical trials of such strategies for PCP intoxication in humans have been carried out to date. Therefore, treatment must be supportive and directed at specific symptoms and signs of toxicity. It is important to remember that especially after oral administration, PCP levels may continue to rise unevenly over many hours or even days. Therefore, a prolonged period of clinical observation is mandatory before concluding that no serious or life-threatening complications will ensue.

Neurologic Toxicity

The majority of patients intoxicated with PCP manifest nystagmus, which may be horizontal, vertical, or rotatory. Nystagmus is one of the crucial signs that can help distinguish PCP intoxication from a naturally occurring psychotic state. Coma can occur at any point during intoxication. There is a dose-dependent neuronal hyperexcitability ranging from increased deep tendon reflexes through opisthotonos to seizure states, generalized or focal, up to status epilepticus. Focal neurologic findings may arise on the basis of cerebral vasoconstriction. Seizures are managed with intravenous benzodiazepines.

Behavioral Toxicity

As noted earlier, a schizophrenia-like psychotic state can be observed after extremely low doses of PCP. In fact, such cognitive and emotional alterations are the threshold effects of this drug. Clinically urgent behavioral complications of PCP abuse stem not from the "core" psychotic symptoms themselves but rather from behavioral disinhibition, which can be coupled with severe anxiety, panic, rage, and aggression. Such reactions are more common with somewhat higher doses, at which some degree of delirium, as well as neurologic symptoms and other medical derangements, can be observed. The behavioral manifestations can severely compromise the clinician's ability to treat the medical complications.

The disruption of sensory input by PCP causes unpredictable, exaggerated, distorted, or violent reactions to environmental stimuli. A cornerstone of treatment is therefore minimization of sensory inputs to PCP-intoxicated patients. Patients should be evaluated and treated in as quiet and isolated an environment as possible. Precautionary physical restraint is recommended by some authorities with the risk of rhabdomyolysis balanced by the avoidance of violent or disruptive behavior.

Drug Treatment

Because no specific PCP antagonist is available, the goal of drug therapy for PCP-induced behavioral toxicity is sedation. This can be accomplished by using benzodiazepines or neuroleptics. There is no convincing evidence that either class of compounds is clinically superior to the other. Benzodiazepines are effective via either oral or parenteral (intramuscular) routes. Diazepam (Valium) is effective via the oral route but may be poorly or erratically absorbed intramuscularly. Lorazepam (Ativan) may be given via either route of administration. Haloperidol (Haldol) is the neuroleptic most commonly used for this indication. Because of the anticholinergic actions of PCP, neuroleptics with potent intrinsic anticholinergic properties should be avoided.

Other Toxic Effects

Severe hyperthermia has been observed in PCP intoxication, which can arise in a delayed fashion and can be of fatal proportions. The anticholinergic properties of PCP can dose-dependently evoke a full-spectrum atropine-like toxicity and can be managed accordingly when life threatening. Mild hypertension may be seen even in minimal PCP intoxication. At higher doses hypertension may be severe and hypertensive crisis with CNS complications has been reported. Finally, rhabdomyolysis may arise from multiple sources. First, PCP in high doses has a direct excitatory action on the muscle end plate. Second, the behavioral toxicity of high doses of PCP frequently leads to muscle trauma. This combination of factors can lead to severe rhabdomyolysis, myoglobinuria, and renal failure.

Conclusion

PCP stands as the prototype of a unique category of drugs—NMDA channel blockers—that have high abuse potential and severe adverse medical effects if abused. The epidemic of PCP abuse in the late 1970s and early 1980s, in focusing scientific attention on the basic mechanisms by which these drugs exert their singular combination of psychotomimetic, cognitive, and abuse-promoting effects, played a key role in advancing research in a major new area of neuroscience. Future scientific progress in elucidating mechanisms of NMDA receptor function may lead to specific pharmacotherapeutic approaches to treatment of PCP abuse and toxicity.

Suggested Readings

Javitt DC. Glutamate as a therapeutic target in psychiatric disorders. *Mol Psychiatry*. 2004;9: 984–997.

Millan MJ. *N*-Methyl-D-aspartate receptors as a target for improved antipsychotic agents: novel insights and clinical perspectives. *Psychopharmacology*. 2005;179:30–53.

Morris BJ, Cochran SM, Pratt JA. PCP: from pharmacology to modeling schizophrenia. *Curr Opin Pharmacol*. 2005;5:101–106.

Zukin SR, Sloboda Z, Javitt DC: Phencyclidine (PCP). In: Lowinson JH, Ruiz P, Millman RB, et al., eds. *Substance abuse: a comprehensive textbook*, 4th ed. Philadelphia: Lippincott Williams & Wilkins; 2005:324–336.

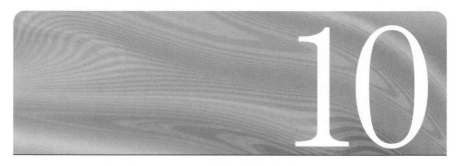

INHALANTS

With the advent of the use of anesthetics in the mid-1800s, chloroform and ether parties occurred, and these substances are still used. Another anesthetic, euphemistically called "laughing gas," accurately describes one of the recreational uses of another anesthetic, nitrous oxide, which also originated in the late 1800s. With the increased use of gasoline at the turn of the 20th century, many more substances became available through the process of petroleum "cracking" and distillation, and were included in many types of solvents, cleaners, degreasers, and glues.

The practice of "sniffing," "snorting," "huffing," "bagging," or inhaling to get high describes various forms of inhalation. If the substance is glue or some other dissolved solid, the user will empty the contents of a can (or a gas) into a plastic bag and then hold the bag to the nose and inhale ("bagging"). Another method is to soak a rag with the mixture and then stick the rag in the mouth and inhale the fumes ("huffing"). A simple but more toxic approach is to spray the substance directly into the oral cavities. This allows these abusers to be identified by various telltale clues, for example, organic odors on the breath or clothes, stains on the clothes or around the mouth, empty spray paint or solvent containers, and other unusual paraphernalia. These telltale clues may enable one to identify a serious problem of solvent abuse before it causes serious health problems or death.

Epidemiology

Prevalence

Individual states and the US national government began to evaluate the extent of the problem of inhalant abuse in the late 1960s and early 1970s. Use of drugs for mind-altering purposes varies by substance and extent of use. It is still reasonable to say even today that more than 1 in 10 have used solvents/gases to get special feelings. It is difficult, of course, to identify which volatile component is most desired in any aerosol. However, the popularity of "cigarette lighter gases" (which contain only these gases) during the 1980s and later makes it clear that these gases are effective mind-altering substances. One substance worthy of note is nitrous oxide. Its use has been increasing in the young adult population. Just like ecstasy, it has been used at concerts and in various youthful parties. There is great concern about any inhalation of gases/solvents by younger age groups (e.g., seventh and eighth graders) because of their lack of understanding of the problem, both what is meant by getting "high" and the resulting consequences of this habit. This emphasizes the need for increased education for children and, especially, their parents, about the nature and dangers of this problem.

Sociocultural Factors

Many solvent abusers, more than other drug users, are poor, come from broken homes, have lower self-esteem, and do poorly in school. Although these characteristics are often observed in African Americans, reports generally indicate a lower-than-expected use of inhalants in this population. Some Hispanic groups, especially recent immigrants from Latin American countries, and Native Americans on reservations have a higher percentage of inhalant users than the population as a whole.

The users of inhalants are categorized into three groups: (a) inhalant-dependent adults, (b) polydrug users, and (c) young inhalant users. Inhalant-dependent adults have the most serious health problems because they have used heavily for a long time; the young inhalant users are those for whom treatment is most desirable to keep them from progressing to the other groups and for whom there may be hope for successful intervention. Although all inhalant abusers use other drugs or alcohol, the first group predominantly uses inhalants, even though other drugs are available. The second group infrequently uses inhalants primarily because they cannot get their drug of choice; their problems arise more from the use of other drugs and are less related to those outlined in this chapter. The young inhalant users, however, are in the experimentation period of solvents, having started with either tobacco, alcohol, or possibly even marijuana, as well as inhalants. Before any of this group matures into the first group, intervening behavioral modifications are very important.

One trait that is often associated with sniffers is disruptive behavior. Some report them to be more violent. Cognitive measures of these groups support the antisocial and self-destructive nature of inhalant abusers. In some instances, examination of school records indicates that cognitive deficits probably occurred before inhalant use began. Although it is uncertain how inhalant abusers became dysfunctional, it is very likely that inhalants prevent their continued growth and development.

Substances Inhaled

Despite the widespread availability and inhalation of these substances, it was not until the 1950s that nationwide attention by reporters and by judicial action focused on what was euphemistically called "glue sniffing." The term is still widely used today to describe a myriad of substances that now include special shoe polishes, glue, gasoline, thinners, solvents, aerosols (paint, cooking lubricant spray, deodorant, hair spray, electronic cleaners, and others), correction fluids, cleaning fluids, refrigerant gases (e.g., fluorocarbons and the newer incompletely halogenated replacements), anesthetics, whippets (whipped cream propellants), room odorizers (organic nitrites), and even cooking or lighter gases. It is important to keep in mind that there are many different chemicals in most of these different products, all of which have different physiologic effects and different toxicities, as well as different chemical properties. Sometimes, the substances are listed on the container, with or without the proportion of each.

No study to date answers the perplexing question: What attracts young people to certain specific substances/products? Some consider the odor, color, or type of product to be important; others believe that the feeling one gets is most important. Yet, it is difficult to say what substances are preferred.

Toxicology of Inhalant Abuse

Acute Intoxication

To understand the solvent abuser, one can conceive of the intoxicated state as a quick "drunk," as many of the symptoms resemble alcohol intoxication. An evaluation of these individuals provides several symptoms, such as initial excitation turning to drowsiness, disinhibition, lightheadedness, and agitation. With increasing intoxication, individuals may develop ataxia, dizziness, and disorientation. In extreme intoxications, they may show signs of sleeplessness, general muscle weakness, dysarthria, nystagmus, and, occasionally, hallucinations or disruptive behavior. Several hours after, especially if they have slept, they are likely to be lethargic, or hung over with mild to severe headaches. Chronic abuse is associated with more serious complications including weight loss, muscle weakness, general disorientation, inattentiveness, and lack of coordination.

Most reports have described the acute intoxication in heavy users of toluene vapors. Acute intoxication with toluene produces headache, euphoria, giddiness, and cerebellar ataxia. At lower levels (just over 200 ppm), fatigue, headache, paresthesia, and slowed reflexes appear. Exposure at levels approaching 1,000 ppm causes confusion or delirium, and euphoric effects appear at or above that level. Although solvent abusers have favorites, they often use an unpredictable array of solvents. Multiple components in the mixtures may enhance the net toxicity in a synergistic or additive manner.

Death can occur during the course of primary intoxication. When it does occur, it is usually the result of asphyxia, ventricular fibrillation, or induced cardiac arrhythmia following high exposures to various solvents. *Cerebral anoxia associated with VSA [volatile substance abuse] fatalities may be related to multiple factors including asphyxia, cerebral and pulmonary oedema, cardiac arrhythmias and arrest, terminal unconsciousness, hyperpyrexia and others.* It is not as evident, but the results of several cases link fibrillation and other cardiac insufficiencies to the use of halocarbons. Some cardiac arrhythmias have also been reported following abuse of substances containing toluene; this includes the only reported nonfatal respiratory arrest of an inhalant abuser.

In evaluating any patient suspected of inhaling solvents either accidentally or to get "high," it is important to determine as precisely as possible not only the solvent(s) but also other contributing factors (including other drugs, such as alcohol, cigarettes, or marijuana; malnutrition; or respiratory irritants, such as fumes or viruses) before beginning treatment.

Recognition of and Criteria for Defining Neurotoxicity

The nervous system may be affected at many levels by organic solvents as well as other neurotoxic substances. As a general rule, resultant syndromes are diffuse in their manifestations. Because of their nonfocal presentation, neurotoxic disorders may be confused with metabolic, degenerative, nutritional, or demyelinating disease. This principle is illustrated in the setting of chronic toluene abuse, which clinically may resemble the multifocal demyelinating disease, multiple sclerosis, in the findings on neurologic examination. As a result, mild cases of intoxication may be very difficult to diagnose.

In general, neurotoxic injuries rarely have specific identifying features on diagnostic tests such as computed tomography (CT), magnetic resonance imaging (MRI), or nerve conduction studies. Because many neurotoxic effects are reversible and some chronic neurotoxic injuries of the brain may not be associated with structural damage sufficiently large to be detected within the spatial resolution of current MRI scanners and imaging sequences, brain imaging studies are primarily used to rule out other disorders. However, recent studies of chronic solvent inhalant abusers suggests that MRI may be the most sensitive and specific method of detecting the brain injury associated with the high dose setting of the inhalant abuser.

Acute, high-level exposure to most, if not all, solvents will induce short-lasting effects on brain function, most of which are reversible. Acute incidents that are irreversible probably act by producing secondary systemic effects such as cerebral hypoxia or a metabolic acidosis, and none of these acute incidents is proven to act by inducing an irreversible functional abnormality. In general, both acute high-level and low-level exposure to organic solvents are associated with full reversibility, and the acute toxicity with high-level exposure in no way predicts whether chronic low-level exposure will lead to an irreversible neurologic disease.

Chronic high-level exposure to organic solvents occurs only in the inhalant abuse setting, where levels several 1,000-fold higher than the occupational setting frequently occur. Chronic neurotoxic injury related to solvent abuse is slowly and incompletely reversible, and usually does not progress after cessation of exposure. Both acute and chronic neurotoxicity from organic solvents are functions predominantly related to the dose and duration of exposure.

Treatment of the Inhalant Abuser

There is no accepted treatment approach for inhalant abusers. Many drug treatment facilities refuse to treat of the inhalant abuser, because many believe that inhalant abusers are resistant to treatment. Longer periods of treatment are needed to be able to address the complex psychosocial, economic, and biophysical issues of the inhalant abuser. When brain injury, primarily in the form of cognitive dysfunction, is present, the rate of progression in the treatment process is even slower. The inhalant abuser typically does not respond to the usual drug rehabilitation treatment modalities. Several factors may be involved, particularly in situations of the chronic abuser, where significant psychosocial problems may be present.

Drug screening may be useful in monitoring inhalant abusers. Routine urine screens for hippuric acid, the major metabolite of toluene, performed two to three times weekly, will detect the high level of exposure to toluene usually seen in inhalant abusers. It should be noted that the metabolism of any one compound may be modified by the presence of another, either increased (following inducement by drugs, e.g., barbiturates) or decreased (benzene metabolism reduced in the presence of toluene).

Neuroleptics and other forms of pharmacotherapy are usually not useful in the treatment of inhalant abusers. However, as alcohol is a common secondary drug of abuse among inhalant abusers, a monitored program for alcohol abuse may be necessary.

Neurologic Sequelae of Chronic Inhalant Abuse

Organic solvents are widely prevalent compounds and inadvertent exposure, primarily industrial, as well as volitional abuse, occurs primarily by inhalation, with significantly less absorption occurring via skin or gastrointestinal routes. These compounds are highly lipophilic, which explains their distribution to organs rich in lipids (e.g., brain, liver, adrenal). Unexpired solvents absorbed by the tissues are then eliminated through the kidneys following metabolism of the solvents to more water soluble compounds. In addition, metabolism of some solvents may create additional compounds that are sometimes more toxic than the parent chemical.

Although most organic solvents produce nonspecific effects following absorption of extremely high concentrations (i.e., encephalopathy), a few produce relatively specific neurologic syndromes with low-level, chronic exposure. Major neurotoxic syndromes occurring in individuals chronically exposed to select organic solvents include a peripheral neuropathy, ototoxicity, and an encephalopathy. Less commonly, a cerebellar ataxic syndrome, parkinsonism, or a myopathy may occur alone or in combination with any of these clinical syndromes.

Compounds of Interest

The organic solvents described in detail below represent those organic solvents that are more commonly associated with abuse or where clear neurotoxicity is associated with exposure.

n-Hexane and Methyl Butyl Ketone

These two organic solvents are classified together because both *n*-hexane and methyl butyl ketone (MBK) are metabolized to the same neurotoxin, 2,5-hexanedione (2,5-HD) and produce an identical clinical syndrome characterized by a peripheral neuropathy. Clinically, the peripheral neuropathy begins with symmetrical, distal sensory loss in the lower extremities, which may progress, if the abuse continues, and eventually produce distal motor weakness.

Methyl Butyl Ketone

MBK had limited industrial use until the 1970s when it became more widely used as a paint thinner, clearing agent, and a solvent for dye printing. Soon afterward, numerous outbreaks of polyneuropathy associated with chronic exposure to MBK were being reported. The route of exposure is usually inhalation, but exposure has also occurred by the oral route by ingesting contaminated food in work areas and by cutaneous contact.

The clinical syndrome is characterized by the insidious onset of an initially painless sensorimotor polyneuropathy, which begins several months after continued chronic exposure. Even following cessation of exposure, the neuropathy may develop or may continue to progress for up to 3 months. In severe cases, an unexplained weight loss may be an early symptom. Sensory and motor disturbance begins initially in the hands and feet, and sensory loss is primarily small fiber (i.e., light touch, pinprick, temperature) with relative sparing of large-fiber sensation (i.e., position and vibration). Electrophysiologic studies reveal axonal polyneuropathy, pathologically multifocal axonal degeneration and multiple axonal swellings, and neurofilamentous accumulation at paranodal areas. Overlying the axonal swellings, thinning of the myelin sheath occurs. These findings are typical of a distal axonopathy or "dying-back" neuropathy described in other toxic and metabolic causes of peripheral neuropathy.

Prognosis for recovery correlates directly with the intensity of the neurologic deficit before removal from toxic exposure, with mild to moderate residual neuropathy seen in the most severely affected individuals up to 3 years after exposure.

n-Hexane

Until the 1970s, *n*-hexane was considered an innocuous solvent. *n*-Hexane is used in the printing of laminated products, in the extraction of vegetable oils, as a diluent in the manufacture of plastics and rubber, in cabinet finishing, as a solvent in biochemical laboratories, and as a solvent for glues and adhesives.

Cases of *n*-hexane polyneuropathy have been reported both after occupational exposure and after deliberate inhalation of vapors from products containing *n*-hexane, such as glues. Clinically and pathologically, the neuropathy occurring with *n*-hexane is that of a distal axonopathy, indistinguishable from that associated with MBK.

Another major component of these glues has been toluene. However, polyneuropathy does not occur from inhalation of toluene alone, and in previous reports of *n*-hexane neuropathy, the neuropathy did not appear until the subject switched to a product containing *n*-hexane. In contrast to toluene, *n*-hexane does not usually induce significant signs of central nervous system (CNS) dysfunction, except with high-level exposures where an acute encephalopathy may occur.

Both clinical and experimental studies provide evidence of CNS effects from *n*-hexane. Clinically, cranial neuropathy, spasticity, and autonomic dysfunction occasionally occur. Abnormalities on electrophysiologic tests of CNS function, including electroencephalography, visual evoked responses, color vision testing, *and* somatosensory evoked responses, are also seen. In spite of these findings, clinical effects of chronic low-level exposure to *n*-hexane is restricted to the peripheral nervous system.

Toluene (Methyl Benzene)

Toluene is one of the most widely used solvents and is employed as a paint and lacquer thinner, as a cleaning and drying agent in the rubber and lumber industries, and in the motor and aviation fuels and chemical industries. It is a major component in many paints, lacquers, glues and adhesives, inks, and cleaning liquids. As with other solvents, inhalation is the major route of entry, although some absorption occurs percutaneously. Of all the solvents, toluene-containing substances seem to have the highest potential for abuse.

Experience is still not sufficient to determine the incidence of chronic effects of toluene and other volatile hydrocarbons. The neurologic pattern, however, is very clearly delineated, with effects only on the CNS. Syndromes of persistent and often severe neurotoxicity include cognitive dysfunction, cerebellar ataxia, optic neuropathy, sensorineural hearing loss, and an equilibrium disorder.

Neurologic abnormalities varied from mild cognitive impairment to severe dementia, associated with elemental neurologic signs such as cerebellar ataxia, corticospinal tract dysfunction, oculomotor abnormalities, tremor, deafness, and hyposmia. Cognitive dysfunction was the most disabling and frequent feature of chronic toluene toxicity and may be the earliest sign of permanent damage. Dementia, when present, was typically associated with cerebellar ataxia and other signs. One patient had pyramidal and cerebellar signs without cognitive impairment. Oculomotor dysfunction, deafness, and tremor were seen only in severely affected individuals. Cranial nerve abnormalities were confined to olfactory and auditory dysfunction.

Although MRI has been very useful in attempting to understand the CNS effects of toluene abuse, an additional study using the functional imaging technique of brain SPECT (single-photon emission computed tomography) was recently published.

Neuropathology

The neuropathology of chronic inhalant abuse is poorly described, but recent studies have begun to shed some light on possible pathogenetic mechanisms.

Trichloroethylene

Trichloroethylene (TCE) is an important organic solvent used extensively in industry in metal degreasing, in extracting oils and fats from vegetable products, in cleaning optical lenses and photographic plates, in paints and enamels, in dry cleaning, and as an adhesive in the leather industry. Although its use in recent years has diminished somewhat as a result of concern that it could be a human carcinogen, the National Institute for Occupational Safety and Health (NIOSH) estimates the total number of individuals exposed to TCE to be in excess of 3.5 million. TCE has been recognized for over 50 years as an industrial hazard with neurotoxic properties.

Its major neurologic manifestation is related to a slowly reversible trigeminal neuropathy, although involvement of other cranial nerves and peripheral nerves has also been described.

Methylene Chloride (Dichloromethane)

Methylene chloride is widely used in industry for paint stripping, as a blowing agent for foam, as a solvent for degreasing, in the manufacture of photographic film, as the carrier in rapid-dry paints, and in aerosol propellants. It is estimated that nearly 100,000 individuals are exposed to methylene chloride in the workplace alone. The evidence suggests that methylene chloride does not produce permanent neurologic sequelae except with massive acute exposures that are associated with hypoxic encephalopathy. No evidence exists that chronic low-level exposure causes any long-term CNS injury.

1,1,1-Trichloroethane

1,1,1-Trichloroethane is widely used as an industrial degreasing solvent and, compared with other solvents, is less toxic, although several reports of severe toxicity and deaths exist in the literature. Its acute toxicity has made it unsuitable as a volatile anesthetic, and its use as a carrier in aerosols was abandoned in the United States in 1973.

In those cases where postmortem examination of the brain was undertaken, the pathologic changes suggested cerebral hypoxia either primary to CNS depressant effect or secondary to cardiac or respiratory arrest. 1,1,1-Trichloroethane is postulated to act on either the autonomic nervous system or on central sleep apnea. Chronic cardiac toxicity is also a possible mechanism of 1,1,1-trichloroethane toxicity.

Gasoline

Gasoline is a complex mixture of organic solvents and other chemicals and metals. The sniffing of gasoline is common among various solvent abusers, especially on some remote Native American reservations. Leaded gasoline is not now readily available in the United States but still presents a problem in some remote Indian villages. Although some CNS or peripheral neuropathies may occur as a result of the solvents in gasoline, other toxicities may result from tetraethyllead (or its metabolite triethyllead). In cases where high lead levels were observed, various disorders were observed, including hallucinations and disorientation, dysarthria, chorea, and convulsions. The symptoms include moderate to severe ataxia, insomnia, anorexia, slowed peripheral nerve conduction, limb tremors, dysmetria, and sometimes limb paralysis. In most cases, the electroencephalograph (EEG) is normal, but in severe states, an abnormal to severely depressed cortical EEG is observed. Because many of these symptoms in the early stages of the disease can be reversed by parenteral chelation therapy with ethylenediaminetetra-acetic acid (EDTA), British anti-Lewisite (BAL) (dimercaprol), and/or penicillamine, it is important to check the serum lead levels in any chronic inhalant abuser to see if this treatment should be prescribed. This type of therapy has recently been reviewed for gasoline alkyllead additives.

Alcohols and Solvents

One interesting phenomenon has been observed following the exposure to two or more solvents. This might explain the "flushing phenomenon" but may or may not relate to the psychologic dependence on solvents or to the development of thirst. An attempt to study the acute effects of alcohol and toluene, at low exposures in human volunteers, failed to produce any interaction by their behavioral measures. This may be indicative that the interaction takes some time and/or high levels of exposure to develop.

Methanol neurotoxicity is well known and exemplified by a recent case, where necrosis of the putamen region of the brain was noted. Methanol intoxication was identified in an individual intoxicated on a spray can of carburetor cleaner containing toluene (42%), methanol (23%), and methylene chloride (20%). Although mild acidosis did occur, the main concern was the high blood level of methanol. Ethanol therapy was used to prevent formation of high levels of formic acid. The above mixture is abused and is very similar in composition to paint thinner; yet the repercussions of prolonged use are unclear.

Nitrous Oxide

Nitrous oxide is a commonly used anesthetic and has been noted for some unusual toxicities. This substance is used as an anesthetic, as a propellant for whipped cream, and as an octane booster. In early studies, it was shown that central and peripheral nerve damage resulted following high levels of N_2O exposure, even in the presence of adequate oxygen and even in short-term use when nitrous oxide was used as an anesthetic. Patients with vitamin B_{12} deficiencies are especially sensitive. The symptoms include numbness and weakness in the limbs, loss of dexterity, sensory loss, and loss of balance. The neurologic examination indicates sensorimotor polyneuropathy. There is also a combined degeneration of the posterior and lateral columns of the spinal cord that resembles vitamin B_{12} deficiencies. Studies focusing on the mechanism of action indicate that cobalamins (vitamin B_{12}) are inactivated by N_2O; more recent studies have focused on the methionine synthase enzyme that needs vitamin B_{12} to function. Vitamin B_{12} (or folinic acid) did not aid recovery from this disease in some patients, but did in others. Rehabilitation proceeds with abstinence from nitrous oxide exposure and is relative to the extent of neurologic damage.

In regard to the dependence on nitrous oxide, animal studies on mice, selectively bred for alcohol dependence showed a cross-dependency on nitrous oxide. Handling-induced convulsions were also observed shortly after cessation of nitrous oxide, which could be prevented by either alcohol or nitrous oxide. This might indicate a physical dependence on nitrous oxide that needs to be dealt with in the treatment of patients in this drug abuse state. Approaches to reducing alcohol consumption should also be considered during treatment.

Psychiatric Disturbances in Organic Solvent Abuse

Psychiatric disorders related to solvent abuse are rare, if existent. Psychiatric morbidity is highest in those referred to psychiatric hospitals and lowest in clinics dealing exclusively with volatile substance (VS) (solvent) abuse. The psychiatric diagnoses of these patients do not appear to differ in type or frequency from those given to well-matched populations of nonabusers, and there is little evidence to suggest that specific or persistent psychiatric disability results from this practice. On the other hand, there is little doubt that personality disorders of an antisocial type are common in VS abusers. Hallucinations are often associated with inhalant abuse. This seldom is seen or identified in studies of groups of inhalant abusers.

Non-nervous System Toxicity of Inhalant Abuse

Most of the adverse clinical effects of inhalant abuse are on the nervous system. There are, however, other significant adverse effects on other organ systems, including kidney, liver, lung, heart, and blood.

Renal Toxicity

Currently, spray paints are widely abused substances, at least in the United States. The abuse of these substances occurs not only among polydrug users but also by painters. The exposure to these and similar substances has resulted in the hospitalization of inhalant abusers for various kidney disorders.

Renal Toxicity in Pregnancy

One must especially be alert for nephrotoxicity in pregnant women who abuse solvents. Numerous pregnant women have presented with renal tubular acidosis.

Hepatotoxicity

Chlorohydrocarbons (e.g., trichloroethylene, chloroform, halothane) have been known for years to produce hepatotoxicities. Any individual who is chronically exposed to these compounds would expect to develop hepatorenal toxicities, depending on the dose and length of exposure.

The recent increase in the inhalation of correction fluids, which contain trichloroethylene and trichloroethanes or tetrachloroethanes, for "pleasure" increases the likelihood of observing more of these toxicities in inhalant abusers. Even during occupational use, exposure to chlorocarbons in poorly ventilated areas is considered to lead to hepatotoxicity.

Pulmonary Toxicity

Despite the likelihood that solvents irritate the lungs, there are few cases noted where the pulmonary system is severely compromised. Solvents have, nevertheless, been noted to cause pulmonary hypertension, acute respiratory distress, increased airway resistance, and residual volume and restricted ventilation. A recent *outbreak of respiratory illness* was associated with changes in solvents/propellants of a leather conditioner. This product produced tachypnea, pulmonary edema, and hemorrhage in rats. Respiratory problems would therefore be expected in inhalant abusers using these or similar products. In addition, increased airway resistance or residual volume may be more clearly noted following an exercise challenge. Additionally, response to an aerosolized bronchodilator is suggestive of an airway involvement perhaps induced by habitual inhalation of hydrocarbons. Although solvents irritate the pulmonary system, it is not at all clear from the limited case studies reported, to date, how extensive or what types of pulmonary damage occur that can be primarily caused by solvent exposure and not to other inspired substances that are dissolved in the solvents.

Cardiotoxicity

Many solvent abusers may die from direct or indirect cardiotoxic actions of solvents without note in any public or private record. More specifically, several recent reports identified ventricular fibrillation and cardiac arrest in hospitalized patients. Some of the subjects had inhaled trichloroethylene- or trichloroethane-containing solvents and were additionally compromised by anesthesia (e.g., halothane). Recent reports have linked glue sniffing to arrhythmias, myocarditis, and cardiac arrest. However, the linkage of arrhythmia to glue sniffing is not well supported by animal studies. The somewhat different cardiotoxicities noted above are not all easily explained, but congenital or other environmental causes are not ruled out.

Hematologic Toxicity

There are three areas of concern in regard to solvent inhalation and the hematopoietic system. First, methylene chloride exposure can increase the carboxyhemoglobin levels, a change that also occurs with cigarette smoking. The levels of carboxyhemoglobin may become sufficiently high to cause brain damage or death. A second group of substances, the organic nitrites, produce methemoglobinemia and hemolytic anemia. A third substance, benzene, causes aplastic anemia, acute myelocytic leukemia, and other hematopoietic cancers. Benzene is present in thinners, varnish removers, and other solvents, and in varying proportions in gasoline.

The nitrites are usually not considered toxic during inhalation because of syncope (fainting). Methemoglobinemia is the major identified toxicity and is the cause of several deaths. There is a specific treatment for nitrite overdose. The high and slowly reversible reduction of methemoglobin can be aided by the use of methylene blue. Organic nitrites also produce bradycardia, reduce killer cell activity, produce allergic reactions, and are potentially carcinogenic.

Heavy organic nitrite use is a risk factor for the development of acquired immune deficiency syndrome (AIDS) and of Kaposi sarcoma. The ability to produce nitrosamines has fueled the speculation that nitrites are carcinogenic. Yet, in contrast to sodium nitrite, organic nitrites produce methemoglobin instantly *in vitro* and may therefore not be around long enough to produce nitrosamines. Thus, the rapid oxidation of organic nitrites by hemoglobin and the fact that detectable levels of organic nitrites in blood are noted only briefly after administration may alter the outcome of carcinogenesis. Although mutagenicity appears possible under special conditions, carcinogenicity is far from proved.

Neonatal Syndrome

There is increasing evidence that solvent inhalation during pregnancy produces a "fetal solvent syndrome." There are numerous cases of infants of mothers who chronically abuse solvents diagnosed with this syndrome. These mothers inhaled paint reducer, solvent mixtures from paint sprays, and drank various quantities of alcohol. Whether toluene (often noted as the major solvent) alone, other solvent components, and/or these components in combination with alcohol or other environmental factors are responsible is still unsubstantiated by laboratory studies, yet toluene appears to be a major contributor. Toluene embryopathy is compared to the better-recognized fetal alcohol syndrome. The infants present with growth retardation, some dysmorphic features, including microcephaly, as well as distal acidosis, aminoaciduria, ataxia, tremors, and slurred speech, and has been considered a human teratogen.

Suggested Readings

Dinwiddie SH. Abuse of inhalants—a review. *Addiction.* 1994;89:925–939.

Jones HE, Balster RL. Inhalant abuse in pregnancy. *Obstet Gynecol Clin North Am.* 1998;25(1): 153–167.

Ludolph AC, Spencer PS. Toxic neuropathies and their treatment. *Baillieres Clin Neurol.* 1995;4(3): 505–527.

Rosenberg NL, Grigsby J, Dreisbach J, et al. Neuropsychologic impairment and MRI abnormalities associated with chronic solvent abuse. *J Toxicol Clin Toxicol.* 2002;40(1):21–34.

Sharp CW, Rosenberg NL: Inhalants. In: Lowinson JH, Ruiz P, Millman RB, et al., eds. *Substance abuse: a comprehensive textbook*, 4th ed. Philadelphia: Lippincott Williams & Wilkins; 2005:336–666.

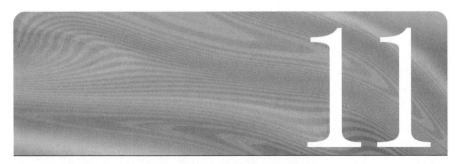

MDMA/DESIGNER DRUGS

The term "designer drug" suggests a level of precision and specificity that may not be reflected in the process or product for the person making a desired compound. However, the term has gained general usage, and hence is used here. Although this chapter is primarily devoted to a review of methylenedioxymethamphetamine (MDMA), other compounds, such as opioid analogues and methcathinone, are also addressed as examples of drugs for this general category of abused substances.

MDMA
Historical Background

MDMA was first synthesized in 1912 by chemists working for Merck Pharmaceuticals in Germany, who were attempting to create a new medication to stop bleeding. As an intermediate step in the synthesis of the styptic medication hydrastinine, MDMA itself was of little interest and was only included in the patent application as a secondary chemical compound. The Merck patent was approved in 1914, and has long since expired. In the early 1950s, as part of systematic U.S. Army Intelligence research on potential psychotropic drug applications to espionage and counterespionage endeavors, MDMA once again came to the attention of researchers. MDMA was administered to a variety of animals for standard median lethal dose (LD_{50}) screening. Plans to initiate human trials with MDMA were abandoned, however, following the tragic and untimely death in 1953 of a subject enrolled in a U.S. Army contract study at the New York State Psychiatric Institute who had received "forced injections" of EA-1298, or methylenedioxyamphetamine (MDA), an analogue and an active metabolite of MDMA.

MDMA remained largely unknown to psychedelic enthusiasts and would not be examined until the mid-1970s when University of California Berkeley biochemist and toxicologist Alexander Shulgin, acting on the suggestion of a student who claimed to have successfully alleviated a severe stutter with the drug, synthesized and self-administered 120 mg of the compound. He would later describe MDMA as evoking "an easily controlled altered state of consciousness with emotional and sensual overtones, and with little hallucinatory effect."

Highly impressed with the apparent capacity of the drug to induce heightened states of empathic rapport, a critical component of successful psychotherapy, Shulgin introduced several psychiatrist and psychologist acquaintances to the unusual profile of action of MDMA. Their responses, both to their own subjective experience, as well as responses from patients who had received the drug, were an unequivocal endorsement of the apparent capacity of MDMA to facilitate the process of psychotherapy. For the remainder of the 1970s, a quiet underground of psychotherapists, particularly on the West Coast of the United States, conducted thousands of MDMA-augmented treatments with what at that time was still a legal and uncontrolled substance. Although, unfortunately, no methodologic research was conducted to substantiate the alleged efficacy of MDMA in alleviating psychologic distress and modifying maladaptive personality structures, testimonials to its therapeutic range of action abounded.

Sensitive to the fate suffered in the 1960s by proponents of psychiatric research and treatment with psychedelics once word of their highly unusual effects had been disseminated to the culture at large, knowledge of MDMA remained a tightly guarded secret among practitioners of its use and their patients for several years. By the early 1980s, however, word of MDMA had filtered out, abetted by media accounts of a new psychotherapeutic "miracle medicine" and the spread of an alternative recreational drug on some college campuses (particularly in California and Texas), where, for a period of time, MDMA replaced cocaine as the new drug-of-choice. First popularly called Adam during its early phase of use among psychotherapists, to signify "the condition of primal innocence and unity with all life," it soon acquired the alternative appellation of "ecstasy," the name by which it is popularly known to this day.

By 1984, with growing use on college campuses and increased media attention and embellishment, political pressure was placed on federal regulators to establish tight controls on what was still a legal drug. Consequently, in 1985 the U.S. Drug Enforcement Agency (DEA) convened hearings to determine the fate of MDMA. These highly publicized hearings achieved the unintended effect of further raising public awareness of MDMA, as well as interest in experimentation. Media accounts further polarized opinion, pitting enthusiastic claims of MDMA by proponents against dire warnings of unknown dangers to the nation's youth. Public debate was further confounded by the frequent confusion of MDMA with 1-methyl-4-phenyl-1,2,3,6-tetrahydropyridine (MPTP), a dopaminergic neurotoxin that had recently been revealed to induce severe Parkinson-like disorders in users seeking synthetic heroin substitute highs. With growing concern over the dangers of new "designer drugs," public discussion took an increasingly discordant tone. The DEA director ruled that MDMA be placed in Schedule I in the late 1980s. Since then, with the exception of a 3-month period in early 1988 when it was briefly unscheduled as a result of a court challenge, MDMA has remained classified as a Schedule I substance.

In the years following the MDMA scheduling controversy, patterns of use have undergone a marked shift. With the failure to establish an official sanction for MDMA treatment, most psychotherapists who had used the drug adjunctively in their work ceased to do so. In the wake of the highly publicized scheduling hearings, however, use among young people escalated. By the late 1980s, interest in MDMA had spread from the United States across the Atlantic to Europe, where it became the drug of choice at marathon dance parties called "raves." Although use in the United States diminished in the early 1990s, by the end of the decade and into the new century its popularity surged. In Europe, and particularly the United Kingdom, MDMA use among young people has consistently maintained high levels. With multiple illicit laboratories, including pharmaceutical manufacturers in former iron curtain countries, the European youth market appears to have become saturated with the drug in recent years.

Epidemiology

Although various estimates have been given on the extent of current illicit MDMA use in the United States and Western Europe, the exact prevalence remains unknown. A Harris Opinion Poll for the BBC in Great Britain presented data that 31% of people between the ages of 16 and 25 years admitted to taking MDMA, most often at "dance clubs," and that 67% reported that their friends had tried the drug. In a survey of school children across the whole of England, 4.25% of 14-year-olds and, in another survey, 6.0% of those aged 14 and 15 years, were reported to have taken MDMA.

In the United States, reported use of ecstasy has increased significantly, doubling between 1998 and 2001. By the early 21st century, 12% of high school seniors admitted to having taken ecstasy. A study of Stanford University undergraduate students reported that 39% had taken MDMA at least once in their lives, and a Tulane University survey revealed that 24.3% of more than 1,200 students questioned had experimented with the drug.

Potential Treatment Applications

Beginning in the late 1970s, proponents of drug-enhanced psychotherapy began to investigate the therapeutic potential of the still-legal MDMA. Compared to LSD, the prototype psychedelic of the 20th century, MDMA was judged to possess distinct advantages as a therapeutic adjunct. MDMA was described as being a relatively mild, short-acting drug capable of facilitating heightened states of introspection and intimacy along with temporary freedom from anxiety and depression, yet without distracting alterations in perception, body image, and sense of self. Patients were reported as losing defensive anxiety, feeling more emotionally open, and accessing feelings and thoughts not ordinarily available to them. Lasting improvement was often reported in patients' self-esteem, ability to communicate with significant others, capacity for achieving empathic rapport, interest in and capacity for insight, strengthened capacity for trust and intimacy, and enhanced therapeutic alliance.

A variety of treatment applications were explored prior to the scheduling of MDMA in the mid-1980s, including the physical pain and emotional distress associated with severe medical illness, posttraumatic stress disorders, depression, phobias, addictions, psychosomatic disorders, and relationship (marital) problems.

Before the value of MDMA as a treatment modality could be subjected to a rigorous, methodologic research evaluation in the United States, the drug was placed on Schedule I status. From the mid-1980s until the early 21st century, efforts to conduct clinical trials with MDMA were not permitted, although approved phase I investigations of physiologic and psychologic effects in normal volunteers with prior MDMA experience were approved at three research centers in the United States.

Consequently, because clinical patient populations have never been subjected to formal examination with MDMA, only anecdotal case reports are available for examination. In addition to accounts of treatment outcome, the experiences of long-term users of MDMA have also been systematically examined. One study, which subjected 20 psychiatrists with past personal histories of MDMA use to extensive semistructured interviews, reported that 85% had increased ability to interact with or be open with others, 80% had decreased defensiveness, 65% had decreased fear, 60% had decreased sense of separation or alienation from others, 50% had increased awareness of emotions, and 50% had decreased aggression. Half of these psychiatrists with MDMA use experience also reported long-term improvement in social and interpersonal functioning.

Adverse Clinical Effects

When examining adverse effects of MDMA, it is important to distinguish between relatively benign, transient effects experienced by healthy, occasional users ingesting relatively moderate dosages versus more dangerous sequelae reported to occur in a small minority of individuals taking MDMA, often in the context of significant premorbid pathology, adverse settings, polysubstance use, and excessive dosing. Common short-term side effects of MDMA have been reported to be similar to effects induced by amphetamines, including trismus, bruxism, restlessness, anxiety, and decreased appetite. Other investigators have reported tachycardia, palpitations, dry mouth, and insomnia.

With substantial alterations in patterns of use over the past decade, from occasional use for therapeutic and spiritual purposes to frequent, repeated ingestion at large rave dances, the reported risks have increased significantly. Although earlier investigations had concluded that MDMA was a drug with a relatively low potential for abuse and for which persistent use patterns were described as extremely rare, the likelihood of individuals frequently ingesting higher dosages of MDMA, often in association with other drugs or alcohol, appears to be increasing. MDMA possesses nonlinear pharmacokinetics, implying that relatively small increases in the dose of MDMA ingested can induce disproportionate increases in plasma concentrations of MDMA, thus exposing individuals to greater risk of developing acute toxicity.

Over the last several years an increasing number of reports of adverse effects attributed to ecstasy have appeared in the medical literature. It is also critical to note that given the clandestine (and often amateur) context within which MDMA is manufactured for the escalating mass market, the available black market drug is often not necessarily what it is advertised as being. Besides escalating degrees of overt drug substitution, ecstasy also often contains contaminants and adulterants. As was the case with psychedelics in the 1960s, following the transition over time from limited and legal use by relatively well-educated aficionados to mass-market consumption for illicit purposes by youth, the purity and quality of MDMA has progressively declined, while the associated risks to the user have climbed.

Given the extent to which MDMA has been subject to widespread use and abuse, it is somewhat surprising that more instances of serious adverse effects have not been reported. Particularly within a context of grave concerns raised over potential risks, fueled by media publicity, only a relatively small number of fatal reactions to the drug have made their way into the medical literature. Nevertheless, serious attention needs to be accorded the potential for catastrophic medical reactions, because they have occurred and are likely to continue to occur particularly in individuals with pre-existing vulnerabilities (both medical and psychologic) who take the drug under circumstances that accentuate the risks.

The first reports of fatalities associated with MDMA ingestion occurred in the United States in 1987, and consisted of five cases of individuals who had precipitously died; postmortem toxicologic screens were positive for MDMA or N-ethyl-methylenedioxyamphetamine (MDEA), an MDMA analogue. One of these cases was an individual who was electrocuted while under the influence of MDMA, whereas the other four were all associated with individuals who sustained fatal cardiovascular events. Three of these individuals apparently had pre-existing severe cardiac or respiratory disease that was felt to have played a primary role in their sudden death. Alcohol and drugs, in addition to MDMA, were also associated with the four cases of death induced by cardiovascular collapse.

The development of prospective investigations on the effects of pure MDMA administered to human subjects has yielded important information on the range of cardiovascular response. Studies have reported that higher dosages of MDMA can induce marked increases in heart rate, blood pressure, and myocardial oxygen consumption, thereby highlighting the heightened degree of risk for individuals with underlying cardiovascular vulnerabilities.

Several cases have also been reported over the last few years in the medical literature of severe cerebrovascular accidents apparently induced by MDMA. Pre-existing neurologic vulnerabilities appear to accentuate the risks for devastating cerebrovascular events. Associated polysubstance and alcohol use also appears to potentiate the dangers of MDMA use, inducing injury to central nervous system structures. Damage to subcortical structures through a mechanism of vasoconstriction brought on by enhanced serotonin neurotransmission has also been suggested as the pathogenesis of some strokes associated with MDMA.

With increasing use of MDMA, often of indeterminate quality and excessive quantity, cases of apparent hepatotoxicity have begun to emerge, particularly in Great Britain. Whether the liver damage in these cases was caused by an idiosyncratic reaction to MDMA or to some contaminant ingested along with it is not known. Although such case reports emphasize the need to inquire about MDMA use histories in young people presenting with unexplained jaundice and hepatomegaly, they do appear to be extremely rare, even in the context of increasing usage of an often impure, illicit compound. The mechanism underlying the reported liver damage remains to be determined.

A severe medical complication of taking MDMA in the context of vigorous prolonged exercise, environmental crowding, lack of sufficient hydration, and high ambient temperature is the induction of a catastrophic hyperthermic reaction leading to disseminated intravascular coagulation (DIC), rhabdomyolysis, acute renal and hepatic failure, seizures, and, on occasion, death. Virtually all such reported cases have occurred in the rave dance club setting, and were associated with prolonged vigorous dancing in poorly ventilated environments and inadequate fluid replacement.

Although maintenance of adequate hydration is a critical component of harm reduction efforts, published case reports reveal that excessive consumption of fluids in association with MDMA administration may provoke severe and potentially fatal hyponatremia induced by the syndrome of inappropriate antidiuretic hormone secretion (SIADH). A prospective study conducted in the United Kingdom demonstrated that the administration of a modest dose of MDMA induced significant elevations of antidiuretic hormone (vasopressin) in human research subjects. Several well-publicized deaths have occurred secondarily to apparent water intoxication.

Given that the degree of MDMA use has climbed well into the millions, initially in Europe, and more recently in the United States, it is not surprising that cases of psychiatric disturbance have been reported. Reported adverse psychiatric events include panic disorder, paranoid psychoses, and depression. High and frequent dosages of the drug had been consumed by many of those individuals who have experienced adverse psychiatric sequelae. By the early 21st century, the Drug Abuse Warning Network (DAWN) in the United States reported that MDMA taken concomitantly with other dangerous drugs was becoming an increasingly dangerous phenomenon, accounting for 86% of all medical and psychiatric emergencies associated with MDMA. Indeed, alcohol was associated with almost half of all MDMA-implicated medical and psychiatric emergencies, whereas cocaine was associated with nearly one third of cases. In the face of significant premorbid psychopathology, and often in combination with other drugs or alcohol, frequent use of high-dose MDMA does appear to heighten risks for deterioration of psychiatric status. The evidence, however, for occasional, low-dose MDMA use, taken in controlled settings without additional drugs or alcohol by individuals with negative histories for psychiatric disorders, appears to be considerably lower.

An additional concern over the uncontrolled use of recreational MDMA has been the potential risks of dangerous interactions with prescription drugs. MDMA is metabolized primarily by the CYP2D6 and CYP3A4 hepatic systems. MDMA might influence or be influenced by other drugs metabolized by the same cytochrome P450 isozymes. Drugs also possessing prominent 2D6 metabolism, including the selective serotonin reuptake inhibitor (SSRI) antidepressants fluoxetine (Prozac) and paroxetine (Paxil), as well as the illicit drug cocaine, inhibit MDMA metabolism in human liver, thus posing the risk of impaired degradation and protracted exposure to high levels of MDMA. Because 7% of whites are poor CYP2D6 metabolizers, these subjects might be at higher risk for development of drug interactions and toxic side effects.

Neurotoxicity

Unlike other amphetamine-like compounds, which exert comparable effects on both serotonergic and dopaminergic neurons, the predominant target of MDMA is the serotonin system (although dopamine systems also can be affected, particularly at high doses). Effects of serotonin systems in laboratory animals subjected to administration of large dosages of MDMA are divided into short-term and long-term effects. Some of the acute effects of MDMA, including the rapid release of intracellular serotonin, are presumed to mediate the behavioral and psychologic profile observed in humans, whereas in animals, the neurotoxic effects are not manifested until days later. It would appear that neurotoxicity is not inextricably linked to the acute effects of the drug. Administration of fluoxetine prior to, or up to 6 hours after, MDMA administration blocks or attenuates the development of neurotoxicity, whereas some acute effects of MDMA (e.g., behavioral, neuroendocrine, and temperature) occur within minutes and peak within a few hours.

The majority of work on MDMA has revolved around its neurotoxic effects and the mechanisms by which these effects are produced. Rats administered multiple doses of MDMA undergo serotonergic neurotoxic changes that can last for many months before neurochemical recovery occurs, although there can be considerable interanimal variability in the degree of neurotoxicity, as well as in the extent of recovery, from the same dosage regimen. The mechanisms underlying MDMA-induced serotonin neurotoxicity are thought to occur by the uptake of MDMA into serotonin nerve terminals, causing an initial reduction of serotonin levels. A second phase of serotonin reduction follows, possibly as a consequence of the formation of neurotoxic metabolites or by generation of free radicals, which causes degeneration of serotonin terminals (and in some cases axons) for weeks to months, depending on the species and dosage regimen employed. Additional data indicate that dopamine also plays a role in the mechanism underlying the neurotoxic effects of MDMA on serotonin neurons, as does glutamate, because N-methyl-D-aspartic acid (NMDA) antagonists can inhibit or attenuate MDMA-induced neurotoxicity. In addition to pure neurochemical modulators, temperature appears to be another variable in the mediation of MDMA neurotoxicity. Because MDMA neurotoxicity is evidently dependent on high core temperatures, preventing the development of hyperthermic states in experimental animals will reduce the loss of serotonergic terminals.

Whereas multiple studies establish and reconfirm that MDMA provokes profound changes in brain serotonin systems of laboratory animals, evidence that functional or behavioral abnormalities are induced remain limited. Similarly, minimal data are available addressing the issue of whether normal function is restored following biochemical recovery. It has long been demonstrated that at least in some species serotonin and other monoaminergic neurons can undergo extensive regeneration following neurotoxin-induced degenerative change. Although it is not known to what extent regenerated (or sprouted) fibers are able to re-establish original synaptic contacts, some data suggest that the observed patterns of reinnervation are abnormal. The degree to which such biochemical alterations affect functional normality is a question still awaiting elucidation. Indeed, it appears that it is the specific "damage" to serotonin fibers, (primarily serotonergic axonal terminals originating from the dorsal raphe), induced by neurotoxins causing significant declines in serotonin levels, that ultimately reactivate latent developmental signals in the brain.

Efforts to extend the neurotoxicity hypothesis to human populations have met with mixed results. Measurements of neurotransmitter metabolites in the cerebrospinal fluid (CSF) of MDMA users were assessed in one early study as being within normal limits. A subsequent study, which reported lower levels of CSF 5-hydroxyindole acetic acid (5-HIAA) in MDMA users, is difficult to interpret because the control population employed was a group of patients with chronic back pain. However, serotonergic mechanisms are involved in pain control as well as the known association of increased levels of CSF 5-HIAA in patients suffering from chronic nonmalignant and malignant pain. The most methodologically sound retrospective evaluation of human MDMA users, although finding no differences between prolactin secretion induced by an L-tryptophan challenge test, did find significantly lower levels of CSF 5-HIAA in MDMA users compared to controls. Surprisingly, however, and confounding expectations inferred by the neurotoxicity hypothesis, these same MDMA subjects with relatively low levels of CSF 5-HIAA were also assessed as having significantly lower scores on personality measures of impulsivity and hostility; opposite results were expected.

Finally, a decrease in stage II sleep and sleep time has been reported in subjects with a history of MDMA. This is both an interesting and perplexing observation. Given the prominent role that serotonin plays in the regulation of both slow-wave and rapid eye movement (REM) sleep, one would have expected that these sleep electroencephalograph (EEG) measures might have been most affected by MDMA. In summary, most, if not all, of the observed changes reported thus far are compatible with a general effect of MDMA on serotonin neurotransmission independent of neurotoxicity, although the latter effect cannot be ruled out.

An additional area of controversy is the impact of MDMA use on mood and cognition, presumed clinical sequelae to suspected serotonin neurotoxicity. One study conducted in the United Kingdom described persistent dysphoria and mild memory impairment experienced by rave participants during the week following their weekend of drug-fueled dancing. These "mid week lows" were significantly more severe for MDMA users who were also regular users of cocaine and amphetamines. Only 2% of this MDMA-using subject cohort were not polysubstance users. A particularly confounding phenomenon is the increasing popularity among ravers of ketamine (Ketalar), a dissociative anesthetic, known to induce strong frontal lobe effects and cognitive dysfunction. Similarly, cannabis, which is consumed by a high proportion of recreational MDMA users, may also cause alterations in neuropsychologic function, further challenging MDMA research methodologies. Unfortunately, many studies fail adequately to take into account the contributory role of other commonly used drugs when assessing the clinical effects of recreational MDMA use.

The role of MDMA as a recreational drug for millions of young people worldwide is worrisome, particularly within the context of ill-prepared and vulnerable individuals consuming an illicitly manufactured and marketed drug of dubious quality in unpredictable and often dangerous settings. Nevertheless, for a true appreciation of the range of effects of MDMA, it is imperative that objective investigations be conducted in a fair and honest scientific environment. One hopes the future will provide the opportunity for well-controlled and methodologically sound investigations to probe the full range of effects of MDMA, and begin to answer the as-yet-unanswered questions surrounding the capacity of the drug to cause harm versus its potential under optimal conditions to facilitate beneficial outcomes.

Opioid Analogues

Fentanyl Analogues

In 1979, a series of unusual deaths occurred in Orange County, California. The fatalities occurred in heroin injectors and resembled heroin overdose but toxicologic analysis was negative. By the end of 1980, 15 such fatalities had been recorded. The toxin was later identified as an analogue of the legal opioid fentanyl, alpha-methyl-fentanyl. It had been promoted in street sales as "China White" (sometimes a name for purported high-quality heroin). Between 1981 and 1984, at least three other analogues were identified in street drug samples and in the bodily fluids of overdose victims: alpha-methyl-acetyl-fentanyl, 3-methyl-fentanyl (TMF) and para-fluoro-fentanyl. TMF is approximately 6,000 times as potent as morphine. By the end of 1984, an apparent decline in use of these products had occurred as had the number of deaths, although perhaps 10 even more unusual analogues were identified.

Potency

Although it is likely that any marketed controlled substance analogue will be relatively potent, a potent opioid has particular dangerous significance. Many users of street heroin do not attain significant levels of tolerance even though previously low-quality, adulterated street heroin has improved. Additionally, "regular" injectors of heroin spend much time not using and may often be susceptible to overdose with any potent material. It is not that fentanyl or its profoundly potent analogues cause a better high or more respiratory depression than heroin, it is that they do it in such a small volume of white powder.

MPTP

The opiate 1-methyl-4-phenyl-4-propionoxypiperidine (MPPP), a close relative of meperidine, had previously been tested as an analgesic but possessed insufficient activity. The synthesis is particularly likely to be contaminated with the MPTP congener under conditions of inadequate control of temperature and pH. In 1982 in California, a number of injectors who had purchased street heroin developed parkinsonian symptoms and subsequent analysis of the product used identified both MPTP and MPPP. The scientists who described this phenomenon reported that the description of the synthesis of MPPP had been carefully excised from journal pages in the Stanford Medical School library. Primates given MPTP develop a parkinsonian syndrome secondary to destruction of dopaminergic neurons in the substantia nigra. MPTP may cause occupational Parkinson disease. One reported case involved a chemist who had conducted repeated synthetic reactions involving MPTP. Exposure may have occurred through accidental inhalation or skin contamination. Follow-up studies indicate that susceptibility to the toxicity is variable. All exposed to MPTP do not necessarily become ill.

Mechanism of Action

The neurotoxicity is not caused by MPTP itself but by a toxic metabolite. MPTP binds with high affinity to neural monoamine oxidase B and is converted to methylphenyldihydropyridine (MPP+). Interference with conversion by prior treatment with a monoamine oxidase inhibitor will prevent experimental toxicity. MPP+ is taken up by sensitive cells in the substantia nigra, reaches high intramitochondrial concentration, interferes with oxidative phosphorylation, and causes cellular death.

Nexus

The DEA has placed 4-bromo, 3,4-dimethoxy-phenethylamine in Schedule I. This drug, often called *nexus* or *2-CB*, has MDMA-like properties in much lower doses (0.1 to 0.2 mg/kg) but is not widely distributed.

4-Methylaminorex

4-Methylaminorex (4MAM or "U4Euh") was the first example of a controlled substance analogue stimulant. Currently, there is little evidence of widespread use, and its clinical importance is unassessed. The widespread availability of cocaine and synthetic methamphetamine may deter attempts to manufacture stimulant controlled substance analogues. 4 MAM has generally been sold in illicit markets as U4Euh. This product was first synthesized by McNeil Laboratories in the 1960s and, like MDA, evaluated as an anorectic. It is illicitly synthesized from the widely available over-the-counter drug phenylpropanolamine. It is associated with one fatality and was moved to Schedule I by the DEA. This drug was never marketed, but a nonmethylated version (aminorex) was marketed in Europe as an appetite depressant in 1965. It was frequently associated with severe pulmonary hypertension and was withdrawn in 1968. Reportedly, aminorex itself has recently appeared in illicit trade in America. Structurally, it most resembles the relatively mild prescription stimulant pemoline. At oral doses of 10 to 20 mg, 4 MAM reportedly provokes a smooth episode of enhanced intellectual energy lasting 10 to 12 hours. Its advocates claim that work is facilitated not only without agitation but with a diminution of anxiety.

Methcathinone

A number of possible stimulant compounds appear in the khat plant (*Catha edulis*). It is now believed that cathinone is the chief active ingredient producing amphetamine-like effects when the leaves are chewed in the khat ceremony. In the 1950s, Parke-Davis conducted studies on an analogue of cathinone, methcathinone. There are no available human data but animal studies revealed a series of effects closely parallel to those of *d*-amphetamine. Methcathinone, like amphetamines displaces [³H]dopamine from rat cells in the caudate nucleus.

Methcathinone (called ephedrone) emerged as a marketed illicit drug in Russia. It was predominantly used by heroin injectors in a "speedball" combination. Reportedly, Russian users would also use the drug alone in intravenous binges resembling a methamphetamine pattern first reported in the United States in the late 1960s.

The drug appeared in commerce in rural Michigan in 1991, reportedly having been manufactured in clandestine laboratories in the upper peninsula of that state. It was quickly placed into Schedule I of the Controlled Substances Act in 1992. Snorting reportedly is followed by euphoria and excitement with enhancement of visual perception. Such use produces 5 to 8 hours of enhanced energy, feelings of toughness and invincibility, and increased sexual desire. Subsequent doses are said to push users from "speeding" to "tripping" with more visual effects and even hallucinations. Use can be accompanied by headaches, abdominal cramps, sweating, and tachycardia.

Conclusion

It is unclear how often and with what impact new synthetic chemicals will emerge onto the illicit psychoactive market. It is also unclear how toxic such products are likely to be, and assessments of toxicity can be difficult because of the overheated character of media and police reports that may occur when such products appear. However, the creation and use of existing designer drugs illustrates that this somewhat diverse category of substances can pose unique challenges in understanding effects and risks associated with their use. It is hoped that future research will provide an evidence base for determining effects and risks associated with these and other designer drugs that may be used illicitly.

Suggested Readings

Grob CS, ed. *Hallucinogens: a reader.* New York: Tarcher/Putnam; 2002.

Grob CS, Poloand RE. MDMA. In: Lowinson JH, Ruiz P, Millman RB, et al., eds. *Substance abuse: a comprehensive textbook,* 4th ed. Philadelphia: Lippincott Williams & Wilkins; 2005:374–386.

Lieb R, Schuetz CG, Pfister H, et al. Mental disorders in ecstasy users: a prospective-longitudinal investigation. *Drug Alcohol Depend.* 2002;68:195–207.

Morgan JP. Designer drugs. In: Lowinson JH, Ruiz P, Millman RB, et al., eds. *Substance abuse: a comprehensive textbook,* 4th ed. Philadelphia: Lippincott Williams & Wilkins; 2005:367–373.

Parrott AC. Human psychopharmacology of ecstasy (MDMA): a review of 15 years of empirical research. *Hum Psychopharmacol Clin Exp;* 2001;1:557–577.

Simon NG, Mattick RP. The impact of regular ecstasy use on memory function. *Addiction.* 2002;97:1523–1529.

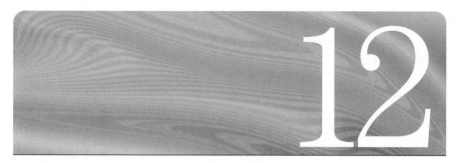

NICOTINE

Nicotine is one of the most widely abused substances in America. An estimated 25% of the US population smokes, making nicotine addiction a critical public health problem in terms of morbidity, mortality, and economic costs to society. It is well documented that smoking substantially increases the risk of coronary heart disease, cancer, and more than 40 other medical diseases. Even in the face of negative health consequences, smokers continue to use tobacco and quit unsuccessfully, attesting to the high addictive potential of nicotine. Current scientific literature clearly establishes the actions of nicotine within the central nervous system that lead to acute positive reinforcement, the development of dependence, and withdrawal symptoms. Other factors that contribute considerably to the highly addictive potential of nicotine include the efficient drug-delivery system of the cigarette, its high level of availability, the small number of legal and social consequences of tobacco use, and the sophisticated marketing and advertising methods used by tobacco companies. This chapter reviews the extent and impact of nicotine use, its addictive properties, and currently available pharmacologic and behavioral treatments.

Extent and Impact of Nicotine Use
Prevalence

According to the Centers for Disease Control and Prevention (CDC), an estimated 46.5 million adults (23.3%) are current smokers. Smoking prevalence is significantly higher among men (25.7%) than among women (21.0%). Among ethnic groups, Asians (14.4%) and Hispanics (18.6%) have the lowest smoking rates, whereas Native Americans/Alaska Natives (36.0%) have the highest. Across education levels, rates are highest for adults who earned a General Educational Development (GED) diploma (47.2%) and lowest for those with advanced degrees (8.4%). Adults living below the poverty level (31.7%) have higher smoking rates than those at or above this income level (22.9%). Among age groups, persons age 18 to 44 years have the highest smoking rates and those age 65 years or older, the lowest. An estimated 44.3 million adults (22.2%) are former smokers, and among current smokers, 70% report that they want to quit completely.

Health Consequences

Smoking is the leading cause of premature death in the United States, resulting in more than 440,000 deaths each year. Illness related to smoking costs the adult smoker an average of 13.2 (female) and 14.5 (male) years of life. Cigarette smoking significantly increases the risk of lung cancer, ischemic heart disease, chronic airway obstruction, and perinatal complications. The health benefits of quitting smoking are substantial, including a decreased risk of lung cancer, other cancers, cardiovascular disease, chronic lung disease, and infertility. Exposure to environmental tobacco smoke (ETS), a known human carcinogen, also increases the risk of cancer and is associated with the deaths of almost 40,000 nonsmokers each year. The economic costs of smoking are tremendous, with each pack of cigarettes sold in the United States resulting in costs of $7.18 in medical care expenses and lost productivity. Further, it is estimated that $75.5 billion is spent each year on smoking-related personal medical care.

Nicotine as an Addictive Drug

Addictive Properties

Nicotine is recognized as the primary compound in tobacco smoke that meets criteria for abuse potential and dependence. First, it has centrally mediated, psychoactive effects that are reliably discriminated from placebo. Second, nicotine produces pleasurable or euphoriant effects, as rated subjectively by smokers on drug "liking" scales. Third, nicotine functions as a positive reinforcer. Both animals and human smokers will self-administer nicotine over placebo. Fourth, tolerance to the effects of nicotine develops after repeated administration. Finally, an abstinence syndrome is observed when regular nicotine administration is discontinued.

A host of smoking-related stimuli influence smoking reinforcement. Many of the behavioral and sensory components of the act of smoking provide cues that become reinforcing through their association with the pharmacologic effects of nicotine. Studies involving denicotinized tobacco cigarettes, that is, cigarettes that resemble normal cigarettes in taste, but deliver one tenth of the nicotine, confirm the important role of nonnicotine factors in smoking reinforcement. Recent observations point to possible gender differences in the role of nonnicotine influences on smoking reinforcement. Women may be reinforced less by nicotine intake and more by other, nonnicotine factors, relative to men.

A subpopulation of smokers (5% to 10%) appears to be resistant to nicotine dependence (termed "chippers" or occasional nondependent smokers). These individuals smoke fewer than five cigarettes per day for many years and stop smoking without experiencing withdrawal symptoms. Like dependent smokers, chippers absorb equal amounts of nicotine, eliminate nicotine at equal rates, and show similar cardiovascular responses to smoking. Thus, smoking patterns in chippers seem to be more influenced by situational factors than are the smoking patterns in dependent smokers.

Determinants of Use

Neurochemical Actions

Actions of nicotine on the neurochemical system appear to be involved in mediating the acute positive reinforcing effects of nicotine. Nicotine activates nicotinic acetylcholine receptors (nAChRs) in the mesocorticolimbic dopaminergic system that projects from the ventral tegmental area (VTA) to the nucleus accumbens and the prefrontal cortex. It is the diversity of nAChRs that may explain the multiple effects of nicotine in humans. When activated, there is a cascade of reinforcing effects, particularly dopamine release. To date, the preponderance of data points to the critical role of the midbrain *dopamine* system in nicotine reinforcement processes. It should be noted, however, that other neuronal pathways, including those involving glutamate, γ-aminobutyric acid (GABA), opioid peptides, and serotonin, appear to contribute to the reinforcing properties of nicotine-induced dopaminergic neurotransmission.

Whereas initial acute nicotine exposure stimulates the nAChR, the effects of nicotine after chronic exposure appear paradoxical in that further exposure leads to receptor desensitization and inactivation. Decreases in dopamine output in the nucleus accumbens have been observed during nicotine withdrawal. Additionally, upregulation of nicotine binding sites during cessation is thought to play a role in the intensity of the early withdrawal symptoms and the likelihood of relapse. Alterations in other neurotransmitter systems also may play a role in nicotine withdrawal.

In summary, preclinical studies have been useful in establishing some of the neuronal mechanisms related to the reinforcing effects of nicotine and chronic nicotine use.

Pharmacokinetic Dynamic Properties of Nicotine

The pharmacokinetic properties of nicotine also enhance its abuse potential. Inhaled nicotine is directly absorbed through the pulmonary capillaries into the pulmonary venous circulation and then to the left side of the heart. It is the arterial concentration of nicotine that first encounters the central nervous system and other tissues, driving acute pharmacologic effects. These high concentrations of nicotine in the arterial circulation produce a host of acute pharmacodynamic effects. In particular, nicotine induces release of epinephrine from the adrenal medulla, which acts, in part, to activate the sympathetic nervous system. Sympathomimetic effects of nicotine include heart rate acceleration, transient increase in blood pressure, increased cardiac output, and some constriction of blood vessels. Tolerance develops to some, but not all, of the cardiovascular effects of nicotine.

Additionally, the absorbed *dose* of nicotine is a determinant of its actions. In general, it has been shown that nicotine produces dose-related effects on cardiovascular, electroencephalographic, appetitive, emotional, and cognitive responses. Other variables that affect nicotine absorption and plasma concentrations during smoking include the interval between cigarettes, the frequency and degree of inhalation, and the nicotine content of the cigarette.

The *speed* at which a drug reaches the brain and central nervous system is critical to understanding its potential reinforcement and abuse liability. Rapid delivery systems have much higher abuse liability, or reinforcing efficacy, than slower delivering systems. Inhalation of nicotine via cigarette smoking produces the most rapid delivery of nicotine to the brain, with drug levels peaking within a few seconds of inhalation, similar to other drugs that have high abuse potential.

In contrast to cigarette smoking, less-rapid release of nicotine, such as via transdermal nicotine, produces slower and lower peak arterial nicotine concentrations, resulting in a relatively steady level of nicotine and significantly less pharmacologic and behavioral reinforcement. The of nicotine absorption from other delivery systems, such as nicotine gum, nasal spray, and inhaler, is more rapid than the patch, but slower than with cigarette smoking. Of the different nicotine replacement systems, the nasal spray has a pharmacokinetic profile closest to cigarettes.

Clinical Aspects of Tobacco Dependence

Development of Dependence

Only one third to one half of individuals who experiment with cigarette smoking become nicotine dependent. The development of dependence involves a progression through a series of stages. Initial use is largely driven by psychosocial motives or non-pharmacologic factors, whereas later use is motivated more by pharmacologic factors, including positive nicotine effects and withdrawal relief. Identifying which adolescents in the early stages will proceed to become established nicotine addicts. Beliefs and attitudes related to smoking appear to be important predictors of the transition from experimentation to established smoking, along with exposure to other smokers and perceived school performance. There may be gender differences in determinants of smoking and nicotine dependence. For girls, a strong need for social interaction influences smoking development, whereas for boys, higher levels of depression symptoms are more influential. For girls, smoking onset and continuation may be influenced by concern for weight and body shape.

Vulnerability to nicotine dependence may be related to individual differences in sensitivity to nicotine, starting with initial exposure. Along these lines, two somewhat contrasting models have been put forth to explain why some people who experiment with tobacco go on to smoke regularly, whereas others do not. According to the "exposure" model of tolerance or dependence, more sensitive individuals, that is, those who encounter aversive effects on initial use, are less likely to engage in further experimentation, whereas people with less sensitivity to nicotine experience fewer unpleasant effects and, as a consequence, are more likely to continue. Social reinforcement, typically peer pressure, serves to further maintain early self-administration of nicotine. Beyond initial sensitivity, the level of continued exposure to nicotine presumably leads to a degree of tolerance and dependence. If the prevailing environment is facilitating or permissive of smoking, nicotine dependence is likely to develop.

In contrast, the "sensitivity" model of dependence proposes that dependent smokers are those who are constitutionally *more* sensitive to nicotine. For them, initial exposure to smoking produces aversive and rewarding effects, with continued exposure associated with a decrease in sensitivity as tolerance develops. Accumulating evidence favoring the sensitivity model of dependence includes research on the genetics of nicotine dependence. Heritability estimates for smoking initiation from various large sample twin studies fall within the range of 46% to 84%, with approximately 30% of the variance accounted for by shared environmental influences.

Dependence

Characteristic features of dependence include persistent use despite knowledge of medical problems related to smoking, withdrawal symptoms upon cessation of use, and unsuccessful efforts to stop. The majority of regular smokers meet the DSM-IV-TR diagnostic criteria for tobacco dependence. Dependent smokers report desirable and useful effects derived from nicotine.

Cotinine, the primary proximate metabolite of nicotine, is present in the blood of smokers in much higher levels than is nicotine. The half-life of cotinine is considerably longer than that of nicotine (average 16 hours vs. 2 hours). Recent findings from a study of cotinine in abstinent cigarette smokers suggest that cotinine is behaviorally active. It has been shown that cotinine, compared with placebo, produced significant changes in (reversal of) subjective parameters of withdrawal, including restlessness, anxiety/tension, insomnia, sedation, and pleasantness. Whereas previously thought to have minimal pharmacologic activity, these data underscore the potentially important role of cotinine in the complex process of nicotine dependence.

Withdrawal

Diagnostic criteria for nicotine withdrawal according to the DSM-IV include at least four of the following signs occurring within 24 hours of abrupt cessation of nicotine use or reduction in the amount of nicotine use: (a) dysphoric or depressed mood; (b) insomnia; (c) irritability, frustration, or anger; (d) anxiety; (e) difficulty concentrating; (f) restlessness; (g) decreased heart rate; and (h) increased appetite or weight gain. Craving for nicotine, although no longer listed as a diagnostic criterion, is considered to be an important element in nicotine withdrawal. Craving and impaired concentration are two of the most frequently reported symptoms of nicotine withdrawal. It is well documented that nicotine deprivation can impair psychomotor and cognitive abilities and that smoking reverses these performance deficits.

Traditional models of drug dependence posit withdrawal to be centrally involved in motivating drug use and relapse. In support, a number of studies show a relationship between the presence and severity of nicotine withdrawal symptoms and the probability that a smoker attempting to quit will relapse. More recently, however, the withdrawal phenomenon has been challenged based on reported inconsistency in the interrelationship of dependence severity, withdrawal, and relapse. Smokers frequently do not identify withdrawal as precipitating relapse, and relapse often occurs long after cessation, when, presumably, withdrawal symptoms have abated. Using newer and more sensitive approaches to the study of withdrawal, it showed that withdrawal profiles, consisting primarily of affect, urge, and sleep/energy dimensions, vary by individual and over time. Moreover, smokers having "atypical" withdrawal profiles, defined as those with unremitting symptoms peaking late after cessation, are more likely to relapse than other smokers having more common withdrawal patterns. Affective components of the withdrawal syndrome have shown the strongest relations with relapse. There is a robust link between depression, negative affect, and smoking relapse. That smokers exhibit higher rates of major depressive disorder than nonsmokers is established, as is the prediction that smokers with past depression will have greater withdrawal-related increases in anger and depression during the first week of quitting and be more likely to relapse. It is not so clear, however, whether negative affect in abstinent smokers constitutes a nicotine-induced withdrawal response or the emergence of an affective disorder. Thus, the effect of nicotine on mood and negative affect is complex and in need of further research.

Withdrawal symptoms are believed to be primarily caused by nicotine deprivation. Nevertheless, other nonpharmacologic factors of tobacco smoking, such as conditioning and expectancy, influence aspects of behavior during nicotine withdrawal. Smoking denicotinized cigarettes can significantly reduce acute tobacco withdrawal symptoms and craving scores, pointing to the apparent contribution of sensory and environmental factors in nicotine withdrawal effects. That nicotine replacement strategies, which presumably suppress withdrawal, do not entirely correspond with their ability to produce abstinence may be explained by the important role of factors other than nicotine in tobacco withdrawal.

Treatment of Nicotine Addiction

Given the substantial negative consequences of smoking, and the finding that 70% of smokers report wanting to quit, the goal of making effective treatment options available to all smokers has become a public health priority. In primary health care settings, however, fewer than one third of smokers are asked about their smoking status, encouraged to quit, or offered assistance quitting smoking. This is unfortunate given the evidence that even brief smoking cessation interventions can be efficacious and cost-effective. To address this problem, the Agency for Health Care Policy and Research published *Treating Tobacco Use and Dependence Clinical Practice Guideline* (the *Guideline*). The purpose of the *Guideline* is to identify effective smoking cessation interventions and provide treatment recommendations applicable to a wide array of clinical settings and patient populations.

According to the *Guideline* treatment model for clinical settings, tobacco use status (current, former, or never) should be assessed and documented for each patient. Current smokers should be advised to quit and their motivation to do so should be assessed. For those willing to make an attempt to quit, counseling and/or pharmacotherapy should be used, either through a brief intervention or referral to more intensive treatment, keeping in mind that there is a strong dose–response relationship between treatment intensity and its effectiveness. Smokers unwilling to quit should be offered a brief motivational intervention designed to encourage an attempt to quit. Recent quitters should receive an intervention to prevent relapse.

Pharmacologic Interventions

The *Guideline* identified five first-line and two second-line smoking cessation pharmacotherapies. First-line pharmacotherapies are those that reliably increase long-term smoking abstinence rates; are safe and effective for the treatment of tobacco dependence; and are approved for this purpose by the U.S. Food and Drug Administration (FDA). These medications have been empirically tested for efficacy and are recommended, unless contraindicated for reasons such as pregnancy/breastfeeding or smoking fewer than 10 cigarettes per day. Second-line medications also have demonstrated efficacy but are not FDA approved and therefore play a more limited role in treatment. Because there is greater concern about potential side effects, second-line pharmacotherapies should only be considered after first-line treatments have proved ineffective.

First-line pharmacotherapies include bupropion SR (Zyban) and four types of nicotine replacement therapy (NRT): nicotine gum, nicotine inhaler, nicotine nasal spray, and nicotine patch. Second-line medications are clonidine (Catapres) and nortriptyline (Pamelor). Tobacco users should be encouraged to use one or a combination of these medications. In addition, most studies reviewed by the *Guideline* combined medication with some type of counseling or behavioral intervention; therefore, a multicomponent approach is recommended.

Bupropion

Bupropion (SR) is the first nonnicotine FDA-approved medication for smoking cessation. Its mechanism of action is presumed to relate to its ability to block the reuptake of dopamine and norepinephrine, with no clinically significant effects on serotonin. The *Guideline* included results from multicenter studies comparing bupropion SR to placebo, with findings indicating that the medication approximately doubles long-term abstinence rates.

Nicotine Replacement Therapy

Four different nicotine replacement products are FDA-approved medications for the treatment of tobacco dependence. Results, based on a review of 47 studies, indicate that nicotine gum, inhaler, nasal spray, and transdermal patch appear to be equally effective, with use of these products approximately doubling long-term abstinence rates when compared to placebo. Further, combination NRT (e.g., combining the patch with nicotine gum or nasal spray) appears to be more effective than use of a single form of NRT.

Clonidine

Clonidine is used primarily as an antihypertensive medication. The FDA has not approved its use as a smoking cessation medication, and no specific dose regimen for this purpose has been established. The five studies included in analyses for the *Guideline* revealed that clonidine approximately doubled abstinence rates when compared to placebo. The medication remains a second-line treatment because of dosing questions and the potentially high incidence of adverse events on abrupt discontinuation of clonidine.

Nortriptyline

Nortriptyline, typically used as an antidepressant, does not have FDA approval for smoking cessation. It remains a second-line medication because of potential side effects and limited evidence to support its efficacy. Recently, it has been found that there is no significant differences in abstinence rates between bupropion and nortriptyline, but both were more effective than placebo.

Other Nicotine Replacement Therapies

Since publication of the *Guideline*, several new methods of delivering NRT have been examined. For instance, 2-mg and 4-mg nicotine lozenges and found both to significantly increase rates of smoking cessation compared to a placebo lozenge at 1 year post–quit date. Comparison of nicotine sublingual tablet to placebo which showed and found significant treatment effects at 6 months post–quit date (33% vs. 18%, respectively). Both of these NRT methods provide effective treatment alternatives for smokers.

Other Medications

A number of additional medications have been evaluated for use with smoking cessation; however, support for their efficacy is lacking. Results of two placebo-controlled trials revealed no significant effect of naltrexone either alone or when combined with the patch. Fluoxetine (Prozac), paroxetine (Paxil), and sertraline (Zoloft) have been tested in combination with NRT and/or behavioral treatments for smoking cessation. None is associated with a significant treatment effect. The *Guideline* also reviewed research on mecamylamine (a nicotine antagonist), diazepam (Valium) and buspirone (Buspan) (anxiolytics), and propranolol (Inderal) (a β-blocker), concluding that evidence was insufficient to recommend their use for smoking cessation.

Behavioral Interventions

The characteristics of behavioral interventions for smoking cessation vary widely. The *Guideline* examined four of these characteristics: advice to quit, intensity, treatment format, and type of clinician, as well as specific elements of various types of counseling and therapy.

Overall results revealed a strong dose–response relationship between treatment intensity (i.e., session length, total contact time, and number of sessions) and treatment effectiveness. However, evidence also indicated that physician advice to quit smoking significantly increases long-term abstinence rates, even with a modal intervention length of 3 minutes or less. Analysis of different treatment formats demonstrated that telephone, group, and individual counseling all improve smoking abstinence rates compared to no intervention.

Types of Behavioral Therapies

In a review of 62 studies examining the effectiveness of different types of counseling and behavioral therapy, four treatment types resulted in significant increases in abstinence rates as compared to no-contact control conditions: (a) providing practical counseling (e.g., skills training approaches), (b) providing intratreatment social support, (c) helping to increase social support outside of treatment, and (d) using aversive smoking procedures.

ALTERNATIVE BEHAVIORAL THERAPIES
Several studies have examined the effectiveness of alternative interventions for smoking cessation, such as hypnosis, physiologic feedback, exercise, and acupuncture. In the *Guideline*, data regarding hypnosis and physiologic feedback were insufficient to address the efficacy of these methods. Findings related to exercise and acupuncture are generally mixed.

ALTERNATIVE TREATMENT GOALS
Harm reduction has been recently suggested as an alternative treatment goal. Harm reduction strategies attempt to change, rather than eliminate, nicotine use so that its harmful effects are reduced. Smokers' views on such strategies are mixed. Several methods for achieving harm reduction have been suggested, including decreased use of tobacco, use of low tar/nicotine cigarettes, or use of nicotine replacement products. However, there are concerns related to some methodologies.

Special Populations

SMOKING AND DEPRESSION

Smokers exhibit higher rates of depression than do nonsmokers, and depressed, as compared to nondepressed, smokers experience greater difficulty quitting. Even subclinical levels of depression are associated with a decreased latency to first cigarette following an attempt to quit. Some pharmacotherapies, such as bupropion SR and nortriptyline, demonstrate efficacy for both smoking cessation and depression, and thus may be ideal for treating the depressed smoker. Attempts to establish the efficacy of other antidepressants for smoking cessation have generally been less successful.

SMOKING AND SCHIZOPHRENIA

Some recent studies examined the efficacy of bupropion in smokers with schizophrenia. For instance, one evaluated... George et al. evaluated outpatients with schizophrenia who received behavioral group therapy for smoking cessation and either bupropion SR 300 mg per day ($n = 16$) or placebo ($n = 16$) for 10 weeks. Bupropion SR significantly increased abstinence rates at the end of treatment, but no group differences were apparent at 6 months posttreatment.

SMOKING AND OTHER CHEMICAL DEPENDENCE

Rates of smoking among abusers of other drugs are higher than those in the general population, with estimates ranging from 75% to 90%. Alcoholic smokers tend to smoke more heavily and experience less success achieving abstinence than their nonalcoholic counterparts. Despite the fact that nicotine continues to be one of the most common drugs of dependence among patients with alcohol and drug problems, and that many substance abusers express a desire to quit smoking, an optimal treatment for smoking cessation in this population has yet to be established. The *Guideline* recommends that smokers with comorbid chemical dependency should be treated with the same smoking cessation interventions proven to be effective in the general population.

WOMEN

Women tend to experience less success quitting smoking than do men. Clinical trials evaluated in the *Guideline* revealed that, although the same smoking cessation treatments are effective for both women and men, certain interventions (e.g., NRT) are less efficacious in women. This may be related to the different stressors and barriers to quitting that women face. For example, women tend to have lower confidence in their ability to quit, a greater likelihood of depression, and greater weight control concerns, and thus may benefit from addressing such issues in treatment.

PREGNANT WOMEN

Despite adverse effects of cigarette smoking on pregnancy outcomes, smoking cessation during pregnancy and postpartum relapse prevention remain significant treatment challenges. Evidence presented in the *Guideline* indicates that extended or augmented interventions should be offered to pregnant smokers whenever possible; in studies reviewed, these produced significantly higher rates of smoking cessation than did usual care conditions. The use of pharmacotherapy is recommended only if a pregnant woman is otherwise unable to quit and if the benefits of quitting outweigh the risks associated with the medication. Additional studies reveal some successful outcomes, but most report no treatment effects. Comparisons of postpartum relapse prevention counseling to standard care, nicotine patch to placebo patch, and telephone counseling to self-help materials plus brief physician advice all failed to demonstrate significant treatment effects. Taken together, these findings support the use of augmented behavioral interventions and suggest that increased social support, financial incentives, and relapse prevention counseling delivered both pre- and postpartum may be especially effective.

ADOLESCENTS

After increasing throughout most of the 1990s, smoking rates among adolescents have declined significantly since 1997, yet remain high. Findings from the National Youth Tobacco Survey indicate that current tobacco use ranges from 15.1% among middle school students to 34.5% among high school students. Each day in the United States more than 6,000 children and adolescents try their first cigarette. This represents a 30% increase between the years 1988 and 1996 in initiation of first use; over the same time period the incidence of first daily use has increased 50%. Teens who smoke are three times more likely than nonsmokers to use alcohol, 8 times more likely to use marijuana, and 22 times more likely to use cocaine.

Despite that more than half of student smokers have expressed a desire to quit, most attempts to quit are unsuccessful. These findings underscore the need to identify effective prevention and treatment programs for use with this population. The *Guideline* makes four recommendations based on available evidence: (a) clinicians should screen pediatric and adolescent patients, as well as their parents, for tobacco use, and they should strongly emphasize the need to abstain from tobacco use; (b) behavioral interventions with demonstrated efficacy for adults should be considered for children and adolescents after content is made developmentally appropriate; (c) bupropion SR and NRT are also treatment options, given the lack of evidence that these medications are harmful to children; and (d) in pediatric settings, clinicians should offer advice and information regarding smoking cessation to parents to limit exposure of children to secondhand smoke.

Conclusion

Cigarette smoking, once referred to as a "habit," meets established medical criteria for drug dependence. Nicotine is the drug in tobacco that causes dependence or addiction. Significant progress has been made in understanding the relationships among the behavioral, subjective, physiologic, and neuroregulatory effects of nicotine. Moreover, this type of scientific research on nicotine dependence has led to improved techniques for reducing tobacco use. Based on a wealth of clinical trial data accumulated over the past decade, the efficacies and approval of five different pharmacotherapies have been established. These and other evidence-based treatments are recommended in a recent Public Health Service report that provides a comprehensive and authoritative guide to the treatment of tobacco dependence. *Guideline* researchers conclude that first-line medications, including bupropion and NRT should be used in conjunction with behaviorally based counseling to produce optimal outcomes in smoking cessation. Despite the development of new medications and their increasing availability over the counter, treatment challenges remain. It has been suggested that as the proportion of smokers in the population declines, those who continue to smoke are likely to be those individuals who are most entrenched in their smoking behavior and, therefore, more difficult to treat. For example, the prevalence of smoking is declining slowest among individuals with comorbid psychiatric and substance abuse disorders, as well as among the poor and less-educated smokers. Thus, the need for brief, broad-based community interventions must be balanced against the need for more intensive and individualized smoking cessation treatments. With a changing population of smokers comes the pressing need to find new ways to help the most dependent smokers to quit.

Suggested Readings

Acton GS, Prochaska JJ, Kaplan AS, et al. Depression and the stages of change for smoking in psychiatric outpatients. *Addict Behav.* 2001;26(5):621–631.

Benowitz NL. Pharmacology of nicotine: addiction and therapeutics. *Annu Rev Pharmacol Toxicol.* 1996;36:23–29.

Fiore M, Bailey WC, Cohen SJ, et al. *Treating tobacco use and dependence clinical practice guideline.* Rockville, Md: U.S. Department of Health and Human Services, Public Health Service; 2000.

Pich EM, Pagliusi SR, Tessari M, et al. Common neural substrates for the addictive properties of nicotine and cocaine. *Science.* 1997;275:83–86.

Schmitz JM, Dehaune KA. Nicotine. In: Lowinson JH, Ruiz P, Millman RB, et al., eds. *Substance abuse: a comprehensive textbook*, 4th ed. Philadelphia: Lippincott Williams & Wilkins; 2005:387–403.

True WR, Heath AC, Scherrer JF, et al. Genetic and environmental contributions to smoking. *Addiction.* 1997;92:1277–1287.

13

CAFFEINE

1,3,7-Trimethylxanthine (caffeine) is the most widely used mood-altering drug in the world. Caffeine is found in more than 60 species of plants and is the best-known member of the methylxanthine class of alkaloids. The dimethylxanthines, which include theophylline and theobromine, are structurally related compounds that are also found in various plants. Caffeine ingestion is woven so intricately into social customs and daily rituals that it is often not perceived as a drug, despite its well-documented pharmacologic effects.

Caffeine can produce tolerance and a characteristic withdrawal syndrome, and heavy use (>400 mg/day) is associated with increased risk for various health problems. Caffeine can cause discrete psychopathology (e.g., caffeine intoxication, caffeine-induced anxiety disorder), exacerbate existing psychopathology (e.g., anxiety, insomnia), and interfere with the efficacy of some medications (e.g., benzodiazepines). This chapter reviews empirical data on the pharmacologic, behavioral, and clinical effects of caffeine.

History

Caffeine has been ingested in one form or another throughout various parts of the world for thousands of years. Tea was first cultivated in China, coffee in Ethiopia, guarana, cocoa, and maté in South America, and kola nut in West Africa. With the development of worldwide trade routes during the 17th and 18th centuries, caffeinated products spread rapidly from their indigenous environments to other parts of the world. The introduction of caffeine into societies often inspired moral outrage and attempts to ban use. Failed efforts to suppress the use of caffeine-containing foods, usually in the form of coffee or tea, have been documented worldwide.

Therapeutic Uses

As a mild central nervous stimulant, caffeine is commonly taken as an energy and alertness enhancer. Studies clearly demonstrate that caffeine is effective at restoring performance that has been degraded by fatigue. Caffeine is also used to enhance athletic performance because of its ergogenic effects. There is evidence to suggest that caffeine functions as an analgesic adjuvant, and it is added to a wide variety of over-the-counter and prescription analgesics used to treat various types of pain including headache. Caffeine, a cerebral vasoconstrictor, is the most effective treatment for caffeine-withdrawal headaches, which are likely caused by rebound cerebral vasodilation in response to the absence of caffeine. Likewise, prophylactic administration of caffeine prevents postsurgical caffeine-withdrawal headaches. Caffeine is used to treat neonatal apnea and has been administered prior to electroconvulsive therapy to increase seizure duration. Because of its lipolytic and thermogenic effects, caffeine is also used in some over-the-counter weight-loss preparations.

Sources of Caffeine

Caffeine occurs naturally in a variety of plant-based products including coffee, tea, cocoa, kola nut, guarana, and maté. Significant amounts of caffeine may also occur in foods such as coffee ice cream, coffee yogurt, and dark chocolate. In recent years, soft drinks and energy drinks made with guarana have become increasingly popular in the United States and elsewhere. Caffeine is added to cola and noncola soft drinks, as well as to other common food items, including gum, mints, water, and energy drinks. Caffeine is also added to thousands of prescription and over-the-counter medications, including stimulants, analgesics, weight-loss supplements, and nutritional supplements.

In the United States, coffee and soft drinks are the major dietary sources of caffeine. The Food and Drug Administration limits the amount of caffeine that can be added to soft drinks to 0.2 mg per mL, or 71 mg for a 12-oz serving.

Epidemiology

Of children and adults in North America, 80% to 90% report regular use of caffeinated products. Mean daily intake among adult caffeine consumers in the United States is approximately 280 mg, with higher daily intakes estimated in Denmark and the United Kingdom. Subgroups that have been identified as heavy caffeine consumers include psychiatric patients, prisoners, smokers, alcoholics, and individuals with eating disorders. More than 50% of adults consume coffee every day and drink an average of 3.3 cups per day.

Estimating actual caffeine exposure in the population is challenging because in many widely used products, both the caffeine concentration and the serving sizes can vary over a wide range. Estimating caffeine exposure is also difficult because caffeine is present in such a vast number of products, and many consumers may be completely unaware of whether a given product contains caffeine.

Genetics

Genetic factors account for some of the variability in the use and effects of caffeine. Monozygotic twins have more similar coffee consumption than dizygotic twins, with heritability coefficients for coffee drinking ranging between 36% and 51%. Total consumption, caffeine intoxication, tolerance, and withdrawal had greater co-occurrence in monozygotic twins than dizygotic twins, with heritabilities ranging between 35% and 77%. There is also evidence that common genetic factors underlie the use of caffeine, cigarette smoking, and alcohol.

Pharmacokinetics

After oral consumption, caffeine is rapidly and completely absorbed. Caffeine enters the brain rapidly, which accounts for the quick onset of mood-altering effects. Peak caffeine blood levels are generally reached in 30 to 45 minutes, but can be delayed by recent food consumption. Caffeine is highly lipid soluble and is widely distributed throughout all body tissues and fluids, including amniotic fluid, breast milk, and semen. Saliva caffeine concentrations are highly correlated with plasma caffeine concentrations and are often used as an alternative to measuring serum levels.

Caffeine metabolism is complex and more than 25 caffeine metabolites have been identified in humans. The primary metabolic pathways involve the P450 liver enzyme system, which carries out the demethylation of caffeine to three pharmacologically active dimethylxanthines: paraxanthine, theophylline, and theobromine. The half-life of caffeine is typically 4 to 6 hours; however, the rate of caffeine metabolism is quite variable among individuals and can vary more than 10-fold in healthy adults. Tobacco smoking increases the metabolism of caffeine as a consequence of stimulation of liver enzymes, with smokers metabolizing caffeine about twice as fast as nonsmokers. Caffeine metabolism is slowed in pregnant women and in individuals with liver disease. The liver enzyme systems of infants are not fully developed until about 6 months of age and thus caffeine metabolism in infants is very slow, with a half-life of 80 to 100 hours. Numerous compounds decrease the rate of elimination of caffeine, including oral contraceptive steroids, cimetidine (Tagamet), and fluvoxamine (Luvox). Caffeine decreases the rate of elimination of the antipsychotic clozapine (Clozaril) and the bronchodilator theophylline (Accurbron).

Neuropharmacology

Adenosine

The primary mechanism of action of caffeine is believed to be competitive antagonism at A_1 and A_{2A} adenosine receptors. This is consistent with the observation that most of the effects of caffeine are opposite to those produced by adenosine. A_1 receptors are found in most brain regions, with the highest densities in the hippocampus, cerebellar cortex, cerebral cortex, and areas of the thalamus. The highest densities of A_{2A} receptors are found in dopamine-rich areas of the brain, including the caudate/putamen, nucleus accumbens, and the tuberculum olfactorium.

Dopamine

There is solid evidence that some of the behavioral effects of caffeine are mediated by dopaminergic mechanisms. Caffeine blocks the effects of adenosine at receptors that are colocalized and that functionally interact with dopamine receptors, thus stimulating dopaminergic activity.

Physiologic Effects

Caffeine produces effects on a wide variety of organ systems. At moderate dietary doses, caffeine increases blood pressure and tends to have no effect or to reduce heart rate. Caffeine-induced blood pressure increases tend to be small; however, such increases may be clinically significant for individuals with borderline hypertension. Both caffeinated and decaffeinated coffee contain lipids that significantly raise serum total and low-density lipoprotein (LDL) cholesterol. Similar to the methylxanthine theophylline, caffeine dilates bronchial pathways. Caffeine is also a respiratory stimulant and has been used therapeutically to treat apnea in neonates and infants. Caffeine stimulates gastric acid secretion and colonic activity. There is no clear association of caffeine use with peptic or duodenal ulcers. Although coffee consumption exacerbates gastroesophageal reflux, this effect appears to be caused by coffee constituents other than caffeine.

Caffeine has a strong diuretic effect and increases urine volume 30% or more for several hours after caffeine ingestion. Caffeine also increases detrusor instability (i.e., unstable bladder) in patients with complaints of urinary urgency and detrusor instability. Several studies show that caffeine causes increased urinary calcium excretion. It has been suggested that caffeine may have a negative effect on calcium balance, but the clinical significance of such an effect is unclear. Caffeine produces dose-related thermogenic effects and is ergogenic during exercise. Caffeine increases plasma epinephrine, norepinephrine, rennin, and free fatty acids. Some studies show that caffeine increases adrenocorticotropin hormone (ACTH) and cortisol levels.

Although caffeine has been shown to have mutagenic and carcinogenic effects in cultured cells *in vitro* at extremely high doses, it is consistently concluded that mutagenic and carcinogenic effects of caffeine are extremely unlikely to occur in humans. Although findings are inconsistent and are difficult to interpret, maternal caffeine use may be associated with increased rates of spontaneous abortion and lower birth weight.

Subjective and Discriminative Stimulus Effects

Acute doses of caffeine in the typical dietary dose range (i.e., 20 to 200 mg) produce a number of positive subjective effects, including increased well-being, happiness, energy, alertness, and sociability. Negative subjective effects typically emerge at higher doses. Acute doses of caffeine greater than 200 mg are associated with increased reports of anxiety, jitteriness, upset stomach, and insomnia. Individual differences in sensitivity and caffeine tolerance seem to play an important role in the likelihood and severity of negative subjective effects. Individuals with higher anxiety sensitivity, panic disorder, or general anxiety disorder tend to be particularly sensitive to the anxiogenic effects of caffeine. The negative subjective effects of caffeine tend to be relatively mild and short-lived. However, very high doses of caffeine are associated with clinically significant distress and psychopathology (e.g., caffeine intoxication).

Caffeine Intoxication

The most common features of caffeine intoxication include nervousness, restlessness, insomnia, gastrointestinal upset, muscle twitching, tachycardia, and psychomotor agitation. Fever, irritability, tremors, sensory disturbances, tachypnea, and headaches have also been reported in response to excess caffeine use. DSM-IV-TR diagnostic guidelines require that the diagnosis be dependent on recent consumption of at least 250 mg of caffeine, but much higher doses (>500 mg) are usually associated with the syndrome.

Although caffeine intoxication can occur in the context of habitual chronic consumption of high doses of caffeine, it most often occurs after consumption of large doses in infrequent caffeine users, or in regular users who have substantially increased their intake. Caffeine intoxication usually resolves spontaneously after caffeine use has ceased, consistent with the 4-hour to 6-hour half-life of caffeine. Treatment of caffeine intoxication may consist of short-term management and support of the patient until symptoms resolve. Although there are generally no long-lasting consequences of caffeine intoxication, caffeine can be lethal at very high doses (e.g., 5 to 10 g), and there are documented cases of suicide by caffeine overdose.

Individual differences in sensitivity to caffeine and tolerance most likely play a role in vulnerability to caffeine intoxication. It has been reported that caffeine intoxication can occur in chronic caffeine users with no prior apparent caffeine-related problems. Although the occurrence of individual symptoms of caffeine intoxication is fairly common (e.g., nervousness), caffeine intoxication serious enough to require medical attention is considered relatively rare.

Caffeine and Anxiety

The anxiogenic effects of caffeine are well established. Acute doses of caffeine generally greater than 200 mg have been shown to increase anxiety ratings in nonclinical populations, with higher doses sometimes inducing panic attacks. Abstention from caffeine has been shown to produce improvements in anxiety symptoms among individuals seeking treatment for an anxiety disorder. Interestingly, individuals with high caffeine consumption have greater rates of minor tranquilizer use (e.g., benzodiazepines) relative to those persons with low to moderate caffeine consumption, although the mechanism underlying this association has not been established.

Caffeine-induced anxiety disorder is characterized by prominent anxiety, panic attacks, obsessions, or compulsions etiologically related to caffeine use.

Caffeine and Sleep

It is well documented that caffeine increases wakefulness and inhibits sleep onset. Perhaps the most widely accepted therapeutic use of caffeine, which has been widely studied, is that caffeine increases wakefulness and decreases performance decrements produced by sleep deprivation. Of course, caffeine also has detrimental effects on planned sleep (i.e., insomnia). Caffeine ingested throughout the day or before bedtime has been shown to interfere with sleep onset, total time slept, sleep quality, and sleep stages. The effects of caffeine on sleep appear to be determined by a number of factors, including dose, the time between caffeine ingestion and attempted sleep, and individual differences in sensitivity and/or tolerance to caffeine. The effects of caffeine on sleep appear to be dose dependent, with greater amounts of caffeine causing greater sleep difficulties. Furthermore, acute abstinence after chronic caffeine consumption increases daytime sleepiness and increases nighttime sleep duration and quality.

The DSM-IV-TR includes a diagnosis of caffeine-induced sleep disorder, which is characterized by a prominent sleep disturbance that is etiologically related to caffeine use. Caffeine-induced sleep disorder is diagnosed when symptoms of a sleep disturbance (e.g., insomnia) are greater than would be expected during caffeine intoxication or caffeine withdrawal. There are no specific data on the prevalence or incidence of caffeine-induced sleep disorder.

Performance

Many studies have examined the effects of caffeine on human performance. Data support the conclusion that caffeine improves performance that has been degraded under conditions such as sleep deprivation, fatigue, prolonged vigilance, and caffeine withdrawal. Studies of the effects of caffeine on nondegraded performance are inconsistent.

There is a growing body of literature on the effects of caffeine on exercise performance. Compared to placebo, caffeine increases endurance for long-term (30 to 60 minutes) exercise and improves speed and/or power output in simulated race conditions.

Reinforcement

Caffeine functions as a reinforcer in humans (i.e., caffeine maintains self-administration or choice behavior). There is quite a bit of individual variability in the reinforcing effects of caffeine. Across studies, the overall incidence of caffeine reinforcement in normal caffeine users is approximately 40%, with a higher incidence (i.e., 80% to 100%) of reinforcement under conditions of repeated caffeine exposure.

Caffeine physical dependence potentiates the reinforcing effects of caffeine. For example, caffeine consumers were more than twice as likely to show caffeine reinforcement if they reported caffeine withdrawal symptoms after drinking decaffeinated coffee. There is also evidence that avoidance of caffeine withdrawal determines caffeine consumption to a greater extent than the positive effects of caffeine.

Recent studies have used a conditioned flavor preference paradigm as an indirect measure of caffeine reinforcement. Subjects who are repeatedly exposed to a novel flavored drink paired with caffeine tend to show increased ratings of drink pleasantness, whereas subjects receiving placebo-paired drinks show decreased ratings of drink pleasantness. It seems plausible that such conditioned flavor preferences in the natural environment play an important role in the development of consumer preferences for different types of caffeine-containing beverages.

Tolerance

Tolerance refers to a decrease in responsiveness to a drug after repeated drug exposure. High doses of caffeine (750 to 1,200 mg/day spread throughout the day) administered daily produce "complete" tolerance (i.e., caffeine effects are no longer different from baseline or placebo) to some, but not all of the effects of caffeine. The degree of caffeine tolerance is likely to depend on a number of factors including dose, amount, and frequency of administration, as well as individual differences in elimination.

Studies show complete tolerance to blood pressure and other physiologic effects (plasma norepinephrine and epinephrine and plasma rennin activity) of high doses of caffeine (e.g., 250 mg t.i.d. for 4 days), but only partial tolerance to blood pressure and middle cerebral artery velocity at somewhat lower doses (i.e., 200 mg b.i.d. for 7 days). Substantial but incomplete tolerance has been shown to the sleep-disruptive effects of high doses of caffeine (400 mg t.i.d. for 7 days).

Physical Dependence and Withdrawal

Physical dependence on caffeine is demonstrated by the occurrence of a withdrawal syndrome (i.e., time-limited biochemical, physiologic, and behavioral disruptions) that occurs after cessation after a period of regular caffeine consumption. Other caffeine-withdrawal symptoms in roughly decreasing order of occurrence include fatigue, drowsiness, dysphoric mood, difficulty concentrating, work difficulty (lack of motivation), irritability, depression, and cognitive or behavioral task impairment. Occasionally, individuals experiencing caffeine withdrawal also report flulike symptoms, which may include nausea or vomiting, muscle aches or stiffness, hot and cold spells, and heavy feelings in arms and legs.

Withdrawal symptoms typically emerge 12 to 24 hours after the last dose of caffeine and tend to peak within 48 hours. Symptoms can persist from 2 days to 1 week or more. Caffeine withdrawal symptoms are usually alleviated quickly after caffeine re-exposure. Caffeine withdrawal can be suppressed by caffeine doses well below the usual daily dose (e.g., 25 mg caffeine suppressed withdrawal after daily doses of 300 mg). Caffeine withdrawal can occur after relatively short-term exposure to daily caffeine (e.g., 3 to 7 days of exposure). The incidence and severity of caffeine withdrawal tends to increase as a function of daily maintenance dose. The daily caffeine dose necessary to produce withdrawal is surprisingly low, with significant withdrawal symptoms observed in individuals using as little as 100 mg caffeine per day.

Although most withdrawal research has been with adults, there is evidence that children and adolescents who use caffeine also experience caffeine withdrawal symptoms upon abstinence. It is possible that children may be even more susceptible to experiencing withdrawal episodes because they likely have less control over the regular availability of caffeine-containing products. More research is needed in this area.

In the DSM-IV-TR, caffeine withdrawal is defined by caffeine withdrawal symptoms (i.e., headache and one or more of the following: marked fatigue or drowsiness, marked anxiety or depression, nausea or vomiting), that cause "significant distress or impairment in social, occupational, or other important areas of functioning."

Caffeine Dependence

Substance dependence is characterized by a cluster of cognitive, behavioral, and physiologic symptoms indicating that the individual continues use of a substance despite significant substance-related problems. It is important to make the distinction between physical dependence and a clinical diagnosis of substance dependence. Whereas the empirical evidence for the occurrence of caffeine physical dependence (reflected by withdrawal) is overwhelming, there is less information available about the ability of caffeine to produce other clinically meaningful characteristics of a substance dependence syndrome.

More research is needed to determine the applicability of substance dependence criteria to caffeine, the prevalence of the disorder, and the utility and clinical significance of the diagnosis. Meanwhile therapeutic assistance should be made available for those who feel that their caffeine use is problematic but have been unable to quit on their own.

Caffeine and Other Drugs of Dependence
Tobacco Smoking and Nicotine

Epidemiologic studies show that cigarette smokers consume more caffeine than non-smokers, and experimental studies show that cigarette smoking and coffee drinking covary temporally within individuals.

Cigarette smoking significantly increases the rate of caffeine elimination, an effect that may partially explain increased caffeine use among smokers. Smoking abstinence produces substantial increases in caffeine blood levels among heavy caffeine consumers. It has been speculated that symptoms of caffeine intoxication caused by increased caffeine blood levels may interfere with smoking quit attempts and/or be misinterpreted as nicotine-withdrawal symptoms; however, the clinical significance of such an effect has not been demonstrated.

Alcohol

There is an association between heavy use and clinical dependence on alcohol and heavy use and clinical dependence on caffeine. Alcohol detoxification in alcoholics is associated with substantial increases in coffee consumption. In a study that identified individuals who met DSM-IV-TR criteria for substance dependence on caffeine, 57% also had a lifetime history of alcohol abuse or dependence. Preclinical studies suggest that caffeine can promote alcohol self-administration. Although it is widely believed that caffeine can reverse the impairing effects of alcohol, animal and human studies have not shown this to be a reliable effect. The available data suggest that the reversal by caffeine of impairment caused by alcohol is generally incomplete and inconsistent across different types of behavioral and subjective measures.

Benzodiazepines

Benzodiazepines are commonly used to treat anxiety disorders and insomnia. There is evidence from animal and human behavioral studies that suggests a mutually antagonistic relationship between benzodiazepines and caffeine. Although caffeine can interact at the benzodiazepine receptor, the lack of uniform antagonism across behavioral measures suggests that the antagonism is functional in nature.

One study showed that heavy caffeine users are almost twice as likely to use benzodiazepines than are low and moderate caffeine users. An important clinical implication is that, although individuals with anxiety disorders tend to use less caffeine than controls, caffeine use should be carefully evaluated when benzodiazepines are being considered for the treatment of anxiety and insomnia.

Cocaine

There is little epidemiologic data on the co-occurrence of caffeine and cocaine use. One study reported that the prevalence of caffeine use among cocaine abusers is lower than the general population. Interestingly, in that same study, cocaine users who consumed caffeine reported using less cocaine than those who do not regularly consume caffeine.

Caffeine and Health

The possibility that caffeine may pose health risks is of great interest to the general public and scientific community, and has been the focus of numerous studies. There is no evidence for nonreversible pathologic consequences of caffeine use (e.g., cancer, heart disease, congenital malformations). In general, there is a lack of evidence to support the conclusion that moderate caffeine use causes significant health risk in healthy adults. However, some groups may be considered at risk for potential adverse health effects of caffeine including, individuals with generalized anxiety disorder, panic disorder, primary insomnia, hypertension, and urinary incontinence; women who are pregnant or trying to become pregnant; and caffeine users who consume inadequate amounts of calcium. In addition, caffeine use can be associated with several distinct psychiatric syndromes: caffeine intoxication, caffeine withdrawal, caffeine dependence, caffeine-induced sleep disorder, and caffeine-induced anxiety disorder.

Clinical Implications

Given the wide range of symptoms produced by excessive caffeine use and withdrawal, as described throughout this chapter, caffeine use should be routinely assessed during medical and psychiatric evaluations. Caffeine use or intoxication should be assessed in individuals with complaints of anxiety, insomnia, headaches, palpitations, tachycardia, or gastrointestinal disturbance. Caffeine intoxication should be considered in the differential diagnosis of amphetamine or cocaine intoxication, mania, medication-induced side effects, hyperthyroidism, and pheochromocytoma. Likewise, caffeine withdrawal should be considered when patients present with headaches, fatigue, dysphoric mood, or difficulty concentrating. Caffeine withdrawal should be considered in the differential diagnosis of migraine or other headache disorders, viral illnesses, and other drug-withdrawal states.

Caffeine users who are instructed to refrain from all food and beverages prior to medical procedures may be at risk for experiencing caffeine withdrawal. Caffeine withdrawal has been identified as a cause of postoperative headaches, and caffeine supplements during surgery are effective in preventing withdrawal.

Caffeine interacts with a number of medications. Caffeine and benzodiazepine-like drugs, for example, diazepam (Valium), alprazolam (Xanax), triazolam (Halcion), are mutually antagonistic and thus caffeine use may interfere with the efficacy of benzodiazepines. Caffeine may also interfere with the metabolism of the antipsychotic clozapine as well as the bronchodilator theophylline to an extent that may be clinically significant. Case studies suggest that caffeine withdrawal may be associated with increased serum lithium concentrations and lithium toxicity. Numerous compounds decrease the rate of elimination of caffeine, including cimetidine, fluvoxamine, and oral contraceptive steroids.

Is Caffeine a Drug of Abuse?

Caffeine is a widely used mood-altering drug that shares some features with classic drugs of abuse (e.g., use despite harm, difficulty stopping use, withdrawal, tolerance). Therefore, it is not surprising that caffeine is sometimes labeled a drug of abuse or addiction. Objections to this classification include the observations that caffeine is widely used, has relatively subtle psychologic effects, produces less social and physical harm than classic drugs of abuse, and is less likely to be associated with craving. However, definitions of drug abuse and addiction are complex and controversial, as reflected in the not so distant debate about whether nicotine should be considered a drug of addiction. One approach to deciding if it is appropriate to label caffeine as a drug of abuse is an analysis of reinforcement and adverse effects. In this type of analysis, the relative abuse potential of a drug can be considered to be a multiplicative function of the degree of drug reinforcement and the degree of adverse effects. As discussed earlier, caffeine functions as a reinforcer under a more limited range of conditions than classic stimulant drugs of abuse, such as amphetamines. Caffeine produces some adverse psychologic and physical effects; however, in contrast to classic drugs of abuse, life-threatening health risks from caffeine at usual dietary doses have not been conclusively demonstrated. Although caffeine has these two defining features of drugs of abuse, the modest reinforcing effects and modest adverse effects documented to date suggest that caffeine has a low abuse liability relative to classic drugs of abuse. However, this type of analysis would also predict that if future research were to demonstrate significant adverse effects of caffeine, societal perceptions of caffeine as a drug of abuse would be radically altered.

Treatment

Reduction or elimination of caffeine is advised for individuals who have caffeine-related psychopathology or when it is believed that caffeine is causing or exacerbating medical or psychiatric problems, or interfering with medication efficacy. A surprisingly large percentage of caffeine users in the general population (56%) report a desire or unsuccessful efforts to stop or reduce caffeine use.

There are no published reports of treatment interventions designed to assist individuals who would like to completely eliminate caffeine. Several reports suggest the efficacy of a structured caffeine reduction regimen (i.e., caffeine fading) for achieving substantial reductions of caffeine intake.

Given the limited number of treatment strategies that have been evaluated for reducing or eliminating caffeine consumption, a reasonable approach is to draw from validated behavioral techniques used to treat dependence on other drugs (e.g., tobacco dependence). Effective behavior modification strategies include coping response training, self-monitoring, social support, and reinforcement for abstinence. Substance abuse treatment strategies, including relapse prevention and motivational interviewing, could also be readily applied to the treatment of caffeine dependence. Some individuals may not readily accept the idea that caffeine is contributing to their problems (e.g., insomnia, anxiety). Such individuals should be encouraged to engage in a caffeine-free trial. There is some evidence that withdrawal symptoms may thwart attempts to quit. Gradually reducing caffeine consumption may help attenuate withdrawal symptoms, although there has been no systematic research to determine the most efficacious reduction schedule. In general, reduction schedules over the course of 3 to 4 weeks are effective. No data about the probability of relapse are currently available, although relapse after caffeine reduction has been reported.

Suggested Readings

Carrillo JA, Benitez J. Clinically significant pharmacokinetic interactions between dietary caffeine and medications. *Clin Pharmacokinet.* 2000;39:127–153.

James JE. Acute and chronic effects of caffeine on performance, mood, headache, and sleep. *Neuropsychobiology.* 1998;38:32–41.

James JE. *Understanding caffeine.* Thousand Oaks, Calif.: Sage Publications; 1997.

Juliano LM, Griffiths RR. Caffeine. In: Lowinson JH, Ruiz P, Millman RB, et al., eds. *Substance abuse: a comprehensive textbook*, 4th ed. Philadelphia: Lippincott Williams & Wilkins; 2005:403–421.

Miller WR, Rollnick S. *Motivational interviewing: preparing people to change addictive behavior.* New York: Guilford Press; 1991.

Nawrot P, Jordan S, Eastwood J, et al. Effects of caffeine on human health. *Food Addit Contam.* 2003;20:1–30.

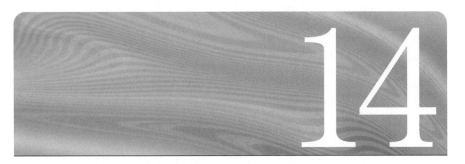

ANABOLIC–ANDROGENIC STEROIDS

The first use of anabolic–androgenic steroids (AASs) as performance enhancers purportedly dates to World War II, when they were administered to German soldiers prior to combat. AASs were used for those injured in World War II and for concentration camp survivors to promote weight gain. Use in sports, which began in the 1940s, first brought AASs widespread public attention. During the Cold War, the intense international Olympics competition between Eastern Bloc and Chinese communist nations and Western democratic nations led to an official program of steroid development and use for athletes in the communist nations. Soviet weightlifters reportedly used steroids in the 1952 and 1956 Olympics. Because of limitations of analytic technology, testing of athletes for AAS use did not begin until the 1976 Olympic Games, when eight samples that had screened positive by a newly developed radioimmunoassay technique were confirmed by gas chromatography-mass spectroscopy.

This chapter uses the term *anabolic–androgenic steroid* to denote all steroids exhibiting myotrophic actions and that also promote the expression of male sexual characteristics in any ratio, and includes both endogenous animal or human hormones and synthetic derivatives of testosterone. The discovery of a new class of noncontrolled nonsteroidal androgen receptor agonists promises new opportunities for research and therapeutics, as well as abuse.

Physiology and Pharmacology

AASs affect somatic, sexual, and neural cell chemistry and function. Testosterone is produced in males by Leydig cells in the testes in response to luteinizing hormone, a gonadotropin secreted by the pituitary. The complex mechanisms of action of AASs, particularly at supraphysiologic doses, include consequences of individual interactions with other steroid receptor systems, including those for estrogens, progestins, and glucocorticoids. AASs augment the release of growth hormone alpha.

Epidemiology and Usage Patterns
Incidence and Prevalence

The spread of AAS use has been largely a silent phenomenon, yet the estimate from the U.S. Substance Abuse and Mental Health Services Administration (SAMHSA)

National Household Drug Abuse Survey published in 1995 is that 1,084,000 Americans had ever used AASs and that 312,000 (29%) of those had AASs used in the prior year. Prevalence is higher in males than in females: lifetime estimates from population and school-based surveys are 1.8% to 11% in males and 0.2% to 3.2% in females in the United States. Athletes, particularly weightlifters, have a greater prevalence of use than do nonathletes everywhere, but the difference is surprisingly small in some studies, pointing to the importance of other factors in the decision to use AASs.

Reasons for Illicit Use

Direct pharmacologic actions of AASs result in euphoria and a subjective "high" in some individuals. Withdrawal symptoms also can become important factors in continued use. AASs seem to have a greater long-term effect on most users, rather than the immediate rush and alteration of mood, reward, or sense of well-being seen with other drugs of abuse. Yet some AAS users compulsively self-administer ever-increasing doses of AASs in the face of adverse consequences, are more likely to self-administer other drugs of abuse, and experience a withdrawal syndrome when AASs are discontinued. The highly addictive behavioral components of AAS use, that is, use ritual, injection ritual, sensation, and peer approval, provide immediate rewards, are important factors in sustaining use, and probably contribute to the withdrawal syndrome.

Bodybuilders generally start AAS use seeking psychologic rewards from attention to, and admiration of, a muscular physique. Athletes use AASs seeking to improve their performance; this performance enhancement may be a result of objective effects of increased muscle mass, or because of subjective effects such as increased levels of aggression or increased confidence. Female-to-male (FTM) transgendered individuals without access to appropriate medical care may self-medicate with AASs in an effort to increase secondary male characteristics and decrease female attributes.

Disorders of Body Image

Dissatisfaction with body image, specifically the perception of being too small or insufficiently muscular, is common in AAS users, and is associated with AAS dependence. In one study of males, bodybuilders were at greater risk than martial artists or runners for problems often seen in eating disorder patients: body dissatisfaction, thinness seeking, muscle bulk desiring, bulimia, self-esteem problems, depression, maturity fears, and perfectionism. Disorders of body image associated with AASs are also found in women.

Patterns of Use

To obtain maximum increases in lean muscle mass, body weight, and strength, AAS abusers practice "stacking," using three or more kinds of AASs, which may be administered by different routes. In an attempt to minimize deleterious side effects, abusers alternate between cycles of abuse and nonuse. Typical cycles may run 4 to 18 weeks on AASs and 1 month to 1 year off. Bodybuilding and weight training are typically done in phases; AASs are commonly and heavily used during the muscle build-up phase, rather than during the training or maintenance phases that follow. Cycles that involve building up to a peak dose and then tapering down are called "pyramids." Administration of multiple steroids in increasing and tapering doses is known as "stacking the pyramid". Users often meticulously plan and record their use of AAS, and may be able to give detailed histories of use. The patterns of cyclic use, variable doses, simultaneous use of multiple AASs that have differing physiologic effects, and use of grossly supratherapeutic doses makes extrapolations from therapeutic and experimental data problematic.

Other Performance-Enhancing and Physique-Modifying Drugs

Athletes who use AASs also may employ drugs from among a wide variety of psychomotor stimulants, including ephedrine, caffeine, phenylpropanolamine, pseudoephedrine, methoxyphenamine, cocaine, and methamphetamine. Although some of these may be abused for their psychoactive properties, this class of drugs is accepted by segments of the athletic community as performance enhancing, that is, "ergonomic" or "ergogenic."

Human growth hormone (Hgh) is anabolic and is been used by AAS users. A variety of substances purported to increase release of endogenous Hgh are also abused, notably γ-hydroxybutyrate. Somatotropin and insulin-like growth factor I are anabolic; increased production of these hormones through gene therapy may be undertaken to increase athletic performance in the future. The β_2-adrenergic agonist clenbuterol was observed to increase the deposition rate of lean mass and to retard adipose gain in animal husbandry. Based on this information, clenbuterol entered into use by athletes as an anabolic agent. Other agents reportedly abused to enhance performance include salbutamol, deprenyl, β-adrenergic antagonists, levothyroxine, erythropoietin, and darbepoetin. An early example of botanicals employed to enhance performance is yohimbine bark. Yohimbine bark still is promoted as an alternative to AAS to enhance athletic, as well as male sexual, performance.

Drugs Taken to Ameliorate Side Effects

Diuretics are used by bodybuilders to counter the fluid retention caused by AASs and to increase muscle definition—to create a more "ripped" or "cut up" look with increased definition of superficial vasculature, muscular shape, and muscular striations. Hemoconcentration with hematocrits of up to 71% has been reported in AAS abusers, possibly because of coadministration of diuretics that AASs users take to control secondary edema, increase muscle definition, and decrease total weight; the resulting increase in blood viscosity may increase the risk for thromboembolic phenomena. Diuretic-induced electrolyte derangements, particularly of potassium, create a serious potential for dysrhythmias. Supplemental potassium may also be taken, leading to a risk of hyperkalemia, particularly when potassium-sparing diuretics are used.

Estrogenic effects of AASs and their metabolites can lead to gynecomastia. The partial estrogen antagonists tamoxifen and clomiphene are used to prevent and treat this complication of AAS abuse.

Human chorionic gonadotropin (hCG) stimulates androgen production by the interstitial cells of the testes. hCG is used to counter the profound suppression of production of endogenous testosterone and testicular atrophy caused by exogenous AASs.

The testosterone 5α-reductase inhibitor finasteride significantly reduces the level of dihydrotestosterone (DHT) in both serum and skin, where human androgen receptors are found, even at low doses. Because DHT in puberty is responsible for some male sexual characteristics of skin, it may have utility in preventing the emergence of male sexual characteristics in females abusing AASs, including facial hair and baldness, although there are significant teratogenicity concerns. Hence, doping tests for female athletes could include finasteride as an indirect indicator of AAS abuse.

Consequences of Use

Therapeutic Uses

The therapeutic utility of AASs was once limited because there were few indications for use and few patients with those indications. These medications now have an ever-expanding range of indications and patient populations who may benefit from them. They are employed in many fields of medicine for a variety of anabolic, endocrine, hematologic, psychiatric, oncologic, and other uses.

Classic uses of AASs are treatment of delayed puberty and primary and secondary hypogonadism in males. AASs have been recommended as adjuncts for treatment of hypogonadism caused by heroin and opioid abuse. Specific AASs have therapeutic utility in a variety of conditions that result in small stature. Oxandrolone has been employed successfully with Hgh in the treatment of Turner syndrome to increase final height, although this combination also has been reported to be ineffective in patients with Turner syndrome.

There is continued interest in the therapeutic application of AASs to improve nutrition and lower-body muscle strength, and to promote weight gain. AASs, particularly oxandrolone, are widely used with varying success to treat cachexia in patients with cancer, in patients with chronic renal failure, in patients with human immunodeficiency virus (HIV)/acquired immune deficiency syndrome (AIDS), and to improve stasis ulcer healing. There is also interest in their effectiveness for accelerated and improved wound healing in medical, renal, HIV, trauma, surgical, cachectic cancer, and burn patients and in postmenopausal women.

AASs are under investigation for treatment of lipodystrophy in patients with HIV/AIDS taking protease inhibitors and nucleosides. Tibolone and certain other AASs are used to ameliorate the lipodystrophy caused by protease inhibitors. Tibolone dramatically lowers triglycerides and very-low-density lipoprotein (VLDL) cholesterol. However, it also adversely affects serum lipid profiles by lowering high-density lipoprotein (HDL) cholesterol, and apolipoprotein A-I both in rats and in humans.

Despite serious risks associated with long-term use, AASs are used, alone and in combination therapies, for short-term treatment of refractory anemia, especially aplastic anemia; anemia of chronic disease in renal failure; and Fanconi syndrome. Acute intermittent porphyria also responds to AAS–gonadotropin-releasing hormone (GnRH) analogue therapy.

Gynecomastia and Mastodynia in Men

Testosterone and other aromatizable AASs are metabolized in part to estradiol and other estrogen agonists. These estrogen agonists can lead to breast pain in men and gynecomastia. Gynecomastia is one of the most frequently reported side effects of AAS abuse. Affected tissue contains both androgen and estradiol receptors. Gynecomastia is a sufficiently common and permanent adverse effect where staging criteria and techniques for surgical management have been presented.

Breast Health in Women

The impact of anabolic steroids on the female breast is an issue because AASs, especially tibolone, are used internationally to treat the symptoms of menopause and to prevent osteoporosis. At approved therapeutic doses, the consequences to breast tissue are probably minimal; however, long-term high-dose AAS abuse has not been well studied. Anabolic implants in female lambs caused breast cell autolysis and necrosis. In human breast cancer cell lines positive for androgen receptors, AASs show varied effects, with the growth of some cell lines promoted and the growth of others inhibited. Their role in the growth and progression of breast cancer is not well defined and is under study. *In vitro* androstene-3β, 17α-diol (17α-AED) inhibits breast cancer cell proliferation regardless of estrogen receptor positivity or negativity.

Male Genitourinary and Renal Systems

AASs suppress gonadotropins, with variable effects on sexual interest, spontaneous erections, the prostate, the gonads, and fertility. Testicular atrophy has also been documented in a controlled study, and is an expected effect through negative feedback exerted by AASs on the testes. Azoospermia and oligospermia may also follow AAS use, and may resolve spontaneously or require gonadotropin treatment. Androgens are essential for normal prostate physiology. Central prostate volume is responsive to AASs. AASs may be cocarcinogens for adenocarcinoma of the prostate. The development and progression of prostate cancer may be positively influenced by AASs. Antiandrogen therapy and orchiectomy cause regression of prostatic cancer.

Renal failure has been reported, although the etiology was uncertain and possibly related to AAS-induced hypertension. A cluster of two cases of clear cell renal carcinoma are reported in 26-year-old male bodybuilders.

Female Genitourinary

Uterine blood flow in ovariectomized ewes is significantly increased by tibolone, an AAS. This vascular response is mediated via an estrogen receptor-dependent, nitric oxide mechanism. Postmenopausal women treated with tibolone sometimes develop uterine bleeding. In one study of 47 consecutive cases, no anatomic pathologic cause for the uterine bleeding was found in the majority; however, endometrial polyp (11 patients), uterine fibroids (7 patients), thickened endometrium (6 patients), and carcinoma *in situ* (2 patients) were found in the other patients, further emphasizing the mandatory investigation of postmenopausal uterine bleeding, especially in the context of AAS use.

Raised levels of androgens have been implicated in epidemiologic studies of ovarian carcinogenesis, although the causal role and mechanisms are unknown. *In vitro* studies show that ovarian epithelial cells contain androgen receptors. The response of these cells to tibolone is increased DNA expression and a significant increase in proliferation with decreased cell death, important factors in the pathophysiology of ovarian cancer.

Virilization of Women

Supraphysiologic doses of AASs in women lead to virilization, although the effects and rate of development of changes vary with the drug and with the individual. Specifically, women taking AASs have been reported to have voice instability and deepening in both the projected speaking voice and the singing voice, clitoral hypertrophy, shrinking of the breasts, menstrual irregularities, nausea, and hirsutism. In contrast to the cosmetic side effects that occur in males, in females these side effects are largely irreversible.

Conversely, an individual may abuse AASs without obvious side effects such as deepening of the voice or the appearance of acne.

Dermatologic Effects

Striae, acne, and balding are frequently reported stigmata of AAS abuse. Sebaceous gland hypertrophy, cysts, increased skin surface fatty acids, and increased cutaneous populations of *Propionibacterium acnes* put AAS abusers at increased risk for acne vulgaris; there is one case report of injection-related seeding and infection of these bacteria causing spondylodiscitis in an AAS abuser. Acne is a common side effect of AASs, self-reported by 21 of 53 (40%) of AAS abusers in one series and 12 of 22 (55%) abusers in another study. Their high incidence makes cystic acne and pitting scars pertinent findings when screening for use of AASs.

Balding is under study. It occurs in both male and female AAS abusers and is believed to be a consequence of the gradual transformation of active large scalp epithelial hair follicles into smaller dermal vellus follicles via androgen receptors in the mesenchymal dermal papilla. Balding hair follicle cells contain a higher number of androgen receptors than do nonbalding cells. Other dermatologic effects of AAS abuse include linear keloids, striae, hirsutism, seborrheic dermatitis, and secondary infections, including furunculosis.

Central Nervous System Effects

Case reports of adverse effects to the central nervous system cover a wide spectrum of observations. The first case of secondary partial empty sella syndrome with significant pituitary gland atrophy from negative feedback inhibition was reported in an elite bodybuilder with a long history of exogenous abuse of growth hormone, testosterone, and thyroid hormone. AASs exert negative feedback on the hypothalamic–pituitary–gonadal axis and cause predictable depression in follicle-stimulating hormone, LH, and testosterone, unless testosterone is the exogenous AAS being administered. In rats, AASs at doses comparable to human abuse levels reversibly block sexual receptivity, and interrupt the neuroendocrine axis. The first case report of persistent hiccups in an elite bodybuilder abusing AASs discussed the hiccup reflex arc and whether the brainstem is the steroid-responsive locus. There is a case report of permanent central vertigo in a 20-year-old male bodybuilder who abused three AASs for two courses. Insomnia in male AAS abusers is reported, although insomnia in postmenopausal women may improve with administration of AASs. Other central nervous system effects are under investigation.

Other Physical Effects

AASs are associated with a wide variety of other adverse effects, including induction of an attack of coproporphyria, splenic peliosis and rupture, and aggravation of tics in Gilles de la Tourette syndrome. Fluid retention is commonly reported by AAS users and largely drives their use of diuretics, as previously described. Alterations in thyroid function occur, most notably a decrease in thyroid-binding globulin, but the clinical significance is unclear. AASs cause adrenal hyperplasia, and elevated secretion of corticosterone and cortisol in treated female rats; the authors of this text conclude that

AASs administered to animals are stressors that can adversely affect animal welfare. Unexplained increases in serum levels of medications metabolized by cytochrome P450 or cytochrome b5 may warrant investigation for AAS abuse in patients deemed at-risk; these enzymes decreased in rat liver in response to chronic AAS abuse.

Personality Disorders

Prospective controlled studies for the development of personality disorders in AAS abusers have not been done. Small studies evaluating AAS-abusing bodybuilders/weightlifters with self-reported AAS-naïve matched controls, using self-reports and informants for retrospective assessment, have been done. These studies concluded that AAS abusers have similar personality characteristics to controls before AAS use, but unlike controls, develop abnormal personality traits and disturbances which are attributed to AAS use.

AGGRESSION

Endogenous testosterone has long been postulated as mediating aggressive behavior in males through brain AAS receptors. Aggression may be defined as a spectrum of behavior, from less fear or anticipatory anxiety all the way to explosive outbursts in humans and other animals. Adolescents who abuse AASs have nearly triple the incidence of violent behavior. Many case reports lend credence to the hypothesis that exogenous AASs may increase aggressive behavior and violence. Explosive outbursts are well known among AAS abusers who refer to them as "roid rages." Violent behavior can occur in individuals with no prior history or other risk factors and may culminate in fatal and near-fatal outcomes.

SEXUALITY AND GENDER IDENTITY

AASs can have marked effects on sexual function. AASs are used therapeutically to increase libido for postmenopausal women, although animal studies show a decrease in sexual receptivity in oophorectomized females given AASs. There are many case reports of male AAS users experiencing increased libido, decreased libido, and impotence.

ANXIETY, MOOD CHANGES, AND PSYCHOTIC SYMPTOMS

Beyond aggression and libido changes, many other psychiatric effects of AAS use have been reported, including a variety of mood changes and slowed intellectual performance. When considering psychiatric effects of AASs, there are diagnoses for which organic causes, such as AAS use, are exclusion criteria. Per DSM-IV-TR criteria, these diagnoses are then classified as substance-induced disorders. Abundant case reports exist of hypomania and mania, along with reports of irritability, elation, recklessness, racing thoughts, and feelings of power and invincibility that did not clearly meet diagnostic criteria for hypomania or mania. One case of hypomania resolved 3 to 4 days after discontinuation of AAS use and recurred after resumption of AAS use, suggesting a causal relationship. Depressed mood and major depression with psychotic features also have been reported during periods of AAS use, as have paranoia, auditory, and tactile hallucinations.

COGNITIVE CHANGES

Cognitive impairment, including distractibility, forgetfulness, and confusion, has been demonstrated in controlled trials. Improvement in performance of a psychomotor task (a pegboard test) was noted in another controlled trial. Although these changes are usually subtle, there may be significant impairment in a subset of AAS users.

DEPENDENCE

Acute anabolic steroid withdrawal symptoms usually include cravings and depression. In addition, visible changes are seen, including anxiety, aching, elevated blood pressure and heart rate, chills, piloerection, hot flashes, diaphoresis, nausea, anorexia, vomiting, irritability, and insomnia, all suggestive of central nonadrenergic hyperactivity.

Evaluation and Treatment

Screening and Testing

The prevalence of AAS use in competitive athletes, both male and female, is high enough that it should always be considered a possibility. Denial of use, or even negative testing, does not rule out steroid abuse, even in the context of national championships and the Olympics. Patients may not give their physician important history that would assist with diagnosis, treatment, and HIV risk reduction.

As with other drugs of abuse, laboratory analyses of biologic specimens for AASs can be helpful in both diagnosis and treatment. Most testing for AASs occurs in the context of athletic competition, where the object is to "level the playing field" by prohibiting a wide variety of performance-enhancing drugs. This rationale stands in contrast to testing in the workplace where the goal is to detect drug use associated with performance impairment. Ideally, results will be quickly obtainable from simple, rapid, sensitive, specific, and reproducible methodologies that can be conducted on small aliquots of sample. Standards must be established for each type of sample to be tested, for example, urine, serum, saliva, pigmented or unpigmented hair, or stool. In some contexts, it will be important that test methods detect rarely used, synthetic, or even never-marketed AASs, as well as those that are frequently abused. Tests must differentiate between normal variations in endogenous steroid and metabolite levels versus exogenous AASs. In athletic contexts, testing should be done without notice, at random, both during practice and during the regular season.

Because the effects of AASs on musculature and health may persist for months after discontinuation, evaluation for past use may be desirable. In addition to direct assays for the presence of AASs, other tests may provide useful indirect evidence of AAS abuse; unexpectedly elevated hemoglobin and hematocrit, suppressed follicle-stimulating hormone (FSH), decreased luteinizing hormone (LH), increased acid phosphatase, and hyperlipidemia and hypertriglyceridemia, are examples of such indirect indicators of AAS abuse. For males who abuse synthetic AASs there may be profound and persistent suppression of endogenous testosterone production, lasting longer than 10 months in one case report; low, as well as high, levels of testosterone may therefore indicate abuse.

Highly sensitive and specific, rapid, reliable methods for AAS testing on small samples for minute concentrations of unknowns include gas chromatography-mass spectrometry/mass fragmentography, tandem mass spectrometry, high-pressure liquid chromatography (HPLC), and enzyme-linked immunoabsorbent assay (ELISA). New testing methods are being developed. Because specimen collection sites may be at a great distance from AAS testing facilities, the specimen collection, preservation, and shipping conditions must be considered; for example, the use of dried capillary blood on filter paper, shipped through the mail, is highly effective and reproducible for nandrolone and testosterone level determinations by radioimmunoassay. Although testosterone is cleared relatively rapidly, other AASs may be detectable for a month or more after discontinuation. This prolonged half-life of some AASs needs to be considered when evaluating repeatedly positive results in those who deny current use. Metabolites of over-the-counter AAS precursors can be detected in urine, sometimes for 2 to 6 days.

Several points of caution need to be raised when considering which laboratory to employ and how to interpret test results. Even those laboratories that test for some AASs may not test for all of the dozens of different compounds that are abused, nor use techniques that detect picogram amounts, leading to the possibility of false-negative results. Inter- and intralaboratory reliability may be an issue. Researchers at the Biostatistics Branch of the U.S. National Cancer Institute sent split samples of serum to different laboratories to be tested for 10 different endogenous AASs and AAS metabolites. There was poor reliability even within the same laboratory, with tests of different aliquots from the same blood sample usually yielding significantly different results.

Treatment

Although it is estimated that there are more than 1 million AAS users in the United States, the percentage of those who receive treatment for dependence is minute. Tentative treatment recommendations can be made. These are based on treatment of other dependencies, the pharmacology of AASs, and the psychologic characteristics of AAS users. Assessment of psychiatric status is essential; severe symptoms are an indication for inpatient treatment. AAS users may have a variety of relationship problems that merit therapy for the relationship with a qualified family or couples therapist. Because assault may occur in AAS users' relationships, it is important to interview the spouse separately and confidentially, and also to offer the spouse referral both to therapy and to appropriate recovery groups (for survivors of abuse, if indicated, and for partners of drug addicts). This is true in every relationship, both heterosexual and homosexual. Ongoing assessment of sexual function is indicated, as impotence and decreased libido may occur upon discontinuation of AASs and diminished sexual function has reportedly led to relapse. Persistent decrease in an individual's sexual function relative to baseline (i.e., prior to AAS use) is an indication for consultation with an endocrinologist. Depression is another common problem in AAS abstinence syndrome, and can lead to relapse. The recovering AAS addict should be evaluated for depression and treated accordingly.

Psychosocial treatment must include an understanding and acknowledgment of the motivation for continued use. Treatment approaches will differ for individuals whose use persists because of AAS-induced hypomania (an increase in confidence, energy, and self-esteem) or euphoria, versus those who continue to use because they experience depressed mood upon discontinuation, versus those who use it to enhance body image (particularly those with a distorted body image), versus those who use for performance enhancement. The nature and course of AAS withdrawal should be reviewed with the user. Conventional drug abuse treatment is appropriate for those who abuse AASs for their mood-altering effects or who are dependent on additional substances. For people who are engrossed in the bodybuilding culture or who are seeking increased athletic performance, realistic goals with respect to appearance and performance must be set, and a diet and exercise plan should be agreed upon to achieve these goals. Peer counseling by ex-bodybuilders and group support may be of particular value for these users. Nutritional counseling and consultation with a fitness expert may be helpful. Gymnasiums are a frequent locale for acquisition of AASs and need to be avoided until recovery is firmly established. Although a wide variety of individuals can deliver psychosocial treatment to AAS users, those who are physically fit or former AAS users will have certain advantages in terms of relating to the AAS abuser seeking treatment.

The role of pharmacotherapy in treatment of AAS dependence is poorly defined. Although depression, mania, and psychosis may be induced by AAS use or withdrawal, their etiology may be difficult to establish with certainty. Pharmacotherapy for psychiatric symptoms should be based on a consideration of the risks and benefits, including the potential side effects of the medications and the consequences of inaction, which may include problems with retention in treatment. Maintenance and controlled taper have not been reported as therapeutic modalities, and no routine pharmacotherapy is recommended.

Prevention

The development of interventions to reduce the initiation of AAS use is in its infancy. The primary force driving the illicit use of AASs appears to be a strong cultural value placed on sports heroes, physical strength, and large, well-defined muscles, particularly for men, and physical competence and athletic achievement for all. Unless society sends a different message about physical beauty and athletic success, the demand and acceptance of AAS use is likely to persist. Hence it may be difficult for an adolescent to decline an offer of AASs, because AAS use may be seen as a way to achieve highly desired goals. It is important to direct educational programs both to parents and to student athletes, and to include a range of information about steroids, such as the risk of potential early epiphyseal closure in the adolescent skeleton, the association between body dysmorphia and initiation of steroid abuse, the high potential for addiction, and the nature of addiction in graphic detail.

Suggested Readings

Arvary D, Pope HG Jr. Anabolic–androgenic steroids as a gateway to opioid dependence. *N Engl J Med.* 2000;342(20):1532.

Bahrke MS, Yesalis CE, Kopstein AN, et al. Risk factors associated with anabolic-androgenic steroid use among adolescents. *Sports Med.* 2000;29(6):397–405.

Demling RH, DeSanti L. The rate of restoration of body weight after burn injury, using the anabolic agent oxandrolone, is not age dependent. *Burns.* 2001;27(1):46–51.

Eisenberg ER, Galloway GP. Anabolic-androgenic steroids. In: Lowinson JH, Ruiz P, Millman RB, et al., eds. *Substance abuse: a comprehensive textbook,* 4th ed. Philadelphia: Lippincott Williams & Wilkins; 2005:421–459.

Gruber AJ, Pope HG Jr. Psychiatric and medical effects of anabolic-androgenic steroid use in women. *Psychother Psychosom.* 2000;69(1):19–26.

Yoon JM, Lee KH. Gas chromatographic and mass spectrometric analysis of conjugated steroids in urine. *J Biosci.* 2001;26(5):627–634.

Section III

COMPULSIVE AND ADDICTIVE BEHAVIORS

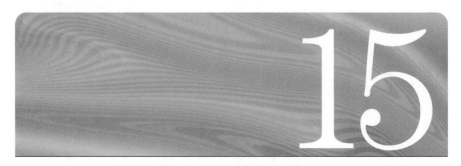

EATING DISORDERS

Eating behavior is complex but it appears that the mesolimbic dopaminergic system (MDS) is activated by food reward. Food is reported to be addicting or extremely rewarding by some patients who complain of compulsive candy, potato chip, or other food consumption. In animals, it appears that food reward depends in part on its palatability or the hedonic component related to the sensory properties of foods. When animals are offered a more palatable diet, most animal species eat more and become obese. Passive drug administration is not addicting whereas active goal-directed behavior seeking and using drugs for euphoria production is addicting. Being stuffed with cake is a markedly different experience from sneaking around and raiding the refrigerator after midnight. Host factors, such as genetic vulnerability at conception or acquired *in utero* or early in life, will play an important role in determining the pathologic reward produced by drugs, food, or some micronutrient, thus underlying the acquisition of a pathologic attachment we call addiction, binge eating, or obesity.

We believe that this primitive reward system is central to the development of both eating disorders and addiction. The numerous associations between eating disorders and drug addictions, including a high comorbidity and recidivism, genetic linkage, and common neurobiologic pathways, modification of drug reward by eating or starvation, lead us to consider the possibility that binge-eating disorders represent a drug-free auto-addiction for a significant subset of the addiction-prone population. In others, it is a trigger leading to a drug or alcohol relapse. Mesolimbic dopamine (DA) activity is but one common thread linking rewarding properties of both food and illicit drugs.

Drug Reward

The MDA system is thought to act as an interface between the midbrain and forebrain. It seems to function as a modulator, integrating emotion into directed behavior. Drug reward also confers importance or significance upon certain behaviors and not others. Many studies demonstrate that species-specific survival drives (feeding, drinking, and copulation) are reinforced or given salience through this system.

Primary Reinforcers

Feeding, like drinking and copulation, is considered a specific species-survival behavior reinforced through the medial forebrain bundle. These survival behaviors are "primary reinforcers"; that is, they have a direct effect on the medial forebrain bundle. Drugs of abuse are also primary reinforcers. Feeding within the arena of eating is also a primary reinforcer. But normal feeding behavior and eating disorders differ in the purpose they serve. Feeding behavior is typically a response to hunger. Hunger may have been a more important reason to eat in our past than it is in the United States today. Hunger is likely generated by depletion of nutrient and energy stores. The reward generated by feeding, paired with the state of hunger and its resolution into satiety, thus positively reinforces feeding behavior in a state of hunger.

Neurobiology of Feeding

The neurobiology of feeding involves a complex interplay of peripheral afferent signaling, central modulation, and nutrient composition. This is a dynamic process of hunger, feeding, satiation, and satiety. The similar effect of food reward and addictive drugs on these regulatory systems may help to explain the relationship between substance abuse and eating disorders. It is becoming apparent that eating and drug disorders share a common neuroanatomic and neurochemical basis. The latter may access brain reward through exogenous, illicit drugs and the former through dietary and environmental manipulations. Understanding this relationship of substance abuse and eating disorders will allow us to create more effective and focused treatment strategies.

The concepts of hunger, satiation, and satiety have variable definitions. They may also be dependent on one's culture and the availability of food. In cultures without starvation and where few individuals eat in response to hunger, eating disorders appear much more common. Hunger can be thought of as both a physiologic drive to eat and as a perceived desire to eat. Satiation is generally recognized as the process that ends eating behavior. Satiety, then, is the state after the completion of eating behavior in which further eating is inhibited. Eating disorders and obesity may be divided into related groups that affect either aspect of the eating process.

Although the precise physiologic mechanisms regulating feeding behavior have not been fully described, research studying the role of various neurotransmitters and neuropeptides has contributed to a greater understanding of this complex process. The overall regulation of feeding includes central nervous system (CNS) integration of peripheral afferent signals; reward; endocrine responses; energy states; drive and mood states; micronutrient intake and supply; neurotransmitter responses; and efferent motor commands. These compose a coordinated system assuring the organism's metabolic needs in the face of more global environmental factors. Our interest focuses on how disruptions in this system give rise to self-perpetuating, maladaptive behaviors. Furthermore, once established, the primitive reward systems seem to function to preserve these maladaptive behaviors. We mainly consider the role of neurotransmitter systems in the pathogenesis of eating disorders and their similarity with substance abuse disorders.

Neurobiology of Eating Disorders and Reward

Recently, the physiologic mechanisms regulating feeding, diet, and weight have been under increasing scrutiny, particularly in light of the unfortunate trends of the increasing prevalence of eating disorders in industrialized nations. The definitive work in this area stems from the results of studies where microinjections of drugs are delivered to specific brain foci. Microdialysis studies of neurotransmitters in conjunction with the microinjection studies have allowed unprecedented access to brain mechanisms and a new understanding of the neurochemistry of addictive and eating disorders. Recently, many new neuropeptides have been discovered with crucial roles in regulating feeding. Furthermore, advances in neuroimaging and immunochemistry have also added to the evolving renaissance of neurobiologic understanding.

Neuropeptides

Many studies of brain lesions, microinjection of drugs, neuropeptides, and microdialysis studies of neurotransmitter levels in freely moving and behaving animals indicate that the control of feeding behavior can be localized to the hypothalamus. The paraventricular nucleus (PVN) seems to be the part of the hypothalamus that is most critical to this process. Lesions of these areas cause obesity, increased parasympathetic tone, and hyperphagia.

A significant amount of data suggests that eating disorders represent dysregulations in the neurotransmitter pathways involving DA, serotonin (5-HT), endogenous opioids, and other neuropeptides. The role of the dopaminergic system in eating disorders links them with the pathway of brain reward in which all the classical addictions appear to converge. This reality seems obvious considering the common desire for a cigarette or coffee after a good meal and the stereotypical use of alcohol before sex and a cigarette afterward. Patients in early alcoholism recovery begin eating ice cream and potato chips, bingeing at night. They note that this behavior calms them down. It seems likely that one of the stimulatory peptides is involved in the release of driven eating. Still, eating is much more complex, involving numerous stimulatory and inhibitory peptides and messengers.

It is believed that DA, norepinephrine, and 5-HT are all involved in eating and satiety. Recently, there has been increased interest in the study of CNS 5-HT function and its general relationship to behavior. This research had produced an array of findings that have been among the most replicated in modern biologic psychiatry. Central to these studies is the finding that a low cerebrospinal fluid (CSF) concentration of 5-hydroxyindole acetic acid (5-HIAA), a measure of CNS 5-HT activity, is correlated with impaired impulse control and with violence toward others and self. Patients with eating disorders exhibit several clinical features and biologic findings indicative of 5-HT dysregulation, including feeding abnormalities, depression, suicide, impulsivity, violence, anxiety, harm avoidance, obsessive–compulsive features, seasonality, and simultaneous disturbances in neuroendocrine and neurochemical systems linked to 5-HT.

Neuropeptide Y

Neuropeptide Y (NPY) is a good place to start as a model for uncontrolled hyperphagia. NPY is one of the most abundant and widely distributed neuropeptides known. It is a member of the pancreatic polypeptide family but has a number of unique actions in the regulation of bodyweight by driving food intake. NPY is involved in the regulation of other hormones and neurotransmitters and appears involved in circadian rhythms. Studies indicate that 5-HT may play an antagonistic role with NPY in the regulation of feeding. 5-HT neurons innervate NPY-containing neurons in the arcuate nucleus. Central injections of 5-HT inhibit food intake through NPY as we might expect selective serotonin reuptake inhibitors (SSRIs) to act. NPY infusions in the hypothalamus decrease 5-HT release. NPY is the most potent activator of feeding behavior yet discovered.

d-Fenfluramine, a potent 5-HT agonist previously used in the treatment of obesity, blocks or attenuates NPY-induced or driven feeding in animals. Acute *d*-fenfluramine administration actually decreases NPY content in the hypothalamus, selectively in the paraventricular and arcuate nuclei. Although the precise mechanism of the effects of fenfluramine on eating is unknown, it does appear that it is an effect dependent on the presence of the medication and related to inducing a NPY store deficiency in the hypothalamus. These are very exciting and important studies because of the basic literature that supports a critical role for NPY. Studies of NPY microinjections into the hypothalamic PVN elicit a binge-type behavior similar to the binges of patients with bulimia, even overriding states of satiety. NPY may be the physiologic signal of the brain that means hunger and is the physiologic signal that drives feeding.

Peptide YY

Another key modulator of food intake is peptide YY (PYY), a neuropeptide cleaved from the larger molecule that includes NPY and pancreatic polypeptide. The substance is released in response to fatty nutrients and acts to inhibit gastric motility and gastric and insulin secretion. Although mainly found in the ileum and large intestine, lower doses have been reported in the mammalian CNS. Receptors have been located throughout the brain with higher density in the thalamic, limbic, and hindbrain nuclei.

It is believed that PYY is an even more potent orexigen than NPY. PYY produces hyperphagia when injected into either of the cerebroventricles, the PVN, and the hippocampus, an extrahypothalamic site not usually associated with ingestive responses. Among all orexigenic peptides and neurotransmitters known, PYY is the most potent acute stimulator of food intake.

Pancreatic Polypeptide

Pancreatic polypeptide (PP) is a 36-amino-acid peptide that belongs to a family including NPY and PYY. PP is produced in the endocrine-type F cells located in the periphery of pancreatic islets and is released into the circulation after ingestion of food and exercise. PP released by food ingestion inhibits further food intake by modulating the rate of gastric emptying during the meal. On the other hand, central administration of PP elicits food intake and gastric emptying via NPY receptors. Therefore, PP actions on food intake may be, in part, attributable to gastric emptying. PP is an anorexigenic signal in the periphery and an orexigenic signal in the CNS.

A recent study in healthy volunteers investigated the effect of intravenous PP on appetite and energy expenditure. The data demonstrate that PP causes a sustained decrease in both appetite and food intake. As expected, appetite and energy intake decreased 2 hours after infusion. More importantly, the inhibition of food intake was sustained, such that the 24-hour energy intake was significantly reduced. These data demonstrate that PP causes a sustained decrease in both appetite and food intake.

Ghrelin

Ghrelin is a neuropeptide, produced in the hypothalamus, which stimulates the release of growth hormone. Ghrelin is also an important regulator of food intake, being released from the stomach in response to fasting. Antighrelin immunoglobulins greatly suppress feeding. Ghrelin also increases NPY gene expression and antagonizes the effect of leptin-induced feeding reduction. In obese individuals, plasma ghrelin is low. Increased fasting plasma ghrelin levels are reported in patients with anorexia nervosa (AN). Specifically, those with the binge–purge variety have a statistically higher level than their restricting counterparts. Patients with bulimia who used vomiting as their purging method also appear to have higher ghrelin levels than their nonpurging peers. Leading hypotheses regarding these results include that vomiting may accelerate the release of ghrelin or damage the ghrelin-producing endocrine cells or influence circulating ghrelin levels via the vagal system. Ghrelin continues to play important roles in the understanding and treatment of eating disorders and obesity.

Behavioral Similarities

Addictions and eating disorders share many common clinical features. Some researchers suggest that classifying eating disorders as addictions based on phenomenologic analogy is an example of overgeneralization and selective reduction. However, it is clear that the commonalties between these disorders are not limited to behavioral observations but involve an array of still to be elucidated neurotransmitter abnormalities that converge in the centers of brain reward. Addiction has been defined as a disease characterized by the repetitive and destructive use of one or more mood-altering drugs that stems from a biologic vulnerability exposed or induced by environmental factors.

If current psychiatric diagnostic categories did not define addiction in terms of a psychoactive substance, would eating disorders qualify? Yes. The phenomenologic similarities between eating disorders and traditionally recognized substance abuse disorders are (a) a higher-than-average family history of alcohol or drug abuse; (b) cravings for food or a psychoactive substance; (c) cognitive dysfunction; (d) the use of food or psychoactive substances to relieve negative affect (e.g., anxiety and depression); (e) secretiveness about the problem behavior; (f) social isolation and maintenance of the problem behavior despite adverse consequences; (g) denial of the presence and severity of the disorder; (h) depression; and (i) experience of a transition where food or the psychoactive substance no longer relieves negative affect but creates the feelings the food or substance was originally used to allay. With the change away from considering tolerance and withdrawal as essential pieces of dependence, eating disorders share many of the most salient features of addictions. In the eating disorders currently classified in the *Diagnostic and Statistical Manual of Mental Disorders*, 4th edition, text revision (DSM-IV-TR), AN, bulimia nervosa (BN), and binge-eating disorder (BED), food is a substance used both repetitively and destructively by either its prolonged restriction or episodic overconsumption.

Eating Disorders

Eating disorders share the primary reward of feeding but differ in the paired stimuli. Feeding in this context is typically not a response that promotes survival, but rather serves to satisfy other paired stimuli. Various classifications of eating disorders abound in the literature. These classifications have established objective diagnostic criteria that are not correlated with neurotransmitter or other medical abnormalities. The recent basic neurobiologic studies show a plethora of neurotransmitter systems are involved in the regulation of feeding, in mood, and in the pathogenesis of psychiatric and addictive disorders. Although we have reported similarities between certain patients with eating disorders and those with addictive illness, others have argued for the inclusion of BN and AN into depressive illness or as an obsessive–compulsive spectrum disorder because of the many similarities between obsessive–compulsive disorder and eating disorders. They even further suggest that these disorders appear to be related to mood disorder, thus the obsessive–compulsive spectrum disorder family may be a subset of an affective disorder spectrum family.

Weight and food preoccupation are the primary symptoms in both AN and BN. Many patients demonstrate both anorexic and bulimic behaviors. Obese, especially morbidly obese, patients describe similar preoccupations. AN appears in restricting and bulimic subtypes. Up to 50% of patients with AN develop bulimic symptoms; significant numbers of patients who are initially bulimic develop anorexic symptoms, and restricting and bulimic subtypes may occasionally alternate in the same patient. The diagnostic process is confusing or confused.

Regardless of the diagnosis, the prevalence of *all* eating disorders appears to be increasing. Age-specific and gender-specific estimates suggest that approximately 0.5% to 1% of teenage females develop AN; up to 5% of older adolescent and young adult females develop BN. However, a recent population-based study by the Commonwealth Fund estimates that 25% of adolescents regularly engage in self-induced purging as a means of controlling their weight. Although there are no reliable population estimates for BED among children and adolescents, clinical experience with obesity in adults suggests that it is at least as common as the other conditions combined. The increase in prevalence rates over time for eating disorders is accounted for primarily by increases in the incidence of BN, increased media attention, improved detection, and less-stringent diagnostic criteria also probably contribute to the apparent "epidemic" of eating disorders.

Eating disorders are not distributed uniformly in the population. More than 90% of patients are female, more than 95% are white, and more than 75% are adolescents when they first develop their eating disorder. Most patients are from middle to upper socioeconomic status families, but patients can be of any gender, race, age, or social stratum. Recent studies suggest that the prevalence of eating disorders among minority females is much higher than previously suspected.

Currently, according to the Obesity Educational Initiative compiled by the National Heart, Lung, and Blood Institute, there are 97 million Americans who are overweight or obese. This is a dramatic increase since 1960. Over the last decade, 54% of adults over the age of 20 years would now be classified as overweight or obese. This increase occurs despite personal trainers, home exercise equipment, and other fitness developments. The specific impact the BED has on this prevalence is not exactly known. However, it is diagnosable in more than 28% of patients who are seen in a weight-loss clinic. A better understanding of the disorder is needed to stop this epidemic.

AN and BN are the two eating disorder syndromes recognized in the current DSM-IV, which was published in 1994. BED, although officially classified as an eating disorder not otherwise specified (NOS), is being considered for acceptance as a distinct diagnostic entity.

Anorexia Nervosa

Although some experts suggest that there are no cases of AN, only starvation, in cultures without food abundance, it appears across the globe in various cultures. In fact, symptoms of anorexia were reported as early as the Middle Ages in female Christian saints. AN is noted, however, to be more prevalent in industrialized societies where "one can never be too rich or too thin." It also occurs in non-Western cultures where weight concern is not apparent and the expressed motivation for food restriction may be epigastric discomfort or distaste for food.

The diagnostic criteria for AN are listed in the DSM-V-TR. The name anorexia is a misnomer because loss of appetite is actually rare. Patients with AN tend to be obsessed with food, and may even hoard food and exercise for hours daily. They become socially isolated and depressed. Despite steady diminution in social and occupational functioning and the appearance of life-threatening physical disturbances, they will typically deny the severity of their symptoms and respond with disinterest and even resistance to treatment attempts. A cognitive distortion develops in which self-worth becomes inexplicably tied to the ability to achieve and maintain an emaciated state. Amenorrhea can appear before noticeable weight loss has occurred. Delayed sexual development in adolescents and poor sexual adjustment in adults is common.

Individuals with anorexia are classified into two subtypes. The restricting subtype limits their weight loss techniques to calorie restriction and excessive exercise. They tend to exhibit obsessive–compulsive behaviors, including, but not limited to, bizarre diet and exercise routines, and express diminished sexual interest. The binge-eating/purging subtype regularly engages in binge eating and purging. Purging methods include self-induced vomiting and the abuse of laxatives, diuretics, or enemas. The presence of binging and purging in individuals with anorexia is associated with impulsive behaviors, such as substance abuse, promiscuity, suicide attempts, self-mutilation, and stealing. Bulimic symptoms occur in 30% to 80% of those with anorexia, and subtypes can alternate in the same patient.

The incidence of AN has increased dramatically in the past 30 years. Eating disorders affect an estimated 5 million Americans every year. Females continue to comprise most of the cases, with only 5% to 15% being male. Prevalence is 0.5% to 1% among late adolescents and adult women with subsyndromal cases even more common. The mean age of onset is 17 years and occurrence is rare in persons older than 40 years of age. Anorexia has an impressive mortality rate of 0.5% to 1% per observational year. Death is a consequence of suicide in 30% to 50% of the cases, with the remaining morbidity secondary to medical complications. There is complete recovery in approximately 40% of patients with anorexia. In another 20% of patients with anorexia there is resolution of the eating disorder, but subsequent emergence of other significant psychiatric pathology, including schizophrenia, bipolar disorder, depression, personality disorders, and substance abuse.

Bulimia Nervosa

Like adolescent alcohol and drug use, although many young men and women experiment with severe diets, starvation, fasting, and self-induced vomiting, few apparently lose control and become anorexic or bulimic. The diagnostic criteria for BN are listed in the DSM-V-TR. The impulse to binge is perceived as irresistible by the person with bulimia. There is a subjective loss of control during the binge, with rapid consumption until the person with bulimia is uncomfortably, or even painfully, full. Because of significant shame engendered by this behavior, binge eating is typically done only in private and stopped if inadvertently discovered. After the binge-eating episode has run its course, the individual can be left with feelings of depression, guilt, or self-disgust.

The compensatory methods in bulimia are categorized as purging and nonpurging. Purging behaviors are self-induced vomiting and abuse of laxatives, diuretics, or enemas. Self-induced vomiting is practiced by 80% to 90% of patients.

BN is more common than AN, with prevalence among women of 1% to 3%. Only 10% to 15% of people with bulimia are men. BN has traditionally been regarded as a disease afflicting middle to upper class white women, but recent reports suggest that its prevalence among ethnically diverse groups, although not as great, is significant. The age of onset ranges from 12 to 35 years of age, with a mean of 18 years of age. It is thought that BN tends to occur in overweight individuals during or following a dieting attempt and up to a third may have previously suffered from anorexia. The body-weight of individuals with bulimia fluctuates but tends to remain in the normal range. There is an increased incidence of mood disorders, specifically dysthymia and major depression; the prevalence of borderline personality disorder in those with bulimia ranges from 25% to 48%. The reported incidence of drug abuse among individuals with bulimia is as high as 46%. Bulimia has a significant relapse rate (31%) within 2 years following treatment, but relapse after 6 months of symptom control is unusual. Relapse occurs more often in patients who are vomiting than in those who are bingeing, but the significance of this fact is unknown.

BN, like AN, is characterized by abnormalities in the regulation of feeding. It has long been known to have a high comorbidity with substance abuse, particularly alcoholism.

Binge-Eating Disorder

Obesity has many possible causes and may be divided into groups including hypothyroidism, diabetes mellitus, or BEDs. BED is perhaps the most common, yet least studied, of the eating disorders. BEDs, like drug addiction, are characterized by a pathologic attachment. Both include obsessive thoughts about food and compulsions to eat more food than most people would eat within similar periods of time and in similar circumstances. Like cocaine addiction or alcoholism, binge eaters cannot take or leave it—they "can't eat just one." The binge episodes generally cause binge eaters much distress, leaving them with feelings of guilt, disgust, and depression.

Higher rates of depression, psychologic distress, and impulsivity have been reported among those who binge than among obese subjects who do not. Preliminary studies did not consistently demonstrate an increased incidence of substance abuse or dependence in individuals with BED. In a study comparing men and women with BED, men appeared to have higher lifetime prevalence for alcohol dependence than the general population. However, the rate of substance abuse among their first-degree relatives was reported to be 49%, greater than the rate of 37% in the first-degree relatives of individuals with bulimia.

Sweet cravings occur with opiate addiction and sweets can sometimes improve opiate withdrawal. Drugs affecting the same neurotransmitter systems have been found to be efficacious in treating both eating disorders and the classical drug addictions. The serotonergic agent fenfluramine, in combination with the weak amphetamine phentermine (Adipex-P) that is currently being used in the treatment of obesity, has been reported to decrease craving and self-reported use in cocaine addicts. Naltrexone, which reduces the frequency of binge eating, reduces craving and relapse in alcoholics. A careful look at the neural events involved in pathologic drug attachment appears essential in links to pathologic eating.

DA involvement in normal and pathologic food intake appears to be related to its role in reward and reinforcement. Although no data are available specifically in the BED population, information is increasing about DA in obese patients. Imaging studies using positron emission tomography implicate low brain DA activity in obese individuals. Specifically, it has been shown that the DA D2 receptor availability was decreased in obese individuals in proportion to their body mass index. It is believed that pathologic eating in obese individuals may serve to increase activation of this underactive system. It is important to note that low levels of DA D2 receptors have also been reported in individuals addicted to various types of drugs, including cocaine, alcohol, and opiates. This reinforces the central role of DA in addictive behavior, be it disordered eating or substance use.

It is known that medications that increase available 5-HT decrease carbohydrate consumption. The use of antidepressants to suppress binge eating in patients with BED is based on their demonstrated efficacy in BN. SSRIs, used in high dosage, and tricyclic antidepressants yield substantially greater reduction in binge eating than placebo.

Several medications are in use for the treatment of substance abuse disorders, as well as eating disorders. As mentioned earlier, naltrexone has been investigated for its potential role in the treatment of cravings in anorexia, bulimia, and BED. Bupropion (Wellbutrin) is an antidepressant that is FDA approved for assisting in smoking cessation. A recent study showed its effectiveness in assisting weight loss in overweight and obese woman during an 8-week trial. These patients were not assessed for a binge pattern being a factor in their current weight.

Two studies (one case series and one open label) of topiramate (Topamax), an anti-epileptic, for BED have been encouraging; both showed a significant reduction in bingeing and subsequently bodyweight in the majority of patients. Topiramate is an antiepileptic medication that facilitates γ-aminobutyric acid (GABA), leading to a decrease in extracellular release of DA in the midbrain. Studies for its use in BED have been encouraging. One case series and one open-label trial have both showed a significant reduction in bingeing, and subsequently of bodyweight, in the majority of patients. Recently, researchers have started to investigate the role of topiramate for the treatment of alcohol dependence. The initial randomized controlled study seems promising, with the study drug being more efficacious than placebo as an adjunct to standardized management. Multicenter trials are under way to elucidate further the role of this medication both in the treatment of eating disorders and substance addiction.

Other Treatment Modalities

We have examined the many similarities between substance addiction and eating disorders. As stated earlier, many of the same psychopharmacologic agents are used in the management of these syndromes. As important to treatment are the psychosocial and behavioral interventions frequently used. Group therapy is one of the most frequently used techniques in both substance abuse and eating disorder treatment programs. It allows communication of feelings, the sharing of frustrations, and offers the experience of closeness. It is a mechanism to provide strength for others who are struggling with control of substances or food. A 40-study meta-analysis with an average follow-up of 1 year suggests that group therapy for bulimia is moderately effective. Although commonly used as a component of their treatment, limited evidence is available for the use of group therapy in patients with anorexia and BED.

Marital therapy and family therapy focus on the maladaptive behaviors of the identified patient and on abnormal patterns of family interaction. It includes family members as active participants in the healing process. With their help, medication compliance and session attendance is ensured. Therapy focuses on improving family dynamics and restructuring poor communication patterns. The goal is the establishment of a more supportive, appropriate environment for the person in recovery. Several well-designed research studies support the effectiveness of behavioral relationship therapy in improving the functioning of families and improving treatment outcomes for individuals with substance addiction, as well as AN.

Cognitive–behavioral therapy (CBT) attempts to alter the cognitive processes that lead to maladaptive behavior, intervene in the chain of events that lead to the disorder, and then promote and reinforce necessary skills and behaviors for achieving and maintaining remission. Research studies consistently demonstrate that such techniques improve self-control and social skills, thus helping to reduce drinking. In patients with eating disorders, the aim is to help patients rethink their eating and exercise habits and find other ways to cope with situations and feelings that induce binges. Many studies have found CBT to be successful in reducing the frequency of binge eating and self-induced vomiting, as well as in improving attitudes toward eating, in patients with bulimia. As expected, this intervention is also being used to help control binge episodes in those with BED. Preliminary results are encouraging.

Self-help groups are defined as *a supportive, educational, usually change-oriented mutual aid group that addresses a single life problem or condition shared by all members.* Twelve-step groups such as Alcoholics Anonymous, Narcotics Anonymous, and Cocaine Anonymous are the backbone of many substance treatment efforts as well as a major form of continuing care.

Importance of Drug State to Behavior

Most current drugs of abuse have profound and important effects on eating and food preference. Alcoholics report appetite loss during intoxication and specific food cravings during abstinence. Nicotine dependence is associated with loss of weight and weight gain with abstinence. Marijuana induces eating and specific eating patterns descried as the "munchies." Cocaine and amphetamines are potent anorexics. Opiates appear to induce and opiate antagonists to decrease eating. Drug abstinence states are referred to in terms of food. Hunger for drugs, the taste of drugs, and cravings are commonplace and can just as easily be heard on an eating disorder ward as an addiction service.

There have been numerous reports of comorbidity between eating disorders and substance abuse. Eating disorders run in addiction families, and vice versa. Eating patterns change among alcoholics and other addicts depending on their drug status. Alcoholics in early abstinence report carbohydrate craving. NPY is a primary mediator of carbohydrate "drive" and norepinephrine is also a possible mediator, but DA is not. Whereas norepinephrine and NPY drive carbohydrate cravings and intake, 5-HT is a primary inhibitor of carbohydrate intake. Although humans have well-developed and highly regulated drives for micronutrients in food, we appear to have poorly developed satiety. If we are deprived of a food or drink that we are accustomed to, the brain increases appetite for nutrients, appetites for specific foods, and/or alcohol ingestion, causing decreased perception of anxiety and stress. NPY appears to reduce anxiety, so carbohydrate or alcohol intake can actually increase self-perceptions of well-being.

Another neuromodulator of eating, galanin, is also known to be a potent analgesic. This suggests that eating, especially eating fat, may reduce pain. Just putting a galanin antagonist in the hypothalamus of animals totally stops the eating of fat. Like opioids and other drugs, the more fat we eat, the more we want. The more eating of fat, the more galanin is found in the brain. In this way, it explains the "drive" for fat and a mechanism for fat craving. The resultant obesity occurs as a consequence of our poor fat satiety control. We eat carbohydrates generally in the morning; we eat fat between lunch and dinner. Alcoholics, in the early abstinence stage, report bingeing not only on fats but also on carbohydrates throughout the day.

Conclusion

The American media have expanded the country's interpretation of addictions and substance abuse. Pop culture has broadened its concept of addictions to encompass other self-destructive, yet seemingly compulsive, behaviors. These include "workaholics," gamblers, compulsive spenders, and food addicts, the self-confessed "food aholics." Although this process may provoke a knee-jerk rejection of commonalties, this chapter has addressed the issue of whether the eating disorders should legitimately be considered as forms of addiction. It appears that this tendency to consider every potentially harmful compulsive or repetitive behavior as an addiction is a major reason for not considering some eating disorders as addictive or autoaddictive disorders. Some believe that the conception of eating disorders as another form of addiction disorder is a "therapeutic dead end." One concern raised is that the addiction-as-disease model is primarily an abstinence model and dieting and food avoidance are risk factors for eating disorders. It must be recognized, however, that with the evolution of our understanding of brain reward systems, the future addiction-as-disease model will include appropriate medication management for relapse prevention. It has also been proposed that patients with eating disorders embrace the suggestion that they have an addiction because then no self-responsibility is involved. However, it is clear that eating disorders are not a result of a lack of self-control. In addition to the neurotransmitter aberrations that have been described on single-photon emission computed tomography (SPECT) imaging, people with bulimia exhibit low or negative changes in regional blood flow to the frontal lobe area. In answer to the initial question of whether eating disorders should be classified as addictions, we propose that both disorders involve similar brain systems and result in similar behaviors and feeling states. Both are important diseases where loss of control and compulsive use are preeminent. Both are diverse groups of people with illnesses of unknown etiology, characterized by a chronic relapsing course without specific pathophysiology or treatment. Both involve the acquired pathologic attachment with the agent(s) of their ultimate compromise and possible destruction. Both may involve host or risk factors that predispose a person to extreme reward after consumption or use thereby making repetition more likely to occur. Both involve denial and reluctance to accept that people are in fact ill and in need of treatment. Both can result in early death. Both generally require early experimentation—one with drugs, the other with dieting. Both can be relapse triggers for each other. Drugs are used to decrease eating and eating is used to decrease drug taking. Both are used to accentuate the other. The similarities are numerous and striking. But as long as the diagnostic scheme is descriptive and not neurobiologic, it will be difficult to identify which patients have one disorder and which have two disorders.

Food is a powerful mood-altering substance that is repetitively and destructively used (or restricted) in eating disorders, and there is considerable experimental evidence of biologic vulnerability. Finally, categorizing eating disorders as addictions also has ramifications for prevention. Epidemiologic studies among high school students show that eating disorders are associated with alcohol use, and that even dieting in adolescents is related to alcohol and tobacco abuse. With our current appreciation of eating disorders as yet another form of dangerous addiction, it is time that educational efforts be targeted to the adolescent population to halt the current burgeoning growth of eating disorders in our society. It is time that individuals with eating disorders are not held "responsible" for a disease process any more than patients with diabetes or heart disease are held responsible. One hopes this is true for other addicts. Experts worry whether such a discussion might lead to gambling or compulsive sexual behaviors being proposed for inclusion as addictions.

Suggested Readings

Batterham RL, Le Roux CW, Cohen MA, et al. Pancreatic polypeptide reduces appetite and food intake in humans. *J Clin Endocrinol Metab.* 2003;88(8):3989–3992.

Gold MS, Star J. Eating disorders. In: Lowinson JH, Ruiz P, Millman RB, et al., eds. *Substance abuse: a comprehensive textbook*, 4th ed. Philadelphia: Lippincott Williams & Wilkins; 2005:469–488.

James GA, Gold MS, Liu Y. Interaction of satiety and reward response to food stimulation. *J Add Dis.* 2004;23:(3):23–39.

Johnson BA, Ait-Daoud N, Bowden CL, et al. Oral topiramate for treatment of alcohol dependence: a randomized controlled trial. *Lancet.* 2003;361(9370):1677–1685.

Nakazato M, Murakami N, Date Y, et al. A role for ghrelin in the central regulation of feeding. *Nature.* 2002;409:194–198.

16

PATHOLOGIC GAMBLING

A long with the human tendency to gamble have come gambling-related problems, including the loss of control of gambling behavior, commonly referred to as compulsive gambling. For the purpose of understanding gambling problems, it is important to define gambling narrowly rather than to use a broad definition. Gambling or wagering involves either playing a game for money or staking something of value (usually money) on an event influenced by chance (e.g., betting on whether a specific set of numbers will be picked in a lottery). To be important to the development of gambling problems, this wagering must be short term, so that a feeling of excitement can be produced while awaiting the outcome. Thus, a long-term financial investment would not be considered gambling for this purpose, although chance may play a role in its gain or loss of value.

The term "gambling problems" is used as an umbrella term for a wide range of problems related to gambling activities, such as underage gambling, illegal gambling, and dishonest games, in addition to personal and family problems related to excessive gambling by an individual. "Problem gambler" is sometimes used to refer to a person whose gambling creates problems, whereas "compulsive gambler" or "pathologic gambler" applies specifically to an individual suffering from the disorder described in the American Psychiatric Association's *Diagnostic and Statistical Manual of Mental Disorders*, 4th ed. text revisions (DSM-IV-TR), as "Pathological Gambling."

Different varieties of currently popular gambling involve differing proportions of chance and skill. Playing chess for money involves significantly more skill than chance. Betting on horse races may involve considerable knowledge of the competitors and skill in handicapping, whereas playing the lottery or roulette relies entirely on chance. Forms of gambling also differ in the immediacy of their payoff. Casino games such as blackjack tend to be short-interval gambling, and slot machines offer an almost immediate payoff. However, little research has been devoted to the impact of different games on gamblers and most ideas about these differences are based on clinical experience.

Diagnosis of Pathologic Gambling

In the current edition, DSM-IV-TR, the disorder is characterized as persistent and recurrent maladaptive gambling behavior, not better accounted for as a component of a manic episode. At least 5 of the following 10 criteria must be present for the diagnosis to be made:

1. "Is preoccupied with gambling (e.g., preoccupied with reliving past gambling experience, handicapping or planning the next venture, or thinking of ways to get money with which to gamble)." Preoccupation is sometimes extreme. Pathologic gamblers have been known to go to the racetrack on their wedding day. Pathologic sports bettors may follow several games simultaneously on two or three radios or television sets.

2. "Needs to gamble with increasing amounts of money in order to achieve the desired excitement." This phenomenon is comparable to the tolerance seen in substance dependence.

3. "Has repeated unsuccessful efforts to control, cut back, or stop gambling." This criterion refers to impaired control.

4. "Is restless or irritable when attempting to cut down or stop gambling." This describes the equivalent of a withdrawal state in substance dependence. Approximately 65% of Gamblers Anonymous (GA) members reported such withdrawal symptoms, which also included insomnia, headaches, upset stomach or diarrhea, anorexia, palpitations, weakness, shaking, sweating, and breathing problems.

5. "Gambles as a way of escaping from problems or relieving a dysphoric mood (e.g., feelings of helplessness, guilt, anxiety, depression)." Female pathologic gamblers often describe such "escape" as a primary reason for gambling.

6. "After losing money gambling, often returns another day to get even ('chasing' one's losses)." Chasing is a common symptom of this disorder. It has no equivalent in alcohol or other drug addictions.

7. "Lies to family members, therapist, or others to conceal the extent of involvement with gambling."

8. "Has committed illegal acts such as forgery, fraud, theft, or embezzlement to finance gambling." Individuals who are normally honest and law abiding often begin to appropriate other people's money when they develop pathologic gambling. They characteristically rationalize this activity as temporary borrowing, but their need for money eventually overpowers their moral standards. Pathologic gambling is closely associated with criminal activity, especially white-collar crime.

9. "Has jeopardized or lost a significant relationship, job, or educational or career opportunity because of gambling." Marital and other family relationships are usually the first to be affected as the gambler becomes preoccupied with gambling activity, although all relationships and activities are eventually damaged by the disease.

10. "Relies on others to provide money to relieve a desperate financial situation caused by gambling." This is generally known as a "bailout" and is often elicited from family or friends without revealing that the indebtedness is caused by gambling. If the donors of the funds are aware of the gambling, they often insist on a promise that the pathologic gambler will give up or reduce this activity.

These criteria have much in common with the criteria for substance dependence and some authors consider pathologic gambling a behavioral addiction. Pathologic gambling is a progressive disease that often has its onset in adolescence, but may begin at any age. Its characteristics may differ with age and sex. Female pathologic gamblers show both a faster progression of the disease and higher comorbidity with anxiety and depression. They are less likely to commit crimes than males and report less indebtedness. Women also more often report gambling to escape from the psychologic distress produced by a painful situation, for example, an abusive relationship or a husband who is often absent. The increasing availability of gambling machines, a form of gambling that particularly appeals to women, at supermarkets, Laundromats, and other places frequented by women, has been pointed out. This increase in exposure may lead to an equalization of gambling problem rates between men and women in the near future. In spite of methodologic differences, studies conducted in North America in the early 1990s generally agreed that the male–female ratio for pathologic gambling was approximately 2:1 in most populations, but a recent general population study of US adults found a male–female ratio close to 1:1.

Epidemiologic and genetic data show that pathologic gambling runs in families and is highly associated with alcoholism; therefore, special attention should be paid to children of problem gamblers and problem drinkers when screening for pathologic gambling.

Epidemiology of Gambling Problems

Prevalence Rates

In spite of varying methodologies, prevalence studies in the United States have reported rates between 1% and 2% for current pathologic gambling among adults, and an additional 2% to 4% for problem gamblers who do not meet criteria for pathologic gambling. To date, only four studies have investigated national samples. One of these is a meta-analysis of state and regional prevalence studies across North America. In its review of this topic, the National Research Council stresses the experience of the states of Iowa, Minnesota, Texas, and Connecticut where repeated surveys demonstrated an increase in prevalence rates after the introduction of legal gambling. Reviewing the evidence one may fairly conclude that the greater the availability of gambling, the greater the prevalence of pathologic gambling.

At-Risk Populations

The picture of the *typical* pathologic gambler emerging from epidemiologic studies is a male subject, married with children, in his 30s, white, from a low socioeconomic stratum, and having a high school education. Nevertheless, more women are gambling now than in previous generations, and the proportion of nonmarried subjects (single, divorced, or separated) is higher among pathologic gamblers than in the general population, suggesting loneliness as an associated factor. Also, a number of studies have reported higher rates of pathologic gambling among ethnic minorities, including African Americans, Hispanics, Native Americans, and other populations. Little is known about the impact of social and cultural variables on gambling behavior. For example, although low socioeconomic status is associated with pathologic gambling, it is not clear whether this may be cause or effect.

Age seems to play an important role in pathologic gambling. Today's youngsters are the first generation to be fully exposed to new societal rules in which gambling is not only accepted, but promoted by federal and state governments and entrepreneurs as a legitimate amusement and source of revenue. Studies conducted in the last 10 years in the United States and Canada show current prevalence rates up to almost 6% for current probable pathologic gambling among students in the 6th to 12th grades, a rate almost six times higher than in the adult population. Studies point out the possibility of artificial inflation of prevalence rates by the use of instruments originally meant for screening in older subjects, but the higher frequency among adolescents and young adults has been so often replicated that it is a legitimate cause for public concern. On the other hand, although pathologic gambling is consistently reported as less frequent among older people, the population segment over the age of 65 years has had the greatest growth in gambling engagement in the last 20 years. The effect of this increase has not yet been fully investigated.

Prevalence rates for pathologic gambling are higher among patients in treatment for substance use disorders than in the general population. Studies conducted at addiction treatment sites report rates of pathologic gambling four to ten times higher for substance abusers and dependents than for the general population. Two telephone surveys and one household survey have replicated the association between pathologic gambling and substance use disorders. The latter was a study conducted in St. Louis, Missouri, a site-specific investigation as part of the broader Epidemiological Catchment Area study. This study showed that the risk for alcohol abuse/dependence and nicotine dependence increased as the severity of gambling rose.

The prevalence of pathologic gambling among other psychiatric patients has also been studied. A lifetime prevalence of 6.7% for probable pathologic gambling in a survey of 105 patients admitted to an acute adult psychiatric service for primary psychiatric problems has been found. Another study reported a prevalence rate of pathologic gambling of 6% among patients presenting to primary care settings.

Reports on comorbidity show substance-related, anxiety, and mood disorders as the main syndromes comorbid with pathologic gambling, but the temporal relationship between pathologic gambling and affective syndromes remains unclear. One epidemiologic study described anxiety and depression symptoms preceding gambling activity suggesting that they could be potential catalysts for problem gambling.

High rates of pathologic gambling have been described among jail and prison inmates. Conversely, high comorbidity with antisocial personality disorder is also reported.

Phenomenology of Pathologic Gambling

Pathologic gambling is currently understood as a disease characterized by an addiction to what gamblers call "being in action." This term describes an aroused state compared by some gamblers to the "high" experienced after using stimulants such as cocaine. A gambler is "in action" while awaiting the result of a significant wager. In some cases, a feeling of altered identity or dissociation is experienced. Both the "high" and the dissociated state afford a relief from dysphoric feelings such as boredom, anxiety, and depression. They allow a reduction in self-criticism, worry, and guilt, and permit the gambler to indulge in fantasies about the next "big win."

Pathophysiology

There are considerable gaps in our knowledge about how gambling affects the brain. The research into gambling neurobiology started timidly in the late 1980s, but grew impressively throughout the 1990s. Different studies found altered regulation of monoamine neurotransmitters such as noradrenaline, serotonin, and dopamine, which, in turn, were related to the regulation of motivated behaviors and impulse control.

It has been proposed that decreased dopamine activity on the mesocorticolimbic circuitry is related to addictions and addiction-like behaviors, the so-called reward deficiency syndrome. Genetic studies relate pathologic gambling to gene polymorphism at dopamine receptors, D1, D2, and D4. Conversely, three studies reported 13 cases of pathologic gambling that started among patients with Parkinson disease after the introduction of L-dopa therapy, noting that hyperactivity of dopamine circuitry could be responsible. The only study addressing the actual impact of gambling on neurotransmitters reported an increase of peripheral norepinephrine at the beginning of a winning streak and an increase of dopamine at the end of it.

A genetic alteration in norepinephrine receptors in pathologic gamblers has been reported, and elevated activity has been suggested by both peripheral and central measures of norepinephrine metabolites.

Both a decreased level of peripheral monoamine oxidase (MAO) and genetic polymorphism for MAO types A and B among pathologic gamblers support the hypothesis that deregulated monoamine activity contributes to altered motivated behavior.

A functional magnetic resonance imaging (MRI) study of normal volunteers identified several brain sites involved in active gambling, for example, ventral tegmental area, orbitofrontal cortex, sublenticular extended amygdala, and the hypothalamus, identified by the authors as areas also involved in brain stimulation by cocaine infusion. A study of event-related potentials in the brain identified an electric activity generated by a medial-frontal region, probably related to the anterior cingulate cortex that reacted to monetary losses, that is, punishment. Overall, both studies show that gambling is a complex behavior that involves different parts of the brain depending on a combination of previous expectancies (expected to win/expected to lose) and actual outcome.

Psychodynamics

Considerable attention has been devoted to the study of psychodynamic factors involved in pathologic gambling. Psychoanalysts stress the role of unconscious conflicts. Gambling enables the satisfaction of unacceptable erotic impulses, while providing masochistic punishment for the guilt caused by such satisfaction. Lately, the roles of narcissism and fantasies about power and control have also been explored. Behavioral psychologists point to the roles of classical and operant conditioning, and the self-reinforcement properties of gambling given its intermittent schedule of payout.

The possibility of predisposing personality features has been difficult to explore because of a lack of consensus about personality models. However, pathologic gamblers tend to score high on measures of impulsivity, and impulsivity assessed during mid adolescence is related to problem gambling at late adolescence.

Course of the Disease

The progressive course of pathologic gambling is usually described in three phases. They are: the winning, losing, and desperation phases. More recently, the hopeless or "giving-up" phase has been added. About a third of probable pathologic gamblers identified in general population studies are female, so it is not surprising that this progression of phases may not be characteristic of all gamblers. Women tend to start their gambling problems later than men, but they progress faster, coming to treatment at roughly the same age as men. This phenomenon, also described for alcohol dependence, has been called the *telescoping effect*.

Winning Phase

In some cases, the career of the pathologic gambler begins with a big win (equal to half the individual's annual earnings or more). For most gamblers, however, the winning phase reflects the time and effort they devote to gambling on skill-related forms of wagering such as horserace betting, playing the stock market, or playing cards. Winning induces a feeling of power, wealth, and omnipotence. As the gambler's involvement with gambling grows, the gambler depends increasingly on the "high" derived from being in action and less on other mechanisms of defense to deal with problems and to counteract negative emotional states. The gambler pulls away from intimate interpersonal relationships and derives a growing proportion of his or her self-esteem from both gambling skill and the feeling of being favored by God, Fate, or Lady Luck. Whereas others must work for a living, the gambler feels empowered to obtain money through magical means. Although pathologic gamblers both win and lose during this phase, they tend to recall and talk about their wins and deny, rationalize, or minimize their losses. For this reason, they are often unable to account for money claimed to be won. The winning phase is more characteristic of pathologic gamblers as opposed to initial "escape-seekers" who begin their gambling involvement as a way to relieve situation-related dysphoria.

Losing Phase

This phase often begins with the kind of unpredictable losing streak experienced by anyone who gambles. Sometimes it begins with a "bad beat" (an unexplained bizarre circumstance that turns an expected win into a loss). For example, a horse approaching the finish line well in front of the pack suddenly drops dead, or a winning horse is disqualified because of a technicality irrelevant to the race itself. The experience of losing would be distressing for the ordinary gambler, but for the pathologic gambler it is experienced as a severe narcissistic blow, and may begin a pattern of "chasing" losses. This experience may be related to the phenomenon described by gamblers as "going on tilt" (an acute deterioration of play). In any case, the gambler now feels compelled to win back money the gambler has lost and begins to gamble less cautiously, thereby compounding losses. As losses mount, gambling becomes more urgent and also more solitary. Lying to cover losses, appropriating assets from family members, taking out loans, and continually searching for money become prevalent activities. Interpersonal relationships are further strained. Family members find themselves isolated and confused by the gambler's behavior and the disappearance of family funds. Spouses sometimes suspect the gambler is having an affair. Even when they know about the gambling, spouses are usually unaware of the extent of the gambler's indebtedness.

Comorbidities, including affective disorders, may become more apparent during this phase, described by some patients and families as "like being on an emotional roller coaster." The gambler both wins and loses during this phase, but money won is only partially used to pay debts. Most of it is gambled.

During this phase the gambler may seek a bailout, promising to cut down or stop gambling in return. The bailout, however, is treated like a "big win," partly gambled, and accepted as further evidence of the gambler's omnipotence.

Desperation Phase

This phase may begin with the gambling away of funds from a bailout or some other grave disappointment. The gambler is now desperate. Immoral and/or illegal acts (e.g., fraud, embezzling, writing bad checks) become a necessity, as does the compensatory belief in a big win "just around the corner." Irritability, mood swings, isolation, escape fantasies, and suicidal ideation or attempts are common. Debts mount. Additional bailouts are sought. The gambler may be arrested and prosecuted.

Most members of GA who come for help reporting they have "hit bottom" do so in this phase. Surveys of GA members have reported severe depression in 72% and suicidal attempts in 17% to 24%.

Giving-Up Phase

Pathologic gamblers who reach this phase no longer cling to the fantasy of "winning it all back." They gamble sloppily. Their goal is just to stay in action.

Comorbid psychiatric conditions have already been mentioned. Depression, bipolar disorder, and suicidal attempts are particularly common, as are substance use disorders. Physical conditions generally thought of as stress related (e.g., hypertension, gastrointestinal problems, respiratory symptoms) are also common at all stages of the disease. Spouses of pathologic gamblers often suffer from a variety of physical and emotional disorders, and may experience several phases in their own reactions, as the disease develops. These have been described as denial (broken through in "cycles of discovery"), stress, and exhaustion. Studies of children of pathologic gamblers have found increased rates of such health-threatening behaviors as drinking, drug use, smoking, overeating, and gambling. These problems are especially evident in children of parents with comorbid conditions such as combined pathologic gambling and substance dependence.

Pathologic Gambling and Substance-Use Disorders: Identification in Clinical Populations

Because of the high prevalence of pathologic gambling among persons suffering from substance use disorders, all such patients should be evaluated for gambling problems. The relationship between substance use and gambling is a complex one. The two activities are often combined. Alcoholic beverages are served in casinos and at sports events. Both licit and illicit gambling activities may be centered at bars, where illicit drugs are also sold. Substance dependence may develop simultaneously with pathologic gambling or may develop before or afterward. It is, therefore, important to assess risk in substance-dependent patients who do not report current gambling problems. Patients with a history of intense interest in gambling before the onset of substance dependence, patients with a family history of pathologic gambling, and patients with a history of gambling problems in remission are at special risk. The altered psychologic state experienced during gambling may lead to relapse in a newly abstinent substance-dependent patient. Alternatively, abstinence from alcohol and drugs may be sustained, but a "switch of addictions" experienced. The action of gambling is easily substituted for the substance-induced "high" in the patient's pattern of dependence, leading to a rapid development of pathologic gambling.

The South Oaks Gambling Screen (SOGS) is available to screen clinical populations. It can be administered as a pencil-and-paper test or a clinical interview. It should be scored with the score sheet because not all questions are counted in the total score. The first few questions, although not scored, give the evaluator a quick survey of the kinds and amounts of wagering done by the subject, and of family history. The amounts wagered must be evaluated relative to the subject's total disposable income. The family history is useful in judging risk. Question 12 is not scored, but acts as a lead-in to question 13. In addition, although questions 16 (j) and (k) are not scored, they provide valuable information to the rater. The maximum SOGS score is 20. Scores of 5 or more are indicative of probable pathologic gambling, whereas a score of between 1 and 4 may indicate some gambling problem. Note that the questions are written in a lifetime mode. Patients who score 5 or more should be evaluated using DSM-IV-TR diagnostic criteria for pathologic gambling, either current or in remission.

The SOGS has been translated into many languages, including Spanish, Italian, German, Turkish, Japanese, Hebrew, and several Southeast Asian languages, and adapted to different cultures.

In addition to screening for pathologic gambling in chemically dependent populations, the SOGS is recommended for patients in mental health and general medical settings and in employee assistance programs (EAPs). Jail and prison populations should also be screened, because pathologic gamblers who complete their sentences are highly likely to resume criminal activity if their disease is untreated.

The SOGS has demonstrated both adequate specificity and reliability in clinical populations but may overestimate when it is used to measure the prevalence of pathologic gambling in general population surveys.

Treatment of Pathologic Gambling

Current treatment for pathologic gambling is in many ways similar to the treatment of substance use disorders. Most of the treatment is delivered on an outpatient basis, with inpatient or residential care reserved for patients in a crisis of some kind, treatment failures, and patients with comorbid disorders.

Modalities employed include psychoeducation, individual and group therapies, and family involvement, either in conjoint family sessions or in separate individual or group therapy for "significant others." Family members can and should be referred for help whether or not the problem gambler accepts treatment.

Referrals to GA and Gam-Anon (a 12-step fellowship for family members) are often made and attendance is encouraged as an adjunct to treatment. GA was established in 1957, based on the 12 steps of Alcoholics Anonymous (AA), as adapted to the recovery of pathologic gamblers. GA has developed several specific strategies in dealing with the extreme financial indebtedness of new members and their initial difficulties in handling money.

Abstinence is the ultimate goal in most treatment programs, although reduction or control of gambling is sought in some programs, presumably for earlier-stage problem gamblers.

Initial Treatment

Patients may begin treatment for a variety of reasons. There is often an external motivation, for example, an arrest or threatened arrest, pressure from the family as a condition of providing a bailout, or job jeopardy. The patient may have been diagnosed through screening while in treatment for a psychiatric or substance use disorder, or there may be a crisis such as a suicide attempt or personal bankruptcy. Initial treatment attempts to prevent gambling from doing further harm. Many clinicians recommend limiting access to money, to credit, and to gambling venues and partners early in treatment. Such a strategy involves some loss of autonomy and patients may resist the idea. Because noncompliance may lead to relapse and treatment dropout, motivational techniques can be useful. Initial treatment also involves educating the patient and family about the nature of the disease and its treatment, and dealing with concomitant psychiatric, physical, and social problems.

Various psychoactive medications have been tried in pathologic gamblers, including mood stabilizers, antidepressants, antipsychotics, and opiate receptor blockers. One single-blind study found both lithium and valproate associated with improvement over a 14-week period. Further investigation is needed to clarify the effectiveness and role of psychopharmacology. It is also important to note that a high initial placebo-response rate has been reported, up to 59%, so that extended studies are required.

Rehabilitation

Continued treatment includes exploring the role of gambling in patients' lives and helping them develop other, healthier means to satisfy these needs. Understanding relapse triggers, learning relapse prevention techniques, and practicing stress management are helpful, as are measures to improve the interpersonal and social functioning of the patient. Family treatment is also critical to rehabilitation. In some patients long-term psychodynamic psychotherapy is required for stable recovery.

Few random controlled trials of treatment for pathologic gambling have been conducted, most of them employing cognitive–behavioral approaches. Cognitive therapy is based on the hypothesis that false assumptions regarding chance events and the laws of probability account for gambling attractiveness. The overestimation of one's skills, fantasies about being able to influence random events, and ideas that deny the independence of chance events (e.g., "odd numbers have come out so many times in a row, that now there will be an even number") feed into fantasies of restitution and the desire to resume gambling. Cognitive therapy asks that the patient keep a log of gambling thoughts, identify those pertaining to the distorted belief system, and challenge these misconceptions with more rational thoughts. Preliminary reports of progressive exposure to gambling machines coupled with response prevention has found this method potentially useful in diminishing cravings elicited by gambling cues.

Long-Term Follow-up

Pathologic gambling is a lifelong disorder. As with substance dependence, patients may relapse after years of abstinence. Therefore, long-term follow-up in GA is helpful, with the availability of professional assistance as needed in times of increased stress or risk of relapse. Likewise, long-term Gam-Anon involvement is helpful for family members. Unfortunately, Gamateen, a self-help, 12-step-based fellowship for adolescent children of pathologic gamblers, is not yet widely available.

Prevention of Pathologic Gambling

In spite of the immense social and personal costs of pathologic gambling, there has been very little research or programmatic attention paid to the prevention of this disorder. Some attempts at prevention have been made through public education (e.g., posting signs in casinos) and the establishment of toll-free referral numbers. However, the shortage of treatment resources and the long waiting lists at many clinics hamper efforts to connect individuals and families in need with professional help.

A comprehensive prevention plan should address both education of those at risk for developing gambling problems, and lowering treatment barriers for those experiencing them already. Informative material for adolescents may be useful to address misconceptions about gambling, but their utility in preventing pathologic gambling is still under investigation. A wider range of treatment options is needed to address different stages of illness. Shame, secrecy, and lonely attempts at financial recovery through gambling have been associated with treatment delay, and should be addressed in messages specifically targeting pathologic gamblers.

A more rapid onset of pathologic gambling among players of computerized games has been described. Because computer games are fast paced and allow immediate rebetting, they enable dysfunctional gambling. Furthermore, computer games reach a greater proportion of the population because they are not as associated with male culture as are more traditional games such as card games and horseracing.

Clearly, the growth of commercial gambling coupled with technologic advances set important challenges for the future. Enhanced societal support for research, prevention, and treatment will be needed if we are to remedy the individual, family, and community devastation produced by pathologic gambling.

Suggested Readings

Blume SB, Tavares H. Pathologic gambling. In: Lowinson JH, Ruiz P, Millman RB, et al., eds. *Substance abuse: a comprehensive textbook*, 4th ed. Philadelphia: Lippincott Williams & Wilkins; 2005:488–498.

Gehring WJ, Willoughby AR. The medial frontal cortex and the rapid processing of monetary gains and losses. *Science.* 2002;295(5563):2279–2282.

Potenza MN. The neurobiology of pathological gambling. *Semin Clin Neuropsychiatry.* 2001; 6(3):217–226.

Stinchfield R. Reliability, validity, and classification accuracy of the South Oaks Gambling Screen (SOGS). *Addict Behav.* 2002;27(1):1–19.

Tavares H, Zilberman M, Beites FJ, et al. Gender differences in gambling progression. *J Gambl Stud.* 2001;17:151–159.

Welte J, Barnes G, Wieczorek W, et al. Alcohol and gambling pathology among U.S. adults: prevalence, demographic patterns and comorbidity. *J Stud Alcohol.* 2001;62(5):706–712.

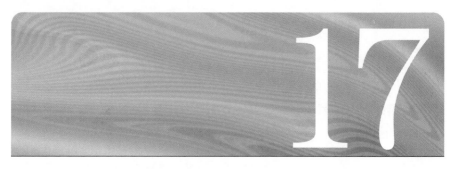

SEXUAL ADDICTION

Diagnosis and Epidemiology

Sexual addiction can be defined as a condition in which some form of sexual behavior is employed in a pattern that is characterized by two key features: (a) recurrent failure to control the behavior, and (b) continuation of the behavior despite significant harmful consequences. A definition tells us what something is, and diagnostic criteria tell us how to recognize it when we see it. Diagnostic criteria for sexual addiction are proposed to be:

> A maladaptive pattern of sexual behavior, *leading to clinically significant impairment or distress*, as manifested by three (or more) of the following, occurring at any time in the same 12-month period:
>
> (1) tolerance, as defined by either of the following:
>   (a) a need for markedly increased amount or intensity of the sexual behavior to achieve the desired effect
>   (b) markedly diminished effect with continued involvement in the sexual behavior at the same level of intensity
>
> (2) withdrawal, as manifested by either of the following:
>   (a) characteristic psychophysiologic withdrawal syndrome of physiologically described changes and/or psychologically described changes upon discontinuation of the sexual behavior
>   (b) the same (or a closely related) sexual behavior is engaged in to relieve or avoid withdrawal symptoms
>
> (3) the sexual behavior is often engaged in over a longer period, in greater quantity, or at a higher level of intensity than was intended
>
> (4) there is a persistent desire or unsuccessful efforts to cut down or control the sexual behavior
>
> (5) a great deal of time is spent in activities necessary to prepare for the sexual behavior, to engage in the behavior, or to recover from its effects
>
> (6) important social, occupational, or recreational activities are given up or reduced because of the sexual behavior

(7) the sexual behavior continues despite knowledge of having a persistent or recurrent physical or psychologic problem that is likely to have been caused or exacerbated by the behavior

Significantly, no form of sexual behavior in itself constitutes sexual addiction. Any sexual behavior has the potential to be engaged in addictively, but constitutes an addictive disorder only to the extent that it occurs in a pattern that meets the diagnostic criteria or accords with the definition. The key features that distinguish sexual addiction from other patterns of sexual behavior are (a) the person is not reliably able to control the sexual behavior; and (b) the sexual behavior has significant harmful consequences and continues nonetheless.

Differential Diagnosis

The hypersexual activity and paraphilic (i.e., perverse or unconventional) sexual behaviors that characterize sexual addiction can occur also as manifestations of underlying organic pathology, and occasionally are its earliest or most prominent symptoms. Paraphilic or hypersexual behavior can be a symptom of a brain lesion, particularly a lesion in the medial basal-frontal, diencephalic, or septal region. Anomalous sexual behavior can occur also in the context of a seizure disorder, especially in association with temporal lobe epilepsy. More broadly, any disorder that is associated with an impairment of cerebral functioning can weaken normal inhibitory controls and thereby allow the expression of sexual behaviors that ordinarily are suppressed. Hypersexual behavior can occur also as a side effect of medication, particularly antiparkinsonian agents. Finally, sexually aggressive behavior has been associated with elevated levels of testosterone. Clues that invite an organic evaluation include onset in middle age or later, regression from previously normal sexuality, excessive aggression, report of auras or seizure-like symptoms prior to or during the sexual behavior, abnormal body habitus, and presence of soft neurologic signs. The diagnostic criteria for sexual addiction are useful also in distinguishing sexual addiction from nonaddictive patterns of exploitative or aggressive sexual behavior that can occur with antisocial personality disorder.

Obsessions and compulsions with sexual content can occur in obsessive–compulsive disorder (OCD). Sexual obsessions are fairly common in OCD, and were reported in 32% of the patients in a large study. The content of these obsessions, however, consisted most often not of sexual fantasies, but of fears of acting on sexual impulses or fears of being a pervert. More generally, symptoms of sexual addiction differ from sexual obsessions and compulsions in that the former are associated with sexual arousal and sexual pleasure, whereas the latter typically are not.

A syndrome that meets the diagnostic criteria for sexual addiction can occur in the context of other psychiatric disorders, including manic–depressive conditions, schizophrenia, personality disorders, and substance dependence. When the diagnostic criteria for both sexual addiction and another psychiatric disorder are met, both diagnoses are warranted, regardless of whether sexual addiction might be secondary to the other psychiatric disorder.

Prevalence

It has been reported that 3% to 6% of Americans suffer from sexual addiction, and that approximately 5% of the population met diagnostic criteria for "sexual compulsivity."

Gender and Age Features

Approximately 80% of sex addicts are male. Gender differences in prevalence are greater for paraphilic than for nonparaphilic sexual addictions. Within the nonparaphilic arena, males tend to focus more on physical sexual gratification, and thus more often engage addictively in masturbation, use of prostitutes, and impersonal sex. Females tend to focus more on the emotional aspects of sexuality and thus more often engage addictively in romantic relationships. Addictive use of sexual behavior typically begins in the teens or early 20s, peaks between the ages of 20 and 40 years, and then gradually declines.

Comorbidity and Familial Patterns

A review of comorbidity findings is prefaced by the observation that little research has actually been conducted specifically with individuals who use sexual behavior addictively. For a variety of reasons, most of the reviewed research studied paraphilic subjects and sex offenders. Although the group of sex addicts overlaps with the group of sex offenders, and overlaps even more with the group of paraphilic subjects, these groups are not identical.

Researchers have noted significant comorbidity among different forms of sexual addiction: that is, individuals who engage addictively in one form of sexual behavior are likely also to engage addictively in other forms of sexual behavior. High frequencies of comorbidity have been observed not only within the category of paraphilic sexual addictions, but also between paraphilias and nonparaphilic sexual addictions. A variety of psychiatric disorders have been reported to be comorbid with sexual addiction at a rate that is higher than their prevalence in the general population. The strongest trend that the research reveals is significant comorbidity of sexual addiction with substance dependence and with other addictive disorders, including pathologic gambling, bulimia, and compulsive buying. Significant comorbidity between sexual addiction and mood disorders, anxiety disorders, attention-deficit disorder, and personality disorders is indicated by the literature as well.

Etiology

Very little research or theory that addresses sexual addiction has been published. Most of the literature that could be relevant explicitly pertains not to sexual addiction but to paraphilias or perversions. Theories of paraphilias or perversions in this discussion of sexual addiction are included here, partly because at least some components of these theories may be applicable also to sexual addiction, and partly because limiting the discussion to theories that were developed specifically to account for sexual addiction would result in an unsatisfyingly brief and narrow discussion. Sexual addiction differs from paraphilia and perversion in that it can occur with behaviors that are socioculturally normal, and in its inclusion of impaired control as one of its defining characteristics. The group of all individuals with sexual addictions and the group of all individuals with paraphilias or perversions overlap, but are not identical.

Biologic Theories

Contemporary biologic approaches to understanding sexual addiction or paraphilias focus on the brain. Some earlier theories had attributed paraphilias to abnormalities of androgen metabolism, but reviews conclude that research results have provided little support for these theories. Brain-oriented approaches can be divided into two groups, one that emphasizes brain anatomy and another that emphasizes brain chemistry. Most studies of the relationship between hypersexual or paraphilic behavior and brain anatomy have focused on the temporal lobes. Temporal lobe epilepsy may be associated with changes in sexual behavior. Most often the results are impotence and loss of libido. However, in other cases, libido increases and, in some individuals with epilepsy, paraphilic or hypersexual behavior appears. The sexual behaviors that have been most frequently associated with epilepsy are fetishism and transvestism, although a wide range of sexual behavior anomalies has been reported.

The biologic approaches that emphasize brain chemistry consider sexual addiction to be part of a "spectrum" of disorders that share a number of clinically significant features. It has been hypothesized that these disorders are parts of obsessive–compulsive or affective disorder spectrums, and that the primary neurobiologic abnormality that is associated with the disorders is a disturbance of the serotonin system. The spectrum disorder theories enhance our understanding of sexual addiction and its relationship to other psychiatric disorders. However, they say little about what actually occurs in the brain of a sex addict, and even less about how sexual addiction differs neurobiologically from other disorders in its spectrum or about how sexual addiction develops.

Sociocultural Theories

A number of publications have addressed the sociocultural contribution to the etiology of sexual aggression from a feminist perspective. They describe the male-centered, power-oriented structure of our society; they identify relationships between sexual aggression and social attitudes toward women; and they criticize the social acceptance and the prevalence of sexual aggression in various forms. Although these characteristics of our society are likely to be correlated with a significant prevalence of sexual aggression against women, such correlations do not necessarily indicate the nature of the relevant causal relationships. Moreover, although almost all males in our society are exposed to much of the same array of sociocultural messages, images, and attitudes, only a limited number of men engage in sexually aggressive behaviors. Sociocultural factors undoubtedly foster and shape the expression of sexually aggressive behavior. However, an adequate understanding of the development of sexual aggression in some, but not all, men in our sociocultural milieu requires that other, more specific factors be considered.

Another perspective is the relationship between addiction in general and the technologic orientation of our society, which idealizes control and promotes a reliance on external, material things that we believe we can control as a means of solving our inner emotional and spiritual problems. These sociocultural hypotheses do not address why some individuals in our society develop clinically significant addictive disorders but most do not.

In short, although sociocultural factors are critical determinants of how sexuality is expressed and of how normal sexual behavior is defined, they are of limited utility in explaining sexual aggression, perversion, or addiction in general. Nonetheless, sociocultural factors are worthy of attention and study.

Sexual Addiction and Childhood Sexual Abuse

The relationship between sexual addiction and childhood sexual abuse has been the focus of considerable attention. For example, it has been found that 39% of 160 male sex addicts and 63% of 24 female sex addicts reported having been sexually abused, as compared to 8% of 78 nonaddicted men and 20% of 98 nonaddicted women. The trend of the research seems to support the claim that childhood sexual abuse is more common in the histories of sex addicts than it is in the general population.

Cognitive–Behavioral Theories

A number of investigators have proposed psychologic theories of sexual addiction, which they identify as cognitive–behavioral. These theories actually go beyond cognitive–behavioral psychology and incorporate elements of social learning, family systems, and psychodynamic approaches, as well as cognitive and behavioral theories.

Psychoanalytic Theories

The psychoanalytic literature includes more material that pertains to sexual addiction than does the literature of all other areas of psychiatry and psychology combined. Although some of the literature was written about driven heterosexual genital intercourse or pathologic hypersexuality—often referred to in colorful terms such as "Don Juanism" and "nymphomania"—most of it was written about perversions. The underlying processes that writers from different decades and orientations hypothesized to account for perversions not only are fairly consistent with each other; they also are fairly consistent with the underlying processes that were hypothesized to account for pathologic hypersexuality. The psychodynamic and etiologic factors in perversion and pathologic hypersexuality can be grouped in two categories: nonspecific factors that promote the development of addictive patterns in general, and specific factors that foster sexualization and thus promote the development of sexual addiction in particular.

The psychoanalytic literature on alcoholism, drug addiction, bulimia, and pathologic gambling describes the development and dynamics of these other disorders in similar terms. Why might someone develop a perversion, rather than alcoholism or bulimia? The key factor seems to be sexualization. Sexualization is a use of sexual behavior and sexual fantasy in which a person's self-protective or self-preservative functions have greater urgency and significance in the person's motivational hierarchy than does sexual drive gratification. A tendency to rely on sexualization begins in childhood, often in early childhood, and when present in the context of the nonspecific factors that potentiate addictive disorders, it can tilt the balance toward perversion.

Treatment

Medication

Two different kinds of pharmacologic treatment may be used in the treatment of sexual addiction: endocrinologic agents and affect-regulating agents. A number of other medications have side effects of decreased sex drive or erectile dysfunction and are, on occasion, used informally, often by patients on their own initiative and sometimes without informed medical direction, in attempts to reduce the symptoms of sexual addiction. These include antihypertensive agents, anticholinergics, antihistamines, disulfiram, antipsychotic medications, and hair growth stimulants. None of these has been studied for use in controlling sexual fantasies, urges, or behavior.

Endocrinologic Agents

Endocrinologic agents are used primarily to reduce the sex drive in paraphilic men. Those that are in use at this time include antiandrogenic agents and gonadotropin-releasing hormone (GnRH) agonists. Estrogens have been studied for use in controlling sexual behavior, but they were found to have too many undesirable effects to be worthy of consideration.

Medroxyprogesterone acetate (Depo-Provera) and cyproterone acetate are the antiandrogenic agents that are being used in the treatment of paraphilias. The latter is not currently available in the United States. Most reviewers agree that antiandrogenic agents do not by themselves constitute adequate treatment for paraphilias, but that they can be a valuable adjunct to behavior modification, group therapy, or individual psychotherapy with some patients, particularly during early stages of treatment.

Analogues of GnRH have been developed that have higher potency and longer duration of action than does naturally occurring GnRH. Initial administration of these agents raises serum testosterone by stimulating pituitary gonadotrope cells to increase production of luteinizing hormone (LH) and follicle-stimulating hormone (FSH), the former of which then stimulates testicular Leydig cells to synthesize more androgens. However, continuous administration of long-acting GnRH analogues produces down-regulation of GnRH receptors on the pituitary gonadotropes, which leads to a decrease in secretion of LH and FSH, and a consequent decrease in the synthesis of testosterone. Four reports of uncontrolled open-label trials of GnRH agonists in the treatment of paraphilias and hypersexual disorders have demonstrated positive effects.

Although these medications do not change the direction of the paraphilic man's sexual interest, they decrease the intensity of his sexual drive, so he is more in control and less likely to act on his paraphilic interest. Their primary therapeutic function is to reduce the sex drive to manageable levels in those individuals whose ability to control their behavioral impulses is so impaired that they are at risk either to injure themselves or others, or to render them unresponsive to psychologic interventions.

Affect-Regulating Agents

A number of reports have provided evidence for the efficacy of affect-regulating agents (primarily antidepressants) in the treatment of paraphilias, even in patients who are not suffering from a major affective disorder. Agents that have been found to be effective include fluoxetine, sertraline, paroxetine, fluvoxamine, nefazodone, imipramine, desipramine, clomipramine, lithium, buspirone, and electroconvulsive therapy. Most studies report a positive response rate in the range of 50% to 90%. Although antidepressant medications, especially the serotonin reuptake inhibitors, can produce decreased libido as a side effect, a number of the studies noted that antidepressants reduced the drive for pathologic sexual behavior, but not the drive for healthy sexual behavior. Such a large number of positive findings is encouraging, but the confidence with which conclusions can be drawn from them is limited by the paucity of controlled studies.

Behavior Modification

Aversion Conditioning

In aversion conditioning, unwanted patterns of sexual behavior are linked repeatedly with unpleasant stimuli, most often electric shock or foul odors. This classical or pavlovian conditioning procedure is intended to transform stimulus features of the sexual behavior into conditioned stimuli or triggers for the aversive responses to the unpleasant stimuli. A number of uncontrolled studies found that aversion conditioning yielded positive results.

Covert Sensitization

Covert sensitization was developed as an imaginary form of aversion conditioning, in which fantasies of paraphilic arousal are paired with fantasies of aversive events to promote a learned association between paraphilic themes and unpleasant feelings. Patients are first led through a relaxation exercise. They then are instructed to visualize themselves engaging in some aspect of their paraphilic behaviors, and they are encouraged to feel personally involved. At that point, patients are told to imagine either an unpleasant event, such as nausea and vomiting, or an aversive consequence that could follow the behavior in reality, such as public humiliation or shame at being discovered. The aversive valence of the imagined noxious scene can be reinforced by the presentation of a nauseating odor. Studies have found covert sensitization to be effective in the treatment of exhibitionism and pedophilia.

Masturbatory Training

Masturbatory training attempts to shift paraphilic patients' arousal patterns in the conventional direction by controlling the fantasies or visual stimuli that they experience while masturbating. The two main forms of masturbatory training are satiation and fading. Satiation involves instructing male patients to masturbate to orgasm with conventional sexual stimuli or fantasies, and then to continue masturbating while visualizing their deviant objects. The idea is that masturbating after orgasm will extinguish erotic arousal to paraphilic fantasies. In the fading technique, paraphilic patients' fantasies are gradually shifted from deviant to conventional during periods of sexual arousal.

Imaginal Desensitization

The technique of imaginal desensitization is based on the theory that, once an individual has developed a sequence of sexual activity that begins with a sexual thought or fantasy and ends with overt behavior, interruption of the sequence results in anxiety, which then motivates completion of the sequence. Imaginal desensitization uses systematic desensitization to diminish the anxiety that is aroused by interruption of that sequence. The procedure begins with patients describing a scene in which they are stimulated to carry out the sexual activities for which they sought treatment. After relaxation is induced, the patient visualizes performing a sequence of behaviors that leads to noncompletion of the act. Relaxation is allowed to develop with each visualized behavior before the patient proceeds to the next behavior in the sequence. The patient is thus trained to visualize not completing the sexual act, while remaining relaxed.

Cognitive–Behavioral Therapies

Cognitive Behavioral Therapy consists of a structured, intensive program that in many ways resembled a traditional chemical-dependency treatment program. A series of lectures and workshops were interwoven with group therapies and homework assignments. The program incorporated principles and methods from the 12-step approach, and participants were encouraged to regularly attend meetings of a 12-step fellowship for recovering sex addicts after they had completed the program. The program also involved members of sex addicts' families, who were invited to participate in special lectures and groups. Finally, the program included relapse prevention techniques. Participants were guided in compiling an inventory of their relapse risk factors, and then in preparing for what could be done before a slip, during a slip, and after a slip had occurred. They learned to anticipate "triggers" that could precipitate a slip, and to devise a series of action steps that could serve to prevent a slip from occurring.

Therapeutic Groups

Many clinicians believe that group therapy and self-help groups are the most effective modalities for the treatment of individuals who use sexual behavior addictively. The types of therapeutic group that have been employed in treating sex addicts include cognitive–behavioral groups, psychodynamic psychotherapy groups, and support groups. Although group therapy can range from highly structured to relatively unstructured, most investigators have concluded that individuals who use sexual behavior addictively seem to do best in groups that are at least moderately structured.

The most widespread and easy-to-access therapeutic groups for individuals who use sexual behavior addictively are the 12-step groups that are based on the model of Alcoholics Anonymous and adapted for sexual addiction. Four 12-step fellowships of recovering sex addicts have been developed: Sex Addicts Anonymous (SAA), Sex and Love Addicts Anonymous (SLAA), Sexaholics Anonymous (SA), and Sexual Compulsives Anonymous (SCA). The primary differences between the four fellowships are in their definitions of sobriety. Sobriety in SAA is defined as no "out-of-bounds" sex. Sex addicts identify the sexual behaviors that are likely to lead to harmful consequences, and then define "boundaries" that exclude these behaviors. In SLAA, sobriety is similarly defined as no "bottom-line" sex: "Define your bottom-line behavior . . . any sexual or emotional act which, once engaged in, leads to loss of control over rate, frequency, or duration of its recurrence, resulting in worsening self-destructive consequences." Sobriety in SA is more strictly defined as no sexual activity other than with a spouse. In SCA, members are encouraged to define sexual sobriety for themselves and to develop sexual recovery plans that are consistent with their own values. The differences between the 12-step fellowships may, however, be less important than the differences between individual groups, and the characteristics of a particular group are determined primarily by the individuals who attend it.

Couple and Family Therapy

The inclusion of couple or family therapy in the treatment of sexual addiction is recommended by psychiatric and psychoanalytic clinicians. Both the cognitive–behaviorally oriented therapists and the psychodynamically oriented therapists, while noting that couple or family therapy can be important in the treatment of sexual addiction, accorded it a supplemental or adjunctive status.

Psychodynamic Psychotherapy

A number of psychoanalytically oriented clinicians have stated that intensive psychodynamic psychotherapy is the treatment of choice for paraphilias. Significantly, researchers who were not primarily oriented toward psychodynamic psychotherapy have observed that the beneficial effect of antidepressant medications in sexual addiction *may only be seen in combination with intensive psychotherapy*, and that the success of behavioral treatments depends to a great extent on the relationship between the patient and the therapist and on how the issues that emerge in the context of this relationship are managed.

The primary focus of psychodynamic treatment is on patients' character pathology, rather than on their pathologic behavior. All the investigators who recommended psychodynamic psychotherapy qualified their recommendations with statements to the effect that the general criteria of suitability for psychodynamic psychotherapy apply to sex addicts as well.

Integrated Treatment

Many investigators have concluded that no single treatment is effective for all patients with paraphilia, and that the best approach for most patients seems to be to provide individually tailored combinations of behavioral, psychosocial, psychodynamic, and pharmacologic modalities. A number of clinicians have presented programs for treating sexual addiction that combine two or more therapeutic modalities. Interestingly, multimodality programs with a cognitive–behavioral core were usually described by their authors as "cognitive–behavioral," whereas multiple-modality programs with a psychodynamic core were described as "integrated."

Relapse Prevention and Other Cognitive–Behavioral Techniques

Relapse prevention consists of three primary components: risk management, urge coping, and slip handling. Relapse-prevention strategies help people who use sexual behavior addictively (a) to recognize factors and situations that are associated with an increased risk of acting out sexually, (b) to cope more effectively with sexual urges, (c) to recover rapidly from episodes of symptomatic behavior, and (d) to use such "slips" as opportunities to learn about how their recovery plans can be improved. "Risk management" teaches the person who uses sexual behavior addictively to be aware of factors that increase the likelihood of symptomatic sexual behavior, and to recognize these factors before they overwhelm an ability to cope with them. "Urge-coping" skills are behavioral and cognitive skills that help people who use sexual behavior addictively to manage these urges without lapsing into symptomatic behavior. "Slip-handling" skills are developed to prevent progression to relapse after an episode of symptomatic sexual behavior, or a slip, has occurred.

Cognitive–behavioral techniques other than relapse prevention have a variable role in the treatment of sexual addiction, depending on the addict's needs and limitations. They comprise directive or didactic procedures that focus not on the symptomatic sexual behavior itself, but on other aspects of a person's life that predispose to reliance on symptomatic behavior as a means of coping with painful affects and unmet needs. Applicable cognitive–behavioral techniques may be divided into two groups: skills training, which helps patients to learn thoughts and behaviors that will result in more effective management of their affects and meeting of their needs (e.g., anger management, assertiveness training), and lifestyle regeneration, which helps patients learn to achieve and maintain a healthy, balanced lifestyle.

Therapeutic Groups

Therapeutic groups can facilitate the development of abilities to make meaningful connections with others and to turn to people in times of need instead of turning to addictive behavior. Treatment in groups is particularly helpful for relapse prevention and for other cognitive–behavioral techniques. Therapeutic groups can provide a variety of beneficial processes, including support, commonality (the "I'm not the only one" experience), empathic bonding, group cohesiveness, and sense of belonging. They also can offer opportunities to learn interpersonal skills while receiving feedback, to develop social confidence, to learn vicariously by identifying with others in the group, and to help others. In therapeutic groups, the emotional energy of the interpersonal connection and consequent transference responses are typically weaker and more diffuse than they are in individual psychotherapy. One consequence of this difference is that character healing is more likely to occur in individual psychodynamic psychotherapy than it is in therapeutic groups, and closeness is likely to be less intense in therapeutic groups than in individual psychotherapy. As a result, groups can often be more rapidly effective than is individual therapy in supplementing members' impaired self-care and self-governance functions.

Unfortunately, treatment groups for sex addicts are typically feasible only in larger clinics or in association with treatment centers, hospitals, or other institutions. Independent practitioners are more likely to integrate relapse prevention and other cognitive–behavioral techniques into individual psychotherapy. Meanwhile, 12-step groups for individuals who use sexual behavior addictively are readily available across the United States and in other countries as well. Such 12-step groups can potentially provide all of the beneficial effects of therapeutic groups. In addition, they offer membership at no charge for as long as a person wishes, round-the-clock support, and connection with a worldwide support network. They present a coherent framework for approaching addictive problems and life in general, including honesty with self and acceptance of limitations.

Treatment Organization and Course of Recovery

Treatment for sexual addiction is most likely to be effective when the treatment plan for each person is individually tailored and evolves as he or she progress through recovery. Recovery from sexual addiction is a developmental process that can be understood to proceed in four overlapping stages: stage I, initial behavior modulation; stage II, stabilization (of behavior and affect); stage III, character healing; and stage IV, self-renewal. Of course, this schema of stages is a heuristic device that oversimplifies the picture. Behavior, affect, character, and self are interrelated dimensions of a person that are together involved at all points in the developmental process. In general, the more concrete and directive treatment modalities (behavior modification, psychiatric pharmacotherapy, cognitive–behavioral therapy) tend to be more prominent during the earlier phases of recovery, whereas the more exploratory, interpersonal, and existential modalities (psychodynamic psychotherapy and spiritual regeneration) tend to be more prominent during the middle and later phases.

Prognosis

Although the long-term response of sexual addiction to various types of treatment cannot at this time be reliably predicted, a number of factors have been identified that seem to influence the prognosis. These factors can be clustered in three groups: (a) illness factors (that tend to worsen the prognosis), which include early age of onset, high frequency of symptomatic sexual behavior, concomitant use of alcohol or other drugs, and absence of anxiety or guilt about the behavior; (b) recovery support factors (that tend to improve the prognosis), which include a stable job, a stable primary relationship, a supportive social network, and availability of appropriate sexual outlets; and (c) personality factors (that tend improve the prognosis), which include intelligence, creativity, self-observatory capacity, sense of humor, capacity to form interpersonal connections, and motivation for change. Prognosis is influenced also by comorbidity with other psychiatric disorders, by the degree of associated character pathology, and by the kind of relationship that develops between the patient and the therapist.

Significant recovery from sexual addiction, as from any other addictive disorder, requires a considerable period of time. Addiction interferes with normal development and corrodes interpersonal relationships. These problems remain after the addictive behavior has ceased, and only then can they begin to be addressed. However much they may have benefited from treatment, most addicts (of any behavioral type) will to some extent remain vulnerable to being overwhelmed by intense affects and loss of self-coherence in situations that would be neither traumatic nor disorganizing for individuals whose self-regulation systems are intact. And sex addicts are particularly likely to experience threats of being overwhelmed by these internal states as urges to engage in sexual behavior. Even after stable recovery has been achieved, ongoing maintenance activity may be required indefinitely to prevent relapse. Sexual addiction is not an acute disease that effective treatment can cure, but a chronic disease that effective treatment can, with the patient's active collaboration, bring into and keep in remission.

Suggested Readings

Black DW. The epidemiology and phenomenology of compulsive sexual behavior. *CNS Spectr.* 2000;5:26–35.

Goodman A. Sexual addiction: nosology, diagnosis, etiology, and treatment. In: Lowinson JH, Ruiz P, Millman RB, et al., eds. *Substance abuse: a comprehensive textbook,* 4th ed. Philadelphia: Lippincott Williams & Wilkins; 2005:504–539.

Goodman A. What's in a name? Terminology for designating a syndrome of driven sexual behavior. *Sex Addict Compulsivity.* 2001;8:191–214.

Kafka M. Psychopharmacologic treatments for nonparaphilic compulsive sexual disorders. *CNS Spectr.* 2000;1:49–59.

Section IV

EVALUATION AND DIAGNOSTIC CLASSIFICATION

CLASSIFICATION, DIAGNOSIS, AND DIAGNOSTIC LABORATORY

The *Diagnostic and Statistical Manual of Mental Disorders*, 4th ed, text revision (DSM-IV-TR) is the diagnostic classification system developed by the American Psychiatric Association. The *International Classification of Disease, Tenth Revision (ICD-10)* is the system used by the World Health Organization. The substance use disorders sections of previous iterations of each classification system differed significantly from each other, though many of the concepts they contained were similar. As a result, considerable efforts were made to make the current versions of these two systems as similar as possible and these efforts were mostly successful. ICD-10 actually has two versions: the clinical and the research. The clinical version is the manual that is used in clinical practice.

Overview

Psychiatric disorders attributable to abusable substances are of two general types: (a) disorders related to the pattern and/or consequences of substance use itself—that is, dependence, abuse (in DSM-IV-TR), and harmful use (in ICD-10)—and (b) disorders produced by the pharmacologic effects of the substances themselves (i.e., intoxication, withdrawal, and substance-induced mental disorders). A major accomplishment of DSM-IV was to place all these disorders into one section, "Substance Related Disorders," consisting of two parts: "Substance Use Disorders," which includes dependence and abuse, and "Substance-Induced Disorders," which includes intoxication, withdrawal, and substance-induced mental disorders. This major change in the organization of DSM-IV, retained in the DSM-IV-TR, has made their overall organization much more similar to that of ICD-10.

Dependence and Its Course Modifiers, Abuse, and Harmful Use

Dependence

DSM-IV-TR has seven criteria items for dependence, and ICD-10 has six. In each classification system, three items are necessary to make a diagnosis of dependence. Specific items are ordered differently in each system.

In DSM-IV-TR, dependence is specified as existing either with or without physiologic features. Dependence with physiologic features is present if there is evidence of tolerance or withdrawal (i.e., criterion item 1 or 2 is present). Dependence without physiologic features is present if three or more items are present but none of these is item 1 or 2. There is no comparable subtyping of dependence in ICD-10.

Both DSM-IV-TR and ICD-10 include course modifiers for dependence. DSM-IV expanded the limited number of course modifiers that were present in DSM-III-R, again resulting in greater consistency between DSM-IV-TR and ICD-10. The course modifiers for both classification systems apply only to dependence and not to abuse or harmful use.

DSM-IV-TR

DSM-IV-TR organizes its course modifiers in terms of stage of remission, agonist therapy, or being in a controlled environment.

REMISSION

A person is not classified as being in remission until that person has been free of all criteria items for dependence and all the "A" items for abuse for at least 1 month. The first 12 months following cessation of problems with the substance is a period of particularly high risk for relapse; thus it is given the special designation of "Early Remission." There are two categories:

- *Early Full Remission:* No criteria for dependence, and none of the "A" criteria for abuse, have been met for the last 1 to 12 months.
- *Early Partial Remission:* Full criteria for dependence or abuse have not been met for the last 1 to 12 months; however, one or two dependence, or one or more of the "A" abuse criteria have been met, intermittently or continuously, during this period of Early Remission.

When 12 months of Early Remission have passed without relapse to dependence, the person is in "Sustained Remission." There are two categories:

- *Sustained Full Remission:* None of the criterion items for dependence and none of the criterion items for abuse have been present in the last 12 months.
- *Sustained Partial Remission:* Full criteria for dependence have not been met for a period of 12 months or longer. However, one or two dependence, or one or more of the "A" criteria for abuse have been met, either continuously or intermittently, during this period of Sustained Remission.

ON AGONIST THERAPY

The person is on prescribed, supervised agonist medication related to the substance, and the criteria for dependence or abuse (other than tolerance or withdrawal) have not been met for the agonist medication in the last month.

This category also applies to persons being treated for dependence using an agonist/antagonist with prominent agonist properties.

IN A CONTROLLED ENVIRONMENT

No criteria for dependence or abuse are met but the person has been in an environment for 1 month or longer where controlled substances are highly restricted.

Examples are closely supervised and substance-free jails, therapeutic communities, or locked hospital units. Occasionally, persons will be on agonist therapy while also in a controlled environment. In such cases, both course modifiers apply.

ICD-10

The course modifiers for ICD are similar but not identical and are as follows:

- Currently abstinent
- Currently abstinent, but in a protected environment (e.g., hospital)
- Currently on a clinically supervised maintenance or replacement regime (controlled dependence) (e.g., with methadone, nicotine gum, or nicotine patch)
- Currently abstinent, but receiving treatment with aversive or blocking drugs, for example, naltrexone (Narcan) or disulfiram (Antabuse)
- Currently using the substance [active dependence]
- Continuous use
- Episodic use [dipsomania]

After publication of the ICD-10 clinical criteria, the ICD-10 research criteria were published. The section on course modifiers in the research criteria were made even more similar to those of DSM-IV-TR.

Abuse and Harmful Use

Although the current ICD and the DSM definitions of dependence are very similar, they differ sharply on the concepts of abuse and harmful use. In DSM-IV-TR, abuse is defined in social terms, that is, problematic use in the absence of compulsive use, tolerance, and withdrawal. ICD has been reluctant to accept criteria items that are defined in terms of social impairment. However, ICD does recognize a nondependent type of substance use disorder. In ICD-10, this disorder is called "Harmful Use" and involves substance use that results in actual physical or mental damage.

Four DSM-IV criteria items were developed for abuse. One (hazardous use) had been part of earlier definitions. Another (use resulting in failure to fulfill role obligations) was moved from a DSM-III-R dependence criterion item to abuse. The third and fourth items (recurrent substance-related legal problems; continued use despite having recurrent social or interpersonal problems) were split from one DSM-III-R dependence item and moved to abuse. Portions of that original item (recurrent substance-related medical or psychiatric problems) remained in a DSM-IV dependence item. Because diagnostic criteria did not change from DSM-IV to DSM-IV-TR, the operationalization of abuse is the same for both.

Substance-Induced Disorders

As described above, intoxication, withdrawal, and the wide range of substance-induced mental disorders are included in a single section in both DSM-IV-TR and ICD-10. DSM-IV-TR provides a brief description of the clinical manifestations of intoxication and withdrawal for each substance; exceptions are those few substances that do not have an identified withdrawal syndrome, such as lysergic acid diethylamide (LSD). ICD-10 provides less detail about each substance but provides general criteria that allow for classification of intoxication or withdrawal according to specific substances.

Comparisons of Differences in Specific Diagnostic Categories

There are a few other important categories that are found in one system but not the other. For instance, DSM-IV-TR has three categories that are not specified in ICD-10: "Polysubstance Dependence," "Other (or Unknown) Substance-Related Disorders," and "Phencyclidine (or Phencyclidine-Like)-Related Disorders." These categories would likely be classified under the ICD-10 heading of "Disorders Resulting from Multiple Drug Use and Use of Other Psychoactive Substances."

ICD-10 has a section (listed as a subsection of "Behavioural Syndromes Associated with Physiological Disturbances and Physical Factors") that is separate from the psychoactive substance use section and that is used for classifying abuse of nondependence-producing substances. This includes problematic use of antidepressants, laxatives, steroids, and hormones. A comparable section in DSM-IV-TR is found under "Other (or Unknown) Substance-Related Disorders."

Diagnostic Laboratory

Alcohol and drug abuse are two major health care problems in America. This has prompted advancement in laboratory methods diagnosing substance abuse in psychiatric patients and suspected drug abusers. Physicians are more knowledgeable today than in the past about the nature of drug abuse, yet uncertainty remains in the use of the diagnostic laboratory. The confusion surrounding drug abuse testing is a result of many variables. Each individual drug is unique, and detectability depends on the type of drug, size of the dose, frequency of use, the type of biologic specimen tested, differences in individual drug metabolism, sample collection time in relation to use, and sensitivity of the analytical method. All these variables make each test request an individual case, and there are no general rules for all drugs and all situations.

Rationale for Testing

Treatment of drug abusers in therapy would be extremely handicapped if testing were not used. Therefore, comprehensive drug testing is important for making precise follow-up evaluations and selecting appropriate treatment. Testing is also important after drug abusers are identified. Treatment strategies are intimately connected to frequent urinalyses to monitor recovering addicts. Negative results support the success of treatment, whereas positive results alert the physician to relapses. Objective testing, therefore, is a necessary component of modern treatment. Drug abuse testing may also be forensic in nature. Parole officers monitor ex-drug abusers after release from incarceration. A positive drug test may signal to law enforcement the parolee's involvement with drugs and may invalidate the parole.

Health professionals such as doctors, dentists, and nurses are afflicted with drug abuse problems. Once involvement with drugs is exposed, professional medical licenses are in danger of suspension. Rehabilitation of addicted health professionals is linked to drug testing as a condition of probation.

Professional athletes often abuse drugs. Staying drug-free is often a prerequisite for athletes to be allowed to compete. Laboratory testing of body fluids for drugs of abuse is the objective technique used to enforce these rules.

Finally, the conduct of business and the public's safety may be endangered by impaired or intoxicated employees. Bankers and stockbrokers who handle investors' money should not be influenced by drugs, especially psychoactive drugs. Drug abuse has been identified among airline pilots, bus drivers, railroad engineers, and police officers. In all these examples, drug abuse testing is advantageous to the drug abuser and the general public.

Abused Drugs Tested

Epidemiologic studies expose the types of drugs used, new trends, and frequency of drug abuse by different populations in specific geographic regions and countries. In effective drug abuse testing, such information is used to help identify drug abusers. The testing of five drugs, selected by the Department of Health and Human Services Substance Abuse and Mental Health Services Administration (DHHS/SAMHSA), is required for accreditation by its National Laboratory Certification Program (NLCP). Panel I testing includes amphetamines, cannabinoids, cocaine, opioids, and phencyclidine. Panel II represents other commonly abused drugs, such as barbiturates, benzodiazepines, methaqualone, propoxyphene, methadone, and ethanol. Interestingly, some powerful hallucinogens seldom are tested routinely. They are listed in Panel III: LSD, methylenedioxyamphetamine (MDA), methylenedioxymethamphetamine (MDMA), psilocybin, and other designer drugs. These drugs are psychoactive in very low doses. Therefore, when they are diluted in total body water, detection is difficult or impossible unless large doses are taken or samples are collected immediately after drug use.

"Designer drugs" are structural congeners of common drugs of abuse. Often they are not yet regulated when sold and used. "Street chemists" occasionally synthesize new and often dangerous drugs. They will operate as long as abusers will try new drugs and their trade remains profitable. The laboratory's role is to develop sensitive methods for the detection of designer drugs in the biofluids of users.

Club Drugs of Abuse

γ-hydroxybutyrate (GHB) is a central nervous system depressant. It is an endogenous substance in human and mammalian tissues at very low concentrations and thought to be a neurotransmitter. It had some clinical use as an anesthetic and hypnotic drug in the past, but now it is used only in research. Some of the pharmacologic effects are amnesia and hypotonia and, at large doses, sleep. This drug is used in date rapes for its amnesia-producing effects. The perpetrator hopes that the victim will have no recollection of the sexual attack after the drug wears off. Detection of GHB is accomplished with analysis by gas chromatography (GC) and/or high-pressure liquid chromatography (HPLC).

Another drug used in clubs and date rapes is flunitrazepam (Rohypnol) a member of the benzodiazepine family of drugs. At low doses it causes sleepiness, and at larger doses, anesthesia. Detection, as for several other benzodiazepines, is performed by screening with an immunoassay and confirmation with GC-mass spectrometry (GC-MS) or HPLC.

Recently ketamine (Ketalar) or "Special K" appeared in clubs. It is chemically related to phencyclidine (PCP) or "angel dust". Both of these drugs were used as rapidly acting dissociative anesthetics. However, in some individuals ketamine and PCP produce exit psychosis with paranoid ideation. Abuse of ketamine results in a diverse set of reactions depending on individual predispositions: numbness, loss of coordination, sense of invulnerability, muscle rigidity, aggressive/violent behavior, slurred speech, blank stare, and an exaggerated sense of strength. Recently, immunoassays were developed for ketamine screening. Positive results are confirmed by GC-MS or GC-tandem mass spectrometry (GC-MS-MS).

Tests Available

Different laboratories have different definitions of the term "comprehensive drug testing." The physician should be familiar with laboratory procedures and menus to ensure effective use of the drug-testing laboratory.

Urine samples are most commonly sent for "routine drug screen." But oral fluid (saliva) testing is becoming more popular because of the ease of collection. Thin-layer chromatography (TLC), mostly used in the past, is not sensitive enough to detect drugs such as marijuana, PCP, LSD, MDA, MDMA, mescaline, fentanyl, among others. Thus, a negative drug screen may mean that the test cut off is too high, the test menu does not contain the drug(s) of interest, or there is no evidence of high-doses and/or recent abuse of drugs commonly detected by the screening method used. Low-level abuse of drugs is not likely to be detected; therefore, "false negatives" are very common for drug screens performed by TLC. More recently enzyme immunoassays (EIA) have replaced TLC as a screening procedure. EIA, enzyme-linked immunoabsorbent assay (ELISA), and fluorescent polarization immunoassay (FPIA) are routinely used with biologic fluids screening such as urine, oral fluid, sweat, and hair.

Currently, screening for prescription drugs and drugs of abuse is performed by EIA, such as the enzyme multiplied immunoassay test (EMIT), ELISA, radioimmunoassay (RIA), or FPIA, and a modern version of TLC, high-performance TLC (HPTLC), which has improved sensitivity over that of conventional TLC systems. In a very few laboratories, drug screening is performed by capillary gas-liquid chromatography (GLC). In a single GLC analysis more than 25 drugs can be identified. This system is advantageous when there is no clue to the identity of the abused substance; however, GLC, HPTLC, and GC-MS are time-consuming, labor-intensive, and usually expensive procedures. In fact, most good laboratories offer a 5-drug or 10-drug panel, with or without alcohol, performed by EIA.

Analytic Methodologies
Alcohol Methods of Analysis

Ethanol is one of the few drugs for which blood levels can be correlated with levels of intoxication or impairment, although large individual variations do exist. Ethanol is analyzed by means of chemical assays and enzymatic and GLC methods. The most specific quantitative method for blood alcohol determination is GLC or "head space" analysis by GLC.

If ethanol analysis is performed on breath by means of a Breathalyzer, or on blood or urine by one of the chemical or enzymatic assays, the results are reliable for general use. Some states allow Breathalyzer results, as acceptable values, to determine legal impairment in driving accidents. In most forensic cases, however, results should be confirmed with a blood specimen using the GLC "head space" method. For clinical purposes, urine alcohol levels can be ordered. The conversion factor is a 1.3 urine–blood ratio.

Thin-Layer Chromatography

TLC is a qualitative method and is the least-sensitive analytic technique for most drugs. Visualization of the spots on TLC is achieved by illumination with ultraviolet or fluorescent lights, or by color reactions of the spots after spraying with chemical dyes.

Radioimmunoassay, Enzyme Immunoassay, and Enzyme-Linked Immunoabsorbent Assay

Antibodies are used to seek out specific drugs in biofluids. In samples containing one or more drugs, competition exists for available antibody-binding sites. The presence or absence of specific drugs is determined by the percent binding.

The specificity and sensitivity of the antibodies to a given drug differ depending on the particular drug assay and the assay manufacturer. Immunoassay can be very specific; however, compounds structurally similar to the drug of interest (i.e., metabolites or structural congeners) often cross-react. Interaction of the antibody with a drug plus its metabolites increases the sensitivity of the assay.

EIA, ELISA, and FPIA are commonly used for drug abuse screening because no complicated extraction is required and the system lends itself to easy automation. EIA is more sensitive for most drugs and detects lower drug concentrations than TLC.

ELISA offers greater sensitivity than some other screening assays. A variety of biologic samples are applicable to ELISA assays such as urine, serum/plasma/blood, and oral fluid or saliva. Depending on the concentration of drug expected in the specimen, sample size can be adjusted accordingly. ELISA assays are available for manual, semiautomated, and fully automated platforms. Analysis time varies between 1 and 2 hours. Cut off levels and limits of detection (LOD) for saliva samples are very low compared with conventional immunoassays: amphetamines 50 ng/mL and 1 ng/mL, respectively; barbiturates 20 ng/mL and 1 ng/mL, respectively; benzodiazepines 5 ng/mL and 2 ng/mL, respectively; cocaine 20 ng/mL and 1 ng/mL, respectively; methadone 5 ng/mL and 1 ng/mL, respectively; opiates 40 ng/mL and 0.25 ng/mL, respectively; PCP 10 ng/mL and 0.5 ng/mL, respectively; tetrahydrocannabinol (THC) 4 ng/mL and 0.1 ng/mL. Also sample volumes are as low as 10 μL per analysis.

The scientific literature supports oral fluid as an excellent alternative to urine and blood for the identification of drug abuse. Because oral fluid collection is convenient, noninvasive, fast, and observable, sample adulteration is not likely to occur.

On-Site Screening Immunoassays

Rapid results are useful for monitoring psychiatric patients, monitoring compliance within a drug rehabilitation program, and supervising parolees. Because these tests are designed to be performed on-site, they may be performed directly in front of the person being tested or, certainly, at the site of collection. This is particularly useful for pre-employment screening, random or probable cause workplace testing, and for workplace accident-related injuries. It may also be important to conduct drug testing on-site in safety-oriented occupations, such as public transportation.

Visually interpreted competitive immunoassays that require no instrumentation have been developed in recent years. These kits are particularly effective because there is no calibration, maintenance, or downtime required, and no special skills are needed to perform these tests.

Gas-Liquid Chromatography and Gas Chromatography-Mass Spectrometry

GLC is an analytic technique that separates molecules by migration as described for TLC.

Not all bonds in molecules are of equal strength. The weak bonds are more likely to break under stress. In the mass spectrometer detector, electron beam bombardment of molecules breaks weak bonds. The exact mass and quantity of the molecular fragments or breakage products are measured by the mass detector. The breakage of molecules results in fragments unique for a drug. They occur in specific ratios to one another; thus the GC-MS method is often called "molecular fingerprinting." GC-MS is the most reliable, most definitive procedure in analytic chemistry for drug identification.

The sensitivity of GLC for most drugs is in the nanogram range, but with special detectors some compounds can be measured at picogram levels. GLC and GC-MS can also be used quantitatively, which provides additional information helping to interpret a clinical syndrome or explain corroborating evidence in forensic cases. MS-MS offers greater sensitivity than GC-MS.

HPLC is used especially for drugs that are not volatile or that cannot be made volatile by derivatization. These drugs are not amenable to analysis by GC-MS or GC. Examples of drugs or drug groups for which HPLC is the analysis of choice are the benzodiazepines, tricyclic antidepressants, and acetaminophen.

Choice of Body Fluids and Time of Sample Collection

Some drugs are metabolized extensively and are excreted very quickly, whereas others stay in the body for a long time. Thus, success of detection depends not only on the time of sample collection after last use, but also on the drug used and whether the analysis is performed for the drug itself or for its metabolites.

When drug abuse detection is the goal, the following questions should be asked: (a) How long does the suspected drug stay in the body, or, what is its biologic half-life? (b) How fast and how extensively is the drug biotransformed? Should one look for the drug itself or its metabolites? (c) Which body fluid is best for analysis, or, what is the major route of excretion? Intravenous use or smoking drugs of abuse provides nearly instantaneous absorption into the bloodstream and excretion of the drug and/or metabolites in urine occurs almost immediately. Inhalation (smoking or snorting) or oral use of drugs will result in slower absorption and excretion in urine may not be detected immediately after use.

Cocaine is rapidly biotransformed into benzoylecgonine and ecgonine methyl ester. Less than 10% of cocaine is excreted unchanged into the urine and is detectable for only 12 to 18 hours after use. Cocaine metabolism and disposition is contrasted with methaqualone, which is also very lipid soluble but has a half-life of 20 to 60 hours as a consequence of slow biotransformation. Thus, either blood or urine tests are effective for many days to detect methaqualone itself.

The collection of urine specimens must be supervised to ensure donor identity and to guarantee the integrity of the specimen. It is not unusual to receive someone else's urine or a highly diluted sample when collection is not supervised or screened by the laboratory for pH, specific gravity, and creatinine levels. As a rule, first morning urine samples are more concentrated; therefore, drugs are easier to detect than in more diluted samples. The decision to use blood or urine must be based on the information needed and the pharmacokinetic and excretion data of the specific drug. Drug levels in urine are higher than in blood; therefore, urine is usually the biofluid of choice for drug detection.

Interpretation of Results

The psychoactivity of most drugs lasts only a few hours, whereas urinalysis can detect some drugs and/or metabolites for days or even weeks. Thus, the presence of a drug (or metabolite) in urine is only an indication of prior exposure, not proof of intoxication or impairment at the time of sample collection.

Drug analysis reports, either positive or negative, may raise questions about the absolute truth of the results. The usual questions are (a) What method was used? (b) Did the laboratory analyze for the drug only, the metabolite only, or both? (c) What is the cut off value for the assay? and (d) Was the sample time close enough to the suspected drug exposure?

False-negative results occur more easily than false-positive results, mainly because once a test is screened negative it is not tested further. Negative reports based on TLC alone are inconclusive because of a lack of sensitivity.

As technology advances, more drugs and chemicals will be analyzed in biofluids at the nanogram and picogram level. Advancement, however, does not mean that modern methodologies are infallible or that they replace clinical judgment.

Forensic Drug Testing

Forensic drug testing has three components: workplace testing, postmortem testing (medical examiner), and criminal justice (correctional and parole) testing.

Historically, forensic drug testing developed from clinical and pathologic testing. Certified laboratories must be able to prove that positive test results are accurate and reliable and that the tests performed were from the individual listed on the report. Weak links in external or internal chain-of-custody procedures or poor standards or quality control in the testing process provides sufficient ammunition to defense attorneys and expert witnesses to contradict the validity of positive results.

"Workplace testing" is performed on subjects at their place of employment. Many industries and governmental agencies mandate testing of individuals performing critical duties. These places of employment have strict drug policies in place, informing employees that drug abuse is not tolerated and that tests are performed to protect the public interest.

Other forms of forensic drug testing requiring "litigation documentation" are "medicolegal cases" and postmortem analysis of body fluids for the presence of drugs, alcohol, and poisons. Another example of drug testing is in "correctional cases" and testing in the prison system. A very large percentage of prisoners' criminal activity is connected either with drug use or drug trafficking.

Testing Drugs in Saliva, Sweat, and Hair

Most drugs enter saliva by passive diffusion. The major advantages of saliva as a test specimen are that it is readily available, collection is noninvasive, the presence of parent drug is in higher abundance than its metabolites, and a high correlation of saliva drug concentration that can be compared with the free fraction of drug in blood.

Sweat is approximately 99% water and is produced by the body as a heat-regulation mechanism. Because the amount of sweat produced is dependent on environmental temperatures, routine sweat collection is difficult because of a large variation in the rate of sweat production and the lack of adequate sweat collection devices. However, cocaine, morphine, nicotine, amphetamine, ethanol, and other drugs have been identified in sweat. A recently developed "sweat patch" resembles an adhesive bandage and is applied to the skin for a period of several days to several weeks.

Testing for drugs in hair is an alternative method to the drug abuse detection technology. Because of the very low concentrations of drugs incorporated in hair, very sensitive methodology must be used. Screening is performed by RIA with ultrasensitive antibodies, or by ELISA, with confirmation by GC-MS or MS-MS.

Ethical Considerations

Legitimate need for drug abuse testing in the clinical setting is indisputable. Denial makes identification of drug abuse difficult; therefore, testing is necessary both for identification of drug abusers and monitoring of treatment outcome. Drug testing in the workplace and in sports is more controversial because positive test results may be used in termination of long-time employees or refusal to hire new ones.

Civil rights must be respected to protect the innocent. Names of subjects should be known only to the medical office where the sample is collected. Testing must follow strict security and chain-of-custody procedures to ensure anonymity and prevent sample mix-up during testing. Many progressive laboratories have instituted barcode labeling of samples and related documents to ensure confidentiality. Barcoding also improves accuracy of reporting and tracking of samples and records. This system ultimately prevents sample mix-up as a consequence of human error during accessioning and processing.

Before issuing certification, governmental agencies require laboratories to adhere to strict standards in personnel qualifications, experience, quality control, quality assurance programs, chain-of-custody procedures, and multiple data review prior to reporting results.

Two nationally recognized agencies protect the rights of individual citizens by assuring proper procedures in forensic drug testing. DHHS/SAMHSA administers its NLCP and the College of American Pathologists runs its Forensic Toxicology Inspection and Proficiency Program. In addition, numerous state and city regulatory agencies, such as the New York State Health Department, inspect and certify drug-testing laboratories.

Good laboratories are easily identified by having current certificates of qualification issued by national and local regulatory agencies.

Suggested Readings

American Psychiatric Association. *Diagnostic and Statistical Manual of Mental Disorders*, 4th ed. Washington, D.C.: American Psychiatric Association; 1994.

American Psychiatric Association. *Diagnostic and Statistical Manual of Mental Disorders*, 4th ed. text rev. (DSM-IV-TR). Washington, D.C.: American Psychiatric Association; 2000.

Cacciola J, Woody GE. Diagnosis and classification: DSM-IV-TR and ICD-10. In: Lowinson JH, Ruiz P, Millman RB, et al., eds. *Substance abuse: a comprehensive textbook*, 4th ed. Philadelphia: Lippincott Williams & Wilkins; 2005:559–563.

Spiehler V. Hair analysis by immunological methods from the beginning to 2000. *Forensic Sci Int.* 2000;107:249–259.

Verebey KG, Meenan G, Buchan BJ. Diagnostic laboratory: screening for drug abuse. In: Lowinson JH, Ruiz P, Millman RB, et al., eds. *Substance abuse: a comprehensive textbook*, 4th ed. Philadelphia: Lippincott Williams & Wilkins; 2005:564–577.

World Health Organization. *Tenth Revision of the International Classification of Disease (ICD-10)*. Geneva, Switzerland: World Health Organization; 1992.

Section V

TREATMENT MODALITIES

DETOXIFICATION

Withdrawal is recognized for the following groups of substances: alcohol, amphetamines and related substances, cocaine, nicotine, opioids, sedatives, hypnotics, and anxiolytics. As signs and symptoms of withdrawal are generally the opposite of those observed in intoxication with the substance; three diagnostic criteria have been established for substance withdrawal: (a) development of a substance-specific syndrome as a consequence of cessation of (or reduction in) substance use that has been heavy and prolonged; (b) the substance-specific syndrome causes clinically significant distress or impairment in social, occupational, or other important areas of functioning; and (c) the symptoms are not a result of a general medical condition and are not better accounted for by another medical or mental disorder.

Detoxification may take place in either inpatient or outpatient settings. Detoxification, or the achievement of substance-free state, is but the beginning of substance abuse treatment and sustained abstinence from alcohol and drugs. This chapter describes the detoxification process for all of the major substances of abuse and dependence, except for nicotine.

Alcohol Withdrawal

Diagnostic Criteria

The essential feature of alcohol withdrawal is the presence of a characteristic withdrawal syndrome that results after the cessation of (or reduction in) heavy drinking and prolonged alcohol use. According to the *Diagnostic and Statistical Manual of Mental Disorders*, 4th ed., text revision (DSM-IV-TR) criteria, the withdrawal syndrome includes at least two of the following symptoms developing within several hours to a few days after the decline in blood alcohol concentration:

1. Autonomic hyperactivity (e.g., pulse rate >100 beats/minute)
2. Increased hand tremor
3. Insomnia
4. Nausea or vomiting
5. Transient visual, tactile, or auditory hallucinations or illusions
6. Psychomotor agitation
7. Anxiety
8. Grand mal seizures

The DSM-IV-TR diagnostic criteria also require that these symptoms cause clinically significant distress or impairment in social, occupational, or other important areas of functioning. Moreover, these symptoms are not caused by another medical condition or mental disorder. Perceptual disturbances, such as auditory, visual, or tactile illusions in the absence of delirium, may accompany the withdrawal syndrome. Differential diagnoses include withdrawal from anxiolytics or sedative–hypnotics and generalized anxiety disorder.

The milder symptoms appear within hours of cessation or reduction of alcohol consumption and remit over several days to a week. Seizures usually appear within 24 to 48 hours of alcohol withdrawal and are either single or as a series. Approximately 30% of those who experience seizures will experience delirium tremens (DTs), which typically manifest 48 to 72 hours after alcohol withdrawal. The five risk factors significantly correlated with alcohol withdrawal delirium are current infectious disease, tachycardia defined as a heart rate in excess of 120 beats per minute at admission; signs of withdrawal accompanied by an alcohol concentration greater than 1 g/L of body fluid; history of epileptic seizures; and history of delirious episodes. A history of multiple previous detoxifications is associated with more severe alcohol withdrawal symptoms.

Measurement

The use of a rating scale to quantify the alcohol withdrawal syndrome provides valuable clinical information. The ideal scale would aid in the diagnosis of the withdrawal syndrome, indicate when drug therapy is required, alert staff to the development of serious withdrawal symptoms requiring more intensive medical input, and reveal when medication can be discontinued and the patient discharged. The clinical institute withdrawal assessment scale–alcohol (CIWA-A) and an abbreviated version, the CIWA-A revised (CIWA-Ar), are among the best known and studied. The CIWA-Ar is not copyrighted and may be used freely.

Pharmacology

Alcohol affects endogenous opiates and several neurotransmitter systems in the brain, including γ-aminobutyric acid (GABA), glutamate, and dopamine. Pharmacologic management of alcohol withdrawal has been attempted with medications ranging from benzodiazepines, anticonvulsants, barbiturates, and neuroleptics to sympatholytics, and even to alcohol itself. Comprehensive reviews of treatment options have all come to the same conclusion—benzodiazepines are the preferred pharmacologic agents for the treatment of alcohol withdrawal. Benzodiazepines alone reduce withdrawal severity, reduce the incidence of delirium, and reduce seizures.

All benzodiazepines appear to be equally efficacious in the treatment of alcohol withdrawal. Some clinical considerations may be of assistance in selection. For example, short-acting benzodiazepines may have a lower risk of oversedation. Long-acting agents may be more effective in preventing withdrawal seizures and can contribute to a smoother withdrawal with fewer rebound symptoms. Other benzodiazepines may have a higher liability for abuse, such as those with rapid onset of action. The main disadvantage of the benzodiazepines is the risk of subsequent dependency, but that risk should be avoided if their use is confined to the withdrawal period.

Other Treatment Options

Anticonvulsants may be an alternative to benzodiazepines in the treatment of alcohol withdrawal. Advantages are threefold: they do not interact with alcohol, they lack abuse liability, and they ameliorate psychiatric symptoms. However, disadvantages of anticonvulsants include their gastrointestinal and other side effects, rare cytopenias, and unproven efficacy in preventing seizures and treating DTs.

Carbamazepine was found to be superior to placebo and equal in efficacy to barbital and oxazepam for patients with mild to moderate withdrawal in several studies. Moreover, it had no significant hematologic or hepatic toxic effects when used in 7-day protocols for alcohol withdrawal, and it reduced psychiatric distress and hastened the return to work more than oxazepam. When compared in a 5-day protocol using lorazepam, carbamazepine-treated subjects had fewer withdrawal symptoms and less relapse to alcohol use. However, dizziness, vomiting, and nausea were common side effects, particularly at the initial 800-mg dose. Carbamazepine has not been evaluated for treating DTs.

Valproate may also reduce symptoms of alcohol withdrawal, based on several open-label studies, as well as two controlled studies. Two double-blind, randomized studies treated patients for 4 to 7 days on 500 to 1,200 mg of valproate and found fewer seizures, less dropout, less-severe withdrawal, and less use of oxazepam than in patients on placebo or carbamazepine.

Adjuvant Treatments

Except as adjuvant treatments most other agents have poor justification as sole medications during alcohol withdrawal. The phenothiazines and haloperidol reduce signs and symptoms of withdrawal, but are significantly less effective than benzodiazepines in preventing delirium and seizures. β-Adrenergic antagonists and clonidine reduce autonomic manifestations of withdrawal, but have no known anticonvulsant activity. Symptoms of early withdrawal or impending delirium may be masked by propranolol. Centrally acting α-adrenergic agonists, such as clonidine, ameliorate symptoms in patients with mild to moderate withdrawal, but reduction of delirium or seizures is unlikely. These adrenergic agents may be used in conjunction with benzodiazepines for patients with certain co-existing conditions, such as coronary artery disease.

Although neither thiamine nor magnesium will reduce delirium or seizures, each might also be administered as part of the pharmacologic management of alcohol withdrawal. Individuals with alcohol dependence are frequently deficient of both thiamine and magnesium.

Administration of thiamine will prevent Wernicke-Korsakoff syndrome, which includes acute encephalopathy characterized by ataxia, dysarthric, and oculomotor paralysis, and then psychologic symptoms, with anterograde amnesia, confabulation, and some degree of retrograde amnesia. A parenteral dose of thiamine, 100 mg, is given initially and then followed by 50 to 100 mg daily by mouth, for 7 days.

Supplementation with magnesium has also been recommended, particularly for elderly patients. Serum magnesium levels are generally unhelpful when trying to decide if magnesium replacement is needed. Magnesium, 2 to 4 mEq/kg intravenously on day 1, and then 0.5 to mEq/kg orally or intravenously on days 2, 3, and 4, is safe in the absence of renal impairment. Patients with hypomagnesemia are at risk for cardiac dysrhythmias and other nonspecific signs and symptoms such as weakness, tremor, and hyperactive reflexes. In contrast to the administration of thiamine, for which there is consensus, routine administration of magnesium is not uniformly endorsed.

Treatment Regimens

There are three treatment regimens for the management of alcohol withdrawal using benzodiazepines. The regimens are fixed dose, front loading, and symptom triggered.

The fixed-dose method relies on the administration of benzodiazepines at predetermined intervals and doses. An example is chlordiazepoxide, 50 to 100 mg given every 6 hours for the first 24 hours, then 25 to 50 mg every 6 hours for the next 2 days. Additional medication is given if needed. This approach may be particularly suitable for patients with a history of DTs or a history of seizures. Pregnant women or people with acute medical or surgical illness might also be appropriate candidates.

The front-loading method relies on high doses of medication given early in the course of withdrawal. An example is 20 mg of diazepam given every 2 hours until there is resolution of withdrawal symptoms. Usually, three doses are required, but at least one dose should be given if an asymptomatic patient has a history of seizures or an acute medical illness. The use of long-acting benzodiazepines provides a self-tapering effect. This method is more labor-intensive at the outset of treatment, but requires less medication and time than the fixed-dosed approach.

The symptom-triggered method gives each patient an individualized treatment regimen that studies have demonstrated to result in less medication and more rapid withdrawal treatment. An example is the administration of 25 to 100 mg of chlordiazepoxide hourly whenever the patient is symptomatic and has a CIWA-Ar score greater than or equal to 8.

Treatment of Seizures and Delirium Tremens

Uncomplicated alcohol withdrawal seizures do not require the long-term use of antiepileptics. The generalized seizures typically resolve spontaneously and are usually single. Severe or repeated seizures can be treated with intravenous diazepam 5 to 10 mg. The development of DTs requires the constant observation offered in a hospital, as well as active treatment to achieve stabilization. Intravenous diazepam is the most effective and safest treatment regimen for DTs.

Anxiolytic, Sedative, or Hypnotic Withdrawal

Diagnostic Criteria

Commonly abused substances in this class include benzodiazepines. The characteristic withdrawal syndrome is precipitated by a marked decrease or cessation of intake after several weeks or more of regular use. According to the DSM-IV-TR criteria, at least two or more of the following symptoms are manifest:

1. Autonomic hyperactivity (e.g., sweating)
2. Increased hand tremor
3. Insomnia
4. Nausea or vomiting
5. Transient visual, tactile, or auditory hallucinations or illusions

6. Psychomotor agitation
7. Anxiety
8. Grand mal seizures

Withdrawal from anxiolytics, sedatives, or hypnotics produces a syndrome similar to that associated with alcohol withdrawal. Perceptual disturbances should be specified if the transient visual, tactile, or auditory hallucinations occur in the absence of delirium. Of individuals undergoing untreated withdrawal, 20% to 30% will experience grand mal seizures.

The half-life of the substance will generally predict the time course of withdrawal. Substances with a half-life of 10 hours or less will produce withdrawal symptoms 6 to 8 hours after decreasing blood levels. The symptoms will then peak by the next day and improve by the fourth or fifth day. Withdrawal may persist until the second week, and subside by the third or fourth week. Chances for a severe withdrawal are increased if the substance has been used at high doses (more than 40 mg of diazepam daily) for a long time.

Measurement

The CIWA-Ar has been adapted for benzodiazepine withdrawal assessment.

Pharmacology

Benzodiazepines cause an increase of GABA inhibitory impulses in the central nervous system (CNS). The benzodiazepine antagonist flumazenil selectively blocks the central effects of benzodiazepines by competitive interaction at the benzodiazepine receptors.

Treatment

Predictors of withdrawal severity from benzodiazepines include both pharmacologic and clinical variables. Pharmacologic variables that increase the risk of severity are higher daily dose of benzodiazepine, shorter benzodiazepine half-life, longer duration of benzodiazepine therapy, and a rapid taper, particularly in the last half. Clinical variables that increase the severity of withdrawal include diagnosis of panic, higher pretaper levels of anxiety or depression, higher levels of psychopathology, and concomitant abuse or dependence of alcohol or other substances.

If the amount of anxiolytic or sedative–hypnotic is known, and there are no additional complicating factors, it may be possible to offer a medically supervised outpatient taper over the course of 4 or more weeks. This may be most effective for low-dose withdrawal, where patients have exceeded recommended doses on a daily basis for more than 1 month. High-dose withdrawal is considered for patients who have been using more than the equivalent of 40 mg of diazepam daily for 8 months. In this case, the patient is tolerance-tested with diazepam, and if dependent, tapered off medications at the rate of 10% per day in a medically supervised setting. Where patients have significant levels of anxiety or depression prior to initiation of a benzodiazepine taper, other pharmacologic or therapeutic measures should be undertaken while the patient continues to take his or her established benzodiazepine dose. Once levels of psychopathology are reduced, then the taper may begin.

Reduced levels of benzodiazepine may be maintained for several months before the final taper is attempted.

If the dose of a sedative–hypnotic is not known, or if the patient may be using several simultaneously, one strategy may be to offer a pentobarbital challenge test, estimate phenobarbital equivalences for drugs of abuse, and then begin a phenobarbital taper. The details of the pentobarbital challenge test can be summarized as follows. An awake patient is given 200 mg of pentobarbital by mouth and carefully observed. If the patient falls asleep, it is most likely that the patient is not dependent on sedative–hypnotics and the diagnosis revised. If the patient appears intoxicated (with nystagmus, ataxia, dysarthria), then the patient's 6-hour pentobarbital requirement is between 100 and 200 mg. If the patient does not appear to be intoxicated, then a 100-mg pentobarbital challenge can be administered every 2 hours until intoxication is achieved or 500 to 600 mg of pentobarbital is administered. The total pentobarbital dose is calculated and then converted to phenobarbital (100 mg pentobarbital = 30 mg phenobarbital). The patient is then stabilized with a standing dose of phenobarbital for 48 hours, after which point the daily dose is decreased by 30 mg, until detoxification is achieved.

Cocaine and Amphetamine Withdrawal

Diagnostic Criteria

The withdrawal syndrome for both cocaine and amphetamine withdrawal is characterized by the development of dysphoric mood and at least two of the following, according to DSM-IV-TR criteria:

1. Fatigue
2. Vivid, unpleasant dreams
3. Insomnia or hypersomnia
4. Increased appetite
5. Psychomotor agitation or retardation

These developments follow a few hours to a few days after the cessation of or reduction in amphetamine or cocaine use that has been heavy and prolonged. Moreover, these symptoms cause significant distress or impairment in social, occupational, or other important areas of functioning. These symptoms cannot be attributable to another general medical or mental disorder.

An episode of intense, high-dose use of amphetamines or cocaine can be followed by a period of acute withdrawal. The individual may experience intense and unpleasant feelings of lassitude and depression, and may need several days of rest and recuperation. Some may experience suicidal ideation or behavior, which would warrant close observation.

Measurement

The Cocaine Selective Severity Assessment is a measure of cocaine abstinence signs and symptoms. The instrument appears to be helpful in predicting early treatment failure.

Pharmacology

Neural circuits of dopamine-containing and dopamine-receptive neurons are altered functionally after repeated intermittent administration of cocaine and its withdrawal in animal models. The neuroadaptive changes are important because they may relate to addictive or withdrawal states associated with cocaine abuse and suggest targets for the development of medications to treat cocaine dependence.

Treatment

The symptoms associated with withdrawal from CNS stimulants are usually transient. Inpatient studies of the acute symptoms of abstinence from cocaine suggest that they are minimal, and not clinically significant. However, ambulatory treatment may be associated with more severe symptoms for any number of reasons, including the psychosocial stressors of everyday life, cocaine availability, and triggers for craving. A prior history of depression might be related to whether or not a cocaine abuser reports withdrawal symptoms. Indeed, suicidal ideation, intent, or plan in the context of CNS stimulant withdrawal should warrant careful evaluation and observation.

Several new approaches to the management of severe cocaine withdrawal have been studied. Amantadine (Symmetrel), an indirect dopamine agonist, might be able to stimulate the release of dopamine and therefore offer particular relief to those with severe cocaine withdrawal symptoms. Propanolol (Inderal), a β-blocker, may have some utility for the treatment of the symptoms of autonomic arousal associated with early cocaine abstinence. Disulfiram (Antabuse), which acts centrally by inhibiting dopamine β-hydroxylase, leading to an excess of dopamine and decreased synthesis of norepinephrine, may blunt cocaine craving, resulting in a decreased desire to use cocaine.

Opiate Withdrawal
Diagnostic Criteria

Commonly abused opioids include heroin, hydromorphone hydrochloride, oxycodone, propoxyphene, meperidine, opium, and codeine. The characteristic withdrawal syndrome can be precipitated by either cessation or reduction of opiate use that has been heavy or prolonged or the administration of an opiate antagonist such as naloxone (Narcan) after a period of opiate use. According to the DSM-IV-TR criteria, three or more of the following, developing minutes to several days after last use or administration of the antagonist, are required:

1. Dysphoric mood
2. Nausea or vomiting
3. Muscle aches
4. Lacrimation or rhinorrhea
5. Pupillary dilation, piloerection, or sweating
6. Diarrhea
7. Yawning
8. Fever
9. Insomnia

These symptoms cause clinically significant distress or impairment in social, occupational, or other important areas of functioning. The symptoms cannot be attributable to another medical condition or mental disorder.

The onset of these withdrawal symptoms depends on the amount and type of opiate abused. Withdrawal from heroin, which has a short half-life, begins 4 to 8 hours after last use, peaks within 24 to 48 hours, and may persist for as long as 2 weeks. Withdrawal from methadone does not begin until 24 to 36 hours after last use, and may go on for several weeks. As uncomfortable as opiate withdrawal may seem, it differs from alcohol or anxiolytic withdrawal because serious complications, such as seizures or DTs, do not typically occur.

Measurement

A measure of opiate withdrawal distress may helpful for both clinical and theoretical reasons. The opiate withdrawal scale (OWS) is a 32-item measure of withdrawal signs and symptoms that has been shortened to a 10-item version.

Pharmacology

Repeated administration of opioids that activate the μ-opioid receptor results in tolerance and dependence. Reduction or cessation of opiate use results in the characteristic, spontaneous withdrawal syndrome. Withdrawal may also be precipitated by the administration of an opiate antagonist such as naltrexone (ReVia) or naloxone. The duration of the precipitated withdrawal will depend on the half-life of the antagonist.

Treatment

No clear guidelines to assist with the choice between detoxification and opioid-agonist therapy exists for the opiate-dependent patient. Specific state and federal regulations govern admission criteria for methadone and levo-alpha-acetylmethadol (LAAM) maintenance. Treatment election should be guided by good clinical judgment informed by patient participation in treatment planning and local regulations.

There are four major categories of opiate detoxification options: (a) detoxification using opiate agonists, (b) detoxification using nonopioid medications, (c) rapid and ultrarapid detoxification, and (d) opioid detoxification in physician offices. Detoxification may be precipitated by a naloxone challenge test to establish actual physical dependence on the opiate.

The general principle of detoxification using opiate agonists is to substitute the opiate being abused with one that will be tapered under medical supervision. Methadone is the most commonly used opiate substitute for this purpose. Buprenorphine (Buprenex) is a partial opiate agonist approved by the U.S. Food and Drug Administration (FDA) for use in detoxification. The total amount of opiate used by an individual in a 24-hour period is estimated and the physical findings of withdrawal are observed. The patient is given an initial dose of methadone, 15 to 30 mg orally. Additional medication can be given on the basis of physical findings consistent with withdrawal. Once the correct daily dose is established, the rate of tapering reflects the planned rate of detoxification (e.g., 5% to 10% per day).

In addition to short-term detoxification, long-term (up to 180 days) detoxification was approved in 1989 as a treatment option for opioid-dependent patients who are ineligible for methadone maintenance or who do not want it.

LAAM is associated with potential cardiovascular complications. Patients maintained on LAAM may experience symptomatic arrhythmia with prolongation of the QT interval. Thus, LAAM is contraindicated in patients with known or suspected QT prolongation, and may be best reserved for appropriate patients who have failed with methadone treatment.

Detoxification with nonopioid medications is also a possibility. Clonidine (Catapres), an α_2-agonist, has been the best studied. The rationale for the use of clonidine is to diminish norepinephrine activity associated with opiate withdrawal. The patient is given up to 1.2 mg in divided doses over a 24-hour period, with careful monitoring of blood pressure. The peak clonidine dose is given on day 3 for detoxification from heroin, and on day 5 for detoxification from methadone. The peak dose is then tapered down over 4 to 7 days by 0.2 to 0.1 mg per day. Variations of clonidine detoxification include combining it with an opioid antagonist or using a transdermal patch.

Rapid and ultrarapid detoxification have been proposed to shorten the time necessary for withdrawal. Rapid detoxification begins by precipitating withdrawal through the administration of an opioid antagonist such as naloxone or naltrexone, followed by naltrexone maintenance and adjuvant medications such as antiemetics, analgesics, sedative–hypnotics, or buprenorphine for withdrawal symptoms. In ultrarapid opioid detoxification, patients undergo withdrawal precipitated by an opioid antagonist while under general anesthesia or heavy sedation. The efficacy of the rapid and ultrarapid techniques needs to be compared with more traditional approaches in randomized trials. The high costs and anesthesia risks of ultrarapid detoxification warrant careful consideration, because detoxification is the not the end of treatment.

The Drug Addiction Treatment Act of 2000 allows qualified physicians to use buprenorphine products for office-based treatment for detoxification or maintenance. Prior to the initiation of office-based treatment, the secretary of Health and Human Services requires notification. Physicians are qualified to offer office-based opiate treatment if they have subspecialty board certification in addiction psychiatry from the American Board of Medical Specialties, addiction certification from the American Society of Addiction Medicine, or completion of not less than 8 hours of training for the treatment and management of dependent patients provided by an approved organization (e.g., American Academy of Addiction Psychiatry). Careful selection of appropriate patients for office-based detoxification is essential. The *Field Review Draft of Buprenorphine Clinical Practice Guidelines* suggests that individuals with comorbid dependence on high doses of alcohol, benzodiazepines, or other CNS depressants; significant psychiatric comorbidity; active or chronic suicidal or homicidal ideation or attempts; multiple previous treatments and relapses; and previous nonresponse to buprenorphine are not optimal candidates for office-based treatment.

The patient must be in early withdrawal before buprenorphine is administered. In the case of a patient dependent on short-acting opioids, 12 to 24 hours should lapse since the last opioid use. Patients dependent on longer-acting opioids must also be in withdrawal prior to initiation of buprenorphine. In the case of methadone dependence, the last dose should be 40 mg or less, 24 hours before initiation of buprenorphine. For LAAM, the last dose should be 40 mg or less, 48 hours before initiation of buprenorphine. The patient is given up to 8 mg of buprenorphine with 2 mg naloxone on the first induction day, after an initial dose followed by at least 2 hours of observation for withdrawal symptoms. The patient should be stabilized on an appropriate dose for 48 hours. If there is a compelling reason for a rapid taper, then buprenorphine can be reduced over the course of 3 to 6 days and then discontinued. If a rapid taper is not necessary, the patient can be stabilized on buprenorphine/naloxone for at least 1 week, after which a taper from the combination therapy over the course of 2 weeks should be initiated. If no withdrawal symptoms emerge, then the taper can continue until the medication is discontinued. If withdrawal symptoms are evident, divided daily doses of the medication can be tried until the medication is discontinued. Patients maintained on buprenorphine are likely to have doses as high as 24 to 32 mg each day and probably should have these doses tapered over several weeks to maximize successful achievement of abstinence.

Marijuana and Hallucinogen Withdrawal

A withdrawal syndrome specific to marijuana and hallucinogens is not formally recognized. Of the limited research available, most has focused on marijuana, which is not commonly perceived to result in a physical withdrawal syndrome when regular use is stopped. A possible explanation is the long half-life of cannabis, which would allow for a "self-tapering" drug effect.

The development of a specific cannabinoid antagonist, SR141716A, however, has advanced the notion that there is a physiologic basis for cannabis dependence. This antagonist has been tested in both animal and human subjects. Rats treated daily with the potent synthetic cannabinoid HU-210 for 2 weeks were then given antagonist SR141716A. The induced withdrawal was accompanied by a marked elevation in extracellular corticotropin-releasing factor concentration and a distinct pattern of Fos activation in the central nucleus of the amygdala, supporting the possibility that long-term cannabinoid administration alters corticotropin-releasing factor function in a manner similar to that observed with other drugs of abuse, and also induces neuroadaptive processes.

Other studies of controlled marijuana administration to known marijuana users have described abstinence symptoms. For example, subject reports of anxiety, irritability, stomach pain, and objectively decreased food intake compared to baseline have followed abstinence from marijuana and tetrahydrocannabinol (THC). Others have described signs and symptoms of cannabis withdrawal as including restlessness, dysphoria, insomnia, muscle tremor, increased reflexes, and autonomic effects.

More rigorous studies, which include control groups, comparable substance administration, and symptom severity measurement, are needed, particularly in light of the prevalence of marijuana use.

Conclusion

Detoxification can take place in either inpatient or outpatient settings. An accurate and competent clinical assessment is essential when detoxification and subsequent treatment plans are formulated, particularly as some patients are dependent on more than one substance. The most appropriate setting for treatment will be determined by clinical judgment, treatment availability, and patient cooperation. Detoxification is but the first step to sustained abstinence.

Suggested Readings

Chang G, Kosten TR. Detoxification. In: Lowinson JH, Ruiz P, Millman RB, et al., eds. *Substance abuse: a comprehensive textbook*, 4th ed. Philadelphia: Lippincott Williams & Wilkins; 2005: 579–587.

O'Connor PG, Fiellin DA. Pharmacologic treatment of heroin-dependent patients. *Ann Intern Med.* 2000;133:40–54.

Pages KP, Ries RK. Use of anticonvulsants in benzodiazepine withdrawal. *Am J Addict.* 1998;7:198–204.

Sees KL, Delucchi KL, Masson C, et al. Methadone maintenance vs. 180-day psychosocially enriched detoxification for treatment of opioid dependence: a randomized controlled trial. *JAMA.* 2000;283:1303–1310.

Williams D, Lewis J, McBride A. A comparison of rating scales for the alcohol-withdrawal syndrome. *Alcohol Alcohol.* 2001;36:104–108.

Williams D, McBride A. The drug treatment of alcohol withdrawal symptoms: a systematic review. *Alcohol Alcohol.* 1998; 33:103–115.

METHADONE TREATMENT

M ethadone is a synthetic narcotic analgesic developed in Germany just prior to World War II. It was patented in 1941 but was not used by German physicians. After the war methadone was studied at the U.S. Public Health Hospital in Lexington, Kentucky, and was found to have effects similar to those of morphine but longer in duration. These initial studies led to the use of methadone for analgesia and for withdrawal from heroin. Although methadone continues to be used for these purposes, its unique pharmacologic properties make it a highly useful medication for maintenance treatment.

As a maintenance medication, methadone has distinct advantages. When administered in adequate oral doses, a single dose lasts between 24 and 36 hours without creating euphoria, sedation, or analgesia. Therefore, the patient can function normally and can perform mental or physical tasks without impairment. Patients continue to experience normal physical pain and emotional reactions. Most importantly, methadone relieves the persistent narcotic craving or hunger that is believed to be the major reason for relapse.

Cross-tolerance, or "blockade," is another important property of the medication. In sufficient doses, methadone "blocks" the effects of normal street doses of short-acting opioids such as heroin. Because tolerance to methadone remains steady, patients can be maintained indefinitely (e.g., in some cases more than 20 years) on the same dose. Finally, methadone is a medically safe treatment medication, with minimal side effects.

Much has been said about the importance of appropriate and adequate dosages of methadone. A series of studies has shown that patients maintained on doses of 60 mg per day or more had better treatment outcomes than those maintained on lower doses. Methadone doses should be determined individually, because of differences in metabolism, body weight, length and amount of heroin use, its purity, and, most importantly, maintenance of appropriate methadone blood levels throughout the 24-hour period.

Methadone Maintenance Pharmacotherapy

The initial dose of methadone is most commonly given at a time when the patient is having both signs and symptoms of opioid withdrawal. The immediate purpose is to relieve the withdrawal and also to establish a dose reference point on which future dose adjustments can be made. The purpose of early induction is to bring the methadone dose to approximate the established opioid tolerance in a prompt but safe manner. If this process is too slow, the patient may continue to use heroin or other unprescribed opioids; if the process is too fast, some degree of intoxication or overdose may result. Induction overdoses can result from exaggeration of tolerance and dependence by the newly admitted patient, overestimation on the part of the clinician, and the failure to consider basic steady-state pharmacology. Because the pharmacology of methadone differs from that of other opioids, the initial dose on the first day should be in the range of 20 to 40 mg, but not more than 40 mg.

Methadone has a half-life of 24 to 36 hours. At 24 hours after the initial dose is administered, about half remains to which the second dose is added. The result is a significant increase in mean methadone levels with no increase in dose. This accumulation process continues until steady state is achieved at 4 to 5 half-lives or days. Thus, the effect of the medication will increase in the absence of a dose increase, and relief of withdrawal may require time before the dose is increased. Both the clinician and the patient should be alert to any sedation on day 1 or 2 as subsequent days may result in overmedication.

The peak serum plasma levels occur between 2 and 4 hours after oral administration of methadone. During early induction when signs and symptoms of withdrawal persist, it is prudent to wait at least 3 hours before additional doses of 5 to 10 mg are provided.

Once the initial relief of withdrawal has been achieved, a more gradual dose adjustment may be indicated to establish an adequate maintenance dose. An example would be the patient who has an initial elimination of withdrawal and craving at 50 mg per day but who is exposed to opportunistic heroin use, suggesting the need to establish a "blockade" level of cross-tolerance, usually requiring doses of 80 mg or more. Once the stabilization dose is achieved, its indefinite administration should ensure continued maintenance of the desired effects. Most patients may remain on a stable dose for decades whereas others, at times, may require some adjustment. However, both patients and clinicians should avoid the tendency to lower the dose simply because the patient is stable and doing well.

Maintenance to Abstinence

Medically supervised withdrawal should be attempted only when desired by the patient with adequate supervision and support. Staff should carefully explore the motivation for withdrawal. In consideration of the high rate of relapse to intravenous drug use and its concomitant medical and social risks, patients who have withdrawn or who are withdrawing should be carefully monitored. In the event of relapse or impending relapse, appropriate intervention should be initiated, including rapid resumption of maintenance pharmacotherapy. The method of withdrawal usually involves a carefully individualized gradual reduction in dose over time.

Use of Plasma Levels of Methadone

Adequate dosing can be based on clinical findings in the majority of the cases, but reliable determination of methadone levels is available and affordable if indicated. Blood levels may be considered to clarify a clinical picture that does not correspond to the dose of methadone, to confirm suspected drug interactions, to ensure adequacy of a given dose, to document or justify the need for a particular dose or schedule, or to determine the need for and the effectiveness of split-dose practices.

Plasma levels of 150 to 200 ng/mL are adequate to prevent most craving and withdrawal. Adequate cross-tolerance or "blockade" is achieved at plasma levels at or above 400 ng/mL. The rate of change in plasma blood levels is critical and can be determined by calculating a peak-to-trough ratio. Ideally, this ratio is 2 or less. Higher ratios indicate rapid metabolism and the possible need for a split dose twice per day.

Side Effects

Tolerance to the opioid properties of methadone (sedation, analgesia) develops within a period of about 4 to 6 weeks. However, tolerance to the autonomic effects, most commonly constipation, libido, and sweating, develops at slower rates. Therefore, it is important to monitor the stabilization process carefully to minimize side effects and withdrawal symptoms. Methadone prescribed in high doses up to 150 mg per day on a long-term basis has no toxic effects and minimal side effects.

The major side effects during methadone maintenance treatment occur during the initial stabilization process. Although these effects are minor and usually subside over time, they can also be reduced or eliminated by an appropriate dose adjustment. In addition to constipation and sweating, the following have been ascribed to methadone: transient skin rash, weight gain, and water retention. Some patients have reported changes in libido. Most women who experienced amenorrhea while addicted to heroin report a return of menses when stabilized on methadone. However, some women complain about irregular menses or continued amenorrhea. To address the issues of side effects, appropriate medications may be prescribed, as well as providing counseling, education about methadone, family planning, and nutritional guidance. However, some of these side effects may be complications of co-existing alcoholism, multiple substance abuse, smoking, advanced age, other medical conditions, diet, and lifestyle.

Methadone maintenance, itself, does not impair the normal functioning of patients. Psychomotor performance tests that measure skills such as reaction time, driving ability, intelligence, attention span, and other important abilities have been administered to patients on methadone, volunteers, and normal college students with no drug history. The performance of patients on methadone did not differ from those of normal volunteers or college students. The mean intelligence quotient (IQ) of methadone patients at the time of entry into treatment has been found to be slightly higher than that of the general population. Ten years later, the same patients show even higher scores, possibly as a consequence of improved quality of life. Based on these studies, it can be concluded that methadone maintenance does not impair normal functioning or intellectual capacity.

Methadone Programs

In the United States, methadone maintenance programs are controlled and regulated by federal and state agencies. In 1972, to establish minimal standards and quality, the Food and Drug Administration (FDA) promulgated regulations governing the use of methadone; the Drug Enforcement Administration (DEA) was established to oversee the security and dispensing of the medication. In 2000, new federal regulations went into effect. The role of the DEA remains, but the FDA no longer is involved with the regulation of methadone. The Center for Substance Abuse Treatment (CSAT) has assumed the oversight of methadone and management of the accreditation process on the federal level. States have the right, and often exercise it, to make their licensing criteria more stringent than federal regulations. They cannot, however, loosen the criteria beyond those permitted on a federal level. These minimum standards regulate admissions, staffing patterns, record keeping, treatment planning, service provision, storage, facility standards, frequency of visits and of urine testing, and dose limitations.

For admission to methadone treatment, federal standards mandate a minimum of 1 year of addiction to opiates as well as current evidence of addiction, although they allow for exceptions such as pregnancy or recent discharge from a chronic care institution or prison. The minimum age for admission is 18 years (or younger with parental or legal guardian consent). Applicants younger than age 18 years must have at least two prior documented treatment episodes, either short-term detoxification or drug-free treatment, before they can be considered for methadone maintenance.

In the United States, methadone treatment has evolved into three phases during the past two decades. The first phase consists of a stabilization period that can last for about 3 months, during which patients adjust to the medication, receive their first annual physical examination, and are oriented to program regulations, expectations, routines, and services offered. Treatment planning begins with a thorough psychosocial history and assessment. Emergency situations and entitlements are addressed. Referrals are made to appropriate medical and social service agencies. New patients must report to the program daily (6 or 7 days per week) during this initial period. During the second phase, the treatment plan is reviewed and revised, if necessary. This often involves implementing vocational goals, such as job training or employment and providing ongoing medical and mental health treatment. For patients with serious medical problems such as HIV/AIDS, hepatitis C, or tuberculosis, or those with serious alcohol or multiple-drug problems, this phase of treatment can be extended as long as necessary. During this phase, patients may receive take-home medication, depending on their progress and adjustment to treatment. The third and final phase of treatment consists of continued methadone maintenance but a minimum of other services. These patients most often are employed and no longer require the intensive services provided in other phases but still require ongoing methadone maintenance. They continue to submit urine specimens for drug screening and ingest a dose of methadone under observation, and they can consult with program staff if necessary. Skilled counseling, an adequate dose, and case management are essential components of an effective program.

A quality program should have clear, cogent, consistent, and humanistic policies and procedures that are known and understood by both patients and staff. There should be a multidisciplinary approach that is flexible in order to provide individualized treatment planning and implementation based on assessed patient needs.

A well-organized methadone maintenance treatment program should provide a clean, safe, and attractive environment that is friendly, cheerful, and accommodating. Although it is difficult to estimate the optimal size of an adequate program, between 15 and 20 sq ft for each patient in treatment should be allotted, based on a patient census of 300.

Each clinic should be organized around the services it provides, and services should flow into each other easily. There must be a methadone dispensing area that is easily accessible to the patients it will serve. Ideally, a nurses' station or dispensing area is constructed adjacent to a comfortable patient waiting area. With the current concern about hepatitis C, HIV infection, and other health issues, the waiting room can be used to impart information about the program and its services, hepatitis C and HIV education, prenatal care, and parenting skills, as well as other important information. Because patients often bring young children with them to the clinic, the area should be safe for young children and out of sight of the actual dispensing area. The medical suite should be organized to ensure privacy and encourage patients to meet with the physician and other medical staff. The examination room must be well equipped and comfortable and there should be an adjacent office for staff to consult with patients. Patient records should be stored in a secure area but should be easily accessible to those who must use them frequently. Appropriate bathrooms are crucial, as programs must collect urine specimens from patients to monitor clinically whether patients continue to take methadone and do not misuse other drugs. The bathrooms should also be clean and neat and allow for privacy. Some clinics turn off the hot water in patient bathrooms to prevent the warming of urine specimens brought from elsewhere.

Programs with clear, cogent policies, procedures, goals, and objectives that are familiar to both staff and patients and consistent with state-of-the-art knowledge will provide the best outcomes. Programs must be operated with flexibility and under-standing of patient behavior, but with clear rules against violence or threats of vio-lence. Patients must see the clinic site as distinct from the hostile environments where they formerly used heroin and understand that different rules apply inside the clinic. The methods used to communicate these basics and the program's policies and proce-dures often can facilitate making the distinction. Patients must always be treated with compassion, dignity, and respect.

Because patient motivation is high upon entry into treatment, it is important that the entire treatment team engage the patient early. The medical history, physical examination, laboratory tests, psychosocial history, and medical, mental health, and social assessments should be completed during the first weeks of treatment. Most important in this process is staff–patient contact and the initial orientation. The initial physician–patient contact gives the doctor an opportunity to establish a relationship of trust, to explain the effectiveness and pharmacology of methadone, and to treat acute medical problems. Patients must learn to respect methadone as a legitimate medication and not regard it as a substitute "street drug." Patients should be educated to dispel destructive myths and misunderstandings about methadone, understand how it is used, its effects and its side effects, how the maintenance dose will be achieved, how to request a dosage change, and how to store methadone safely, if take-home doses are dispensed. They also should be educated about the nature of addiction and the need for long-term treatment. Patients must understand how the program func-tions and be introduced to the program staff. The patient should participate in the development of an individualized treatment plan and clearly understand the goals and objectives of the program and what the program expects. Patients should know the services to which they entitled, what services are provided at the program and, if nec-essary, by referral to cooperating agencies.

Some methadone treatment programs have taken advantage of the fact that patients visit regularly and remain in treatment to offer needed services that are usually difficult to obtain. This model, "one-stop shopping," provides HIV/hepatitis C-related services, services for children and families, services for pregnant and post-partum women, vocational and educational services, primary medical care, mental health services, and an array of substance abuse treatment services to deal with those who continue to abuse drugs and/or alcohol. Counseling and casework, relapse pre-vention techniques, 12-step groups, and other services are offered to patients with these problems.

Methadone Treatment, HIV/AIDS, and Hepatitis C

Several studies have confirmed that continuous methadone treatment is associated with a reduced risk of contracting HIV and may prevent infection of those patients not yet exposed to the virus. Because of the high prevalence of infectious diseases (e.g., HIV/AIDS, hepatitis, tuberculosis) among patients on methadone, many programs have developed research and service delivery systems to deal with the high numbers of infected patients. Staff members with special training in HIV spectrum disease provide risk reduction education, distribute condoms, and assist with referrals to infectious disease clinics. An increase in tuberculosis, especially treatment-resistant tuberculosis, among this group has resulted in tuberculosis case management projects including direct observation therapy (DOT), the provision of medications for prophylaxis and treatment. Some hospitals have developed specific methadone programs for HIV infection.

Hepatitis C is now the most prevalent infectious disease among patients on methadone maintenance with histories of intravenous drug use. The infection is usually acquired during the first year of injection. Therefore, it is estimated that the prevalence of hepatitis C among former injectors who are now in treatment is between 64% and 88% depending on the geographic location. Many clinics provide diagnostic services. However, patients are mostly referred to specialized services for ongoing treatment if the clinic is unable to provide it. In the 1980s, AIDS was the major cause of death among patients on methadone. However, by the late 1990s the death rate from AIDS stabilized and the death rate from hepatitis C had increased; eventually the death rate from hepatitis C may supersede that from AIDS.

Efficacy of Methadone Maintenance Treatment

Despite the differences in goals and policies among programs, methadone maintenance treatment has yielded consistently positive evaluations since it was implemented in 1964. As stated previously, when appropriate doses are provided, illicit opioid use is markedly decreased or eliminated in most patients.

Alcohol and cocaine (crack and cocaine hydrochloride) have been and continue to be major substances of abuse among patients on methadone maintenance. In a review of methadone treatment programs, the U.S. General Accounting Office reported that in 1989, 14% of the patients in the programs surveyed had problems with cocaine or crack. In eight of the programs, up to 40% of the patients used the drug, whereas in 16 programs, cocaine was used by 0% to 15% of the patients. Yet studies suggest that the level of cocaine use decreases from time of admission to methadone treatment. For example, one study found a decrease in cocaine use from 84% at admission to 66% after 6 months in treatment in a population with an exceptionally high prevalence of cocaine use.

Prior to the increase in cocaine use and HIV infection, alcohol and the medical complications of alcoholism were the most serious problems found among patients on methadone, affecting approximately 20% to 25% of the patients. Before 1986, medical conditions related to alcoholism were the major causes of mortality in methadone maintenance treatment. Studies also suggest that when patients leave methadone treatment, their drinking behavior increases.

Many studies have documented a substantial reduction in criminal behavior from pretreatment levels. Like most other treatment variables, reduction in criminal behavior increases with length of time in treatment. These trends have been consistent through-out the more than three decades of methadone treatment and in a variety of settings. Socially productive behavior as measured by employment, schooling, or homemaking also improves with length of time in treatment. It has been shown that methadone-maintained patients have held positions across the spectrum of the job market, includ-ing lawyer, architect, musician, film producer, housewife, chef, construction worker, social worker, secretary, laborer, driver, and doorman.

Research has concluded that program characteristics are a critical factor in suc-cessful outcomes. It has been found that the major factor in outcome is the length of time in treatment. Factors that influence longer retention are adequate dose, well-trained staff, trusting and confidential relationships between the patients and program staff, clear policies and procedures, low staff turnover and high morale, flexible take-home policies, and other pertinent program characteristics. There is a high degree of consistency in the results of studies of patients who leave treatment. The majority of discharged patients revert to use of heroin, other illicit narcotics, and/or alcohol. Ball and Ross found that 82% of the patients had relapsed to intravenous drug use after having been out of treatment for 10 months or more, with almost half (45.5%) relaps-ing after having been out of treatment for 1 to 3 months. Older patients may substitute heavy alcohol use for heroin, and favorable outcome is associated with shorter dura-tion of heroin use, longer duration of treatment, employment, and an absence of behavioral problems while in treatment. Withdrawal from treatment may have fatal consequences. One study found that the death rate for discharged persons was more than twice that of patients still in treatment. The major difference in the causes of death between treatment and posttreatment is the sharp increase in opioid-related deaths after leaving treatment. No evidence was found of opioid-related deaths among properly stabilized patients during methadone treatment.

Methadone maintenance treatment is cost-effective and beneficial to society. Using data from the U.S. Treatment Outcome Prospective Study (TOPS), and after examining the average cost of a treatment day, detailed measurements of criminal activity rates, and the costs to society of various crimes, one study found that methadone treatment yielded a benefit:cost ratio of 4:1. It is clear that methadone maintenance pays for itself, and benefits accrue not only to the patient but to society in general.

Special Issues and New Treatment Approaches

To enhance the traditional outpatient methadone clinic, changing patient needs dic-tate that new and innovative approaches be piloted. Since the 1980s, several such efforts have been implemented. For example, to address homelessness and/or abuse of cocaine and other drugs, residential short-stay methadone treatment programs for patients who are not functioning well (e.g., because of mental illness and substance abuse) have been developed. In New York City's Rikers Island Correctional Facility, the Key Extended Entry Program (KEEP) offers methadone maintenance treatment to opioid-addicted inmates who request treatment upon incarceration. Eligible inmates are those with sentences of no more than 1 year who meet admission criteria. They are maintained while in jail and are referred to a community clinic where they are guaran-teed continued treatment.

Methadone medical maintenance (MMM) is the integration of socially rehabili-tated methadone patients into general medical practice. Patients are treated by internists or other primary care physicians in a private practice setting, indistinguishable from other patients. This program was started in 1983 at The Rockefeller University by Drs. Dole, Nyswander, and Kreek. In 1985, 25 of their stable long-term methadone patients were transferred into the general medical practices of Drs. David Novick and Edwin A. Salsitz at Beth Israel Medical Center. As of July 2004 approximately 225 patients were enrolled in this ongoing project. Two models have been modified by allowing for dispensing of methadone in a commercial pharmacy and in a community primary care setting.

Patients in MMM are seen monthly or, if indicated, more frequently if problems should arise. At the time of the office visit a urine toxicology is obtained, a 28-day or an appropriate supply of methadone diskettes or tablets is dispensed, the physician observes ingestion of a methadone dose, medical problems are treated and addressed, and other problems or issues are discussed. Most patients return every 28 days or more frequently if needed. Fees are collected at the time of the office visit. In the pharmacy project, the physician collects the urine and delivers the methadone order to the pharmacy either electronically or in person. The physician meets with the pharmacist once per month but remains in contact if changes in prescriptions are needed. The patient receives the methadone without observed ingestion but is subject to random callbacks for counting of methadone tablets to assure quality control. The fee for MMM includes the office visit, the urinalysis, an annual physical, and the methadone. However, in the pharmacy program, the patient pays the pharmacy for the methadone.

A 15-year follow-up study of 158 MMM patients showed that 83.5% of the patients had been compliant with the rules and regulations of the program. The projected median retention time for this group of patients was 13.8 years. Noncompliant patients (16.5%) were referred back to their clinics for failure to report as directed and abuse of cocaine/crack. Approximately 8% were able to withdraw from methadone successfully. A total of 12 compliant patients (8.2%) electively withdrew from methadone in good standing, and 1 compliant patient voluntarily returned to the clinic.

MMM is a proven method of methadone treatment. Physicians must be properly trained and not harbor the many and pervasive methadone myths. They must be flexible and sensitive to the patients' needs for confidentiality and changes of appointments. When referrals are made, contact must be made by the MMM physician with the consulting physician to dispel misinformation and educate them about methadone treatment, possible drug interactions, and to ensure that patients receive proper pain management. MMM and office-based prescribing of methadone has been established in New York, Oregon, Maryland, New Mexico, and California.

Treatment Issues: Access, Expansion and Retention

At present, methadone treatment programs in the United States treat approximately 15% to 20% of narcotic addicts at any given time. The cost to society of more than 500,000 untreated opioid addicts is a major public health problem. Mobile vans have been used in the Netherlands, in Baltimore, and in Boston to reach addicts where it has not been possible to establish permanent clinic sites. Such a strategy could be used to introduce treatment to shelters and other social service agencies directly serving addicted people. Pilot projects have been developed in California and New Mexico to expand the intake of untreated heroin addicts into treatment by using vans as clinics and dispensing units, as well as community pharmacies working with private physicians to dispense methadone and become part of the treatment process.

Outreach and harm reduction workers themselves may harbor biases against methadone treatment and, therefore, may not refer untreated addicts to treatment. Heroin addicts also harbor unfounded biases and myths about methadone treatment (e.g. rots the bones) and object to the regulations. Many do not have the necessary identification for entrance into treatment and benefits. Untreated addicts are ambivalent about methadone treatment because of misunderstandings about methadone and its use as a medication to treat addiction. These views and beliefs have adversely influenced their decisions to enter and remain in treatment.

Diversion and Mortality

The major source of methadone found in deaths where methadone is cited in autopsy reports across the United States is from sources outside the methadone clinic system. The majority of deaths where methadone was identified at autopsy were polydrug abuse deaths involving other psychoactive substances. Although data remain incomplete, a National Assessment meeting recommended "creation of case definitions that would make a distinction between deaths caused by methadone and deaths in which methadone is a contributing factor or merely present." The panel noted that increasing numbers of prescriptions by physicians for methadone to treat pain "are paralleling the increase in prescriptions for oxycodone, hydrocodone, and morphine, as physicians prescribe to meliorate chronic pain." Therefore, the panel recommends the inclusion in health care curricula of information about the "diagnosis and treatment of addiction and appropriate pharmacotherapies for pain."

The panel is of the opinion that reports of methadone mentions in deaths involve one of three scenarios: (a) illicitly obtained methadone used in excessive or repetitive doses in an attempt to achieve euphoric effects; (b) methadone, either licitly or illicitly obtained, used in combination with other prescription medications such as benzodiazepines (antianxiety medication), alcohol, or other opioids; or (c) an accumulation of methadone to harmful serum levels in the first days of treatment for addiction or pain, before tolerance is developed.

The director of the CSAT stated, "Methadone continues to be a safe, effective treatment for addiction to heroin or prescription pain killers. While deaths involving methadone increased, experiences in several states show that addiction treatment programs are not the culprits."

Conclusion

Methadone maintenance has proven to be a highly effective treatment and has been recognized throughout the world, as well the by National Institutes of Health and the Institute of Medicine. However, since the early years of methadone maintenance, many new social and health problems have emerged. These have had an adverse effect on methadone patients and the programs that treat them. HIV/AIDS, hepatitis C, problems of an aging patient population, homelessness, chronic unemployment, and destitution have placed methadone programs in the position of assuming ever-wider responsibilities.

The frequency of clinic attendance by patients gives programs the opportunity and the responsibility to provide the medical and social care that a chronic, debilitating, and potentially terminal illness requires. Some programs are now moving in the direction of providing primary care with expanded social services for their patients in addition to methadone treatment. Patients are also educated about the transmission of infectious diseases and are either treated on site or referred to other facilities. Therefore, a quality methadone maintenance treatment program is one that continuously evaluates and assesses the changing needs of its patients and seeks to meet them to the best of its ability. As the public currently demands programs that are cost-effective, it is important that programs develop the capability to evaluate and document their productivity and the improved status of their patients.

Suggested Readings

Amato L, Davoli M, Minozzi S, et al. Methadone at tapered doses for the management of opioid withdrawal. *Cochrane Database Syst Rev.* 2005;(3):CD003409.

Faggiano F, Vigna-Taglianti F, Versino E, et al. Methadone maintenance at different dosages for opioid dependence. *Cochrane Database Syst Rev.* 2003;(3):CD002208.

Lowinson JH, Marion I, Joseph H, et al. Methadone maintenance. In: Lowinson JH, Ruiz P, Millman RB, et al., eds. *Substance abuse: a comprehensive textbook*, 4th ed. Philadelphia: Lippincott Williams & Wilkins; 2005:616–633.

Salsitz EA, Joseph H, Frank B, et al. Methadone medical maintenance: treating chronic opioid dependence in private medical practice—a summary report. *Mt Sinai J Med.* 2000;67(5&6): 388–397. Available at: www.mssm.edu/msjournal.

Strain EC, Stitzer ML. *The treatment of opioid dependence.* Baltimore: Johns Hopkins University Press; 2006.

21

BUPRENORPHINE FOR TREATMENT OF OPIOID ADDICTION

Overview of Pharmacodynamics, Pharmacology, and Pharmacokinetics

Buprenorphine, a derivative of the morphine alkaloid thebaine, has been available in numerous countries as an analgesic for parenteral and sublingual administration since the 1970s, and a parenteral dosage form has been available in the United States since the early 1980s. As an analgesic, buprenorphine is approximately 25 to 50 times more potent than morphine. Typically, 0.3 mg of buprenorphine is considered to produce analgesia approximately equivalent to 10 mg of morphine when both medications are given parenterally.

Unlike methadone and levo-alpha-acetylmethadol (LAAM), which can be characterized as full μ-opioid agonists, buprenorphine may be described as a partial agonist. That is, buprenorphine produces submaximal effects relative to those produced by full μ-opioid agonists when a maximally effective dose of buprenorphine is given. Although this description does not detail the molecular mechanisms involved in the actions of the drug, it does provide a basis for understanding the potential utility and limitations of using buprenorphine as an opioid-addiction treatment medication. Although buprenorphine has a high affinity for the μ-opioid receptor, it also has a low intrinsic activity. This high affinity makes buprenorphine extremely difficult to displace from the receptor by opioid antagonists; the clinical implications of this are discussed later. Furthermore, buprenorphine dissociates very slowly from the receptor and it is very lipophilic, both factors contributing to the relatively long duration of activity of buprenorphine. Buprenorphine also binds with high affinity to the κ-opioid receptor but functions there as an antagonist. Buprenorphine binding at other receptor types has also been demonstrated, but it is its activity at the μ- and κ-receptors that is associated with its unique and often complex pharmacologic profile.

Buprenorphine has poor oral bioavailability, less than 10% compared to that when given intravenously. This is secondary to extensive gastrointestinal and hepatic metabolism. The primary metabolite of buprenorphine is norbuprenorphine, which, as a more polar compound, is associated with less penetration into the central nervous system. Buprenorphine and norbuprenorphine also form glucuronide conjugates. Given the low oral bioavailability of buprenorphine, and a concern that a parenteral dosage form should not be used for the treatment of opioid addicts (so as not to reinforce injection-associated behaviors), the sublingual route of administration has been considered the most appropriate for opioid-addiction treatment.

Initially, in many clinical studies assessing the safety and efficacy of buprenorphine, a sublingual solution was used. This solution was commonly formulated to contain 30% or 40% ethanol secondary to the poor solubility of buprenorphine in a totally aqueous medium. The bioavailability of this solution typically has been reported to be between 30% and 50%. However, there are many factors that could make a hydroalcoholic solution impractical for general use. These include concerns regarding storage requirements and ease (or lack thereof) of dispensing, as well as potential diversion and illicit use.

To obviate these concerns, two sublingual buprenorphine tablet formulations were developed—one containing only buprenorphine and one containing a combination of buprenorphine and naloxone in a 4:1 ratio (to reduce its potential for diversion and illicit use). The bioavailability of the buprenorphine tablet has been reported to be approximately 50% to 65% compared to the sublingual solution. Naloxone itself has poor sublingual bioavailability. Thus, when taken sublingually as directed, naloxone will not interfere with the therapeutic effects of buprenorphine. However, when taken parenterally by opioid-dependent individuals, the naloxone component may be expected to produce signs and symptoms characteristic of opioid withdrawal.

Development of Buprenorphine as a Treatment for Opioid Addiction

The results of a clinical study fostered interest in, and suggested the utility of, buprenorphine for the treatment of opioid addiction. Subsequent studies generally confirmed the initial observations regarding the potential effectiveness of buprenorphine by providing evidence for its patient acceptability, ability to substitute for and block the effects of other opioids, safety, and its utility in maintaining individuals in treatment.

Findings from a number of studies indicate that buprenorphine can substitute for other opioids and decrease illicit opioid use. In one of the first clinical pharmacology investigations, it was reported the results from an inpatient study in which individuals maintained on placebo or buprenorphine could make operant responses to earn money or receive intravenous heroin; those receiving buprenorphine took significantly less heroin. Over the next 20 years, numerous clinical laboratory and treatment–research studies, conducted in a variety of settings over varying periods of time and using various schedules of buprenorphine administration, provided evidence that buprenorphine can be used effectively and safely as an opioid-substitution pharmacotherapy.

Demonstration of the efficacy and safety of buprenorphine for treatment of opioid addiction comes from three basic types of clinical trials: (a) comparisons of buprenorphine to other opioid agonists used for treatment (methadone and LAAM), (b) comparisons of buprenorphine to placebo, and (c) studies providing buprenorphine dose–response data. It must be pointed out that most of the trials were conducted using a sublingual liquid formulation of buprenorphine, not the sublingual tablet formulation of buprenorphine (or buprenorphine-naloxone) that is currently approved for use. Nonetheless, without reviewing in detail each of the trials, certain general observations can be discussed.

It is likely that the maximum agonist effects from higher therapeutic dosages of buprenorphine (approximately 8 mg/day of the sublingual liquid or 16 mg/day of the sublingual tablet) are likely to be comparable to methadone dosages no higher than about 60 mg per day. As a partial agonist, the effects of buprenorphine are dose dependent within a limited range, above which increasing doses to not produce corresponding increases in effect. Thus, patients who have been maintained on higher dosages of methadone (or corresponding dosages of LAAM) may not be good candidates for buprenorphine treatment. Buprenorphine, however, was not developed to replace methadone and LAAM, but rather to provide a treatment alternative for patients and clinicians who could not or would not consider treatment with one of the other available therapies. Furthermore, the same μ-opioid, partial-agonist profile that provides a ceiling to the therapeutic effects of buprenorphine also provides for a greater safety margin for buprenorphine.

Patients initiating treatment may be inducted onto therapy using either buprenorphine or the buprenorphine–naloxone combination. Consideration should be given to the type of opioid the patient has been abusing (e.g., heroin, morphine, methadone), the time since the patient last used opioids, and the current level of the patient's opioid addiction. Generally, the induction process will be easier in patients using shorter-acting (e.g., heroin) than in those using longer-acting (e.g., methadone) opioids; patients experiencing mild withdrawal symptoms will be easier to induct than those who are not (i.e., it is harder if patients have recently used other opioids); and patients with lower levels of addiction will be easier to induct than those with higher levels. Initial doses of buprenorphine will typically range from 4 to 8 mg per day (In the buprenorphine–naloxone combination, the ratio of buprenorphine to naloxone is 4:1). Administering the first day's dosage as two or three individual doses may also be useful. Dosages on subsequent days are then gradually increased to the desired level. For patients transferring to buprenorphine therapy who have been actively maintained on methadone or LAAM, lowering the dose of that medication to the equivalent of no more than 30 to 40 mg per day of methadone will facilitate a smooth transition onto buprenorphine. For individuals maintained on higher doses of methadone, the use of adjunct medications (e.g., clonidine, oxazepam) while rapidly reducing the daily methadone dosage, or administering the first dose of buprenorphine more than 24 hours following the last methadone dose, may be useful.

Although buprenorphine has been used effectively to substitute for other opioids and to suppress the development of opioid withdrawal signs and symptoms, its partial agonist properties are also responsible for its potential to precipitate an opioid withdrawal syndrome under certain conditions. Precipitated withdrawal has been observed or suggested by both preclinical and clinical studies. It may not always be clear in clinical situations, however, whether withdrawal symptomatology is a result of an insufficient or excessive dosage of buprenorphine being administered. Furthermore, for patients being maintained on high dosages of methadone, or addicts using large amounts of heroin or other opioids, there may not be a dosage of buprenorphine that will fully substitute for the other opioid drug. The administration of buprenorphine to these individuals may result in the production of significant opioid withdrawal effects.

Of particular interest with respect to substitution therapy with buprenorphine has been its long duration of action. It was reported in some of the initial studies that at sufficient doses buprenorphine could be effectively administered once daily. Those findings were subsequently supported by results from numerous clinical trials. Later studies indicated that alternate-day, or even less-frequent dosing was possible.

Potential for Abuse

It is obvious that a medication must be acceptable to the targeted treatment population if it is to be effective, and studies assessing the utility of buprenorphine as a treatment agent for opioid addiction have provided evidence of its acceptability. Subjects have reported "liking" and opioid-like effects following its administration. These "positive" subjective effects may be important for initiating and maintaining individuals on buprenorphine.

However, as is true for methadone and LAAM, buprenorphine should be considered to have a potential for abuse. In various drug-discrimination paradigms, buprenorphine has been discriminated by human subjects to be one of various opioid agonists or agonist–antagonists. In a controlled clinical trial, intravenously administered buprenorphine was associated with positive subjective effects in individuals not dependent on opioids and, in another, buprenorphine was self-administered by individuals who were not opioid dependent. The former also indicated that the effects of buprenorphine were not consistently dose related, consonant with the partial agonist profile of buprenorphine. Results from other studies that assessed the effects of buprenorphine in methadone-maintained patients suggest that buprenorphine would have a limited potential for abuse in these individuals, and that the time of buprenorphine administration relative to that of the last methadone dose may be an important determinant of the subjective effects of buprenorphine.

As mentioned previously, the combining of naloxone with buprenorphine is expected to reduce the abuse liability of buprenorphine used clinically. Support for this assertion has been obtained from studies using various ratios of buprenorphine to naloxone (e.g., 2:1, 4:1, and 8:1), various subject populations (e.g., nondependent, methadone-maintained, morphine-stabilized), and various routes of buprenorphine–naloxone administration (e.g., sublingual, intramuscular). Furthermore, a number of studies provide evidence that the naloxone component will not interfere with the therapeutic effectiveness of buprenorphine.

Since 1983, reports of buprenorphine abuse have come from various countries, although its relative availability and the availability of licit and illicit alternatives need to be taken into account when interpreting these reports. Thus, buprenorphine abuse has often been associated with a lower cost and more ready availability than other opioid alternatives.

Safety

The use of buprenorphine has not been associated with an adverse effect profile that would appear to limit its utility as an opioid-addiction pharmacotherapy. Adverse effects reported following the administration of buprenorphine for opioid addiction treatment have included primarily sedation, drowsiness, and constipation, and other effects typical of μ-opioid agonists in general. Tolerance to these effects can be expected to develop during continued buprenorphine therapy. The safety of buprenorphine is, like its pharmacodynamic profile, related to its partial agonist properties. In particular, the potential for severe drug-induced respiratory depression, a concern for medications such as methadone and LAAM, as well as drugs primarily used illicitly, such as heroin, does not appear to be a relevant concern for buprenorphine. Even 32 mg of buprenorphine administered sublingually (approximately 70 times higher, corrected for differences in bioavailability, than a 0.3-mg analgesic dose given intramuscularly) produced only marginal effects on respiratory function in individuals not dependent on opioids, and 12 mg given intravenously (also in individuals who were not opioid addicted) was shown to have a high margin of safety.

The high affinity of buprenorphine for the μ-opioid receptor would also render usual therapeutic doses of naloxone or nalmefene ineffective in the management of respiratory depression secondary to that which might be seen following an overdose of buprenorphine; doses of naloxone ranging from 10 to 35 mg per 70 kg could be required. Buprenorphine has a longer duration of action and greater μ-opioid receptor affinity than either naloxone or nalmefene, such that mechanical support of respiration could be required in an overdose situation.

Deaths have been reported when buprenorphine has been combined with other drugs, particularly central nervous system depressants such as benzodiazepines. These reports come from France, where buprenorphine was approved for use in 1996 and where more patients have received buprenorphine therapy than have in any other country. In these cases, buprenorphine tablets typically have been pulverized and then administered intravenously.

Buprenorphine is widely available in France with minimal regulatory constraints upon its use. However, even with fewer restrictions placed on buprenorphine compared to methadone treatment, buprenorphine appears to be a safe alternative to methadone. From 1994 to 1998, there were an estimated 1.4 times more buprenorphine-related deaths than methadone-related deaths in France. However, for each of those years (except for 1994 when no deaths were reported), the calculated death rate was always *higher* (ranging from 3.5 to 30 times higher) for methadone than for buprenorphine. Considering 1998, for example, buprenorphine was associated with slightly more than three times the number of deaths (13 compared to 4 for methadone), but there were more than 10 times as many patients receiving buprenorphine (55,000) compared to methadone (5,360).

In addition to the obvious drug interactions that may occur when buprenorphine is combined with central nervous system depressants, other potential interactions may occur with medications that either induce or inhibit cytochrome P450 3A4, which catalyzes the dealkylation of buprenorphine to norbuprenorphine. Because patients receiving buprenorphine may also be HIV-positive, potential interactions of buprenorphine with anti-HIV medications is a concern. Although a recent *in vitro* study indicated that ritonavir (Norvir), saquinavir (Fortovase), and indinavir (Crixivan) (all HIV protease inhibitors) competitively inhibited the metabolism of buprenorphine, another study did not indicate that buprenorphine influenced viral load in patients receiving highly active antiretroviral therapy.

Office-Based Treatment with Buprenorphine and Buprenorphine–Naloxone

Since methadone therapy was developed in the 1960s by Dole and Nyswander, methadone has become the prototypical pharmacotherapy for opioid addiction treatment. In the United States, methadone is a Schedule II substance under the Controlled Substances Act and can be used only in a strictly regulated environment. Thus it is taken under direct observation or with limited privileges for take-home dosing. Regulations also govern treatment eligibility criteria, administrative oversight, requirements for mandatory urine testing of participants, and how medication is to be stored and secured.

Unfortunately, although born from concerns related to the possible diversion and illicit use of the treatment medications, the regulations governing methadone treatment also serve as barriers to treatment for certain individuals. Some individuals will not qualify for treatment because they do not meet regulatory criteria. Others may not live within a reasonable proximity to a methadone clinic. Others who could qualify for treatment do not present themselves for it secondary to real or perceived fears regarding the medications themselves. Still others have attempted treatment and failed, sometimes on multiple occasions.

From the standpoint of many clinicians and patients, both regulatory reform and enhanced treatment options were necessary. Some regulatory reform regarding the existing federal regulations covering the use of methadone has recently been adopted. An important part of this reform was a liberalization of the take-home dosing policies for methadone. More dramatic, however, was federal legislation that can literally mainstream addiction treatment and may substantially increase the availability and accessibility of opioid-addiction treatment.

In October, 2000, Public Law 106-310, the Children's Health Act of 2000, became effective. A part of that law, the Drug Addiction Treatment Act of 2000 (DATA), allows qualified physicians in the United States to prescribe medications in Schedule III, IV, or V as part of office-based maintenance or detoxification treatment for opioid addiction. Physicians must also have the capacity to refer patients for counseling and other appropriate ancillary services, and no more than 30 patients may be treated by an individual physician at any one time. Furthermore, individual states may not preclude clinicians from prescribing or dispensing these medications unless a particular state specifically enacts a law prohibiting such activity. Both buprenorphine and the buprenorphine–naloxone combination are currently in Schedule III, and thus may be used for opioid-addiction treatment under DATA.

There are numerous potential advantages regarding the use of office-based addiction treatment including expansion of treatment availability, better matching of treatment services to individual needs, minimizing the stigma that often accompanies drug addition and its treatment, and limiting patients' contact with other substance-abusing individuals.

Conclusion

Buprenorphine is a safe and effective treatment for opioid addiction. Its partial agonist character makes it a potentially safer medication than methadone or LAAM, particularly with regard to drug-induced respiratory depression. The combination product containing buprenorphine and naloxone is expected to decrease the abuse liability of buprenorphine yet provide comparable efficacy. Importantly, buprenorphine and buprenorphine–naloxone may be used for addiction treatment in office-based settings, thereby likely increasing the availability and accessibility of opioid-addiction treatment.

Suggested Readings

Fiellin DA, O'Connor P. Office-based treatment of opioid-dependent patients. *N Engl J Med.* 2002; 347:817–823.

Fudala PJ, O'Brien CP. Buprenorphine for the treatment of opioid addiction. In: Lowinson JH, Ruiz P, Millman RB, et al., eds. *Substance abuse: a comprehensive textbook*, 4th ed. Philadelphia: Lippincott Williams & Wilkins; 2005:634–640.

Johnson RE, Chutuape MA, Strain EC, et al. A comparison of levomethadyl acetate, buprenorphine, and methadone for opioid dependence. *N Engl J Med.* 2000;343:1290–1297.

Ling W, Wesson DR. Clinical efficacy of buprenorphine: comparisons to methadone and placebo. *Drug Alcohol Depend.* 2003;70:S49–S57.

Strain EC. Clinical use of buprenorphine. In: Strain EC, Stitzer MI, eds. *The treatment of opioid dependence*. Baltimore: Johns Hopkins University Press; 2006:230–252.

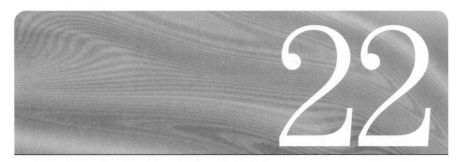

ALTERNATIVE PHARMACOTHERAPIES FOR OPIOID ADDICTION

Nonopioid Treatments: Clonidine and Lofexidine

The acute opioid withdrawal syndrome is a time-limited phenomenon, generally of brief duration. Following the abrupt termination of short-acting opioids such as heroin, morphine, or hydromorphone, withdrawal signs and symptoms usually subside by the second or third opioid-free day. Although uncomfortable for the addict, the opioid withdrawal syndrome, in contrast to the syndrome associated with the withdrawal of other drugs such as benzodiazepines and alcohol, does not pose a medical risk to the individual. Thus, there is a particular appeal for treating this syndrome symptomatically, especially with medications that do not themselves produce physical dependence. It should be recognized, however, that detoxification from opioids is only one of the initial steps in the process of rehabilitating opioid-addicted individuals if complete and permanent abstinence is the treatment goal.

Clonidine is an α_2-adrenergic agonist indicated for the treatment of hypertension. It is useful in the medical detoxification of patients from methadone, as well as from commonly abused opioids such as heroin, morphine, propoxyphene, and meperidine. In particular, it has been shown to be useful in preparing individuals for stabilization onto the opioid antagonist naltrexone. Clonidine has also been reported to be useful in decreasing withdrawal signs and symptoms associated with the cessation of alcohol and tobacco use.

The capacity of clonidine to ameliorate withdrawal-associated effects (e.g., lacrimation and rhinorrhea) is linked to its modulation of noradrenergic hyperactivity in the locus ceruleus. Additionally, clonidine may affect central serotonergic, cholinergic, and purinergic systems. It seems to be most effective in suppressing certain opioid withdrawal signs and symptoms, such as restlessness and diaphoresis. However, clonidine is not well accepted by addicts because it does not produce morphine-like subjective effects or relieve certain types of withdrawal distress, such as anxiety. Sedation and hypotension also limit its utility. Dosages are generally individualized to each patient based on therapeutic response and side-effect limitations.

Interestingly, clonidine abuse by users of illicit opioids and other drugs has been reported since the early 1980s. This abuse may be secondary to a desire to obtain various drug-related effects, such as sedation, euphoria, or hallucinations. Clonidine may also be used to prolong and enhance the effects of heroin or other opioids.

Secondary to an effort to identify an agent with less sedating and hypotensive effects than clonidine, a number of other α_2-adrenergic agonists have been evaluated for their ability to moderate the opioid-withdrawal syndrome. Of these, lofexidine, a clonidine analogue licensed in the United Kingdom for opioid detoxification treatment, has been the subject of much clinical evaluation. Lofexidine has enjoyed widespread usage in the United Kingdom. Lofexidine is suggested to be used for a period of 7 to 10 days at doses ranging from 0.4 to 2.4 mg per day.

Studies conducted in the early 1980s provided initial data indicating that lofexidine could be effective in suppressing some of the signs and symptoms of opioid withdrawal. More recent trials have provided further evidence for the efficacy of lofexidine. When lofexidine was compared to clonidine, both treatments were generally found to produce similar therapeutic effects, but lofexidine typically was better tolerated. For example, when lofexidine was compared to clonidine in an outpatient, double-blind trial, both medications produced positive treatment outcomes, but clonidine was associated with more hypotensive effects and more required home visits by medical staff. In a double-blind, inpatient study, lofexidine and clonidine were reported to be equally effective in treating the withdrawal syndrome. Clonidine, however, was associated with more hypotension, and better treatment retention than was noted for lofexidine. In another double-blind, inpatient study using methadone-stabilized opioid addicts, both lofexidine and clonidine produced a similar suppression of withdrawal symptoms, but lofexidine was associated with less hypotension and fewer adverse events. However, when lofexidine was compared to buprenorphine in an open-label study, patients receiving buprenorphine reportedly had less-severe withdrawal symptoms and were more likely to complete detoxification treatment.

LAAM: An Opioid Agonist Alternative to Methadone

Levo-alpha-acetylmethadol (LAAM) is a derivative of methadone, and like methadone, is a synthetic μ-opioid agonist. LAAM was approved in the United States for the management of opioid dependence in 1993. It was initially developed in the late 1940s by chemists in Germany seeking an analgesic substitute for morphine. Subsequent studies indicated that LAAM would be unsuitable for the treatment of acute pain given its slow onset of effect and extended duration of action. However, the data are mixed concerning the onset of the effects of LAAM. Initial studies indicated that LAAM given orally produced a more rapid onset of effect than when it was given intravenously or subcutaneously, although other data suggest that LAAM produces effects of immediate onset when administered parenterally. Although it was noted early in the development of LAAM that LAAM could alleviate the signs and symptoms of opioid withdrawal, it was also observed that giving LAAM on a daily basis could lead to signs indicative of opioid toxicity, such as severe nausea and vomiting and respiratory depression.

The use of methadone to treat opioid-dependent individuals, which began in the mid-1960s, provided a new and important therapeutic option for managing opioid addiction. Methadone, which has a plasma half-life of about 30 hours, requires administration on a daily basis to be optimally effective. There were concerns related to the potential diversion of this medication to illicit channels when it was dispensed to patients for consumption outside the clinic environment. The opioid effects produced by LAAM and its active metabolites, along with the potential for administering the parent drug on alternate days or on a three-times-weekly schedule (thus eliminating the need for "take-home" doses), fostered interest in its potential use as an alternative to methadone.

LAAM had already been shown to produce effects that were qualitatively similar to morphine and methadone. Also, LAAM is converted to two pharmacologically active compounds (*nor*-LAAM and *dinor*-LAAM) in addition to inactive compounds. The long half-lives of the *nor*-LAAM and *dinor*-LAAM metabolites, 48 and 96 hours, respectively, contribute to the extended duration of activity of LAAM.

Numerous studies provide evidence for the effectiveness of LAAM compared to methadone as an opioid-dependence treatment agent. Outcome measures most often assessed in these studies included treatment retention, patients' illicit use of opioids and other drugs during the course of treatment, social functioning (such as employment history and interactions with the legal system), and general medical and psychiatric parameters, including adverse events potentially related to the treatment medication.

Although these studies have shown that LAAM is effective, concerns that LAAM was associated with serious cardiac adverse events, including torsades de pointes, led to the decision to withdraw LAAM from the European market. It was not removed by the Food and Drug Administration (FDA) in the United States; however, the manufacturer subsequently withdrew it from the US market. Although LAAM is not currently available, it is possible LAAM sales could resume at some point, so further information about its clinical use is provided here

Because LAAM is administered on alternate days or three times weekly, it may provide advantages over methadone for some patients. Some individuals, because of the distance of their place of residence or employment from the treatment program, may find it difficult to receive their methadone doses on a daily basis. Take-home doses of methadone may provide an alternative; however, methadone is sometimes diverted for illicit sale and street use. The use of LAAM eliminates the need for a schedule of daily medication administration.

As with the use of any opioid-dependence treatment medication, patients must be carefully evaluated prior to the initiation of therapy. Close monitoring is especially important during the first few weeks following the beginning of LAAM therapy while a pharmacokinetic steady state is being attained. Although alcohol and illicit drug use should be discouraged throughout the entire course of treatment, this is especially important during the first few weeks of LAAM therapy when the potential for cumulative toxicity with other agents may be particularly difficult to predict. Additionally, because of the nature of the metabolism of LAAM, microsomal enzyme inducers, such as phenobarbital and rifampin, and inhibitors, such as cimetidine or ketoconazole, may have variable effects on the apparent activity or duration of action of LAAM. LAAM, unlike methadone, however, does not significantly affect the pharmacokinetics of the reverse transcriptase inhibitor zidovudine.

Opioid Antagonists

Antagonists help addicts to avoid relapse by occupying opioid receptor sites and blocking the effects of agonists at the cellular level. Relatively pure opioid antagonists, such as naltrexone, are not in themselves addicting and do not have the pharmacologically reinforcing effects of agonists. However, if an individual stabilized on naltrexone administers an opioid agonist, the effects of that drug are effectively blocked. Partial agonists, such as buprenorphine, may block or enhance the effects of other opioids and may have an abuse potential of their own.

Among the opioid antagonists, naltrexone has emerged as the most extensively studied agent. Despite its minimal side effects, naltrexone has not been widely accepted by addicts. This may be a result of several factors, including the risk of precipitating a withdrawal syndrome during naltrexone induction and the absence of reinforcing opioid effects. Many addicts stop taking naltrexone before they learn new, nonopioid methods for controlling anxiety or depression, or before they can recognize cues that can trigger withdrawal symptoms and the urge to use illicit drugs.

Pharmacology of Opioid Antagonists

Opioid antagonists are substances that bind to opioid receptors but do not produce morphine like effects. They compete at the receptors with both exogenous (e.g., morphine) and endogenous (e.g., endorphins) opioid agonists. When an antagonist is given in sufficient quantities, drugs such as heroin are prevented from interacting with their receptors. Opioid antagonists with high receptor affinity also displace agonists from receptor sites, reversing agonist effects. Antagonists also may be used to assess physical dependence, because they precipitate a withdrawal syndrome in chronic opioid users. Failure to respond to an opioid antagonist can be regarded as evidence against current physical dependence on opioids.

The first clinically useful antagonist was nalorphine, which reduced morphine effects, but also produced some direct agonist effects. Because of its potential for increasing rather than decreasing respiratory depression, nalorphine has been replaced by naloxone, which has no agonist effects and is considered to be a "pure" μ-opioid antagonist. Although opioid antagonists could potentially interfere with normal central pain inhibitory systems, consistent experimental evidence of this effect in human subjects has not been produced.

Naloxone has limited utility as a maintenance agent because it is poorly absorbed and has an effective duration of only a few hours following oral administration. Naltrexone, an analogue of naloxone synthesized in 1963, also has a high affinity for opioid receptors. It is well absorbed in the gastrointestinal tract and has antagonist activity for up to 72 hours after oral ingestion.

Formerly opioid-dependent patients have been maintained on effective blocking doses of naltrexone for up to 20 years, and large-scale, short-term studies that included several thousand patients failed to show evidence of naltrexone toxicity or significant laboratory abnormalities. Results from liver function tests in particular were a matter of concern because of the high frequency of hepatitis among addicts. A study of nonaddict groups treated with high doses of naltrexone showed dose-related increases in transaminase levels that were reversible when the medication was stopped. The individuals in that study received naltrexone 300 mg per day, or about six times the therapeutic dose in opioid-dependence treatment. Subsequently, however, measured liver function in response to high doses of naltrexone (up to 400 mg/day) in an eating disorders study, found no adverse clinical or laboratory changes in liver function.

Because medication compliance with the oral preparation of naltrexone has been low, a depot formulation of naltrexone has been developed (with an initial indication for alcohol dependence treatment). A depot form of naltrexone should play a valuable role in the treatment of opioid dependence.

Clinical Studies of Naltrexone

Although the plasma half-life of naltrexone (following oral administration) ranges from about 4 to 10 hours and that of its active metabolite, 6 β-naltrexol, from approximately

10 to 12 hours, the duration of opioid receptor blockade by naltrexone is much longer. The first human studies showing the potential of naltrexone blockade for treating opioid abuse were conducted in the early 1970s. It has been found that 30 to 50 mg of naltrexone administered orally blocked subjective effects of morphine for up to 24 hours. A carefully conducted double-blind study of naltrexone–opioid interactions in human subjects subsequently demonstrated that 150 to 200 mg of naltrexone attenuated heroin or hydromorphone effects for 72 hours, although some patients did report a "rush" or brief high after administration of the agonist.

Recently detoxified patients, particularly those discontinuing methadone maintenance, need to be opioid-free for at least 7 to 14 days to avoid precipitation of a withdrawal syndrome following the first dose of naltrexone. As an added precaution, it is advised that an intravenous or subcutaneous challenge of 0.4 to 0.8 mg naloxone be given prior to administration of naltrexone to ensure that withdrawal signs and symptoms are not produced. If the challenge is negative, patients are usually asymptomatic during naltrexone induction. If positive (i.e., there is evidence of opioid withdrawal), the first naltrexone dose given shortly thereafter is also likely to precipitate a withdrawal syndrome, but of longer duration. After a negative naloxone challenge, patients are given graduated doses of naltrexone, beginning with a 25 mg test dose, followed by 50, 75, and 100 mg on subsequent days. Most patients who tolerate 100 mg without side effects can be maintained on 100 mg of naltrexone on Mondays and Wednesdays and given 150 mg on Fridays.

Patients involved in meaningful relationships, employed full-time, or attending school and living with family members are most likely to benefit from naltrexone treatment. Nonetheless, naltrexone treatment has a very high early dropout rate. Only 20% to 30% of street heroin addicts successfully complete opioid detoxification, "pass" a naloxone challenge test, and begin naltrexone treatment; 40% of them may leave treatment before completing the first month. Only 10% to 20% take naltrexone for 6 months or longer, although addicted professionals and former prisoners on probation have significantly higher rates of accepting naltrexone and remaining in treatment. In one report acknowledging the difficulty in recruiting inner-city patients, only 15 of 300 (5%) offered naltrexone agreed to take it, and only 3 continued on naltrexone for more than 2 months.

Up to 20% of naltrexone patients have more than one treatment episode. During treatment, about a third of the patients will test the naltrexone blockade at least once, although most urine samples collected during treatment are negative for opioids. If patients have a pattern of missing naltrexone doses and using opioids, they soon discontinue naltrexone and relapse to opioid use. No evidence indicates that patients switch to nonopioid drugs while maintained on naltrexone, but those with histories of cocaine or other drug abuse may continue to use other substances. Follow-up of naltrexone-treated patients indicates that 30% to 40% are opioid-free for 6 months after terminating treatment. However, results depend on the population studied and the length of time patients have remained on naltrexone.

Naltrexone has no reinforcing properties of its own and is perceived as a subjectively neutral drug that prevents addicts from getting "high." Because most patients are ambivalent about stopping drug use and miss the reinforcing effects of opioids, many choose very early on to discontinue naltrexone or switch to methadone maintenance. Behavioral therapies using contingency management and reinforcers such as money or vouchers as a reward for opioid-negative urine samples or continued treatment have been used with some success to induce patients to remain longer on naltrexone.

Patients Suited for Treatment with Opioid Antagonists

The best results with naltrexone have been reported in the treatment of health care professionals. For example, in a study of physicians, 74% completed at least 6 months of treatment with naltrexone and were opioid-free and practicing medicine at 1-year follow-up. Another study found that 78% of health care professionals treated for an average of 8 months were rated as "much" or "moderately" improved at follow-up. Both studies involved comprehensive treatment, including medical evaluation, detoxification, psychiatric and family evaluation, and individual and family therapy (as well as confirmation of naltrexone ingestion).

Relapse to drug use and crime after release from prison is common for individuals with drug-related convictions. In efforts to reduce recidivism, naltrexone was studied in former opioid-dependent probationers and parolees. Former addict inmates who volunteered for a work-release program and who were using naltrexone were monitored for illicit drug use by random urine drug screening. Participants were offered additional treatment after their sentences were served. Success rates of former addicts in the work-release program were equal to those of inmates without drug histories. After completing the program, naltrexone-treated individuals had fewer drug arrests than did opioid abusers who did not receive naltrexone treatment. In another study, it has been reported on federal probationers and parolees with a history of opioid addiction who volunteered for a 6-month, randomized, controlled study of naltrexone and brief counseling, which was compared to counseling alone. More than 50% of subjects in the naltrexone-plus-counseling group remained in treatment for 6 months, as opposed to 33% of subjects who received only counseling. Opioid use was significantly lower in the naltrexone group, and fewer naltrexone-treated subjects (26% compared to 56% for the nonnaltrexone treated) had their probation status revoked with a subsequent return to prison during the 6-month period.

Naltrexone as Part of a Comprehensive Drug Treatment Program

Naltrexone treatment retention is enhanced by the presence of family support and supportive or behavioral therapy. Licensed physicians may prescribe naltrexone, but it is recommended that it be used by clinicians knowledgeable about substance abuse. Baseline laboratory tests should include liver function studies, and monthly testing should occur during the first 3 months, and at intervals of 3 to 6 months thereafter. It is recommended that opioid addicts in hepatic failure not be treated with naltrexone, although those with minor liver function abnormalities may receive treatment. After medical and psychosocial assessment, patients physically dependent on opioid agonists must undergo detoxification and a naloxone challenge.

It has been reported that with a procedure using intravenous midazolam and naloxone to shorten the transition time from methadone to naltrexone maintenance, enabling patients to receive therapeutic doses of naltrexone within hours of beginning this procedure. Highly motivated patients were willing to tolerate opioid withdrawal in order to return quickly to their jobs or to a more normal lifestyle. Subsequent studies of rapid detoxification have been conducted with clonidine, lofexidine, buprenorphine, and naloxone; ultrarapid detoxification with naloxone or naltrexone under anesthesia has also been used. These studies produced mixed results, with some describing uncomplicated naltrexone induction and reasonable retention and outcome, whereas others reported complicated induction, with vomiting and aspiration occurring under anesthesia, moderately severe withdrawal discomfort, and early dropout.

Several authors have warned of potential complications of ultrarapid detoxification. It has been found that acute and prolonged effects of ultrarapid detoxification on cardiopulmonary physiology, stress hormones, and clinical outcomes in seven patients inducted onto naltrexone. They found no significant changes in cardiac and pulmonary physiology during the anesthesia phase of ultrarapid detoxification, but plasma adrenocorticotropin hormone (ACTH) and cortisol increased 15- and 13-fold, respectively. During the postanesthesia phase, patients experienced marked withdrawal and tachypnea, and one developed respiratory distress. Withdrawal scores were significantly elevated for 3 weeks following induction, but opioid cravings were reduced. Because of the effects on breathing and stress hormones, the authors recommended further research on ultrarapid detoxification safety and efficacy, and that it be conducted only by experienced anesthesiologists. It has been described in six cases in which patients undergoing an ultrarapid detoxification procedure with subcutaneous naltrexone pellets developed life-threatening complications, including pulmonary edema, prolonged withdrawal, drug toxicity, withdrawal from benzodiazepine and alcohol coaddiction, aspiration pneumonia, and death. It should be noted that the formulation of the pellets used in these patients was *not* the same as the depot formulation.

Following naltrexone induction, compliance with naltrexone ingestion should be verified in the office or clinic, or by significant people in the patient's life. When treatment is progressing well, as determined by treatment engagement, job performance, and absence of illicit drug use confirmed by urinalysis, naltrexone dosing may be reduced to twice weekly. Once patients are stabilized, naltrexone maintenance is associated with few side effects, although nausea, abdominal pain, or headache, and mild increases in blood pressure have been noted. Years of chronic opioid use potentially alter endocrine responses, libido, mood, and pain threshold, so patients may experience rebound effects when opioids are discontinued. Such effects appear to be milder in naltrexone-maintained individuals than in those experiencing the naturally occurring lability of prolonged opioid abstinence without naltrexone. Some individuals taking naltrexone report an increased sex drive, a finding observed in rodents and also seen after patients discontinue methadone and other opioids. Although variable effects on appetite following the administration of naltrexone have been reported, decreases appear to predominate. Long-term opioid-receptor blockade by naltrexone does not appear to lead to alteration in mood, and increases in depression have infrequently been encountered.

Nalmefene: A Long-Acting Opioid Antagonist

Nalmefene is an opioid antagonist that has been approved for use in the management of opioid overdose and for the reversal of opioid drug effects. It is an orally active analogue of naltrexone with a terminal phase plasma half-life of approximately 8 to 9 hours. This is in contrast to the poor oral bioavailability and approximately 1- to 2-hour half-life of naloxone.

Numerous clinical pharmacology and efficacy studies have assessed the antagonist properties of nalmefene in human subjects. A single oral dose of nalmefene 50 mg administered to healthy volunteers blocks for 48 to 72 hours the respiratory depression, analgesia, and subjective effects secondary to intravenously administered fentanyl. A subsequent study confirmed the ability of nalmefene to antagonize respiratory depression induced by multiple fentanyl challenges. In the only study to assess dose effects and duration of opioid blockade in opioid abusers administered oral nalmefene, both the 50- and 100-mg doses blocked various physiologic (e.g., pupillary constriction) and subjective (e.g., morphine-induced euphoria) effects produced by 10 and 20 mg of morphine given intravenously. Nalmefene did not produce noticeable physiologic or subjective effects either alone or in combination with morphine.

Results also indicated that intravenous nalmefene (0.4 mg/70 kg body weight) was comparable to a four times greater dose of naloxone in reversing morphine-induced respiratory depression, and that nalmefene had a longer duration of action. In contrast, it was later reported that nalmefene and naloxone were equipotent in reversing fentanyl-induced respiratory depression following a single, intravenous dose of the antagonist. Other studies have shown nalmefene to be more effective or potent in reversing opioid-induced respiratory sedation and to be effective in the emergency management of opioid overdosage.

Nalmefene has generally been reported to be well tolerated in healthy volunteers. In one study, lightheadedness was the most commonly reported subjective effect following the administration of both single oral nalmefene doses of 50 to 300 mg, and 20-mg doses given twice daily for 7 days. Similarly, the parenteral administration of nalmefene in doses up to 24 mg was also well tolerated, with lightheadedness, dizziness, and mental fatigue being reported. In a study using individuals with a history of opioid abuse, a somewhat different effect profile was reported when nalmefene in single oral doses up to 100 mg was compared to morphine and placebo. Side effects reported only after nalmefene administration included agitation and irritability, muscle tension, abdominal cramps, and a "hungover feeling." Drowsiness or sleepiness was the most common effect reported following each of the treatments. These effects did not appear to be dose related and nalmefene did not produce typical morphine-like effects.

Nalmefene, like naltrexone, apparently does not produce morphine-like subjective effects that could be considered desirable by opioid-dependent or abusing individuals. The successful use of nalmefene, like naltrexone, as an adjunctive treatment for the maintenance of opioid abstinence will probably require highly motivated patients.

Current Status of Antagonist Treatment

Naltrexone treatment currently is limited to a relatively small number of patients. However, selected patients, particularly health care professionals and others with strong social and family support and good jobs, have benefited greatly from naltrexone, and have used even relatively short treatment episodes as a steppingstone toward opioid abstinence. Depot naltrexone may produce better long-term treatment compliance, but problems in recruiting and successfully inducting patients into treatment must be overcome before this type of naltrexone therapy becomes widely accepted. Because opioid dependence is a chronic relapsing disorder, no single treatment may result in long-term abstinence, but a cumulative effect produced by multiple treatments with naltrexone and other modalities may be required.

Conclusion

Various types of pharmacotherapies with different modes of action have been used and continue to be evaluated as treatments for opioid addiction. Because no single medication is appropriate for every individual, it is important that clinicians have a variety of therapeutic agents available to them. Additionally, pharmacotherapy is not a treatment end in itself; other adjuncts to successful treatment may include psychotherapy, social rehabilitation, vocational training, and others. Intraindividual treatment may also change over time as patients cycle through periods of abstinence and drug use. Rational medication therapy begins with an understanding not only of the disease state generally, but also of the specific dynamics of the addiction process that affect the overall success of treatment.

Suggested Readings

Charney DS, Riordan CE, Kleber HD, et al. Clonidine and naltrexone. A safe, effective, and rapid treatment of abrupt withdrawal from methadone therapy. *Arch Gen Psychiatry.* 1982;39:1327–1332.

Fudala PJ, Greenstein RA, O'Brien CP. Alternative pharmacotherapies for opioid addiction. In: Lowinson JH, Ruiz P, Millman RB, et al., eds. *Substance abuse: a comprehensive textbook,* 4th ed. Philadelphia: Lippincott Williams & Wilkins; 2005:641–653.

Gowing L, Farrell M, Ali R, et al. Alpha2 adrenergic agonists for the management of opioid withdrawal. *Cochrane Database Syst Rev.* 2004;(4):CD002024.

Kirchmayer U, Davoli M, Verster AD, et al. A systematic review on the efficacy of naltrexone maintenance for opioid dependence. *Addiction.* 2002;97:1241–1249.

Kreek MJ, Vocci FJ. History and current status of opioid maintenance treatments: blending conference session. *J Subst Abuse Treat.* 2002;23(2):93–105.

Minozzi S, Amato L, Vecchi S, et al. Oral naltrexone maintenance treatment for opioid dependence. *Cochrane Database Syst Rev.* 2006;(1):CD001333.

ACUPUNCTURE

Acupuncture (derived from the word *acus*, meaning a sharp point, and *punctura*, meaning to pierce) is defined as *stimulation, primarily by the use of solid needles, of traditionally and clinically defined points on or beneath the skin, in an organized fashion for therapeutic and/or preventive purposes.* The original acupuncture points (or *acupoints*) are superficial anatomic loci described in traditional Asian texts. Acupuncture points are often palpable as either mild depressions or small, and sometimes tender, subcutaneous nodules. In traditional Asian medicine, these points are stimulated either by puncture and manipulation with solid needles or by local heating. Heating is generally accomplished by the burning of dried, powdered *Artemisia vulgaris* (moxa), referred to as *moxibustion.*

In modern times, new methods of stimulating the acupoints include applications of electric current to needles in the points (electroacupuncture) or skin electrodes over the points, injections into the points, laser light directed onto the points, or finger-pressure massage of selected points, called *acupressure.* In addition, many new points and whole new "microsystems" of points have been described on specific body parts on which an entire homunculus is represented, leading to, for instance, scalp acupuncture, hand acupuncture, and ear acupuncture, also known as auricular acupuncture.

Although acupuncture and related acupoint therapies are most commonly known for their analgesic effects, their medical applications are by no means limited to pain treatment. The World Health Organization (WHO) has listed 42 medical problems that are considered suitable for acupuncture treatment, including the treatment of drug abuse.

Implications from Animal Experiments

The discovery of morphine-like substances (endorphins) in the mammalian brain had a great impact on modern concepts of pain and analgesia. It was soon clear that acupuncture-induced analgesia can be blocked by the opioid antagonist naloxone (Narcan), suggesting the involvement of endogenous opioid substances in acupuncture analgesia. In animal experiments, manual acupuncture or electroacupuncture was shown to accelerate the production and release of endorphins. Interestingly, electrical stimulation of different frequencies can specifically induce the release of different endorphins. For example, low-frequency (2 to 4 Hz) electroacupuncture stimulates release of the enkephalins, whereas high-frequency (100 Hz) electroacupuncture can stimulate the release of dynorphin.

It was natural to think that if acupuncture released endogenous opioids in the brain to ease pain, why not make use of it to relieve opioid withdrawal symptoms? This idea was initially tested in morphine-dependent rats. Withdrawal symptoms were significantly reduced by high-frequency (100 Hz) electroacupuncture administered at the hind limbs. This effect was found to be much greater than that induced by low-frequency (2 Hz) stimulation.

Experimental findings obtained in the rat model had shown that electrical stimulation applied to the surface of the skin could produce analgesic effects similar to that produced by electroacupuncture, as long as the stimulator provided a controlled current (to correct for varying skin resistance in the absence of a penetrating needle electrode). Satisfactory subjective results were obtained for the treatment of heroin withdrawal in humans using the same method of electrical acupoint stimulation via skin electrodes. Subsequent human studies revealed that this form of stimulation could also inhibit the craving for heroin in addiction patients.

Acupuncture and Related Techniques

Manual Needling

Classical acupuncture involves the piercing of the skin by a sharp metallic needle and manipulation by up-and-down and twisting or twirling movements. The traditional purpose of these movements is supposedly to stimulate the underlying anatomic conceptual structures described as meridians or channels (*jing*) and their branches (*luo*). The meridians may represent networks of connective tissue and nerves or may be merely allegorical and/or functional entities that serve as mnemonic aides to point locations. The correct placement of the needle at the acupoint and the optimal manipulation are generally characterized by feedback from the patient concerning a subjective feeling called *de-qi*. This sensation, reported by patients to include heaviness, soreness, numbness, and sense of swelling, occasionally also involves trembling of the local muscle. In the meantime, the operator of the needle often has a feeling resembling that experienced during fishing when a fish is nibbling at or swallowing the bait. This is likely the result of the rhythmic contraction of muscle fibers surrounding the needle. With this approach, the tip of the needle is felt to go deep into the tissue and believed to stimulate the structures to induce maximal *de-qi*. The shortcoming of this method, especially for research purposes, is that it is empirical and subjective in nature, difficult to describe precisely, and by no means easy to replicate by others. According to the traditional acupuncturist, it takes years to master the particular modes of manual stimulation.

Electroacupuncture

The analgesic effect induced by acupuncture can be completely blocked by a local procaine injection deep into the acupoint, but not by its subcutaneous injection, suggesting that the signal of acupuncture originates mainly from nervous tissues (or tissues susceptible to procaine blockade) located in deep structures rather than in the superficial layer of the skin. Using single nerve fiber recording technique to record the afferent impulses of the nerve innervating the site of stimulation, it was found that the nerve fibers responsible for transmission of acupuncture signals belong to the group II (Aβ)

fibers. Strong twisting and up-and-down movements of the needle produces a firing as high as 50 to 80, but no more than 100, spikes per second. Because the analgesic effect induced by manual needling can be totally abolished by local nerve blockade or nerve transection, a neural mechanism is strongly implicated. It is thus rational to use electrical stimulation administered via the metallic needles in lieu of its mechanical movement. This has been called *electroacupuncture*. The advantage of electroacupuncture is that the frequency, amplitude, and pulse width of the electrical stimulation can be determined precisely and objectively. Consequently, it can be replicated by other acupuncturists or experimenters without difficulty. Moreover, the procedure of inserting the needle at a precise skin location, as well as changing the direction and the depth of the needle to an optimal status, can still be performed by an experienced acupuncturist to achieve a maximal *de-qi* for confirmation of placement. It is only at the end of the placement procedure that the needles are connected to the electrical stimulator in place of further manual stimulation.

In addition, because drug addiction patients, especially those who inject, have a high incidence of blood-borne viral infections, it may be more convenient for invasive procedures to be replaced by noninvasive methods that do not produce sharp biohazardous waste.

Han's Acupoint Nerve Stimulator

An alternative to use of the electroacupuncture (insertion of a needle through the skin to deliver electrical stimulation to the underlying tissue) is to use a transcutaneous route of electrical administration. However, because skin has a very high impedance, which is more than 10 times that of the muscle tissue, it is necessary to use a constant current output device to ensure a regular level of stimulation without being affected by the degree of moisture on the skin surface or the change of blood flow rate within the skin. Because the tip of the needle goes several millimeters or even centimeters below the skin, the placement of the skin electrodes should ensure the maximal stimulation of the deep structures underlying the acupoint.

Regarding the frequency of stimulation, it is commonly accepted that conventional transcutaneous electric nerve stimulation (TENS) is based on the gate-control theory that high-frequency (e.g., 100 Hz), low-intensity stimulation is preferable to activate the large-caliber nerve fibers in order to suppress the pain mediated by the unmyelinated small-caliber fibers. On the other hand, "acupuncture-like" stimulation is characterized by low-frequency (e.g., 2 Hz), high-intensity stimulation. The current approach attempts to combine TENS-like and acupuncture-like stimulation to create what is hoped to be an optimal mode of stimulation. A device that possesses these features was designed and named Han's acupoint nerve stimulator (HANS).

Opioid Detoxification

Experimental Studies

Withdrawal syndromes have multiple manifestations. One of the cardiovascular manifestations of the opioid withdrawal syndrome is an increase in heart rate. In a mouse model of morphine dependence induced by injections of increasing doses of morphine for 8 days, the heart rate and blood pressure were measured by the tail cuff method. Morphine abstinence resulted in a 20% increase in heart rate without affecting the blood pressure. Electroacupuncture of 100 Hz or 15 Hz was very effective in bringing down the heart rate to approach the normal level; 2 Hz produced only a mild effect.

Human Observations

To observe the effect of HANS on the withdrawal syndromes in heroin addiction, HANS was used once a day for 30 minutes for a period of 10 days in a drug-addiction treatment center. Aside from the subjective answer to a standard questionnaire, two objective parameters were measured: heart rate and body weight.

Single Treatment

To observe the immediate effect of HANS on the heart rate of patients in withdrawal from heroin, the two pairs of output leads of the HANS were connected to four acupoints in the upper extremities. A "dense-and-disperse" mode of stimulation was administered, in which 2-Hz stimulation alternated automatically with 100-Hz stimulation, each lasting for 3 seconds. The control group received the same treatment of placing skin electrodes, except that the electrodes were disconnected from the electronic circuitry. The average heart rate of the patients in opioid withdrawal was 109 beats per minute before treatment. The dense-and-disperse mode stimulation for 30 minutes significantly reduced the heart rate. Suppression of the tachycardia occurred within the first 5 to 10 minutes. Heart rate continued to fall through minute 20, and leveled at 90 beats per minute for the last 10 minutes. The full effect remained for only 20 minutes after the stimulation; thereafter, heart rate began returning to its original level.

Multiple Treatments

To observe the cumulative effect of multiple daily treatments with HANS, 117 heroin addiction patients were randomly divided into four groups. Three groups received HANS of 2 Hz (constant frequency), 100 Hz (constant frequency), or 2/100 Hz (2 Hz alternating with 100 Hz, or "dense-and-disperse mode"), respectively. The control group received mock stimulation, where skin electrodes were placed and connected to the stimulator with blinking signals, yet the electric circuitry was disconnected. The treatment was for 30 minutes a day and was given for 10 consecutive days. Heart rate was measured with an electrocardiogram before and immediately after the HANS stimulation. For the 2-Hz group, in the first day of observation the heart rate averaged 110 beats per minute, which dropped to 90 beats per minute immediately after the HANS treatment ($p < 0.01$). This trend continued for days 3 and 4. On day 5, no significant difference was found in heart rate before and after the treatment (91 vs. 89 beats/minute), suggesting that the heart rate had returned to "normal" range.

Comparing the effects among the three HANS groups, the 100-Hz group produced a slightly better result than that of 2 Hz. In the 2/100-Hz group, the after-HANS heart rate reached an even lower level (72 beats/minute). Additionally, the heart rate of the 2/100-Hz group returned to "normal" range on day 4, 1 day earlier than the fixed frequency groups. In the control group receiving mock HANS, heart rate did not come down to a level of 100 beats per minute until 8 days after the treatment. These results suggest that repeated daily electroacupuncture treatment is effective in reducing the tachycardia of heroin withdrawal, with an effective order of dense-and-disperse >100 Hz >2 Hz.

Another parameter for measuring the severity of heroin withdrawal is body weight. The heroin-addicted subjects recruited in this study were aged 17 to 35 years; their average body weight was 49 to 51 kg. In the control group receiving mock HANS, body weight showed a reduction of 1 kg at the end of the first week, probably due to the presence of withdrawal distress. In the HANS-treated groups, a significant increase of body weight developed after 4 days of treatment, and continued to increase thereafter. Although the dense-and-disperse mode was significantly better than the fixed frequency groups in ameliorating tachycardia, no significant difference was observed among the three HANS groups in terms of body weight change.

In clinical practice with inpatients, opiate withdrawal symptoms have been significantly reduced, but not totally abolished by the HANS treatment, especially in those who had a history of heroin abuse for more than 5 years. In a study to quantify the role of HANS in a combined HANS/buprenorphine treatment, 28 heroin addiction patients were randomly divided into 2 groups: buprenorphine only, or HANS plus buprenorphine. In the buprenorphine-only group, the total buprenorphine dose requested in 14 days averaged 12.91 ± 1.34 mg ($X \pm$ SEM), whereas the total dosage requested by the HANS-plus-buprenorphine group averaged only 1.01 ± 0.09 mg, which was consumed only in the first 5 days.

Similar observations were made in another group of heroin-addicted subjects using a methadone reduction protocol as control group and HANS (2/100 Hz) plus methadone as the experimental group. The total dose of methadone used in the control group averaged 202 ± 15 mg ($X \pm$ SEM), whereas in the HANS-plus-methadone group the total dose of methadone was only 50.5 ± 8.2 mg ($p < 0.001$).

Prevention of Relapse to Opioid Abuse

Experimental Studies in the Rat

There are several animal models that can be used to study the problem of craving and relapse to drugs of abuse. Conditioned place preference (CPP) is one of the frequently used models. In a two-chamber or three-chamber experimental apparatus, the drug (unconditioned stimulus) is injected in the animal in one of the chambers. Thus, it becomes associated with the environmental stimuli unique to that chamber (color of the surroundings, texture of the floor, etc.). After repeated training, the rat will choose to stay longer on the drug-associated side than in a chamber associated with normal saline injection or no injection. The ratio between the time spent in the drug-associated side and the saline-associated side can be taken as an index for the degree of craving. By using this model, experiments were conducted to test whether acupuncture suppresses the expression of the CPP.

A two-chamber apparatus was used to study the effect of electroacupuncture on morphine CPP in the rat. CPP was established by morphine injection and the rats were trained for 10 days. The rats were then given electroacupuncture at 2 Hz, 100 Hz, or 2/100 Hz (dense-and-disperse mode). CPP was significantly suppressed by electroacupuncture of 2 Hz and 2/100 Hz, but not of 100 Hz. Because the procedure of electroacupuncture consists of keeping the rat in the holder, the insertion of the stainless steel needles into the hind leg points and the administration of electrical stimulation, three control groups of rats received: (a) restraining in the holder for 30 minutes, (b) holder restraining plus needle insertion without electrical stimulation, or (c) intermittent electrical stimulation on the feet (foot shock).

None of the three control groups showed any suppression of the CPP. The results suggest that it is the low-frequency component of the electroacupuncture that suppressed morphine CPP. Another issue deserving attention is that the effect of electroacupuncture can still be revealed 12 hours after the episode of electroacupuncture, suggesting that this effect lasts longer than acupuncture-induced analgesia (which usually disappears within 60 minutes after the end of stimulation).

For simplicity and clarity of analysis, previous studies observed only the effects produced by a single session of electroacupuncture. However, in clinical practice, acupuncture or HANS is delivered daily in consecutive days or even several times a day. To mimic the clinical situation, animal experiments were designed using electroacupuncture on consecutive days. The results showed that not only 2-Hz electroacupuncture, but also 100-Hz electroacupuncture is effective in suppressing morphine CPP. It seems plausible that by optimizing the parameters of electroacupuncture, its utility for the suppression of craving might be further improved.

Effect of HANS on Opiate Craving in Humans

To obtain a quantitative estimate of possible suppression of craving in response to acupuncture, a visual analogue scale (VAS) was used to assess the degree of craving in a group of heroin-addicted patients who had completed the process of detoxification more than 1 month previously. A 10-cm scale was used, with 0 as having absolutely no craving and 10 as having the most severe craving imaginable. A total of 117 subjects were recruited, and were randomly assigned into four groups. Three groups received HANS treatment, each with a different frequency, 2 Hz, 100 Hz, or 2/100 Hz. The intensity was increased from the threshold level of the first day by two or three threshold values in the following days. The fourth group was processed as in the previous groups except that the intensity was minimal to serve as a mock HANS control. There was a very slow decline of the VAS scores in the mock HANS control group. A dramatic decline in the degree of craving was observed in the groups receiving 2-Hz and 2/100-Hz electric stimulation, but not in the group receiving 100-Hz stimulation. Thus, low-frequency HANS was more effective than high-frequency HANS at reducing opioid craving.

Cocaine Abuse

Cocaine addiction is one of the most important challenges for acupuncture treatment of substance abuse for two reasons. First, the incidence of cocaine addiction has surpassed that of heroin in the whole world (13.4 vs. 9.2 million). Second, there is no effective pharmacologic treatment available for cocaine addiction.

Compared with heroin addiction, cocaine addiction shows minimal or no withdrawal syndrome on abstinence; yet more prominent and longer-lasting craving can occur, serving as one of the most important cues leading to relapse. Therefore, an important issue is whether acupuncture can have an effect on cocaine craving.

Experimental Studies

The establishment of cocaine-induced CPP depends on the dose and route of administration, as well as the number of conditioning sessions used. Using an 8-day conditioning paradigm and the dose of cocaine at 1 mg/kg (intraperitoneally) and higher, has permitted the study of the expression of cocaine-induced CPP in rats. High-frequency electroacupuncture (100 Hz) for 30 minutes was found to reduce the CPP significantly, whereas low-frequency (2 Hz) electroacupuncture was without effect. The procedure of electroacupuncture might involve at least three stress factors: restraining, needling, and electric shocking. These possibilities have individually been ruled out by control studies. The results suggest that it is the specific parameter of electroacupuncture rather than a nonspecific stressful condition that played an important role in modulating cocaine CPP.

The effect of electroacupuncture on suppressing cocaine CPP can be blocked by a specific κ-opioid receptor antagonist administered into the nucleus accumbens, but not into the amygdala, suggesting that the nucleus accumbens is one of the sites of action for endogenous opioid peptide, most probably dynorphin, to suppress cocaine CPP. This suggests that cocaine-induced CPP can be suppressed by electroacupuncture in a frequency-dependent manner, being effective at 100 Hz, but not at 2 Hz. The effect of 100 Hz electroacupuncture can be reversed by naloxone at 10 mg/kg but not with lower doses, suggesting the involvement of a κ-opioid mechanism in mediating electroacupuncture effect. These results may suggest a role for 100-Hz electroacupuncture or HANS to reduce cocaine craving and to prevent relapse.

Clinical Trials

Ear acupuncture is often used for the treatment of cocaine addiction in the United States, using the same four to five ear points bilaterally originally developed at Lincoln Hospital for use against opioid addiction and promulgated by the National Acupuncture Detoxification Association (NADA) for general use in addiction programs. In a series of 226 cases of users of cocaine or crack cocaine who had more than 20 visits to the Lincoln Hospital treatment center, 149 (65%) had more than 80% negative urine tests during the entire treatment involvement. Of the remaining patients, 39 (17%) had at least 80% negative urine tests during the 2 weeks prior to data collection. Although there is no control group, the success rate by itself was felt to be quite encouraging.

A randomized, controlled, single-blind, multisite large-scale clinical trial included 620 cocaine-dependent adult patients, 420 of whom used cocaine only and 208 of whom used both cocaine and opiates and were receiving methadone maintenance. Patients were randomly assigned to receive auricular acupuncture (four needles schedule), a needle-insertion control (four needles inserted into the helix of the ear), or a relaxation control. Treatments were offered five times weekly for 8 weeks. Main outcome measures were cocaine use during treatment and at the 3- and 6-month follow-up based on urine toxicology screen and retention in treatment. Analysis of urine samples showed a significant overall reduction in cocaine use but no differences by treatment condition, nor any difference in the rate of treatment retention. The conclusion is that within the clinical context of this study, acupuncture was not more effective than a needle insertion or relaxation control in reducing cocaine use.

Finally, in the planning of future large trials of acupoint therapy for cocaine addiction, attention should also be directed to the results obtained in rat experiments showing that 100-Hz, rather than 2-Hz, stimulation can suppress the cocaine-induced CPP. Recalling that this high-frequency stimulation is quite different from the more closely related low-frequency or manual stimulation, it may be important to include 100-Hz electroacupuncture (and possibly body electroacupuncture or HANS) stimulation in future trials of acupoint therapy for the treatment of cocaine addiction.

Alcoholism

Acupuncture was considered quite promising for the treatment of alcohol addiction in the 1980s. Two consecutive papers were published providing clearly positive results in this regard. The orthodox ear points suggested in the Lincoln Hospital/NADA protocol was used, and points 3 to 5 mm apart were used as nonspecific points for control. The subject size was 54 and 80, respectively, and the observation period was 6 months. The results obtained were in favor of acupuncture treatment, as manifested in the reduced need for alcohol, fewer drinking episodes, fewer subsequent admissions requiring detoxification, less desire to drink, and more people to complete the acupuncture program. However, this result could not be replicated in subsequent studies.

In a recent randomized, placebo-controlled study of auricular acupuncture, Bullock et al. conducted a large-scale clinical trial that included 503 cases. The unique feature of the design of the study for the patient grouping was that, aside from the "specific" ear acupuncture group, "nonspecific" ear acupuncture group, and the conventional treatment group, a fourth group was set using symptom-based acupuncture where the acupuncturists were not constrained to the four ear points stipulated in the other acupuncture treatment group, and point prescription could be changed on a day-to-day basis according to the patients' discomfort. All four groups showed a significant improvement. There were few differences associated with treatment assignment, and there were no treatment differences on alcohol use measures, although 49% of subjects reported that acupuncture reduced their desire for alcohol. These authors concluded that ear acupuncture did not make a significant contribution over and above that achieved by conventional treatment alone in the reduction of alcohol use.

Technical Comments on Using Acupuncture in the Treatment of Addiction

Because of the conflicting opinions regarding the efficacy of acupuncture for substance abuse treatment, the National Institute on Drug Abuse (NIDA) sponsored a technical review in 1991 to discuss this issue in an attempt to propose directions for future studies. A summary report was published, which pointed out four major problems that required a solution: the nonstandard terminology used to describe it, the wide range of procedures that have been called acupuncture, the lack of a clear mechanism to explain the purported benefits of acupuncture treatment, and the lack of systematic clinical research in this area.

Ear Acupuncture versus Body Acupuncture

From an historical point of view, the 14 meridians or channels considered by ancient Chinese physicians as the linkage for acupuncture points, serving as the channel for the flow of "qi," are distributed over the body rather than on the ear. In states that require fully licensed acupuncturists or physicians to administer ear needling, these operators may wish to consider the addition of body points or even additional treatment for other symptoms or complaints while the patient is being treated, concurrently with the NADA ear protocol. In states that have created the category of mid-level "acu-detox technicians" allowed only to administer the ear protocol, this would not be possible unless a fully licensed practitioner were involved. Although training or certification to pierce the skin is not required for the use of a TENS or HANS device, a knowledge of the location of the relevant points is still required.

Needle Staying versus Manual Needling

According to traditional acupuncture practice, a needle inserted into the acupoint can be further processed in at least different three ways: (a) left *in situ* undisturbed for a period of time, which is defined as "needle staying"; (b) manually twisted to obtain maximal *de-qi* sensation; or (c) heated at the shaft of the needle to intensify the therapeutic effect. It is clear that needle staying is the most modest of the three procedures. Moreover, the efficacy of needle staying depends on the site of needle insertion. The ear comprises skin that is covering cartilage, which is quite sensitive to mechanical stimulation and may produce continuous input during the staying of the needle. The situation will be dramatically different if the needle is inserted into soft tissues. When a needle is inserted in most body points, to induce a marked elevation of the pain threshold one has to twist or otherwise stimulate it.

Acupuncture and Electroacupuncture versus Transcutaneous Electric Stimulation

A series of studies showed that the manipulation of the needle triggers a train of nerve impulses transmitted along the afferent nerve fibers to the central nervous system. The physiologic effects produced by acupuncture (e.g., the antinociceptive effect) can be readily blocked by the injection of local anesthetics deep into the point, or along the nerve trunk. If nerve activation accounts for the transmission of the acupuncture signals, then similar effects should be induced whether similar nerve impulses are generated by manipulation of a needle, or directly by electrical impulses through the needles inserted into the point, or even by electrodes on the surface of the skin over the point, that force a current to pass through the same underlying tissue. It is interesting to note that a similar mechanism seems to underlie the two analgesic effects. Thus, no matter the electrical stimulation is delivered via needles or skin electrodes, the opioid antagonist naloxone at a 2 mg per kg dose produced a complete reversal of 2-Hz stimulation-produced analgesia, a partial reversal of 15-Hz stimulation-induced analgesia, and no reversal on 100-Hz stimulation-produced analgesia. In a human study, the analgesic effect induced by manual needling was compared to that induced by transcutaneous electric stimulation. The results indicated that they are essentially the same, if not identical.

In the past, blood-borne virus and anecdotal reports of bacterial infections have been associated with acupuncture. In a 2-year period, cases of acupuncture and relatively alcohol-resistant mycobacteria infection at acupuncture-point-specific locations have been reported. The risk of acupuncture-mediated infection is minimized by strict adherence to the instructions for single use only. For those still concerned, use of skin electrodes rather than needles will reduce this risk from minimal to zero.

How Frequently Should Acupuncture Be Used for Drug Abuse Treatment?

In an inpatient setting, both electroacupuncture and HANS work to suppress the opiate-withdrawal syndrome even if each is administered only once (for 30 minutes) a day. However, for the best results, it is recommended to use it three to four times a day for the first 5 days, followed by a reduction to twice a day for another 5 days, and then once a day for the rest of the time for a total of 2 weeks. Too frequent an application results in a decrease of therapeutic effect because of the development of tolerance. For the treatment of protracted withdrawal syndromes in the period of rehabilitation, once or twice a day is sufficient. The session applied immediately before sleep is critical for the treatment schedule, because this will facilitate a good sleep. It is notable that in rat experiments, the effect of electroacupuncture in suppressing CPP induced by morphine or cocaine bears a long latency of 10 hours and a long aftereffect of at least 24 hours. This may serve as a mechanism for the cumulative effect observed in the treatment of drug abuse with acupuncture.

Conclusion

Acupuncture is an emerging treatment for drug abuse. This new approach is different from that of pharmacologic treatment. From a technical point of view, there is room for improvement and definitive evidence of efficacy remains to be shown. Many patients and providers remain convinced that it has something to add to the treatment package. The complicated network underlying drug abuse can be unraveled only through combined physiologic, neurobiologic, and psychologic endeavors, and acupuncture can play a role at least as one of the tools in a comprehensive approach.

Suggested Readings

Avants SK, Margolin A, Holford TR, et al. A randomized controlled trial of auricular acupuncture for cocaine dependence. *Arch Intern Med.* 2000;160:2305–2312.

Bullock ML, Kiresuk TJ, Sherman RE, et al. A large randomized placebo-controlled study of auricular acupuncture for alcohol dependence. *J Subst Abuse Treat.* 2002;22:71–77.

Gates S, Smith LA, Foxcroft DR. Auricular acupuncture for cocaine dependence. *Cochrane Database Syst Rev.* 2006;(1):CD005192.

Han JS, Trachtenberg AI, Lowinson JH. Acupuncture. In: Lowinson JH, Ruiz P, Millman RB, et al., eds. *Substance abuse: a comprehensive textbook*, 4th ed. Philadelphia: Lippincott Williams & Wilkins; 2005:743–762.

Margolin A, Kleber HD, Avants SK, et al. Acupuncture for the treatment of cocaine addiction. *JAMA.* 2002;287:55–63.

24

INDIVIDUAL PSYCHOTHERAPY

Psychosocial treatment approaches that have originated with treating addictive disorders, such as Alcoholics Anonymous (AA) and therapeutic communities, have emphasized large and small group treatment settings. Although always present as a treatment option, individual psychotherapy has not been the predominant treatment modality for drug abusers since the 1960s, when inpatient 12-step–informed milieu therapy, group treatments, methadone maintenance, and therapeutic community approaches came to be the fixtures of addiction treatment programs. These modalities derived their popularity from the failures of dynamically informed ambulatory individual psychotherapy when it was used as the sole treatment for addictive disorders. There are several reasons this latter approach was poorly suited to the needs of addicts when it was offered as the sole ambulatory treatment.

First, the lack of emphasis on symptom control and the lack of structure in the therapist's typical stance allowed the patient's continued drug or alcohol use to undermine treatment. In addition, another misfit between individual dynamic therapy and addictive disorders is the anxiety-arousing nature of the former coupled with the lack of structure provided by the therapist. Because addicts frequently react to increased affects by resuming substance use, it is important to introduce anxiety-arousing aspects of treatment only after a strong therapeutic alliance has been developed or within the context of other supportive structures.

Individual psychotherapy has become a resurgent approach since the 1980s, as necessary modifications in technique were made to address the factors underlying earlier failures. A major development in recent years has been the growing list of individual psychotherapies for addictive disorders that have demonstrated efficacy in rigorously conducted randomized clinical trials.

Psychotherapy and Pharmacotherapy

The most commonly used pharmacologic approaches to drug abuse are maintenance on an agonist that has an action similar to that of the abused drug (e.g., methadone, nicotine gum), use of an antagonist that blocks the effect of the abused drug (e.g., naltrexone), use of an aversive agent that provides a negative reinforcement if the drug is used (e.g., disulfiram), or the use of agents that reduce the desire to use the substance (e.g., naltrexone, acamprosate). Although these agents are widely used, they seldom are employed without adjunctive psychotherapy.

The shortcomings of pharmacotherapies delivered without psychotherapy were convincingly demonstrated. In a 24-week trial, 92 opioid addicts were randomly assigned to receive one of the following: (a) methadone maintenance alone, without psychosocial services; (b) methadone maintenance with standard psychosocial services, which included regular individual meetings with a counselor; and (c) enhanced methadone maintenance, which included regular counseling plus access to onsite psychiatric, medical, employment, and family therapy. In terms of drug use and psychosocial outcomes, the best outcomes were seen in the enhanced condition, with intermediate outcomes for the standard methadone services condition, and poorest outcomes for the methadone-alone condition.

The results of this study suggest that the majority of patients on methadone maintenance will not benefit from a purely pharmacologic approach, and the best outcomes are associated with higher levels of psychosocial treatments. Psychotherapeutic interventions are needed to complement pharmacotherapy by (a) enhancing motivation to stop substance use by taking the prescribed medications, (b) providing guidance for the use of medication, (c) maintaining motivation to continue taking the medication after the patient achieves abstinence, (d) providing relationship elements to prevent premature termination, and (e) helping the patient to develop the skills to adjust to a life without drug and alcohol use.

Although psychotherapy can enhance the effectiveness of pharmacotherapy, this section would not be complete without considering the role of pharmacotherapy to enhance the efficacy of psychotherapy. These two treatments have different mechanisms of action and targeted effects that can counteract the weaknesses of either treatment alone. Psychotherapies effect change by psychologic means in psychosocial aspects of drug abuse, such as motivation, coping skills, dysfunctional thoughts, or social relationships. Their weaknesses include limited effects on the physiologic aspects of drug use or withdrawal, and effects tend to be delayed, require practice, and repeated sessions. In contrast, the relative strengths of pharmacologic treatments are their rapid actions in reducing immediate or protracted withdrawal symptoms, drug craving, or the rewarding effects of continued drug use. In effect, pharmacotherapies for drug dependence reduce the patients' immediate access to and preoccupation with drugs, freeing the patient to address other concerns such as long-term goals or interpersonal relationships.

Because of the complementary actions of psychotherapies and pharmacotherapies, combined treatment has a number of potential advantages. Although factors such as cost and patient acceptance can limit use of combined approaches, it is important to note that no studies have shown that combined treatments are less effective than either psychotherapy or pharmacotherapy alone.

Individual versus Group Therapy

If psychotherapy is necessary for at least a substantial number of treatment-seeking drug addicts, when is individual therapy a better choice than other modalities such as family therapy or group therapy? Because group therapy has become the modal format for psychotherapy of drug addicts, evaluation of the role of individual therapy should take the strengths and weaknesses of group therapy as its starting point.

An advantage of group therapy is economy. Groups typically have a minimum of six members and a maximum of two therapists, yielding at least a threefold increase in the number of patients treated per therapist hour. Although the efficacy of group versus individual therapy has only rarely been systematically studied with drug addicts, no evidence is available from other populations that individual psychotherapy yields superior benefits.

In addition to the general concept that group therapy can be just as effective as, but less expensive than, individual therapy, there are aspects of group therapy that can be argued to make this modality more effective than individual treatment of drug addicts. For example, given the social stigma attached to having lost control of substance use, the presence of other group members who acknowledge having similar problems can provide comfort. Other group members who are further along in their recovery from addiction can act as models to illustrate that attempting to stop drug and alcohol use is not a futile effort. Moreover, group members frequently can act as "buddies" who offer continued support outside of the group sessions in a way that most professional therapists do not. Finally, the "public" nature of group therapy, with its attendant aspects of confession and forgiveness provides a powerful incentive to avoid relapse. This public affirmation or shaming can be all the more crucial in combating a disorder that is characterized by a failure of internalized mechanisms of control. Drug addicts have been characterized as having poorly functioning internal self-control mechanisms, and the group process provides a robust source of external control.

Given these strengths of group therapy, what are the advantages of individual therapy that can justify its greater expense? First, a key advantage of individual therapy is that it provides privacy. Participation in group therapy always risks a breach in confidentiality, especially in small communities. Although publicly admitting to one's need for help can be a key element of the recovery process, it is a step that is very difficult to take, particularly when the problems associated with substance use have not yet become severe. Public knowledge of drug and alcohol use still can ruin careers and reputations.

Second, the pace of individual therapy allows the therapist more flexibility to address the patient's problems as they arise, whereas group therapy can be out of sync with some members while suiting the needs of the majority. This situation is particularly an issue for open groups that add new members throughout the life of the group, necessitating repetition of many therapeutic elements so as to acquaint new members with the group's history and to address the needs of individuals who have just begun treatment.

Third, from the patient's point of view, individual therapy allows a much higher percentage of therapy time to concentrate on issues that are uniquely relevant to that individual. Members of therapy groups usually have the experience of spending many hours discussing issues that are not problems for them.

Fourth, logistical issues make individual therapy more practical in many settings. Individual therapy is most feasible for many mental health professionals or medical practitioners who do not have a caseload of addicts large enough to conduct group treatment. Unless group therapy is offered in the context of a large clinic or practice with many ongoing groups, scheduling can be very difficult.

Fifth, the process and structure of individual therapy can confer unique advantages in dealing with some kinds of problems presented by patients. For example, individual therapy can be more conducive to the development of a deepening relationship between the patient and therapist over time, which can allow exploration of relationship elements. Alternatively, patients with particular personality disorders, such as borderline or schizoid patients, may be unable to become involved with other group members, as can patients who are so shy that they cannot bring themselves to attend group sessions.

Specialized Knowledge Necessary for Therapy with Addicts

Pharmacology, Use Patterns, Consequences, and Course of Addiction

The principal areas of knowledge to be mastered by the beginning therapist are pharmacology, use patterns, consequences, and course of addiction for the major types of abused substances. It is useful not only to obtain textbook knowledge about frequently abused drugs, but also to become familiar with street knowledge about drugs (e.g., slang names, favored routes of administration, prices, and availability) and the clinical presentation of individuals when they are intoxicated or experiencing withdrawal from various abused drugs. By knowing the natural history of addiction and the course of drug and alcohol effects, the clinician can be guided in helping the patient anticipate problems that will arise in the course of initiating abstinence.

Second, knowledge of drug actions and withdrawal states is crucial for diagnosing comorbid psychopathology and for helping the addict to understand and manage dysphoric affects. Most abused drugs are capable of producing constellations of symptoms that mimic psychiatric syndromes. Many of these symptomatic states are substance induced and resolve spontaneously when such use is stopped. It often is the therapist's job to determine whether presenting symptoms are part of an enduring, underlying psychiatric condition or a transient, drug-induced state.

This need to distinguish transient substance-induced affects from enduring attitudes and traits also is an important psychotherapy task. Affective states are linked closely with cognitive distortions. Because of the tendency for substance-related affective states to color the patient's views, it is important for the therapist to be able to recognize these states so that the associated distorted thoughts can be recognized as such. It is important that the patient also be taught to distinguish between sober and substance-affected conditions and to recognize when, in the colloquial phrase, it is "the alcohol talking" and not the person's more enduring sentiments.

Third, learning about drug and alcohol effects is important in detecting when patients have relapsed or come to sessions intoxicated. It is rarely useful to conduct psychotherapy sessions when the patient is intoxicated. The clinician must rely on his or her clinical skills to determine whether or not the patient is drug free and able to participate in psychotherapy.

Other Treatment and Self-Help Group Philosophies and Techniques

Another area of knowledge to be mastered by the psychotherapist is an overview of treatment philosophies and techniques that are available to substance-using patients. For many addicts, individual psychotherapy is best conceived as a component of a multifaceted program to help the patient overcome a chronic, relapsing condition. Even when the therapist is a solo practitioner, the therapist should know when detoxification is necessary, when inpatient treatment is appropriate, and what pharmacotherapies are available.

A major function of knowing about alternative treatment modalities for addicts is to be alert to the possibility that different treatments can provide contradictory recommendations that may confuse the patient or foster the patient's attempts to sabotage treatment. The individual psychotherapist does not have the option of simply instructing the patient to curtail other treatments or participation in self-help groups while individual treatment is taking place. Rather, it is vital that the therapist attempt to adjust his or her own work to bring the psychotherapy into accord with other treatments.

A commonly occurring set of conflicts arises between the treatment goals and methods employed by professional therapists and those of 12-step self-help movements. For example, the recovery goal for many who use a 12-step approach is a life of complete abstinence from psychotropic medications. This approach may conflict with professional advice when the therapist recommends use of psychopharmacologic treatments for co-occurring psychiatric disorders. Although the 12-step literature supports use of appropriately prescribed medications of all kinds, many individual members draw the line at prescribed psychotropic medications. In the face of disapproval from fellow members, patients may prematurely discontinue psychotropic medications and experience relapse of psychologic symptoms, with consequent return to substance use. To avoid this situation, it is important for the therapist who recommends or prescribes psychotropic medications to warn the patient about the apparent contradiction between the 12-step admonition to lead a drug-free life and the clinician's use of prescribed psychotropic medications.

A second common area of conflict between some forms of psychotherapy and the 12-step philosophy is the role played by family members. The Al-Anon approach tends to suggest that family members get out of the business of attempting to control the addict's use of drugs and alcohol. Separate meetings are held for family members and addicts. In contrast, many therapists encourage involvement of family members. As with the use of psychotropic medications, the major way to prevent a patient's confusion is to anticipate the areas of contradictory advice and to provide a convincing rationale for the therapist's recommendations. In doing so, it is advisable to acknowledge that different strategies appear to work for different individuals.

Common Issues and Strategies

This section reviews issues that must be addressed for individual psychotherapy to be effective. As noted in reviewing the difficulties encountered by early psychodynamic practitioners, the central modification that is required of psychotherapists is to be aware that the patient being treated is an addict. Hence, even when attempting to explore other issues in depth, the therapist should (a) devote at least a small part of every session to monitoring the patient's most recent successes and failures in controlling or curtailing substance use and (b) be willing to interrupt other work to address slips and relapses as they occur.

Implicit in the need to remain focused on the patient's substance use is the recognition that psychotherapy with these patients entails a more active therapist stance than does treatment of patients with other psychiatric disorders, such as depression or anxiety. This need is related to the fact that the principal symptom of substance abuse—compulsive use—is at least initially gratifying, whereas it is the long-term consequences of substance use that induce pain and the desire to stop. In contrast, the principal symptoms of depression or anxiety disorders are inherently painful and alien. Because of this key difference, psychotherapy with addicts typically requires both empathy and structured limit-setting, whereas the need for limit setting is less marked in psychotherapy with depressed or anxious patients.

Enhancing Motivation

Regardless of the treatment type, an early task for psychotherapists is to gauge the patient's level of motivation to stop his or her substance use by exploring the patient's treatment goals. In this task, it is important to challenge overly quick or glib assertions that the patient's goal is to stop using the substance altogether. One way to approach the patient's likely ambivalence is to attempt an exploration of the patient's perceived benefits from use of alcohol or drugs, or the patient's perceived need for them. After the therapist has obtained a clear picture of the patient's perceived needs and desires, it is important to counter these perceptions by exploring the advantages of a drug-free life.

Although virtually all types of psychotherapy for addiction address the issue of motivation and goal setting to some extent, motivational therapy or interviewing makes this the sole initial treatment focus. Motivational approaches are designed to produce rapid, internally motivated change by seeking to maximize patients' motivational resources and commitment to abstinence.

One major controversy in this area is whether controlled use can be an acceptable alternative treatment goal to abstinence from all psychoactive drugs. For illicit drugs of abuse (such as cocaine or heroin), it is unwise for a clinician to take a position that advocates any continued use, because such a stance allies the therapist with illegal and antisocial behavior. The process of arriving at an appropriate treatment goal frequently involves allowing the patient to make several failed attempts to achieve a goal of controlled use. This initial process may be necessary to convince the patient that a goal of abstinence is more appropriate.

Teaching Coping Skills

The most enduring challenge in treating addicts is to help the patient avoid relapse after achieving an initial period of abstinence. A general tactic for avoiding relapse is to identify specific circumstances that increase an individual's likelihood of resuming substance use and to help the patient anticipate and practice strategies (e.g., refusal skills, recognizing and avoiding cues for craving) for coping with these high-risk situations. Approaches that emphasize the development of coping skills include cognitive–behavioral therapy (CBT), in which a systematic effort is made to identify high-risk situations and master alternative behaviors, as well as coping skills intended to help the patient avoid drug use when these situations arise.

Changing Reinforcement Contingencies

Because the typical course of illicit drug use entails initiation of compulsive use between the ages of 12 and 25 years, many patients come to treatment without having achieved satisfactory adult relationships or vocational skills. In such cases, achieving a drug- and alcohol-free life may require a lengthy process of vocational rehabilitation and development of meaningful relationships. Individual psychotherapy can contribute importantly to this process by helping maintain the patient's motivation throughout the recovery process and by helping the patient to explore factors that have interfered with achievement of rewarding ties to others.

Fostering Management of Painful Affects

Many psychodynamic clinicians have suggested that failure of affect regulation is a central dynamic underlying the development of compulsive alcohol or drug use.

Moreover, surveys of psychiatric disorders in treatment-seeking and community populations concur in demonstrating high rates of depressive disorders among drug users. A key element in developing ways to handle powerful dysphoric affects is learning to recognize and identify the probable cause of such feelings. To foster the development of mastery over dysphoric affects, most psychotherapies include techniques for eliciting strong affects within a protected therapeutic setting and then enhancing the patient's ability to identify, tolerate, and respond appropriately to them. Given the demonstrated efficacy of pharmacologic treatments for affective and anxiety disorders and the high rates of these disorders seen in treatment-seeking populations, the individual psychotherapist should be alert to the possibility that a patient may benefit from combined treatment with psychotherapy and medications.

Improving Interpersonal Functioning and Enhancing Social Supports

Gratifying friendships and intimate relationships provide a powerful source of rewards to replace those obtained from drug and alcohol use, and the threat of losing those relationships can be a strong incentive to maintain abstinence. Typical issues presented by addicts are the loss of or damage to valued relationships that occurred when alcohol or drug use became the individual's priority, failure to have achieved satisfactory relationships even before having initiated substance use, and inability to identify friends or intimates who are not engaged in substance abuse.

A major potential limitation of individual psychotherapy as the sole treatment for alcohol or drug dependence is its failure to provide adequate social supports to patients who lack a supportive social network of friends who are not engaged in substance abuse. Approaches that emphasize the development of a strong relationship with persons who are not substance users are traditional counseling, 12-step facilitation, and other approaches that underline the importance of involvement in self-help groups. Self-help groups offer a fully developed social network of welcoming individuals who are understanding and committed to leading a substance-free life. Moreover, a sponsor system is available to provide the recovering person with individual guidance and support. For psychotherapists who working with addicts, encouraging patients to become involved in self-help groups can provide a powerful source of social support that protects the patient from relapse while the work of therapy progresses.

Efficacy Research

Individual Psychotherapy and Opioid Agonist Therapy

Only a few studies have evaluated the efficacy of formal psychotherapy to enhance outcomes with agonist treatments. The landmark study in this area consisted of was when 110 opiate addicts entering a methadone maintenance program were randomly assigned to one of three treatments: drug counseling alone, drug counseling plus supportive–expressive (SE) psychotherapy, or drug counseling plus cognitive psychotherapy. After a 6-month course of treatment, although the SE and cognitive psychotherapy groups did not differ significantly from each other on most measures of outcome, subjects who received either form of professional psychotherapy evidenced greater improvement in more outcome domains than did the subjects who received drug counseling alone. Gains made by the subjects who received professional psychotherapy were sustained over a 12-month follow-up period.

Contingency Management

Several studies have evaluated the use of contingency management to reduce the use of illicit drugs in addicts who are maintained on methadone. In these studies, a reinforcer (reward) is provided to patients who demonstrate specified target behaviors such as providing drug-free urine specimens, accomplishing specific treatment goals, or attending treatment sessions. For example, offering methadone take-home privileges contingent on reduced drug use is an approach that capitalizes on an inexpensive reinforcer that is potentially available in all methadone maintenance programs. change extensive to Extensive extensive work in evaluating methadone take-home privileges as a reward for decreased illicit drug use. In a series of well-controlled trials, these researchers demonstrated (a) the relative benefits of positive (e.g., rewarding desired behaviors such as abstinence) compared with negative (e.g., punishing undesired behaviors such as continued drug use through discharges or dose reductions) contingencies, (b) the attractiveness of take-home privileges over other incentives available within methadone maintenance clinics, and (c) the relative effectiveness of rewarding drug-free urine specimens compared with other target behaviors.

Behavioral Therapies

Naltrexone offers advantages over methadone treatment, including that it can be prescribed without concerns about diversion, it has a benign side-effect profile, and it can be less costly in terms of demands on professional and patient time than the daily or near-daily clinic visits required for methadone maintenance. Most important are the behavioral aspects of treatment, as unreinforced opiate use allows extinction of relationships between cues and drug use.

Naltrexone treatment programs remain comparatively rare and underused. This situation is largely a result of problems with retention. An average of 40% of patients drop out during the first month of treatment and 60% drop out by 3 months. In the 1970s, several preliminary evaluations of behavioral interventions used to address the weaknesses of naltrexone, including providing incentives for compliance with naltrexone and the addition of family therapy to naltrexone treatment, suggested the promise of these strategies. However, the interventions were not widely adopted.

Recent promising data about strategies to enhance retention and outcome in naltrexone treatment have come from investigations of contingency management approaches. Preston et al. found improved retention and naltrexone compliance with an approach that provided vouchers for naltrexone compliance. It has been found that reinforcement of naltrexone compliance and drug-free urine specimens, alone or in combination with family involvement in treatment, improved retention and reduced drug use among recently detoxified opioid-dependent individuals.

Individual Psychotherapy for Cocaine Dependence

Compared with the results of trials evaluating pharmacologic treatment of cocaine dependence, evaluations of behavioral therapies—particularly contingency management, CBT, and manualized disease-model approaches—are much more promising.

Behavioral therapies for cocaine-dependent individuals have focused on key outcomes such as retention and the inception and maintenance of abstinence.

Contingency Management

Perhaps the most exciting findings pertaining to the effectiveness of behavioral treatments for cocaine dependence have been reports by Higgins et al. on the use of behavioral incentives for abstinence. This strategy has four organizing features that are grounded in principles of behavioral pharmacology: (a) drug use and abstinence must be swiftly and accurately detected, (b) abstinence is positively reinforced, (c) drug use results in loss of reinforcement, and (d) emphasis is placed on the development of reinforcers to compete with drug use. In this approach, urine specimens are required three times weekly to detect all episodes of drug use systematically. Abstinence, verified through drug-free urine screens, is reinforced through a voucher system in which patients receive points redeemable for items consistent with a drug-free lifestyle (such as movie tickets and sporting goods).

A series of well-controlled clinical trials have demonstrated high acceptance, retention, and rates of abstinence for patients receiving this approach. Although the strong effects of this treatment decline somewhat after the contingencies are terminated, the voucher system has durable effects. Moreover, the efficacy of a variety of contingency management procedures (including vouchers, direct payments, and free housing) has been replicated in other settings and samples, including cocaine-dependent individuals within methadone maintenance, homeless addicts, freebase cocaine users, and pregnant drug users. These findings are of great importance because contingency management procedures are potentially applicable to a wide range of target behaviors and problems, including treatment retention and compliance with pharmacotherapy.

Nevertheless, despite the very compelling evidence of the effectiveness of these procedures in promoting retention in treatment and reducing cocaine use, the procedures rarely are used in clinical treatment programs. One major impediment to broader use is the expense; average earnings for patients are about $600. Low-cost contingency-management procedures may be a way to bring these effective approaches into general clinical use. Petry et al. demonstrated that a variable ratio schedule of reinforcement that provides access to large reinforcers (but at low probabilities) is effective in retaining subjects in treatment and reducing substance use. Rather than earning vouchers, subjects earn the chance to draw from a bowl and win prizes of varying magnitudes. The prizes range from small $1 prizes (bus tokens) to large $20 prizes (watches), to jumbo $100 prizes (small televisions). This system is far less expensive than the standard voucher system, because only a proportion of behaviors are reinforced with a prize. In a study of 42 alcohol-dependent veterans who were randomly assigned to standard treatment or standard treatment plus contingency management, 84% of the contingency-management subjects were retained in treatment throughout an 8-week period, compared with 22% of standard treatment subjects. By the end of the treatment period, 69% of those receiving contingency-management treatment had not experienced a relapse to alcohol use, but only 39% of those receiving standard treatment were abstinent.

Cognitive–Behavioral Therapies

Another behavioral approach that is effective in treating cocaine abusers is CBT. A number of randomized clinical trials have demonstrated that (a) compared with other commonly used psychotherapies for cocaine dependence CBT appears to be particularly more effective with more severe cocaine users or those with comorbid disorders, (b) CBT is significantly more effective than less-intensive approaches, and (c) CBT is as or more effective than manualized disease-model approaches. Moreover, CBT appears to be a particularly durable approach, with patients continuing to reduce their cocaine use even after they leave treatment.

Manualized Disease-Model Approaches

Until very recently, treatment approaches based on disease models were widely practiced, but virtually no well-controlled randomized clinical trials had evaluated their efficacy alone or in comparison with other treatments. Thus, another important finding emerging from randomized clinical trials that has great significance for the treatment community is the effectiveness of manualized disease-model approaches. One such approach is 12-step facilitation (TSF), a manual guided, individual approach that is intended to be similar to widely used approaches that emphasize principles associated with disease models of addiction and has been adapted for use with cocaine-dependent individuals. Although this treatment has no official relationship with 12-step programs, its content is intended to be consistent with the 12 steps of AA, with primary emphasis given to steps 1 through 5 and the concepts of acceptance and surrender. In addition to abstinence from all psychoactive substances, a major goal of the treatment is to foster active participation in self-help groups.

The findings from studies offer compelling support for the efficacy of manual-guided disease-model approaches. This has important clinical implications because these approaches are similar to the dominant model applied in most community treatment programs and thus can be more easily mastered by clinicians than can approaches such as contingency management or CBT—treatments whose theoretical underpinnings may not be perceived highly compatible with disease-model approaches (although such incompatibility has yet to be demonstrated).

Individual Psychotherapy for Marijuana Dependence

Although marijuana is the most commonly used illicit substance, treatment of marijuana abuse and dependence is a comparatively understudied area to date. Currently, only a few controlled trials of behavioral approaches have been completed. For instance, a study compared a delayed-treatment control group with a two-session motivational approach and to an intensive (14-session) relapse prevention approach, and found better marijuana outcomes for the two active treatments than with the delayed-treatment control group, but found no significant differences between the brief and the more intensive treatment. A replication and extension of that study, involving a multisite trial of 450 marijuana-dependent patients, compared three approaches: (a) a delayed treatment control, (b) a two-session motivational approach, and (c) a nine-session combined motivational/coping skills approach. Results suggested that both active treatments were associated with significantly greater reductions in marijuana use than the delayed treatment control through a 9-month follow-up period. Budney et al. have extended the application of contingency management to marijuana users, and reported that adding voucher-based incentives to coping skills and motivational enhancement improves outcomes during treatment for marijuana dependence.

Psychotherapy as Ancillary Treatment

In considering psychotherapy as part of an ongoing comprehensive program of treatment, it is useful to distinguish between treatment of opioid addicts and alcoholics, for which powerful pharmacologic approaches are available, and treatment of other drugs of abuse, for which strong alternatives to behavioral approaches are not yet available. For alcoholics, naltrexone, acamprosate, and disulfiram have strong potential for improving treatment outcome and reducing relapse rates. However, the effectiveness of disulfiram in the absence of a strong psychosocial treatment is no greater than placebo, and most studies demonstrating the efficacy of naltrexone and acamprosate have been done in the context of a comparatively intense psychosocial intervention. For opioid-dependent patients, the modal treatment approach remains methadone maintenance, whereas an alternative pharmacotherapy, naltrexone, can be highly potent for the minority who choose this approach. Because of their powerful and specific pharmacologic effects, either to satisfy the need for opioids or to prevent illicit opioids from yielding their desired effect, these agents—provided that they are delivered with at least minimal counseling—can be sufficient for many opioid addicts. The choice of those who might benefit from individual psychotherapy may be guided by work that suggests psychotherapy is most likely to be of benefit to those opioid addicts with higher levels of psychiatric symptoms. Because the benefits of psychotherapy can be maximized when instituted relatively soon after treatment entry, assessment instruments such as the Addiction Severity Index can be used to identify quickly those with psychopathology, alerting staff to the need to refer the client for psychotherapy.

For nonopioid drugs of abuse, an active search for effective pharmacotherapies currently is under way. In the interim, the mainstay of treatment for such patients remains some form of psychosocial treatment offered in a group, family, residential, or individual setting. For cocaine use, forms of treatment that currently have the strongest levels of empirical support for cocaine users include contingency management and CBT. However, there is as yet no strong empirical evidence regarding the optimal duration of treatment, nor are there clear guidelines for matching patients to treatment. For other types of drug abuse, in the absence of empirically validated guidelines, the choice of individual psychotherapy can be based on such factors as expense, logistical considerations, patient preference, or the clinical fit between the patient's presenting picture and the treatment modality (e.g., family therapy is ruled out for those without families).

Conclusion

The empirical evidence reviewed here suggests the following:

- To date, most studies suggest that individual psychotherapy is superior to control conditions as a treatment for patients with substance use disorders. This finding is consistent with the bulk of findings from psychotherapy efficacy research in areas other than substance use, which suggests that the effects of many psychotherapies are clinically and statistically significant and are superior to no treatment and placebo conditions.

- No particular type of individual psychotherapy was found to be consistently superior as a treatment for substance use disorders.
- The effects of even comparatively brief psychotherapies appear to be durable among patients with substance use disorders.

Suggested Readings

Budney AJ, Higgins ST, Radonovich KJ, et al. Adding voucher-based incentives to coping skills and motivational enhancement improves outcomes during treatment for marijuana dependence. *J Consult Clin Psychol.* 2000;68:1051–1061.

Carroll KM, Ball SA, Nich C, et al. Targeting behavioral therapies to enhance naltrexone treatment of opioid dependence: efficacy of contingency management and significant other involvement. *Arch Gen Psychiatry.* 2001;58:755–761.

Morgenstern J, Morgan TJ, McCrady BS, et al. Manual-guided cognitive behavioral therapy training: a promising method for disseminating empirically supported substance abuse treatments to the practice community. *Psychol Addict Behav.* 2001;15:83–88.

Petry NM. A comprehensive guide to the application of contingency management procedures in clinical settings. *Drug Alcohol Depend.* 2000;58:9–25.

Rounsaville BJ, Carroll KM, Back S. Individual psychotherapy. In: Lowinson JH, Ruiz P, Millman RB, et al., eds. *Substance abuse: a comprehensive textbook*, 4th ed. Philadelphia: Lippincott Williams & Wilkins; 2005:653–671.

25

GROUP THERAPY

Group therapy has been the primary form of treatment in structured inpatient and outpatient addiction programs for decades. As managed care has moved treatment increasingly from inpatient to outpatient settings, use of outpatient group therapy has risen steadily. A growing trend in recent years is the proliferation of addiction treatment services into office-based practice. Addiction specialists from a variety of professional disciplines have been adding substance abuse services, including group therapy in some cases, to the array of mental health services they already provide in office practice.

Although group therapy is the focus here, it is not touted as the most effective treatment for everyone with an addiction problem. Addiction specialists generally agree that a combination of different approaches works best in most cases and that matching treatment interventions to specific patient needs is the most effective way to produce successful clinical outcomes.

Advantages of Group Therapy

Groups provide patients with opportunities for (a) mutual identification and reduced feelings of isolation and shame; (b) peer acceptance, support, and role modeling; (c) therapeutic confrontation and realistic feedback; (d) peer pressure, social support, structure, and accountability for making positive changes; (e) acquisition of new coping skills; (f) exchange of factual information; and (f) instillation of optimism and hope. The gathering together of people who share a common problem often creates a common bond between them, stemming from a sense of belonging and an expectation of being intuitively understood. The social stigma of addiction and the humiliation of having lost control over one's behavior makes rapid acceptance into a peer group all the more important for newcomers. The group instills hope by giving the person a chance to make contact with others who are getting better and by instantly supplying the individual with a positive support network committed to the pursuit of healthy, shared ideals. Groups provide a broad power base for positive reinforcement (approval) of adaptive behaviors and negative reinforcement (disapproval) of maladaptive behaviors. Because groups typically place high value on self-disclosure, active participation, compliance with group norms (e.g., abstinence, punctuality, attendance, honesty), a spirit of cooperation among group members, and facing rather than avoiding problems, it is difficult for resistant or noninteractive patients to "hide out" in small groups because every member is subjected regularly to the scrutiny of the group. Groups are also an excellent way to facilitate treatment retention and compliance as a by-product of bonding between members.

In addition to clinical benefits, group therapy also has economic advantages. Groups typically have no more than eight to ten members and one or two group leaders. The length of each group session is usually 1 to 2 hours. Accordingly, groups provide a mechanism for treating a larger numbers of patients than would be the case if individual sessions were the only option. Also, because group session fees are usually a fraction of those for individual therapy, groups allow addiction treatment to be more accessible to those who otherwise could not afford it.

Another unique benefit of group therapy is that it serves as an excellent training ground for student therapists who can observe and emulate the clinical skills of an experienced group leader. Finally, from a therapist's standpoint, delivering treatment in a group format is professionally stimulating and rewarding. Addiction recovery groups provide a continuous source of personal and professional growth, even for the most seasoned clinician.

Limitations of Group Therapy

Given the many benefits of group therapy, what are some of its limitations? First, unlike individual therapy where patients enjoy total privacy and confidentiality, group therapy inevitably requires patients to disclose their identity and personal problems to strangers. This can be a problem, especially for patients who live in smaller communities. Although maintaining strict confidentiality regarding group members' identities and the content of sessions is a cardinal rule of group therapy, there is no way to control what group members might say or do outside of group sessions. Despite increasing public enlightenment about addiction as a disorder affecting people from all walks of life, unwanted disclosure of information about an individual's alcohol/drug problem still holds the potential to damage careers, reputations, and relationships.

A second limitation of group therapy is that the content and pace of the treatment is determined by the group as a whole and not by the needs of any one individual. Inevitably there will be times when group therapy is out of step with the needs of some members while focusing on the needs of others. This limitation is most evident in open membership groups where new members are admitted throughout the life of the group. Each time newcomers enter the group, the continuity of treatment is interrupted as attention shifts back to beginner issues. By contrast, individual therapy allows the therapist to address patient's issues as they arise and to spend as much time or as many sessions as necessary to deal with these issues.

A third limitation of groups is that typically only a small portion of the therapy time is devoted to the needs of any one individual. This is offset to some extent by the benefits that patients derive from participating in group discussions focusing on other members' issues. Nonetheless, individual therapy devotes 100% of the therapy time to the needs of one person.

A fourth limitation is that there are practical obstacles to delivering group therapy in certain settings. For example, office practitioners typically do not have an adequate caseload or referral volume of patients needed to both initiate and maintain ongoing recovery groups. It may take the therapist several weeks or longer to gather together enough patients to start a group. While waiting for the group to begin, some patients may change their mind about entering the group, others may enter group therapy elsewhere, and still others may relapse. Even after the group starts, the therapist may not have an adequate referral volume of newcomers to maintain adequate group census as some patients inevitably leave the group. Another practical limitation is that group meeting times are generally inflexible. Groups typically meet one or more times per week on the same days and at the same times of the day every week. Unless there are enough patients to maintain several groups that run at different times of the day many patients who want and need group therapy will be unable to attend because of scheduling conflicts.

A fifth limitation is that group therapy is neither suitable nor appropriate for all patients. Although many, if not most, patients can benefit from group therapy and prefer it to other forms of treatment, others are simply not good candidates for group treatment. Patients with severe borderline personality disorders often find the intense interpersonal interaction and scrutiny in group sessions intolerably stressful. Similarly, patients who are avoidant, shy, or schizoid may be unable to participate actively in group discussions or form meaningful connections with other group members. Apart from psychiatric impairment, some patients simply have no desire or willingness to be in group therapy for whatever reasons. Although further exploration of this unreceptive stance may help to allay certain commonly held fears and misconceptions about group therapy, some patients remain adamant about not wanting group therapy.

Group Therapy versus Self-Help Groups

Group therapy and self-help groups such as, Alcoholics Anonymous (AA), are not good substitutes for one another. Each provides a unique form of help and, ideally, they should be seen as synergistic rather than competing activities. Self-help groups are invaluable, but the in-depth attention given to psychologic and personal issues that takes place in professionally led recovery groups is simply not available in self-help meetings. Moreover, in group therapy sessions members are strongly encouraged to give objective feedback to one another whereas in self-help meetings giving feedback (known as "cross-talk") is strictly prohibited. These are not criticisms of self-help groups, but fundamental differences between these two very different forms of help for people struggling with chemical dependency. Unlike group therapy, self-help meetings are characterized by peer rather than professional leadership, an absence of screening or exclusion criteria, unlimited size of membership, widespread availability of different types of self-help meetings at various times during the day and night especially in highly populated areas, and no time limits on the length of participation, which may extend over a participant's lifetime.

Groups for Different Stages of Recovery
Phase-Specific Groups

The types of therapeutic interventions that work best in the treatment of addiction often depend on phase of recovery or stage of change for the person. Patients progress through a series of phases and many treatment programs offer phase-specific groups that focus on the tasks and goals most relevant to each stage. This may include motivation enhancement or pretreatment induction groups for those who need preparatory work before making an abstinence commitment or entering a formal treatment program; early abstinence groups for those in the process of stopping their use; and relapse prevention or continuing care groups for those in the middle and later stages of recovery. This stratification offers a number of advantages: (a) it focuses the therapeutic work on the specific problems, tasks, and goals relevant to each phase; (b) it provides predefined progress markers that give patients a sense of personal accomplishment as they complete a phase; (c) it makes it is easier for individuals to identify and relate to the content material being addressed within each stage and to bond with others who are dealing with similar issues; and (d) it facilitates patient placement into a group best suited to meet patients' needs at each point in the recovery process. The rationale for stratification is based on the assumption that matching treatment interventions to meet the specific needs of patients as they progress through different stages of recovery is likely to enhance clinical outcomes.

Mixed-Phase Groups

Despite the numerous advantages of phase-specific groups, there are also drawbacks. One significant disadvantage is the disruption caused by members leaving a group in which they have bonded with others and shared intimate details of their personal lives. Another limitation is that private practitioners or small treatment programs may not have sufficient caseloads or staff to maintain different groups for patients in each phase of treatment. In a mixed-phase model, participants stay in a group as long as needed to achieve their treatment goals or as long as their participation in group remains productive. People in recovery move through the process at such different rates that it is not possible to specify in advance how long it will take for a given group member to reach these points. Mixed groups contain a broad array of patients at different phases of recovery. All have an opportunity to interact with one another in a group setting and derive mutual benefits from doing so.

Early Recovery Groups

Early recovery groups focus on issues most relevant to the beginning stages of treatment: helping members to establish initial abstinence; stabilize their overall functioning; acknowledge and accept their addiction problem; work through their initial ambivalence and reluctance about giving up alcohol/drug use; establish a social support network; to become bonded to other members and integrated into the group; overcome early relapses and other setbacks without dropping out; deal effectively with consequences of their addiction; and begin the process of identifying and changing some of the dysfunctional self-defeating cognitions, emotions, and behaviors that perpetuate their addiction. In the absence of strict economic constraints on length of stay, tenure in the group varies according to how quickly patients progress toward achieving their goals, ranging usually from several months to as much as a year, if circumstances permit.

Newcomers struggling to establish or maintain initial abstinence usually need specific guidance from other group members on fundamental issues such as (a) discarding all drug supplies and paraphernalia; (b) avoiding contact with dealers, users, parties, bars, and other high-risk situations; (c) learning how to recognize self-sabotaging behaviors and other "setups" for drug/alcohol use; and (d) learning how to manage urges and cravings. Once initial abstinence is established, the focus predictably shifts to stabilization of the individual's functioning. Often, a profound sense of disappointment emerges in the newly abstinent patient soon after the patient realizes that life is still fraught with problems despite having given up alcohol/drugs. Support and advice from established group members who have "been there" can be extremely helpful at this point.

The issues discussed in early recovery groups are largely patient driven so that members' problems, crises, and issues can be effectively dealt with as they arise. The leader often plays a very active, and at times directive, role in guiding the group discussion by keeping it focused on relevant issues, encouraging participation of all members, and ensuring that members provide helpful therapeutic feedback to one another without lecturing, advice-giving, hostile confrontation, and other unhelpful behaviors.

Relapse Prevention and Continuing Care Groups

The essential tasks and goals of this phase are to strengthen the commitment to abstinence, work through residual ambivalence about giving up alcohol and drugs, and learn and practice relapse prevention strategies including identification of relapse warning signs, as well as behavioral coping and affect-management skills as alternatives to alcohol/drug use. Although relapse prevention is the primary aim of this phase, the group does not focus exclusively on substance use but on a wider range of issues in greater depth (e.g., repairing damaged relationships, forming new ones, working toward resolving the lingering impact of developmental and trauma issues, enhancing self-esteem, and creating a reasonably satisfying lifestyle that is free of alcohol and other drugs).

Relapses that occur after abstinence has been firmly established and practiced for at least several months are frequently caused not so much by environmental triggers as by failure of the patient to cope adequately with negative emotions generated by interpersonal conflicts and other types of life problems and stressors. Among the many topics addressed in this phase of treatment are how to identify negative feelings, how to manage anger, how to avoid impulsive decision making, how to relax and have fun without drugs, how to give and receive constructive criticism, how to be assertive without being aggressive, and how to deal with problems in interpersonal relationships. It is also important to sensitize patients to relapse warning signs so that appropriate measures can be taken to "short-circuit" what is often a progressive backsliding in attitudes and behaviors.

The relapse prevention group should also address psychologic issues that promote relapse. This involves exploring the inner emotional life of each group member and interpersonal problems that repeatedly give rise to the compulsive desire to use alcohol/drugs. Patients with long, destructive histories of substance use often lack the ability to identify, manage, tolerate, and appropriately express feelings. The ultimate goal here is not merely the acquisition of self-knowledge and insight, but fundamental change in the individual's characteristically maladaptive patterns of thinking, feeling, behaving, and interacting. At an appropriate time the group should also address members' problems that may stem from parental alcoholism, physical/sexual abuse, or other developmental and life traumas. Coordination between individual and group therapy is especially vital.

Practical Considerations in Setting Up Groups

Group Size and Member Selection

The optimal group size is usually eight to ten members and the optimal length of group sessions is usually 90 to 120 minutes. When groups are longer than 2 hours and/or exceed ten members, it often becomes difficult to for the discussion to remain focused and for all to remain involved. In a large group, more vocal members tend to dominate the discussion while the more passive members sit quietly as spectators content that the action is not focusing on them.

There is no reliable formula for choosing the optimal mixture of candidates for group membership. As a general rule, however, the composition of a group should be neither too heterogeneous nor too homogeneous. Groups function best when there is a reasonable degree of diversity among members in terms of age, gender, race, socioeconomic status, educational level, and other relevant variables. Ideally, newcomers should be placed in groups where they have an opportunity to identify readily with at least one or two other members. Single "outliers" who are different from all other group members in an important respect (e.g., one woman among all men, one gay person among all heterosexuals, one seriously impaired patient among all highly functional people) are likely to feel out of place and to drop out. In addition to differing demographics, wherever possible there should be diversity among group members with regard to substances of choice. Group membership should not be based on the patients' primary drug of choice because it is the addictive disorder not the drug that is the focus of treatment. It is therapeutic for patients to realize that different types of substances can all lead to the same disorder and that the types of changes required to recover successfully are the same regardless of a person's substance of choice.

Open versus Closed Membership

The choice of open versus closed membership is often decided on purely practical grounds. Open membership groups allow new members to enter as others leave, whereas closed membership groups do not. In addition to the difficulty of assembling an entire cohort of patients to start group therapy all at the same time, some patients inevitably will leave the group before completing treatment no matter what measures are taken to prevent this from occurring. Thus, in nearly all addiction treatment settings open group membership is the norm.

In open groups, the dynamics of the group change significantly whenever new members arrive. Usually, a certain degree of initial discomfort and readjustment is created by the entry of new members, but with proper management by the group leader the potential benefits of adding new members usually outweigh the drawbacks. New members add new points of view, new problems, new ideas, and a new set of life experiences, all of which can broaden the scope and effectiveness of the group experience for its members.

Urine Drug Testing

Urine drug testing is a valuable treatment tool that should be a standard feature of group therapy in outpatient settings. Drug testing helps to establish and maintain the integrity of the treatment environment by establishing behavioral accountability for substance use. It also serves as an objective marker of clinical progress and as a tool that helps patients resist their impulses to use or deny that use has actually occurred. Most patients respond positively to the introduction of urine testing because they intuitively recognize its therapeutic value. Not having secrets about using can prevent a patient who is struggling to maintain abstinence from devaluing the treatment. And with urine monitoring, family members and employers can breathe a little easier and be more supportive of the patient's recovery when they no longer feel the need to scrutinize his or her behavior vigilantly for possible signs of intoxication. (Because alcohol cannot be reliably detected in urine by most testing methods, a breath or saliva test is typically used instead.)

Group Management Considerations

Leadership Roles and Responsibilities

Among group leaders' most important functions are (a) to establish and enforce group rules in a caring, consistent, nonpunitive manner to protect the group's integrity and progress; (b) to screen, prepare, and orient potential group members to ensure suitability and proper placement in the group; (c) to keep group discussions focused on important issues and to do so in ways that try to maximize the therapeutic benefit of these discussions for all members; (d) to emphasize, promote, and maintain group cohesiveness and reduce feelings of alienation, wherever possible; (e) to create and maintain a caring, nonjudgmental, therapeutic climate in the group that both counteracts self-defeating attitudes and promotes self-awareness, expression of feelings, honest self-disclosure, adaptive alternatives to drug use; (f) to handle problem members who are disruptive to the group in a timely and consistent manner to protect the membership and integrity of the group; and (g) to educate patients about selected aspects of drug use, addiction, and recovery.

Effective group leadership demands that the leader adopt a certain posture in the group that differs significantly from that of traditional psychotherapy groups, particularly in the early stages of recovery. In traditional groups, the therapist gently guides and focuses the attention of group members on matters pertaining to group process, group dynamics, and the complicated interpersonal interaction among group members. With the exception of carefully timed comments, the therapist may remain passive, quiet, and nondirective in the customary mode of psychodynamic psychotherapy. By contrast, in early abstinence groups the therapist must work actively to keep the group focused on concrete here-and-now issues that pertain directly to addiction-related issues. The therapist plays a very active and directive leadership role that includes questioning, confronting, advising, and educating group members on relevant issues. The therapist keeps the group task oriented and reality based, and serves as the major catalyst for group discussion. Addressing substance-related issues is always the number one priority of the group, and the therapist must be sure always to keep the group focused on this task.

It is not the group leader's role to direct the group per se, but rather to facilitate a process whereby members learn how to interact with one another in an increasingly open, honest, empathetic manner that promotes positive changes in attitude and behavior. When the group is working properly the leader functions as a group manager staying in the background while the group takes full responsibility for the therapeutic work. When the group is not working properly the leader is doing a lot of talking or spending a lot of time exhorting members to participate in the group discussion. This requires deliberate and persistent intervention by the group leader to return maximum responsibility for what goes on in the group to the group. As compared to early recovery groups, where the group leader plays a much more active role, later-stage groups should be helped to focus increasingly on group process and become reliably self-correcting when the discussion strays off track or becomes unproductive.

Preparing New Members for Group Entry

Preparing new patients for group entry involves not only orienting them to group rules, but also establishing realistic goals and expectations. Before admitting new patients, the group leader should meet individually with the prospective newcomer for at least one or two sessions to assess motivation, clarify myths and misconceptions about group therapy, and address resistances to group participation. Patients should also be informed about how the group works, how to give useful feedback, and how to refrain from unhelpful group behaviors. Before newcomers attend a first group meeting they should agree in writing to adhere to the group rules. They also must be notified that violation of any of these rules is potential grounds for termination from the group. One useful way to enhance the induction of newcomers into the group is to arrange an orientation meeting between the newcomer and a more advanced group member.

A vital prerequisite for entering an early recovery group is for prospective new members to achieve at least 1 to 2 weeks of continuous abstinence from all psychoactive substances just prior to attending their first group session. This is important because it provides the time that may be needed to recover from the acute aftereffects of recent alcohol/drug use, and just as importantly, concretizes the patient's motivation and ability to comply with the group requirement of total abstinence.

Introducing Newcomers into the Group

It is essential to introduce newcomers into the group in a manner that fosters mutual identification and bonding with existing members. The following techniques can be used for introducing new members to the group at their first session. First, ask each group members to give a 2- to 3-minute synopsis of how and why they came to the group, including a brief overview of their addiction/treatment history, what issues they have been working on in the group, and what role group therapy has played thus far in their recovery. Second, ask the newcomer to describe the circumstances surrounding his or her entry into the group, a brief overview of his or her addiction and treatment history including any prior group therapy or experience with self-help programs, and what he or she expects to get out of being in the group. Third, encourage group members to offer feedback to the newcomer based on what they heard thus far and where possible to identify with selected aspects of the newcomer's experiences.

Because outpatient group therapy can be effective only if patients actually show up, integrating newcomers into the group quickly is absolutely critical. This process can be facilitated by asking one or more established group members to maintain daily contact with the newcomer outside the group, including accompanying him or her to local self-help meetings. Newcomers must be helped to see as quickly as possible that their punctual attendance at all group sessions is essential to their recovery and to healthy functioning of the group. When patients miss a group session, it is critical that group members and the group leader call to express concern and communicate that the patient's presence definitely was missed. One such phone call may go a long way toward preventing precipitous dropout in a newcomer who assumes, incorrectly, that "no one really cares."

Managing Peer Confrontation and Feedback

Peer confrontation by fellow group members can be extremely effective in helping others achieve a more realistic assessment of their maladaptive attitudes and behaviors. But heavy-handed, excessive, and poorly timed confrontation can be countertherapeutic and even damaging. Some patients enter groups with the mistaken idea that humiliation and aggressive confrontation are acceptable ways to force resistant members of the group to face reality. Sometimes harsh confrontations are rationalized as attempts to be "truly honest" with members who violate group expectations and norms. Group members typically have less tolerance for negative attitudes and obfuscations than do group leaders, especially when these attitudes are reminiscent of their own. The group leader must never allow unpopular, frustrating, resistant, or severely troubled group members to be verbally scapegoated and bludgeoned by their peers, even when the content of what is being said is entirely accurate. Harsh or excessive confrontation must not be used as a means to push unpopular or troubled members out of the group and discourage them from coming back.

Managing Common Problems

The most common problems that arise in group therapy include the following: chronic lateness and absenteeism, hostility and other disruptive behaviors, lack of active participation, superficial presentations, proselytizing and hiding behind AA, and playing cotherapist.

Lateness and Absenteeism

An atmosphere of consistency and predictability is essential for group therapy to be effective. Because most patients have histories of irresponsible behavior during active addiction, when this type of behavior arises in the group it should not be ignored. A pattern of repeated lateness and/or absenteeism adversely affects group morale and cohesion. It is almost always a sign of ambivalence about being in the group and should be addressed as such.

Hostility and Other Disruptive Behaviors

Sometimes the content of what is said in group is less important than the way it is said. The group leader must attend continuously to the affect, body language, voice intonation, and overall communication style of group members. Some members are chronically antagonistic, argumentative, and sarcastic. They repeatedly devalue the group, complain about how poorly it is run, point out minor inconsistencies, and reject advice or suggestions offered by other group members or the group leader. The group leader must not allow these types of negative behaviors to go by unnoticed and unaddressed. An appropriate intervention by the group leader might be: "I wonder if anyone else is experiencing Tom's remarks as hostile and devaluing? Can someone offer him feedback about how he's coming across and how it is affecting the atmosphere in the group?" The group leader should guide the ensuing discussion to make sure that group members do not use this as an opportunity to assault and demean the problem group member for "bad" behavior, but rather help him to see the self-defeating nature of his actions as well as the negative impact of his behavior on the entire group.

Silence and Lack of Participation

Some group members sit quietly on the sidelines as observers of the group discussion glad to have the focus of attention not be on them. Silent members may secretly harbor intense feelings of ambivalence, resentment, and annoyance about being in treatment, and doubt whether they need to be in the group or if it is useful for them. Some members are just shy and need gentle coaxing and encouragement from the group to open up. An example of how to address a silent group member is as follows: "I've noticed that Dale has not participated at all during the past two or three group sessions. Maybe the group can try to find out what's holding her back and perhaps encourage or make it easier for her to join in the discussion?"

Superficial Presentations

Terse or superficial presentations that focus on facts rather than feelings and reveal little or nothing about the presenter are another form of resistance to the group's therapeutic work. In these situations, the group leader can intervene by saying something like, "I've noticed that when Jason talks about himself his statements are very brief and factual. They tell us very little about what's on his mind or what he is actually feeling. I'm wondering if others share my observations and concerns?" Similarly, some group members present lengthy stories recounting external events and circumstances full of irrelevant details and devoid of emotional content. This is often indicative of a member who is just going through the motions of being in treatment to satisfy a spouse, employer, or mandate. The group leader might intervene by saying, "Jeff, you've just given the group a very long and detailed account of the events of last week, but we heard very little about how you were feeling these past few days on the heels of your recent relapse. I'm wondering if other group members are getting the type of information from you that they would need to give you meaningful feedback. I notice that some group members look bored and uninterested. How are you all feeling right now?"

Proselytizing and Hiding behind Alcoholics Anonymous

This is a one of the most difficult problems to address in group therapy for addiction. In almost every recovery group there are likely to be some members solidly linked into AA or other 12-step programs who insist with absolute conviction that AA is the one and only pathway to successful recovery. They may be intolerant of others in the group who do not embrace AA, and take it as their mission to proselytize the benefits of AA in the hopes of converting nonbelievers. These patients will often polarize the group into opposing factions: those who embrace AA enthusiastically and wholeheartedly versus those who are more tempered in their posture toward AA or reject it completely. If this polarization is not addressed, it ultimately will destroy group cohesion, create an unsafe climate in the group, divert valuable attention from other important issues, and stall the group's therapeutic work. (It is important for group leaders to acknowledge that although AA can be extremely helpful to people struggling with addiction, many are not receptive to it at first and should be coaxed not coerced into giving AA a try. Moreover, no single method of recovery is best for everyone with an addiction problem.) A potentially helpful intervention may include something like, "Well group, we could probably debate the pros and cons of AA here for many sessions and still not reach agreement among everyone in the room. I think it would be more useful to talk about how group members feel that there is a serious split among you on this issue and how it is affecting what we do here in the group."

Playing Cotherapist

Some group members play the role of therapist's helper, which serves (unconsciously) as a diversion or smokescreen for dealing with their own issues. They often perform certain of the group leader's functions such as keeping the group discussion on track, confronting other members on inappropriate behaviors, and reinforcing group norms. Because their input is often very helpful to the group it is easy for other members and sometimes the group leader to overlook the fact that the self-appointed "cotherapist" spends so much time being a helper that the cotherapist fails to address his or her own issues. An appropriate intervention might include a statement like, "Robert, you've been extremely helpful to other group members and it's very clear that everyone here values your input. But I'm wondering if the group can take some time to get to know you a little better and try to help you identify what you want to work on here."

Responding to Relapses

When group members report that they have used alcohol/drugs since the last session, the group must give top priority to addressing this issue. In doing so, the group leader should portray a leadership style that models clear, consistent, and nonpunitive behavior. The group leader's task is to help the group use the discussion of member's relapse as an opportunity to learn something useful. Suggested guidelines for dealing with a relapsed group member are as follows: (a) Ask the patient to give the group a detailed account of the sequence of feelings, events, and circumstances that led up to the relapse. (b) Invite others to ask the patient about early warning signs, self-sabotage, and other factors that may have preceded the actual substance use. (c) Ask others to share any suggestions or feedback they can offer the patient about the relapse and how to prevent it from happening again. Also ask them to share their feelings about the relapse, reminding them to avoid any tendency they may have to scapegoat the patient or to act out feelings of anger and frustration with negative comments. (d) With the patient's active participation, ask the group to develop a list of suggested strategies and behavioral changes to guard against the possibility of further substance use.

Although most group members respond supportively to a member's relapse, there is a limit as to how often relapsing members can expect this type of supportive response. When a group member who is having trouble remaining abstinent shows little evidence of using previous suggestions about how to prevent further relapses, other members frequently become intolerant and feel that the person may be jeopardizing the integrity of the group. Peer confrontation can become very intense when dealing with relapse issues and the group leader must guard vigilantly against the group's tendency to scapegoat or ostracize the relapsed member.

Conclusion

This chapter discusses practical considerations involved in providing group therapy for addiction in outpatient treatment settings. Because it is both clinically effective and cost-effective, group therapy has become the treatment of choice for addiction. Nonetheless, group therapy is not the best or only treatment option for everyone with an addiction problem. Group therapy should not be used as a stand-alone treatment, but as one component of a more comprehensive treatment approach. Group therapists face many challenging tasks including deciding which patients to bring together in a group, keeping group discussions focused and on track, and handling various types of clinical and behavior problems that arise during group sessions. In addition to its therapeutic benefits for patients, groups provide a valuable source of personal and professional growth even for the most seasoned clinician.

Suggested Readings

Washton AM. Group therapy with outpatients. In: Lowinson JH, Ruiz P, Millman RB, et al., eds. *Substance abuse: a comprehensive textbook*, 4th ed. Philadelphia: Lippincott Williams & Wilkins; 2005:671–680.

Washton AM. Outpatient groups at different stages of substance abuse treatment: preparation, initial abstinence, and relapse prevention. In: Brook DW, Spitz HI, eds. *The group therapy of substance abuse*. New York: Haworth Medical Press; 2002:99–119.

Washton AM. Group therapy: a clinician's guide to doing what works. In: Coombs RH, ed. *Addiction recovery tools: a practical handbook*. Thousand Oaks, Calif.: Sage Publications; 2001:239–256.

Weiss RD, Jaffee WB, de Menil VP, et al. Group therapy for substance use disorders: what do we know? *Harv Rev Psychiatry*. 2004;12:339–350.

26

FAMILY/COUPLES APPROACHES TO TREATMENT ENGAGEMENT AND THERAPY

For many years, substance abusers, especially drug addicts, were viewed as "loners," as people who were cut off from primary relationships and living a kind of "alley-cat" existence. It was not until researchers began inquiring about addicts' living arrangements and familial contacts that the picture began to shift. The realization began to emerge that most substance abusers are closely tied to their families or the people who raised them.

In general, the findings are that 60% to 80% of adult drug abusers either live with their parent(s), or are in regular contact (e.g., four to seven times/week) with at least one parental figure; 75% to 95% are reported to be in at least weekly contact with one or both parents.

Questions of family-of-origin contact have received very little attention in regard to alcohol-dependent individuals. This, despite what the first author has observed during 35 years of treating alcoholics: A male drinker's wife typically voices a complaint something like, "I don't see him during weeknights because he's in the bars, and I don't see him during the weekend because he's over at his mother's putting up storm windows or something." In other words, present-day perception of this issue among professionals and researchers is analogous to that which existed in the drug abuse field 35 years ago: nobody asked, so nobody knew.

Of course, living with or regularly contacting parents is not in and of itself pathognomonic; such practices are the rule in some ethnic groups. We emphasize such patterns of connectedness here because (a) they are often overlooked by treatment programs and (b) they underscore that family members are important to substance abusers, and substance abusers are important to their families. Furthermore, as discussed in the section on treatment/self-help engagement, family members can be a tremendous resource toward convincing reluctant substance abusers to seek help.

Some Relevant Family Dynamics

There is an extensive body of literature, covered by a number of reviews on the family and marital/couples aspects of substance abuse. Some highlights are presented below.

Deaths, Losses, and Disruptions

A number of researchers have documented that both the initial onset of, and subsequent relapses to substance abuse are commonly tied to unexpected or disruptive losses—such as a sudden death, forced immigration, even an undesired retirement—within a substance abuser's family-of-origin and extended family. Extending the well-established finding with children that events occurring with parents are more likely to predict child symptoms than are the child's own life events (such as moving to a new school), it has been found that (a) a family stress event preceded an adolescent's initiation of drug abuse in 94% of cases, and (b) there was an average of 3.5 family stress events—particularly major family losses such as a death or disruption (e.g., onset of a life-threatening illness in a parent, a parent getting laid off)—in the year prior to onset. Furthermore, a Chicago study with opiate addicts found that the initial onset of drug abuse, as well as subsequent overdoses, were precipitated 80% of the time by such major family losses or disruptions.

In another example, a recent study reviewed the literature on early deaths/losses and subsequent addiction, and presented data on such questions, with 592 adult, out-of-treatment, intravenous drug users. It found that the regularity with which these participants injected heroin and engaged in other risks related to human immunodeficiency virus (HIV) (e.g., needle sharing, unprotected sex) was significantly correlated ($p < 0.001$) with both (a) the number of their close family members who had died suddenly when the respondents were age 15 years or younger, and (b) the extent to which they and their families had effectively mourned those losses (e.g., very little manifestation of mourning of someone "close" to a participant was regarded as "inadequate" mourning). The canonical correlations between risk taking and measures of inappropriate or inadequate mourning were 0.55 for the total sample and 0.70 for the subsample who experienced early and sudden family deaths. Findings from this and other studies are consistent with the conclusion that the addicted person often serves as a "revenant," or "replacement," for a deceased loved one. The addict is thus held onto in an enmeshed, overattached way as a means of retaining—or perhaps even symbolically "bringing back"—the lost family member. This is undoubtedly a factor in the aforementioned high levels at which most substance abusers maintain contact with their families of origin.

Other Patterns and Dynamics

Although genetics can play a role in many cases, a number of other family factors can also have direct bearing on the genesis and remediation of addiction. For example: (a) parental modeling of drug and alcohol taking is important; (b) the substance abuse may help to maintain family homeostasis, or even serve as a means for getting the drug abuser's parents into treatment; and (c) family members can engage in "enabling" behaviors that perpetuate the substance abuse of a member.

A particularly cogent process is the "family addiction cycle." A cyclical, homeostatic pattern has been described in families of addicts in which, when the addict improves in some way, the parents begin to fight and to separate emotionally from each other. When the addict "fails," such as by taking drugs or losing a job, the parents shift attention from their couple problem and address the addict's problem. Thus, the family becomes, in a sense, "unified." In this way, the addict's behavior serves a purpose of keeping the family together, at least temporarily. Furthermore, from this viewpoint the chemical taking is simply one event within an interpersonal sequence of behavior. It is not an independent phenomenon occurring in a vacuum, but a response to a series of others' behaviors that precede (and succeed) it. That is the reason for the term *family addiction cycle*. Professionals who are not attuned to these kinds of sequences taking place in a client's life put themselves at a disadvantage. They run the risk of being constantly mystified by onset and cessation of chemical taking.

Implications for Prevention

Family dynamics and patterns have also emerged as important in the prevention of substance abuse. Of the six protective factors identified by the U.S. National Institute on Drug Abuse (NIDA) as key to prevention of drug abuse, four (such as strong and positive parental bonds, parental monitoring, clear and consistently enforced rules of conduct) are family related, as are four of the eight most important risk factors (e.g., chaotic home environment, ineffective parenting). Further, of the ten evidence-based drug abuse prevention programs endorsed by NIDA, seven involve parents/family, four very strongly so. As an example, parent–family interventions in the "Project Family" randomized prevention trial have been shown to hold up over a 4-year period. And, regarding alcohol, working with parents reduces drinking and related consequences in college students.

Family/Couples/Network Approaches to Convincing Substance Abusers to Engage in Treatment/ Self-Help

A major concern in the addiction field is that, in any given year, 90% to 95% of drug-dependent and/or alcohol-dependent persons do not enter either treatment or self-help groups. This disturbing finding underscores the need to find new and better ways to help these individuals. Family members and significant others can be major sources of energy, competence, and motivation for addressing this problem.

At least 11 approaches have been developed, ten of which have been examined in at least 19 outcome studies involving 1,501 cases, regarding the means for helping family members or significant others convince a reluctant substance-abusing person to enroll in treatment or to begin attending a self-help group such as Alcoholics Anonymous or Cocaine Anonymous. All the approaches start with what has been termed a "concerned other" person or a "concerned significant other," who is the person who contacts a treatment program to obtain help for a substance abuser. The concerned other might be a family member or relative, a spouse/partner, a friend, a member of the clergy, or anyone else who is motivated and connected enough to have some influence on the substance abuser.

The various approaches fall into two general categories: dual-purpose approaches and engagement-primary approaches. Dual-purpose methods tend to work with one person, most commonly a spouse/partner or an immediate family member such as a parent. The term "dual" refers to the two goals subscribed to by the approach. The first goal is to get the substance abuser engaged in treatment or self-help. The second goal is to help the concerned other to cope more effectively with both the substance abuser and (through counseling and educational material) the patterns that attend the addictive process itself, for example, to cease enabling, nagging, or escalating to the extreme. In this way, the approach resembles a form of personal counseling for the concerned other. Hence, the number of sessions conducted with the concerned other can range from six to thirty six over a period of 3 to 6 months, depending on the particular model applied (the exception being Cooperative Counseling, which involves one to six sessions).

Engagement-primary approaches are pitched almost wholly toward the task of getting the substance abuser to enter treatment or self-help; they do not include an additional counseling component *per se*. The earliest and best known of these approaches is the Johnson Institute's "Intervention," although at least four other engagement-primary approaches have been subsequently developed.

Overall Engagement Rates and Time Period Comparisons

Some of the general findings and conclusions, particularly regarding the intent-to-treat rates/proportions of substance abusers who were engaged within 6 months from concerned other intake, are as follows:

1. As might be expected, later (after 1994) studies tended to achieve higher engagement rates (overall mean = 69%) than earlier (1983 to 1990) studies (52%), partly because the former had the advantage of being able to build on and refine the work of their predecessors.

2. As a group, the engagement experimental conditions performed significantly better (65%) than both wait-list controls (6%) and self-help conditions (17%). Experimental conditions in later studies also outperformed "engagement-as-usual" comparison groups (69% vs. 52%), whereas those in earlier studies obtained an identical rate of 52%.

3. The overall engagement rate with adolescents was 83%, which differed significantly from the overall rate of 59% for adults. However, this is confounded by substance of abuse, in that all the adolescent studies were with drug abusers, whereas there were no studies with adolescent alcohol abusers. A comparison between adolescent and adult drug abusers yielded figures, respectively, of 83% and 78%, and those rates did not differ significantly.

4. Following from the above, the aforementioned 78% rate for adult drug abusers, all of which were from later studies, was significantly higher than the 49% rate for later study alcohol abusers, implying that higher rates can be expected with the former group. However, this difference may be confounded by age, because the alcohol abuser sample appeared (based on incomplete data) to be older.

Comparison of Dual-purpose and Engagement-Primary Approaches

The two groups did not differ significantly, overall, in the design quality of their studies. Nor did dual-purpose and engagement-primary approaches differ significantly in their overall engagement rates with adult problem drinkers, that is, 40% versus 45% (identical 49% rates for later studies). However, among the six experimental conditions (within five studies) with adult drug abusers the engagement-primary approach attained a significantly higher engagement rate than did the dual-purpose approach (88% vs. 69%).

Note was also made of the fact that, although the additional counseling provided by dual-purpose approaches appears, in and of itself, to be of clear value to the concerned others who participate in it, such a requirement is not indicated for a certain proportion of concerned others. For some sorts of concerned others who may call in to obtain help for a substance abuser (e.g., employers, work associates, friends, clergy, second-degree relatives), the quasi-personal counseling component may not be appropriate. Additionally, others who do seem appropriate may still refuse such an option, especially if, or because, it requires a significant number of individual sessions.

Other Conclusions

Additional conclusions emerging from Stanton's work were the following:

1. The four groups of investigators who examined them determined that heavily confrontational approaches, such as the traditional form of the Johnson Intervention, are not indicated in most cases, particularly because the majority (70% to 100%) of concerned others to whom they are offered refuse to carry them out because of the stressful nature of the confrontation, the secretiveness involved, and the potential damage to the relationship. Although in recent years several less-aggressive versions of intervention have been developed, none of them has been examined in engagement outcome studies.
2. Involving parents, not only with adolescents but also with adults, appears to increase the likelihood of substance abuser engagement.
3. Involving greater numbers of significant others in the endeavor may produce better engagement results for less professional effort.

Clinical Options

In light of the above, thinking clinicians are likely to ask, "What are the 'better edge,' manual-guided options if one wants to get an substance abuser into treatment or self-help?" Based on the existent studies in this still-evolving field, below are the first recommendations for engaging seven particular clinical subgroups. This is not meant to imply, incidentally, that approaches not mentioned here have no value, but rather that the research evidence indicates that those listed appear, generally, to be more likely to succeed.

Dual-purpose Preferred Options

If the intent is to help the concerned other both to participate in counseling to cope better with the substance abuser (and perhaps to benefit personally) and to get the substance abuser to enter treatment or self-help, the following are recommended.

Adults with Substance Use Disorder (Drug Abuse)

The Community Reinforcement and Family Training (CRAFT) approach, with its rigorous research underpinnings, is clearly the best option here. CRAFT is a behaviorally oriented, problem-focused, skill-based approach using role-play techniques, and involves, in its latest version, an average of ten to twelve sessions. The overall mean engagement rate for drug abusers across three experimental conditions in two studies was 71%, with some indication that engagement may be additionally improved by providing the concerned other with group aftercare sessions.

A credible second choice to CRAFT is another behaviorally based method known as Community Reinforcement Training (CRT). A nonconfrontational approach averaging 12 to 13 sessions over an 8 to 9 week period, CRT provides motivational training, encourages independence from the substance abuser, and provides training in contingency management. It attained an engagement rate of 64% (56% of those randomized) with adult drug abusers.

Adults with Alcohol Use Disorder

Based on its high-quality outcome research, CRAFT is the first choice here, too. A study with adult problem drinkers, in which concerned others attended an average of 10 to 11 sessions, achieved a 64% engagement rate.

Engagement-Primary Preferred Options

If engagement of substance abusers in treatment/self-help is, in and of itself, the clinical or programmatic goal, the recommendations are as follows.

Adolescents with Substance Use Disorder (Drug Abuse)

CRT-influenced Intensive Parent and Youth Attendance Intervention appears to be the most cost-efficient mode, especially if engagement of the youth is the goal. In particular, its cost-effectiveness, that is, its high rate of return for only 2 hours of professional effort, sets it apart. It involves a standardized handling of the first call, the setting of a parent plus youth intake appointment within 2 to 7 days, and preparatory calls to both parent and adolescent 2 to 3 days prior to the appointment.

Adolescents with Substance Use Disorder (Drug Abuse) and Their Families

Adding family engagement to the agenda evokes the Strategic Structural Systems Engagement (SSSE) option. One of the two best-researched methods, SSSE is particularly effective with Hispanic families. The procedure is to use from (on average) 2.5 to 5.3 "contacts" (phone calls, home visits, office sessions) with the concerned other and resistant family members (including, of course, the substance abuser) in applying techniques such as "joining" and family "restructuring" in an effort to overcome the family's resistance to engagement. Its success rate across two experimental conditions with youthful drug abusers was 87%.

Adults with Either Substance Use (Drug Abuse) or Alcohol Use Disorder

An approach called A Relational Intervention Sequence for Engagement (ARISE) is the most cost-effective choice here. It combines rapid results and a relatively low demand on staff time (an average of 1.5 total hours/case) to attain high rates with both categories of disorder. The approach involves up to three stepped stages: (a) starting with the concerned other's first call (which is pivotal, and involves the message, "You can't do this alone"), (b) holding one or (if necessary) more sessions with significant others (to which the substance abuser is also invited), and (c) culminating in a modified, less-confrontational Johnson Intervention for the small proportion (2% to 3%) of cases that require it. Outcome results yielded an 87% rate with adult drug abusers, and a 77% rate with adult alcohol abusers. Of those who engaged, most (76%) did so within 2 weeks from the first call.

Mothers with Substance Use Disorder (Drug Abuse)

The Engaging Moms approach, with its uniquely tailored protocol, has carved out a distinctive niche in the engagement of women under such circumstances, that is, in which either a mother or her infant tested positive for cocaine. An integrative approach, using techniques from several family and women's treatment models, it entails an average of 15 family, individual, and case management contacts (not necessarily "sessions"), averaging about 7 to 8 total hours, over an 8-week period. The approach obtained an 88% treatment engagement rate with such women.

Family/Couples Treatment Considerations

About Family/Couples Treatment

Fundamentally, family therapy is a way of thinking about human problems that suggests certain actions for their alleviation, rather than a modality of treatment *per se*. The term *systems therapy* actually is preferred by many family therapists, but most agree that it is too late to change the tag. Indeed, it is the systemic (relational, interactional) manner of their thought and interventions that defines the approach, not the attention to the social unit called a "family." Family therapists work with families because the family is one of the systems in which human problems can be most easily understood, and because families often provide a significant resource for solving problems. Furthermore, the term *family therapist* applies to *all* professionals who "think family" in their clinical work, including psychiatrists, psychologists, social workers, counselors, nurses, and clergy, as well as, of course, professional marriage and family therapists. Indeed, family and marital/couples therapy traces its beginnings to pioneers in all of these various fields.

Treating Families with a Substance Abuse Problem

The case can be made that family/couples therapy is appropriate and helpful throughout the process of recovery. This includes, in addition to the substance abuser engagement effort described above, both outpatient and residential treatment contexts. All are fitting settings for the family and its members to learn new ways to continue their lives without chemicals of abuse.

Taking this point further, the converse is also true: A lack of family-oriented services in substance abuse treatment can have calamitous consequences. In fact, without concurrent treatment for nonabusing members, families have been known (in order to preserve the familiar and perhaps avoid the illumination of other problems) to attempt to sabotage treatment efforts when those efforts begin to succeed. Examples of this are commonly reported in the literature; they range from a spouse slipping beer to a recovering alcoholic, to the parents who refuse to work together in maintaining rules for their out-of-control adolescent.

Sometimes it is difficult to convene the whole family of a substance abuser for therapy. Fathers of substance-abusing young people, in particular, often appear threatened by treatment and defensive about their contributions to the problem. Because many have drinking problems themselves, they may also fear discovery, being blamed for the problem, or that their own addiction will be challenged.

Recognizing such hesitancies, family therapists try to recruit families into therapy. Sometimes they ask other family members to help with recruiting, but they are cognizant that this approach may not be sufficient. Thus, they extend personal invitations to the reluctant members. In less seriously disturbed families, one telephone call may enable a therapist to reassure family members that their contributions are important to the solution of the substance abuse. In more disturbed families, it may be necessary to meet family members on "neutral turf" (such as at a restaurant), or to write multiple letters, or even to pay family members for participation in treatment. There are many standardized and creative techniques for involving families of drug or alcohol abusers in treatment.

Involving Parents in Decisions

Parents should be involved in all decisions about treatment when a substance abuser is an adolescent or a young adult. This includes decisions about hospitalization, medication, and drug tests. Family therapists make the parents part of the treatment team because it helps to get the couple working together and because the responsibility for the resolution of the problem is correctly theirs. When the parents of a young abuser are divorced or unmarried, the same holds true; adult caretakers must be encouraged to work together to help their children.

Detoxification at Home

Physical dependence on alcohol or other drugs must, of course, be assessed and managed early in treatment. When dependence exists, the client may be hospitalized for detoxification, especially if the dependence is on sedative hypnotics such as alcohol or barbiturates. However, for some other substances, and given medical backup, the family may attempt, following certain procedures, to conduct the detoxification at home. In fact, home detoxification appears to be a cost-effective option in many cases, with savings of 70% to 85% of the cost of hospitalization.

Dealing with Intergenerational Losses and Patterns

Stemming from the earlier discussion regarding how major losses within a substance abuser's extended family can lead to unresolved mourning, or to the family's otherwise becoming "stuck" in an intergenerational pattern of addiction, a conceptual model of how such patterns develop within a family is already available. By using a genogram covering at least four generations, the method starts by asking, "When, in this family's history, was the family so stressed that it had to change its relational patterns or organization and develop a drinking or drug problem?" That information is then used therapeutically, taking the family back to the point of loss and symbolically "going through" it again from a present-day vantage point. This joins the poles of past, present, and future—spanning the family's generations. The process also depathologizes those members from the past who had problems, and reinstates them, instead, as people who may have been pained and besieged. By granting the forebears their honorable place, honor is also bestowed on the living, their descendants. Such uncovering and rebuilding gives the family members the kind of information that can free them to make a choice: whether to keep, revise, or replace the scripts—the intergenerational instructions—that have been carried down. In other words, it helps them acquire flexibility in coming to grips with the question whether, and how, to move on in life. In experience with several thousand cases, as well as more systematic qualitative study with more than 200 clinical and nonclinical families, the method shows great promise in bringing about long-term change in the intergenerational family addiction pattern.

An Integrative View

More than two dozen books have been written specifically about family/couples therapy with substance abusers. Similarly, many different modalities of family treatment have been described, including marital/couples therapy; group therapy for parents or relatives; concurrent parent and index patient therapy; therapy with individual families, both inpatient and outpatient; sibling-oriented therapy; multiple-family therapy; social network therapy (including friends, neighbors, other therapists, social agents, and, often, systems external to the family); and family therapy with one person. To bring greater coherence to this multifaceted and expanding field, an integrative model of the stages of family/couples therapy with substance abusers has been set forth. The model synthesizes the relevant literature for both alcohol- and drug-dependent adults, as well as for substance-abusing adolescents. It emphasizes the consensus among the various authors in the field, and offers a rich collection of the clear and specific family therapy methods they have developed.

Suggested Readings

Carr A. Evidenced-based practice in family therapy and systemic consultation: I. Child-focused problems. *J Fam Ther.* 2000;22:29–60.

Carr A. Evidenced-based practice in family therapy and systemic consultation: II. Adult-focused problems. *J Fam Ther.* 2000;22:273–295.

Dakof GA, Quille TJ, Tejeda MJ, et al. Enrolling and retaining mothers of substance-exposed infants in drug abuse treatment. *J Consult Clin Psychol.* 2003;71(4):764–772.

Liddle HA, Hogue A. Multidimensional family therapy for adolescent substance abuse. In: Wagner EF, Waldron HB, eds. *Innovations in adolescent substance abuse interventions.* New York: Pergamon/Elsevier Science; 2001:229–261.

O'Farrell TJ, Fals-Stewart W. Marital and family therapy. In: Hester R, Miller WR, eds. *Handbook of alcoholism treatment approaches*, 3rd ed. Boston: Allyn & Bacon; 2002:188–212.

Stanton MD, Heath AW. Family/couples approaches to treatment engagement and therapy. In: Lowinson JH, Ruiz P, Millman RB, et al., eds. *Substance abuse: a comprehensive textbook*, 4th ed. Philadelphia: Lippincott Williams & Wilkins; 2005:680–690.

27

COGNITIVE AND BEHAVIORAL THERAPY

Psychotherapies that focus primarily on individuals' thoughts and behaviors are generally known as cognitive–behavioral therapies (CBTs). There have been many different CBT approaches; some have attended mostly to cognitive processes, some have attended mostly to behavioral processes, and others have been equally attentive to both. CBT is typically active, structured, directive, focused, and oriented to the present.

Early applications of CBT were to depression, anxiety, and various other problems, including anger, stress, somatic disorders, sexual dysfunction, and pain. More recently, CBT has been applied to such complex problems as personality disorders, schizophrenia, crisis intervention, and suicidal behavior. Consistent with this focus on more complex problems, CBT has increasingly been applied to substance abuse. This chapter reviews three theories of CBT for substance abuse, discusses principles of treatment, and describes techniques.

Cognitive–Behavioral Theories of Substance Abuse

The application of cognitive–behavioral theory to substance abuse is relatively recent. For most of the 20th century until the mid-1980s, the field of psychotherapy largely ignored substance abuse, viewing it as a superficial symptom of more important underlying problems. As substance abuse became more widely recognized, interest in developing effective treatments increased.

This section describes three major cognitive–behavioral theories of substance abuse: *relapse prevention*, *cognitive therapy*, and *behavioral learning theory*. These theories provide the conceptual foundation for treatment strategies discussed later in the chapter. All of these theories make the following assumptions:

1. Substance abuse is mediated by complex cognitive and behavioral processes.
2. Substance abuse and associated cognitive–behavioral processes are, to a large extent, learned.
3. Substance abuse and associated cognitive–behavioral processes can be modified, particularly by means of CBT.
4. A major goal of CBT for substance abuse is to teach coping skills to resist substance use and to reduce the problems associated with substance abuse.

5. CBT requires comprehensive case conceptualization that serves as the basis for selecting specific CBT techniques.
6. To be effective, CBT must be provided in the context of warm, supportive, collaborative therapeutic relationships.

Relapse Prevention

Most CBT is derived at least in part from the work of Marlatt and Gordon. Their relapse prevention model is important for several reasons: it was the first major CBT approach to substance abuse; it provides practical, flexible interventions that can be applied by a wide range of clinicians; it can be used adjunctively with other treatments; and it provides a straightforward conceptual model for understanding substance abuse. Some popular relapse prevention techniques include the identification and avoidance of high-risk situations, exploration of the decision chain leading to drug use, lifestyle modification (e.g., choosing friends who do not use), and learning from "slips" to prevent future relapses. Originally developed for substance abuse, relapse prevention has since been adapted for a variety of psychologic problems.

Cognitive Therapy of Substance Abuse

Cognitive therapy of substance abuse is based on the same basic principles as cognitive therapy for other problems, such as depression, anxiety, and personality disorders. In cognitive therapy of substance abuse, the focus is on the complex behaviors that derive from substance-related beliefs, automatic thoughts, and facilitating beliefs. Complex behaviors involve the consumption of substances as well as actions to avoid the negative consequences of substance abuse (e.g., lying about drinking to avoid conflicts with a spouse). Substance-related beliefs involve positive ("anticipatory") beliefs about the effects of substance use (e.g., "Nothing feels as great as getting stoned!"), as well as negative ("relief-oriented") beliefs about the effects of refraining from substance use (e.g., "If I quit now, I'll get the shakes.") Automatic thoughts are brief ideas that spontaneously flash across a person's mind. Some automatic thoughts manifest themselves as sharp visual images, like frozen frames from a movie, such as the image of an ice-cold beer on a hot summer's day. Facilitating beliefs involve permission to use despite prior commitments to stop using (e.g., "I'll just have one drink.")

"Triggers" are an important concept in cognitive therapy for substance abuse and other models such as relapse prevention. From the cognitive therapy perspective, substance use is initiated by activating stimuli ("high-risk situations"). Activating stimuli can be either internal or external. Internal cues may include negative feelings (e.g., anxiety, boredom), positive feelings (e.g., joy, excitement), memories (e.g., flashbacks of being abused), and physiologic sensations (e.g., cravings, pain). External cues include interpersonal conflicts, sights and sounds (e.g., seeing a wine advertisement), other substance users, problems at school or work, and celebration times such as parties and holidays.

In response to internal and external cues, people use psychoactive substances because they believe they will either increase positive feelings (pleasure), or they will alleviate negative feelings (pain). These anticipatory and relief-oriented beliefs lead to automatic thoughts and images (e.g., "I need a drink," "I want a hit") that result in craving for the substance. Following these cravings, individuals may give themselves permission to use (e.g., "I'll quit soon," "Just one is okay"). Permissive beliefs lead to action plans, which eventually lead to continued use or relapse.

Behavioral Learning Theories of Substance Abuse

Behavioral theories contend that human behavior is learned and shaped via complex contingencies. Thus, behavioral theories of substance use are based on the assumption that the primary goal of treatment is to help patients unlearn old, ineffective behaviors and learn more adaptive ones. These theories suggest several ways that learning to use substances may occur.

Social learning theory emphasizes the importance of modeling; that is, learning occurs by observing other people's behavior and its consequences. In terms of substance use, modeling can occur indirectly through cultural norms and prescriptions (e.g., media depictions of substance use) as well as directly through family and peer socialization (e.g., children observing their parents using alcohol to cope with problems). Such modeled behaviors become translated into attitudes, expectancies, and beliefs about substance use (e.g., the belief that alcohol enhances social interactions). Given the vicarious nature of social learning, much learning about substance use can take place, such as in childhood, before an individual ever consumes any.

A second way that learning may occur is through operant conditioning. Operant learning takes place when a behavior serves an instrumental function and, as a result, is reinforced by its consequences. A positive reinforcer strengthens any behavior that produces it, whereas a negative reinforcer strengthens any behavior that reduces or terminates it. The use of substances is established and maintained by both positive and negative reinforcers. Positive reinforcement occurs when substance use is rewarded by, for example, increasing social confidence, enhancing positive affect, and facilitating entry into social groups of substance-using peers. Conversely, substance use is negatively reinforced when it allows escape from aversive stimuli such as negative affect or the physiologic symptoms of withdrawal. The positive and negative reinforcers of substance use vary widely among individuals and it is important for clinicians to assess the specific reasons that any given person uses substances.

A third form of learning is classical conditioning. The first type of learning to be studied within the behaviorist tradition, classical conditioning, was originally researched by Pavlov in the 1920s. In Pavlov's experiments with dogs, he found that repeated pairings of a conditioned stimulus (i.e., a bell ringing) with an unconditioned stimulus (i.e., food) would eventually cause the unconditioned response (i.e., salivating) to occur at the presentation of the conditioned stimulus. When applied to substance use, classical conditioning suggests that substance use may become paired with a variety of stimuli that reliably precedes consumption of substances (e.g., drug paraphernalia, sights and smells associated with substance use, people, places, times of day, and negative emotions). Eventually, exposure to these stimuli may come to elicit a variety of substance-related conditioned responses such as intense cravings, physiologic changes (e.g., increased heart rate), and substance-related thoughts.

Basic Principles

Regardless of specific therapeutic techniques, certain principles are important to all CBT substance abuse treatments. These principles include case conceptualization, collaboration, psychoeducation, structure, attending to the multiple needs of patients, and monitoring substance use.

Case Conceptualization

Case conceptualization involves the assessment of patients' backgrounds, presenting problems, psychiatric diagnoses, developmental profiles, and cognitive–behavioral profiles. Furthermore, case conceptualization should include information about the unique variables responsible for the development and maintenance of substance use by the individual. This case formulation process may be facilitated by the use of standardized assessment instruments.

The therapist's selection and timing of therapeutic techniques should follow directly from the case conceptualization. For example, after conducting a functional analysis of an individual's substance use, treatment planning can focus on the specific skills necessary to intervene in the unique chain of events that lead to substance use for that individual. This approach reflects the CBT emphasis on adapting treatment to individuals, rather than expecting individuals to adapt to treatment. Other ways to individualize treatment include structuring sessions to include time for patient-driven material, repeating topics if patients have difficulty understanding a concept, and offering examples provided by the patient when presenting a new skill or topic.

Collaboration

CBT for substance abuse is highly collaborative, supportive, and empathetic. Collaboration is important because it creates a trusting atmosphere that supports the difficult work of changing addictive behaviors. In addition, substance abuse patients have notoriously high treatment dropout rates and general therapeutic strategies aimed at cultivating rapport, collaboration, and alliance can help to maximize retention. Substance abusers tend to evoke more negative responses in therapists than many other patient populations. Some therapists feel frustrated, angry, or helpless because they are unable to stop patients, substance use. Many find that they cannot compete with substances that provide more intense and immediate effects than therapy. Some therapists feel frustrated because they cannot relate to the chronically impaired lives of such patients.

Cognitive–behavioral therapists are strongly encouraged to confront their thoughts directly about patients who abuse substances. For example, rather than thinking, "This drug addict will never change," therapists are taught to think, "If I am patient, this person may eventually make some important changes." Therapists are also encouraged to use effective communication skills with patients.

Psychoeducation

CBT usually incorporates significant psychoeducational efforts, particularly early in treatment. The complexity of biologic, behavioral, cognitive, and spiritual problems associated with substance abuse requires that CBT therapists be well informed about these areas. Psychoeducation is a delicate process. Just as individuals vary in their readiness to change, they also vary in their readiness for educational interventions. Both timing and style of delivery determine the value of psychoeducational presentations. Rather than randomly lecturing patients, CBT therapists elicit knowledge from patients in areas relevant to their circumstances and needs. Therapists offer opportunities for patients to learn more by means of brief lectures, written materials, videotapes, or work-books on a variety of topics. Long lectures are inappropriate. ("too long" is defined as the point at which patients become bored or distracted). Areas for education might include the physiologic effects of particular substances, high-risk behaviors, the impact of substance use on the family, dual diagnosis, and psychologic models for understand-ing substance abuse.

Structure

Most CBT is quite structured. In cognitive therapy of substance abuse, for example, the structure includes setting the agenda, checking the patient's mood, bridging from the last visit (including a review of substance use, urges, cravings, and upcoming trig-gers), discussion of problems (including potential coping strategies and skill-building activities), frequent summaries, the assignment and review of homework, and feed-back from the patient about the session. In the Seeking Safety model of CBT for the dual diagnosis of substance abuse and posttraumatic stress disorder (PTSD), the structure includes a check-in, a brief inspiring quotation to engage patients emotion-ally, distribution of handouts to help instill new learning, and a check-out to end the session on a positive note (e.g., "Name one thing you got out of today's session").

Attention to the Multiple Needs of Patients

CBTs for substance abuse recognize that patients typically suffer from serious life problems, including health, legal, employment, family, and housing problems. In some cases, these are the result of substance use, for example, a heroin abuser who has con-tracted human immunodeficiency virus (HIV) by sharing needles. In other cases, these life problems may have led to substance abuse, for example, a teenage girl who uses alcohol to cope with childhood sexual abuse. Actively addressing these real-life issues is a necessary component of CBT.

There are numerous opportunities for CBT therapists to provide case manage-ment services. For example, they might refer patients for specialized assistance (e.g., medical, legal, family, or vocational counseling), give patients listings of sober houses, help patients fill out welfare forms, provide referrals to and basic information about self-help groups (e.g., Alcoholics Anonymous or other 12-step programs), review newspaper job listings during sessions, monitor patients' important visits to their physicians, help patients complete domestic abuse restraining orders, or call detoxifi-cation hospital units to determine whether beds are available. Thus, therapists must be familiar with community resources, including legal services, detoxification centers, HIV testing sites, and self-help groups.

In treating dually diagnosed patients, the most important step is the initial assess-ment and monitoring of symptoms throughout treatment. It is important to understand the relationship between psychiatric symptoms and drug use, cravings, and withdrawal. Following initial assessment, patients with deficits in coping skills are taught new skills for managing their lives. Whereas previously many patients were told to become absti-nent first before comorbid disorders could be addressed (e.g., "First get clean, and then we'll talk about your depression"), most CBT models support integrated treatment (i.e., simultaneously addressing multiple disorders). Several CBT dual-diagnosis treatments have been developed and empirically evaluated for PTSD, personality disorders, bipolar disorder, and schizophrenia. When clinicians cannot directly provide dual diagnosis treatment, referral to adjunctive treatments is recommended.

Monitoring Substance Use

CBT therapists actively monitor the types, quantities, and routes of recent substance use at each treatment session. There are various methods for monitoring substance use. Although self-report is the most common, urine and breathalyzer tests provide more objective data. Regardless of the method chosen, asking patients about substance use at each session is an essential component of CBT and the accuracy of self-reports is enhanced when confidentiality is assured.

Specific Treatments and Techniques

CBT for substance abuse comprises a wide range of specific treatments and techniques that focus on general substance use disorders as well as specific substances of abuse. Despite their diversity, there are several strategies common to most CBT approaches to substance abuse. These strategies include conducting functional analyses and providing training in coping skills to better manage the identified antecedents and consequences of substance use. Examples of these strategies are briefly described in this section.

Functional Analysis of Substance Use

Virtually all CBT attempts to identify the chain of cognitive, behavioral, and emotional events that precede and follow incidents of substance use. This process, referred to as *functional analysis* (or chain analysis), is defined as *the identification of important, controllable, causal functional relationships applicable to a specified set of target behaviors for an individual client.* The goal of functional analysis is to understand the variables that are controlling the target behavior (i.e., substance use) and to use this information to provide a focus for coping skills training.

Accordingly, the initial step is to conduct a functional analysis to help the patient recognize what factors tend to trigger and reinforce episodes of substance use, and to determine what skills they will need to learn to intervene in this process.

Functional analysis requires a careful assessment of the circumstances surrounding episodes of substance use and is often addressed through open-ended exploration of patients' substance abuse history (e.g., determinants of substance use, patterns of substance use, common thoughts and feelings associated with urges to use, reasons for using substances). Standardized assessment instruments may also be useful in this process, such as the Inventory of Drinking Situations.

Coping Skills for Managing the Antecedents of Substance Use

Once antecedents of substance use have been identified via functional analysis, coping skills are taught to manage these triggers in an effort to break their connection to substance use. A number of different types of antecedents may be involved in triggering substance use, including social, environmental, emotional, cognitive, and physical factors.

Social Antecedents

Social antecedents for substance use include any social situations or interactions the patient may encounter in which they are at increased risk for substance use. Many substance users consume substances in social contexts and thus have developed networks of family, friends, dating partners, and coworkers with whom they have used substances in the past. These people may trigger urges to use directly by pressuring the individual to engage in substance use or indirectly by their conditioned association with substance use. Social triggers may also include attending social events such as parties or celebrations at which people are using substances.

LIFESTYLE CHANGES

One strategy for coping with social antecedents is to make lifestyle changes that help patients avoid exposure to social situations that trigger substance use. Lifestyle changes may range from informal discussions of lifestyle options to formal planning of and participating in activities together. Other techniques include contracting to engage in new activities that are incompatible with substance use (e.g., exercise, meditation), referring patients to external resources to develop alternative pursuits (e.g., helping patients sign up for volunteer work), and identifying healthy activities.

ENHANCING SOCIAL SUPPORT

Another strategy is to encourage the development of social networks that are supportive of abstinence. Often patients' social networks include many people who use substances and, thus, may trigger urges to drink or use drugs. Strategies include minimizing contact with people who use substances and developing a new social support network that is supportive of abstinence. In network therapy, for example, family or close friends are invited to attend sessions with patients and actively become involved in treatment contracting. In other treatments, such as cognitive therapy, family sessions are provided to enable family members to learn about the treatment and support patients' efforts.

REFUSAL SKILLS

Virtually all CBT includes training in substance-refusal skills to help patients cope with social pressure to use substances. Techniques include role playing to practice refusing offers of substances; educating patients about passive, aggressive, and assertive communication styles; anticipating consequences of refusal; and paying attention to body language and nonverbal cues.

Environmental Antecedents

Environmental antecedents to substance use include any external cues that are associated with substance use for an individual and increased urges to use. These include substance-related cues (e.g., advertisements for alcohol, the smell of alcohol) and general cues that have come to be associated with substance use through classical conditioning (e.g., money, times of day).

CUE EXPOSURE

Drawing from classical conditioning theory, cue exposure treatment (CET) seeks to diminish conditioned responses to substance use cues by repeatedly exposing patients to these cues in the absence of actual substance use. CET involves repeated exposure to the environmental cues associated with substance use (e.g., drug-related paraphernalia, photographs of high-risk locations, and depictions of actual drug use), with the goal of decreasing responsivity (e.g., cravings, substance-related thoughts) to these stimuli.

DECISION-MAKING SKILLS

One strategy for managing environmental triggers of substance use is to train patients in decision-making skills that help them to decrease exposure to these stimuli. Relapse prevention models of substance use focus on the decision chain leading to drug use, including identifying "seemingly irrelevant decisions" that increase the risk of relapse, such as, "I can get a job as a bartender." Training in decision-making skills can help patients to interrupt these decision chains before substance use occurs. Strategies include identifying examples of poor decisions (e.g., keeping substances in the house), recognizing associations between decisions and exposure to high-risk situations, challenging cognitive distortions that encourage risky decisions, and practicing safe decision making.

Emotional Antecedents

Negative emotions such as anger and anxiety can be a common triggers of relapse, and substance use often functions as a way to decrease or avoid these aversive emotional states. Conversely, positive affect (e.g., joy, excitement) can also trigger substance use, as it can remind patients of enjoyable times with others and pleasurable emotions they have experienced when using substances. CBT strategies for coping with emotional triggers focus on how to regulate and tolerate emotional states to decrease the risk of substance abuse.

CHANGE STRATEGIES

CBT for substance abuse includes many emotion regulation strategies that are focused on changing negative affect. Cognitive strategies include challenging distorted thoughts that fuel negative affect, completing daily thought records, and using positive coping statements (e.g., "I can handle these feelings without using"). Behavioral strategies include activities to decrease the intensity of negative affect such as distraction, engaging in pleasurable activities, self-soothing, acting opposite of emotions, and relaxation strategies.

ACCEPTANCE STRATEGIES

In contrast to techniques aimed at changing negative affect, acceptance strategies focus on increasing tolerance for negative emotional states, decreasing emotional avoidance, and encouraging acceptance of emotional experiences. One common technique is mindfulness meditation. Mindfulness is a cognitive strategy that focuses attention on emotions by observing them in an objective, nonjudgmental way, rather than avoiding or suppressing them.

Cognitive Antecedents

Cognitive antecedents of substance of abuse include drug-related beliefs (e.g., "Using drugs improves my mood"), automatic thoughts (e.g., "Smoke!"), and facilitating beliefs (e.g., "I can handle just one hit") that increase the risk of use or relapse. These cognitions often derive from core beliefs about the self (e.g., "I'm vulnerable") and resulting rules that a person has developed for survival (e.g., "If I let myself feel my emotions, I'll fall apart").

MODIFYING AUTOMATIC THOUGHTS AND DRUG-RELATED BELIEFS

An initial step in cognitive therapy for substance use is to help patients identify their automatic thoughts and drug-related beliefs and to recognize that they may not be completely accurate. Patients are taught to identify logical errors in their thinking that may trigger substance use (e.g., ignoring evidence that substance use is becoming problematic, exaggerating their ability to quit, overemphasizing the positive aspects of substance use, devaluing friends and activities that are not related to substance use, and believing that life without substance use is boring). A variety of cognitive restructuring techniques can be used to modify distorted automatic thoughts and drug-related beliefs, including examining the evidence, considering the alternatives, keeping daily thought records, using a cognitive continuum, surveying others, and the double-standard technique. In addition, patients can create flash cards on which they write their common automatic thoughts and effective challenges to them. Patients can refer to the flash cards when confronted with high-risk situations that trigger these cognitions.

MODIFYING CONDITIONAL ASSUMPTIONS AND CORE BELIEFS

A later step in cognitive therapy for substance use is to identify and modify patients' conditional assumptions and core beliefs that are fueling negative automatic thoughts. A variety of techniques are available for identifying core beliefs, including the downward arrow technique, looking for central themes in patients' automatic thoughts, recognizing core beliefs that are expressed as automatic thoughts, Socratic questioning, and the what-if method. Once patients' core beliefs have been identified, strategies for modifying these beliefs include examining advantages and disadvantages, historical tests, keeping a daily log of evidence that supports and contradicts the core belief, and conducting behavioral experiments to test the conditional assumptions associated with core beliefs.

Physical Antecedents

Physical antecedents to substance use typically involve cravings and withdrawal symptoms. In addition, individuals may use substances to cope with other types of physical symptoms that may be unrelated to cravings or withdrawal (e.g., headaches, fatigue, nausea).

DISTRACTION

Perhaps the most common technique for managing cravings is distraction. This involves engaging in activities that distract attention from the craving experience (e.g., physical exercise, talking with someone, snapping a rubber band on their wrist, relaxation strategies). Another version is thought-stopping wherein patients silently say "stop!" when experiencing cravings. Patients can create a coping card containing a list of distraction techniques to help them manage future cravings.

URGE SURFING

Similar to mindfulness techniques for coping with negative affect, urge surfing (going with the craving) involves letting cravings occur, peak, and pass without either fighting them or giving in to them. Urge surfing is done by focusing attention on the experience of craving and describing the physical sensations, feelings, and thoughts associated with it in an objective way. Urge surfing aids in increasing acceptance of craving as a time-limited, normal experience that patients can manage without using substances.

FOCUS ON CONSEQUENCES

Patients often overemphasize the positive aspects of substance use and ignore the negative consequences. Conversely, patients tend to minimize the benefits of abstinence and focus only on its disadvantages. One strategy for correcting these errors is to conduct an advantages–disadvantages analysis to identify the pros and cons of abstinence and continued use. Another strategy involves recalling the negative consequences of past substance use in order to make the disadvantages of giving in to the craving more salient. This can be done by having patients carry a reminder card that lists past negative effects of their substance use and having them review this card whenever cravings occur.

Coping Skills for Managing the Contingencies of Substance Use

In addition to providing training in coping skills for managing the antecedents of substance use, CBT also attempts to help patients manage the contingencies (i.e., positive and negative reinforcers) of their substance use. Examples of strategies for managing contingencies are briefly described here.

Contingency Management

Using principles of operant conditioning, contingency management techniques implement reinforcement to strengthen the incentive to become abstinent and weaken the incentive to continue using substances. Such reinforcement can be either positive (i.e., rewarding patients for abstinence) or negative (i.e., withdrawal of rewards for substance use). Less frequently, treatments have investigated the use of punishment in decreasing substance use (e.g., inducing nausea).

Substituting Alternative Behaviors

Another behavioral strategy for addressing the reinforcers of substance use is to substitute the use of substances with functionally equivalent and more adaptive behaviors. It involves identifying both the positive and negative contingencies of substance use and finding less destructive behaviors that could serve the same function. For example, if substance use decreases negative affect, it could be substituted with emotion regulation strategies (e.g., distraction, self-soothing). If substance use serves a relaxation purpose, functionally equivalent alternative behaviors might include relaxation or meditation.

Conclusion

Over the past decade, numerous CBT approaches to substance abuse have been developed. These structured, focused, collaborative approaches have been based on the assumption that substance abuse is mediated by complex cognitive–behavioral processes. In this chapter, an overview of cognitive–behavioral substance abuse theories and techniques has been presented. These approaches have been among the most productive of the last quarter century with respect to the advancement of empirically validated knowledge of the origins and treatment of substance use disorders.

Specifically, cognitive–behavioral therapists should (a) be knowledgeable about a wide variety of psychoactive drugs, addictive behaviors, and traditional treatment modalities; (b) communicate and collaborate with other addiction treatment personnel; (c) understand and address the role of substances in mood regulation; (d) conceptualize and treat coexisting psychopathology; (e) explore the development of all patients' substance abuse problems; (f) address therapeutic relationship issues; (g) confront patients appropriately and effectively; (h) stay focused in sessions; (i) use techniques appropriately and sparingly; and (j) never give up on addicted patients. Many more lessons will likely be learned as CBT continues to be applied to substance abuse.

Suggested Readings

Linehan MM, Dimeff LA, Reynolds SK, et al. Dialectical behavior therapy versus comprehensive validation therapy plus 12-step for the treatment of opioid dependent women meeting criteria for borderline personality disorder. *Drug Alcohol Depend.* 2002;67:13–26.

Najavits LM. Assessment of trauma, PTSD and substance abuse: a practical guide. In: Wilson JP, Keane TW, eds. *Assessment of psychological trauma and PTSD.* New York: Guilford Press; 2004.

Najavits LM. Seeking Safety: a new psychotherapy for PTSD and substance abuse. In: Ouimette P, Brown PJ, eds. *Trauma and substance abuse: causes, consequences and comorbid conditions.* Washington, D.C.: American Psychological Association; 2002:147–170.

Najavits LM. *Seeking safety: a treatment manual for PTSD and substance abuse.* New York: Guilford Press; 2002.

Najavits LM, Liese BS, Harnod MS. Cognitive and behavioral therapies. In: Lowinson JH, Ruiz P, Millman RB, et al., eds. *Substance abuse: a comprehensive textbook*, 4th ed. Philadelphia: Lippincott Williams & Wilkins; 2005:723–732.

van den Bosch LMC, Verheul R, Schippers GM, et al. Dialectical behavior therapy of borderline patients with and without substance use problems: implementation and long-term effects. *Addict Behav.* 2002;27:911–923.

28

ALCOHOLICS ANONYMOUS

For more than six decades Alcoholics Anonymous (AA) has influenced, guided, and shaped the treatment of alcoholism. The appeal of its "Twelve Steps" program has been extended to other disorders, including drug addiction (Narcotics Anonymous), eating disorders (Overeaters Anonymous), and gambling (Gamblers Anonymous).

What is Alcoholics Anonymous?

AA is a fellowship, that is, a "mutual association of persons on equal and friendly terms; a mutual sharing, as of experience, activity, or interest." AA is open to all men and women who want to do something about their drinking problems. Interestingly, members need not consider themselves alcoholics or seek abstinence. AA is nonprofessional, self-supporting, nondenominational, apolitical, and multiracial. There are no age or education requirements.

At the start of an AA meeting the "AA preamble" is usually read. The preamble is a concise description of AA:

> Alcoholics Anonymous is a fellowship of men and women who share their experience, strength, and hope with each other that they may solve their common problem and help others to recover from alcoholism. The only requirement for membership is a desire to stop drinking. There are no dues or fees for AA membership; we are self-supporting through our own contributions. AA is not allied with any sect, denomination, politics, organization, or institution; does not wish to engage in any controversy, neither endorses nor proposes any causes. Our primary purpose is to stay sober and help other alcoholics to achieve sobriety.

Program of Alcoholics Anonymous

The program of AA consists of studying and following the 12 s of AA. In addition, AA groups are careful to adhere to the "Twelve Traditions" of AA. The 12 steps offer the alcoholic a sober way of life. This program is presented and discussed in AA meetings. Meetings may be "open" or "closed." Closed meetings are for AA members only or prospective AA members, whereas open meetings are for nonalcoholics as well. AA meetings usually last 1 hour and are preceded and followed by informal socializing. There are different types of meetings: In speaker meetings, AA members tell their "stories." They describe their experiences with alcohol and their recovery—what it was like, what happened, and what it is like now. In discussion meetings, an AA member briefly describes some of the member's experiences and then leads a discussion on a topic related to recovery. Step meetings usually are closed meetings and consist of a discussion of the meaning and ramifications of one of the 12 steps.

AA groups are autonomous. Some groups provide proof of attendance that may be required by a court or probation office, whereas other groups choose not to sign court slips. Sponsorship is an essential function of AA. Each person who joins AA is encouraged to obtain a sponsor, that is, another AA member willing to offer person-to-person guidance in working the AA program. A sponsor typically is a person who has a substantial period of sobriety and who has studied and worked the 12 steps. The sponsorship relationship is informal, and the styles of sponsorship vary greatly.

That AA is a fellowship distinguishes it from professional treatment or programs. Alcoholism provides a bond between one AA member and another. In contrast, professional relationships establish a boundary between doctor and patient or therapist and client. The clinician, when confronted with an alcoholic patient, uses the diagnosis of alcoholism to erect a boundary from which role relationships are carefully defined. From the structure of the professional relationship the clinician applies his or her skills and technologies. There is no mutual sharing of experience or any pretense of equality in the relationship.

What Alcoholics Anonymous Does Not Do

Part of appreciating the role of AA in the recovery of alcoholics is understanding what AA does not do. AA does not: (a) furnish initial motivation for alcoholics to recover, (b) solicit members, (c) engage in or sponsor research, (d) keep attendance records or case histories, (e) join "councils" of social agencies, (f) follow up or try to control its members, (g) make medical or psychologic diagnoses or prognoses, (h) provide drying-out or nursing services, hospitalization, drugs, or any medical or psychiatric treatment, (i) offer religious services, (j) engage in education about alcohol, (k) provide housing, food, clothing, jobs, money, or any other welfare or social services, (l) provide domestic or vocational counseling, (m) accept any money for its services, or any contributions from non-AA sources, (n) provide letters of reference to parole boards, lawyers, court officials.

The Growth of Alcoholics Anonymous

The birth date of AA is given as June 10, 1935. On this date Dr. Bob Smith, the Akron surgeon who cofounded AA with Bill Wilson, had his last drink. The official founding of AA was established with that event. About $2^{1}/_{2}$ years later, "Dr. Bob" and "Bill W." estimated that as a result of their combined efforts in both Akron and New York City, there were nearly 40 sober recovering alcoholics. The cofounders knew they were onto something (one alcoholic talking to another) and continued the struggle of carrying their hope, strength, and experience to other alcoholics. Most of those they contacted, however, were neither maintaining sobriety nor had any interest in their ideas. But by the end of 4 years, membership was estimated to be about 100, and by the end of 1941, 8,000 members could be counted. By 1968, 170,000 members were estimated.

In spite of early periods of discouragement, the growth of AA has been phenomenal and continues today, exceeding 1 million members worldwide.

Composition of Alcoholics Anonymous

Approximately 7,500 members in the United States and Canada were surveyed in 2001. The average age of an AA member is 46 years; 75% of members are between the ages of 31 and 60 years. Women make up 33% of the membership and whites make up 88% of the membership; 37% of members are married, 31% single, and 24% divorced. The average AA member has 7 years sobriety and attends two AA meetings per week. An interesting trend is the percentage of AA members reporting addiction to drugs. In 1977, 18% reported drug addiction, but by 1989, 46% were reporting a history of drug addiction. Women and younger people in AA were more likely to report a history of drug addiction.

The Origins of Alcoholics Anonymous

Carl Jung played a role in the first of four founding moments in the development of AA, through his extended and frustrating treatment of an American businessman. Jung eventually advised this man (Roland H.) that medicine and psychiatry had no more to offer. Only a spiritual change or awakening, however unlikely, could be expected to release the continuing compulsion to drink. Roland H. proceeded to join the Oxford Group, a popular nondenominational religious group that sought to recapture the essence of first century Christianity and was interested in alcoholics. Roland H.'s successful conversion and abstinence constituted the first founding moment.

Roland H.'s experience was shared with an old friend and alcoholic, Edwin T. ("Ebby"). He, too, found the evangelical efforts of the Oxford Group sufficient to release him from further drinking (at least, temporarily). Ebby, a friend of Bill Wilson, called on Bill in November 1934. Wilson was at his home in New York City, drinking. Ebby refused a drink, stating, "I don't need it anymore. I've got religion," and described his recent success in giving up alcohol. This conversation was the second founding moment. In spite of Bill's disdain for his friend's newfound "religion," he couldn't shake the image of his friend—sober and confident. Bill was influenced through his conversation with Ebby to try again. Bill had himself admitted to the Charles B. Towns Hospital under the care of a psychiatrist, Dr. William Silkworth.

During this hospitalization Bill became increasingly depressed. Concomitant with his worsening condition there occurred one of those inexplicable events described as a spiritual experience. Wilson experienced "ecstasy." He couldn't describe it, and he feared that it indicated brain damage. Dr. Silkworth re-assured him concerning the latter, and Bill began to read James's *Varieties of Religious Experience* in an effort to understand what had happened to him. The spiritual experience, the influence of James's writings, and the recognition of the utter hopelessness of his drinking were the third founding moment.

Bill then imagined that conversations between one alcoholic and another, such as his with Ebby, could lead to a "chain reaction" among alcoholics. Months later, in May 1935, an opportunity occurred in Akron, where Bill, a stockbroker, was on a business trip. A deal had fallen through, and Bill felt a mounting urge to drink. It was late Saturday afternoon, the day before Mother's Day. He consulted a church directory, reached an Oxford Group minister, and ultimately was referred to a woman who was receptive to his need to talk to another alcoholic. Mrs. Henrietta Sieberling arranged for Bill to come to her house and meet with Dr. Bob Smith, a deteriorating alcoholic surgeon. Dr. Smith was reluctant to accept this invitation but went with his wife to meet Bill W. Their historic meeting, the fourth founding moment, is described as follows:

> . . . here was someone who did understand, or perhaps at least could. This stranger from New York didn't ask questions and didn't preach; he offered no "you musts" or even "let's us's." He had simply told the dreary but fascinating facts about himself, about his own drinking. And now, as Wilson moved to stand up to end the conversation, he was actually thanking Dr. Smith for listening. "I called Henrietta because I needed another alcoholic. I needed you, Bob, probably a lot more than you'll ever need me. So, thanks a lot for hearing me out. I know now that I'm not going to take a drink, and I'm grateful to you." While he had been listening to Bill's story, Bob had occasionally nodded his head, muttering "Yes, that's like me, that's just like me." Now he could bear the strain no longer. He'd listened to Bill's story, and now, by God, this "rum hound from New York" was going to listen to him. For the first time in his life, Dr. Bob Smith began to open his heart. Bill Wilson and Bob Smith became the cofounders of AA. Wilson went on to develop the fellowship of AA and to provide a remarkable chapter in the social history of twentieth century America. Bill W. learned to weave a careful course between religious dogma, on the one hand, and a humanistic liberal psychology on the other. The AA program was successful in incorporating the concepts of "surrender," "powerlessness," and appeal to a "Higher Power." These elements reflect its roots in the evangelical Christianity of the Oxford Group. Yet Bill W. avoided the Oxford Group's focus on attaining "Four Absolutes": absolute honesty, absolute purity, absolute unselfishness, and absolute love. He was aware of the psychological vulnerability of the alcoholic to strive for "absolutes," and, when the mark is missed, to indulge in self-castigation, self-hatred, and, finally, drunkenness.

The AA program counters pathologic narcissism by assisting the alcoholic to be "not-God," to accept limitations, and to serve others. Furthermore, the AA program provides a means for overcoming guilt, for example, by taking a personal inventory and making amends without triggering harsh superego responses. Although the origins of AA are rooted in the sacred and the religious, it has widened its appeal by cloaking the program in spiritual and secular garb.

Affiliation with Alcoholics Anonymous

The 2001 AA General Services Office survey reports that of the factors most responsible for people coming to AA, 32% of newcomers were referred by treatment facilities. A further 33% were attracted to AA by an AA member, and 33% reported being self-motivated.

Gradually, AA is receiving greater emphasis from physicians. Historically, things got off to a slow start with doctors. The first edition of *Alcoholics Anonymous* was published in 1939. AA members were enthusiastic about reaching out to the medical community and sent 20,000 announcements of the *Big Book*. Only two orders for *Alcoholics Anonymous* were received. Since then, of course, physicians have become much more aware of AA; one study from Great Britain reports that 65% of general practitioners believed that AA had something to offer beyond what could be obtained through medical efforts. The 2001 General Services Office Survey reports that 38% of members were referred to AA by a health care professional and that 73% of members' doctors know they are in AA.

Once someone enters AA, what are the chances that person will stay? Figures from AA General Services Office surveys indicate that only 50% of those who come to AA remain more than 3 months. In a review of the literature, dropout rates from AA varied from 68% before 10 meetings were attended to 88% by 1 year after discharge. It has been found that counseling or other related treatments influence AA affiliation as 74% of AA members who received treatment report that it played an important part in their going to AA.

The "dropout" problem raises the question of who is likely to make a stable affiliation with AA. Most alcoholics have the possibility of making an affiliation with AA. Only those whose goal is not to abstain from alcohol would be seen as exceptions. Demographic variables such as education, employment, socioeconomic status of the alcoholic or of the parents, social stability, religion, and measures of social competence are unrelated to the affiliation process. Age favors, although not consistently, older alcoholics making a positive affiliation. Marital status (married) and gender (male) also show some positive relationship to affiliation. Alcoholism variables bear little relationship to making a positive affiliation. For example, loss of control, quantity drunk daily, age at first drink, degree of physiologic dependence, and drinking style bear no consistent relationship to affiliation. It is best to accept as unpredictable who will affiliate with AA, which again emphasizes the importance of recommending AA to all possible members.

Alcoholics Anonymous Outcome

Many efforts have been made to assess the effectiveness of AA attendance. Measurement of "outcome" typically is limited to abstinence or lack of abstinence from alcohol. In studies of AA from the 1940s to the early 1970s, sampling difficulties and other methodologic problems were immense. Nevertheless, the findings indicated that thousands of AA members had achieved sobriety. A review of survey studies found that 35% to 40% of respondents reported abstinence of less than 1 year, with 26% to 40% reporting abstinence of 1 to 5 years, and 20% to 30% having been sober 5 or more years. Overall, 47% to 62% of active AA members had at least 1 year of continuous sobriety.

AA involvement correlates favorably with a variety of outcome measures. Those patients who attend AA before, during, or after a treatment experience have a more favorable outcome in regard to drinking. In the few studies available that assess the outcome on other variables, AA involvement is associated with a more stable social adjustment, more active religious life, internal locus of control, and better employment adjustment. Increased ethical concern for others, an increased sense of well-being, and increasing dependence on a higher power with less dependence on others also have been described. Outcome is more favorable for those who attend more than one meeting per week and for those who have a sponsor, sponsor others, lead meetings, and work Steps 6 through 12 after completing a treatment program. Taking Step 4 or 5 is not consistently related to outcome, nor is telling one's story or doing 12-step work.

Dynamics of Alcoholics Anonymous

The reasons for the effectiveness of AA may be as varied as the individuals involved. At the most basic level, the program works because one follows the 12 steps. It may be that these deceptively simple steps provide a concrete, tangible course of action; they may trigger cognitive processes previously unformed, unfocused, or abandoned; and they may encapsulate powerful dynamics capable of having an impact on craving, conditioning, and character. The AA program revolves around the 12 steps, and most members would offer the commonsense explanation that working the steps keeps them sober. This sentiment is reflected in the *Big Book* chapter on how it works: "Rarely have we seen a person fail who has thoroughly followed our path."

Group Process

The utility of the slogan "keep it simple" is well known to AA members, but need not deter further inquiry into the process or dynamics of the effectiveness of AA. Any effort to understand the efficacy of AA must take into account the ubiquitous group process that is operating.

1. *Hope* is provided by associating with other alcoholics who are not drinking and who apparently are happy, satisfied, or, indeed, grateful not to be drinking.
2. *Universality* is formed through sharing stories and experiences involving alcohol.
3. *Information* is provided informally through conversations, through literature published by AA, and through the topics and content of the meetings themselves.
4. *Imitation* is a very prominent aspect of the group process. Phrases are repeated and rituals followed.
5. *Learning* occurs at multiple levels and includes how sober alcoholics view their disease, how they relate to others, and what they do to stay sober.
6. *Catharsis* can occur. The opportunity is provided (but not demanded) through discussion, speaker, and step-study meetings. One's experiences are appreciated and not subjected to condemnation or judgment.
7. *Cohesiveness* follows from the ability to identify, usually quickly, with the viewpoints and experiences of fellow members. Cohesiveness is also facilitated by participating in the informal socializing characteristic of AA meetings.

The beneficial aspects of group process may be found in many settings, for example, group therapy, religious groups, and organizational activities. The dynamics operative in coherent group settings cannot fully account for the impact of AA on alcoholics. If group process variables were the key to the transformation from inebriety to sobriety, substantial progress in arresting alcoholism could have been expected before the establishment of the AA program. Equal success might have been expected from a variety of group approaches. This has not been the case. It is necessary to look further.

An Empathic Understanding of the Alcoholic

In a series of classic papers, Bean provides a description of the mechanisms of the effectiveness of AA, integrating its phenomenologic and psychodynamic aspects: AA has "accomplished a shift from a society-centered view of alcoholism to an abuser-centered one." For the bereft or discouraged alcoholic, this shift is a startling, powerful encounter. AA provides the alcoholic with a protected environment. After years of feeling debased and worthless, the alcoholic is offered an environment free from the conventional view of drunken behavior. The alcoholic discovers that his or her experience is of value and even interesting to others. Furthermore, the alcoholic's experiences may be useful to someone else, and others thank him or her for sharing it. As Bean explains, "This idea, that a person's experience is of value, is gratifying to anyone and is especially heady stuff to the chronically self-deprecating alcoholic."

Along with the shift in how alcoholism is viewed, AA provides a shift in what is expected of the alcoholic. First, the alcoholic is not asked to admit that he or she is an alcoholic. AA simply asks that one have a sincere desire to stop drinking. There is no effort to point out the error of one's ways or the evils of drink. In fact, the attraction of alcohol and the pleasure of alcohol are openly acknowledged but linked with the statement that "we couldn't handle it." The alcoholic who comes to AA is not asked to change, only to listen, identify, and keep coming back. The style of interpersonal contact is nonthreatening. Last names are not given, attendance is not taken, the setting is casual, and humor and friendliness abound. Nevertheless, the meeting is serious. Each member conveys that there is a lot to lose, regardless of how much has actually been lost, but also that there is much to gain—sobriety. Sobriety is the focus, and remains so, unvaryingly. Not drinking is the coin of the realm. Relapses or "slips" do not represent a failure on the part of the alcoholic or of AA. Rather, slips are further demonstration of the power of alcohol and, therefore, the necessity of AA as a counterforce.

As the alcoholic advances in recovery, self-esteem is protected by abstinence but threatened by remorse over the past. According to Bean, AA techniques to handle this aspect of recovery are as follows:

1. The decision not to drink—repent and reform to build upon the wreckage of the past
2. Place blame on the illness, not the alcoholic
3. Avoid censure
4. Reward good behavior—this is done by dispensing 30-day, 60-day, 90-day, or 1-year "chips" as milestones in sobriety are achieved.
5. Allow expression of low self-esteem in nondestructive ways rather than by drinking

AA does not ask the alcoholic to get a job, be a better family member, or become more responsible. Sobriety is the goal from which other desirable efforts may emerge. The "depressurization" techniques of AA ("one day at a time," "keep it simple," etc.) and the social dimension—sharing "experiences, strength, and hope"—are, from Bean's perspective, critical components of the AA experience.

Accepting Limitations

The writings of Kurtz provide not only a definitive history of AA but also critical insights into the effectiveness of AA. The core dynamic of AA therapy, according to Kurtz, is "the shared honesty of mutual vulnerability openly acknowledged."

An essential insight of AA for the alcoholic is its recognition and acceptance that one is "not-God." With this term Kurtz is referring to the necessity for the alcoholic to accept personal limitation. The First Step of AA communicates to the alcoholic: "We admitted we were powerless over alcohol and that our lives had become unmanageable." The acceptance of personal limitation—a condition of existence for all—is a life or death matter for the alcoholic. AA, in teaching that the first drink gets the alcoholic drunk, implies that the alcoholic does not have a drinking limit, the alcoholic is limited. To experience limitation is tantamount to experiencing shame. As painful as the shame is, it is an affect pivotal to recovery. Acceptance of shame distinguishes the alcoholic who, complies rather than surrenders. Compliance is motivated by guilt, is superficial, and ultimately is useless to extended recovery. Surrender involves recognition of powerlessness. Through surrender the alcoholic becomes open to the healing forces within AA. The AA program treats shame by enabling the alcoholic to accept his or her need for others, by promoting the acceptance of others as they are ("live and let live"), and by valuing and reinforcing traits of honesty, sharing, and caring.

Spiritual Dimension

Mechanisms or explanations have been reviewed in the effort to understand better the dynamics of AA. Among these explanations are the impact of AA on ego functions and pathologic narcissism, its understanding of the alcoholic and alcoholism from the viewpoint of the alcoholic, its confrontation of the powerlessness and loss of control of the alcoholic, and its ability to shift the alcoholic from self-centeredness to self-acceptance. These analyses of the effectiveness of AA (like examination of group process variables) contribute to our understanding of the AA program but are incomplete in their capture of the AA process. The dimension of spirituality must be introduced and considered in the equation of our understanding.

Spirituality rarely is part of the lexicon of the mental health professional but is a dimension of the AA program understood by those who work and live the 12 steps. The spirituality of the AA program is distinct from religious dogma and may be understood as a series of overlapping themes. The first theme is release. Release refers to the "chains being broken"—freedom from the compulsion to drink. The experience of release is a powerful and welcome event for the alcoholic and seems to occur naturally or to be given rather than achieved. A second theme of spirituality is gratitude. Gratitude may flow from the feeling of release and includes an awareness of what we have—for example, the gift of life. The third theme is humility. Humility conveys the attitude that it is acceptable to be limited, to be simply human. The alcoholic's awareness of powerlessness over alcohol engenders humility. Finally, a fourth theme or component to spirituality is tolerance. A tolerance of differences and limitations fosters the serenity often experienced by AA members.

These themes of spirituality are very similar to the healing process in mystical traditions. According to Deikman, the process of attaining higher psychologic development involves renunciation, humility, and sincerity. Renunciation refers to an attitude, that is, a giving up of the attachment to the things of the world. The alcoholic's giving up alcohol would demonstrate renunciation. Humility, according to Deikman, is "the possibility that someone else can teach you something you do not already know, especially about yourself," and sincerity simply refers to honesty of intention. It is apparent that the alcoholic working the 12 steps is involving himself or herself in the processes of renunciation, humility, and sincerity.

In addition to these spiritual themes, an additional healing dynamic may be significant: forgiveness. The seeking of forgiveness is implied, not directly expressed, in the 12 steps. For example, Steps 6 and 7 ask God to remove defects of character and remove shortcomings. The behavior of AA members toward newcomers (welcoming, accepting, friendly, caring) communicates forgiveness. Forgiveness is neither asked for nor offered at AA. The word itself may or may not be heard at AA meetings, but its meaning pervades the transactions of the meetings.

Forgiveness may be a precondition for the dynamic forces described to be operative. For example, forgiveness precedes hope. Hope is necessarily very tenuous for a newcomer to AA and requires a future orientation, an orientation minimized by the emphasis by AA on "one day at a time." Forgiveness is experienced in a moment and may be the foundation for a growing sense of hope. To be forgiven, to feel forgiven implies being accepted, a common description of the AA experience. The experience of shame as a pivotal affect and the treatment of shame in AA may become possible only if preceded by a sense of being forgiven.

The concepts of spirituality, including forgiveness, are put forth only as one further effort to explain the impact and mechanisms of the AA program. Perhaps what is effective in the AA program varies considerably from member to member. An AA member may have limited awareness of (and equally little interest in) the dynamic forces accounting for the effectiveness of AA. But, possibly, for some, the program may be a secular expression of the Christian concept of grace—an unmerited gift from God.

Limitations of Alcoholics Anonymous

AA is predominantly a white, middle-class organization consisting of middle-aged married men. This broad demographic characterization of AA does not indicate a limitation of the AA program itself but may impose some barriers for those out of the mainstream. AA does attract a young population. About 11% of members are 30 years of age or younger. The percentage of women is 33%. Adoption of the AA program by minorities has been slower to occur. Yet, most urban areas have several meetings with a predominantly African American or Hispanic population. African American affiliation with AA is growing stronger and may exceed white affiliation on some variables.

Psychiatric comorbidity may impede AA affiliation for some alcoholics. Personality disorders of the schizoid, avoidant, or paranoid type may not adapt well to the interaction and emotionality of AA meetings. At times, a patient on medications is thrown into conflict by AA members who may advise against the use of any drugs. AA as an organization does not hold opinions on psychotropic medications, but occasionally an AA member may inappropriately influence a fellow member who requires specific psychiatric treatment. An alcoholic persuaded to discontinue lithium or neuroleptics may relapse into psychosis, at great personal expense. As more alcoholics are reaching AA through rehabilitation programs, the AA member under psychiatric treatment will be less likely to experience conflict and inappropriate advice. However, in one study, 29% of AA members reported feeling pressure to stop medication, but 89% of these continued their medications. Only 17% of 277 surveyed AA members believed that medications should not be used.

Should AA be recommended only for certain alcoholics? There is no empirical base from which such a decision-making process could follow. AA generally seems to accommodate a wide variety of personalities and backgrounds. On a case-by-case basis, social or psychodynamic factors may deter the efficacy of AA use, but that can be ascertained on an individual basis only. It is recommended that anyone concerned about drinking be referred to AA.

Apart from the issue of whether every alcoholic should be referred to AA, there are specific limitations to the AA method. These are that AA is rigid, superficial, regressive, inspirational, fanatical, stigmatizing, and focuses only on alcohol. The rigidity is more likely to lie in individual members than the AA program itself. Questioning and intellectualizing are discouraged, but this seems more a means to hold back the ever-present threat of denial than a commitment to absolute dogma. The criticism of superficiality is appropriate if one's goals are to unravel the complex etiologies of alcoholism or to understand the dynamics of behavior change. AA chooses to put its energy into abstaining from drinking and into simultaneously providing and tolerating a system that fosters dependency (hence the criticism of being regressive). AA certainly is inspirational rather than reflective, but again, the alcoholic early in recovery cannot be expected to obtain or use insight. Morale is of critical concern, and the emotional pitch of AA strikes a respondent chord in the demoralized. Unfortunately, fanaticism or zealotry may form part of the operation of AA loyalty. Such members are repellent to some newcomers, who may feel that their emotional needs are not understood or validated. Some charismatic AA members convert many alcoholics but alienate others, including the professionals to whom they relate in a condescending manner. Is there a stigma about attending AA? If there is, it is less than in past years, because acclaim for AA is easily found in popular literature and the media.

AA, like all other therapies for alcoholism, is limited. Considering our current state of knowledge, the clinician is obligated to become conversant with the purpose, principles, and utility of the AA program. By gaining an understanding of the 12 steps program, the clinician will be prepared to motivate and advocate AA to his or her alcoholic patients. This understanding is gained best by attending AA meetings, discussing AA with experienced members, and reading widely, including the AA literature as well as professional writings on AA. From this effort the physician can inform each patient appropriately of the advantages of AA as well as any potential drawbacks he or she may encounter.

Conclusion

This chapter outlines the origins of AA and describes its growth and basic situations. AA works. How well and for whom remain unsatisfactorily researched.

The clinician would be remiss to overlook, ignore, or disparage the value of AA for any patient with a substance use disorder. Familiarity with AA can be obtained by attending open AA meetings, developing friendly relationships with AA members, and insisting that one's patients meet with AA members for an initial, informed introduction to AA. Such efforts can facilitate an alliance with the AA community and foster the development of mutual respect. Such grassroots efforts, however, do not dispel conceptual differences between AA and the treatments offered by the mental health field.

Suggested Readings

Kurtz E. Not-God: A History of Alcoholics Anonymous. Center City, MN: Hazelden, 1979.

McKellar J, Stewart E, Humphreys K. Alcoholics anonymous involvement and positive alcohol-related outcomes: cause, consequence, or just a correlate? A prospective 2-year study of 2,319 alcohol-dependent men. *J Consult Clin Psychol.* 2003;71:302–308.

Moos RH, Moos BS. Participation in treatment and Alcoholics Anonymous: a 16-year follow-up of initially untreated individuals. *J Clin Psychol.* 2006;62:735–750.

Nace EP. Alcoholics Anonymous. In: Lowinson JH, Ruiz P, Millman RB, et al., eds. *Substance abuse: a comprehensive textbook,* 4th ed. Philadelphia: Lippincott Williams & Wilkins; 2005 587–599.

Thomassen L. AA utilization after introduction to treatment. *Subst Use Misuse.* 2002;37(2):239–253.

Timko C, Moos RH, Finney JW, et al. Long-term outcomes of alcohol use disorders: comparing untreated individuals with those in alcoholics anonymous and formal treatment. *J Stud Alcohol.* 2000;61:529–540.

29

THE THERAPEUTIC COMMUNITY

The therapeutic community (TC), which traces its origin to the late 1950s as a homespun approach to the problem of heroin addiction in the United States, has now grown into a worldwide movement under the banner of the World Federation of Therapeutic Communities (WFTC). It has affiliates in six regional federations in North America, Latin America, Europe, Central and Eastern Europe, Asia, and Australasia. The TC treatment treatment philosophy with its approach to the problem of addiction has taken root in diverse cultural and socioeconomic settings, spawning a global network of TCs uniquely adapted to local conditions.

The TC, as a treatment framework, has such wide appeal because it draws from universally practiced social and spiritual values that form part of its community standards and behavior norms. In fact, many of the TC approaches to behavior and psychologic change not only result in improvements in psychosocial functioning of the ex-addict, but also promote a prosocial lifestyle. Furthermore, treatment experience in the TC often results to an increase in self-awareness and a sense of responsibility for oneself and for the welfare of others. Its vigorous method of shaping attitudes and behaviors, as important determinants of sobriety and a safe lifestyle, offers a meaningful approach for influencing both high-risk and drug-using behaviors.

To determine how responsive the TC is to the needs of its clientele and to assess its efficacy in treating clients with various needs and backgrounds, new research has focused on developing tools to measure the treatment processes of the TC. Various outcome studies have been conducted to investigate the efficacy of the TC for funding purposes and accountability. For program developers and clinicians who are seeking to improve the delivery of services and to identify factors that contribute to successful outcome, studies that look into therapeutic processes are equally important. Research on best treatment practices was conducted to identify treatment aspects that contribute to program effectiveness.

Worldwide Growth of the Therapeutic Community

Most of Europe traces the development of the present-day European TCs to two major influences. First is the democratic TC that evolved from the innovations in social psychiatry for the treatment of mentally ill patients. Second is the influx of ideas that originated from the concept-based TC pioneered by Synanon in California to treat narcotic addicts. The politics of social and health service delivery in Western Europe exerted tremendous influences on how the concept-based TC was adapted in an environment that is historically tolerant to drug maintenance. The medical profession played an important role in dispensing or regulating drug maintenance. Traditionally, Western Europe is more inclined to the more liberal democratic TC in contrast with the hierarchical model of the largely American concept-based TC. Whereas the European TC developed along these two lines of kindred, but distinct, treatment philosophies, the Asian, and to a similar extent the Latin American TCs, adopted the concept-based TC as practiced currently in Daytop and in most of North America. The first TC in Asia, established in 1971 by Drug Abuse Research (DARE) Foundation of the Philippines, was patterned after the Daytop model. The same TC model was later transported to Malaysia in 1974, and to Thailand in 1979. These initial isolated outgrowths of the TC led to the establishments of TCs in Singapore, Indonesia, Vietnam, China, Hong Kong, Pakistan, India, Sri Lanka, Nepal, the Maldives, and South Korea. Today, most, if not all, of the Asian TC programs in private or community-based treatment settings, prisons, juvenile detention homes, and parole and probation programs are established along the traditional concept-based TC that was pioneered by Synanon and later adopted by the second-generation TCs such as Daytop Village and Phoenix House.

Similar developments of TC occurred in several countries in Latin America. Countries such as Colombia and Argentina received training assistance in the past from the Italian TC program, Centro Italiano di Solidarieta (CEIS), but had also engaged actively in developing their TCs along the Daytop model. The CEIS TC program had been largely influenced in the beginning by Daytop, which provided staff trainers to develop the Italian TC in the 1980s. In recent years, Daytop, through grants from the Bureau for International Narcotics and Law Enforcement Affairs (INL) of the U.S. Department of State, has been able to assist in developing the TC as part of the drug demand reduction programs in Peru, Ecuador, Brazil, Argentina, and in most parts of Asia, as well as in some parts of Eastern Europe.

The Therapeutic Community in Prisons

The cycle of drug use and crime has resulted in a worldwide trend of overpopulation in prisons. The overrepresentation of substance abusers among prisoners and parolees prompted the California legislature to appropriate $94 million since 1995 for the expansion of TC prison-based substance abuse programs. Of the total inmates in California's 33 prisons, 28% were incarcerated for drug-related offenses and another 21% were incarcerated for property offenses, which are generally related to drug use. The rest of the major U.S. state prisons follow a similar trend in their prisoner profiles.

In England and Wales, there has been a significant rise in recent years in the proportion of offenders in the criminal justice system who are drug abusers, while treatment services offered to them have been inadequate. It was found that 11% of male and 23% of female prisoners were drug dependent prior to their incarceration in 1989. In a frank look into incidents of drug misuse in English prisons, the prison service, in 1995, acknowledged pronounced drug misuse in prisons and drafted the strategy document, "Drug Misuse in Prison." This document provided the framework for reducing the supply of drugs in prison and for reducing drug demand by establishing several pilot, prison-based TCs in 19 prisons in England and Wales.

It is, however, in Asian prisons that the proliferation of TC outside of the United States is happening dramatically.

Drug Abuse and the Prison Situation in Asia

In Asia, the incidence of drug-related offenses among convicted prisoners is no different and, perhaps, even worse. The Thai Department of Corrections reports that there are 137 prisons and correctional institutions across the country with an approximate capacity of 90,000 inmates. Drug offenders compose a staggering 63% of the total prison population. The overcrowding of prisons was the direct result of the imposition of severe penalties for drug offenses in response to the raging amphetamine epidemic in Thailand and the rest of Asia, as well as the increase in crimes spawned by drug abuse.

The picture of the drug and prison situation in the Philippines is similar. Overcrowding is the norm in all the national prisons and jails operated by the Bureau of Corrections (BUCOR) and the Bureau of Jail Management and Penology (BJMP). In the medium-security prison of the National Penitentiary in Manila, 38% of inmates were convicted of drug-related offenses, and 38% of 648 inmates who had undergone diagnostics and assessment were found to have a history of drug abuse. It is estimated that between 50% and 60% of all inmates in provincial, municipal, or city jails are facing drug-related charges.

In 2000, one estimate puts the number of drug addicts in Malaysia to be 300,000, which does not account for the young people who are abusing amphetamine-type substances. These figures translate into a mushrooming in the number of inmates convicted for drug-related offenses, a fact observed in the statistics of drug offenders referred to the government-operated drug rehabilitation centers or boot camps.

The use of illegal drugs and crime go hand in hand. In far too many cases in Bangladesh, drug users will literally do anything to obtain drugs. During the last few years, because of an increased incidence of drug abuse, there has been a significant rise in crime rate. In Peshawar, located in northwestern frontier of Pakistan, where drug incidence is alarming, records show that 44% of prison inmates are charged with drug-related offenses.

Against this backdrop, the prison-based TC, applying the U.S. concept-based model, offered a much-needed treatment technology to stem the rising tide of drug abuse among prison inmates in Asia. What began in the prisons of Thailand and Malaysia in 1992 is now unfolding in the Philippines and Singapore, with TCs operating to serve criminal justice clients both in prisons and in the community. The successful adaptation of the TC for criminal justice clients in the aforementioned countries has prompted prison agencies in Indonesia, Sri Lanka, Nepal, the Maldives, Bangladesh, and Pakistan to express their interest in developing their own prison-based TCs.

Implementation and Operational Issues in the Prison-Based Therapeutic Community

The implementation and development of the prison-based TC are often both exciting and frustrating to TC professionals: exciting because it presents a radical opportunity to use the TC in a different setting that is full of new challenges; frustrating because the world of "corrections" with its massive institutions and traditional doctrines clashes with the optimistic and humanistic culture of the TC. One is steeped in a largely retributive philosophy with heavy emphasis on security and total control of its inmates. The other is focused on providing treatment for its "residents" and the provision of services that allow the processes of change to take place. Two contrasting cultures require reconciliation of their differences in order to work toward a common goal, yet not willing to give up an inch of what they hold as their primary functions. These realities experienced by the pioneers of the prison-based TC initiatives in the United States are the very same hurdles and challenges encountered by the innovators of the TC within the prison systems of Asia. Adaptive changes have since been made by both the prison authorities and the treatment staff to establish viable TCs within the prison system. The constraints that the prison system and its special population of prisoners impose on the TC implementers might look daunting but should not deter anyone willing to try.

The experiences and observations of prison-based TCs, such as Project REFORM in New York, were instructive as they declared that (a) prison-based treatment efforts were most likely to be effective when carried out jointly between correctional and treatment staff (TC-trained staff), (b) the primary focus of these programs must be the reduction of criminal recidivism, (c) successful in-prison TCs must include a seamless continuum of care for graduates paroled in the community, and (d) evaluation outcomes must include objective measures such as urine monitoring, infractions, and official arrest records.

The following are common systemic and treatment issues encountered in prison-based TCs:

1. Collaboration and communication between the prison administration and prison-treatment personnel are often hampered by the contrasting ideologies of the correctional and treatment system. Whereas the treatment system views drug abuse as a chronic treatable disorder, the correctional system views drug abuse as a crime and the prescription for controlling it is through punishment and incarceration.
2. Departments of corrections, by and large, are bureaucratic organizations that require strict adherence to the policy and procedure manual as standard operating procedure for its personnel. This fact, coupled with the underlying philosophies and objectives of the correctional system, supports and reinforces a firmly established culture that puts emphasis on safety, security, and strict adherence to established policies and procedures.
3. The continued availability of sufficient resources properly directed to maintaining adequate treatment facilities and quality services is essential to ensuring treatment effectiveness. This includes the training and hiring of adequately trained drug treatment staff.
4. For prison-based TCs that use prison officers as TC personnel, assignment to the TC project could be perceived as a slower track for career advancement, especially if the project is not given due priority.
5. The TC is an intensive form of substance abuse treatment that costs money to deliver. In addition, not every substance-abusing offender needs the TC treatment modality. This requires judicious identification of substance-abusing offenders whose treatment needs match the TC admission criteria.
6. The TC requires the full immersion of the members into the community environment and its culture in a seamless 24-hour structure. However, because of conflicting programming priorities, the members may be required by prison authorities to spend several hours in profit-producing cottage industries to meet business demands.
7. There is a high rate of comorbidity among substance-abusing prisoners that requires prison-based TCs to have a well-established assessment and diagnostic procedure to assess residents' clinical needs and determine those who are appropriate for the TC.

Transfer of Therapeutic Community Technology to Other Cultures and the Role of Training

The Therapeutic Community Philosophy and Culture

TC has been defined as a treatment environment wherein members, who suffer from addiction or companion problems, consent to live together in an organized and structured setting that facilitates the process of change and the acquisition of a lifestyle free from any form of substance abuse. It is a microcosmic representation of the larger society, where everyone fulfills distinctive roles and lives by established community norms that facilitate residents' re-integration into the larger society. In short, it is helping oneself while helping others in the therapeutic process. Each resident takes responsibility for achieving personal growth, acquiring prosocial values, nurturing a meaningful and responsible life, and protecting the integrity of the community.

The TC vary in several ways as it adapts itself to different conditions. There are, nevertheless, fundamental principles or elements that must be maintained. The most important of these is the philosophy and its belief system. The TC believes in the inherent goodness of the individual, in the individual's capacity to change, in helping others to help themselves, in a power greater than oneself, and in human values. The philosophy and the beliefs pervade the community and serve as reminders for the members as to the purpose for living as a community.

Elements of the Therapeutic Community

Defining the essential elements of the TC is a crucial first step in conducting training and adapting the TC to other cultures. TC program fidelity represents an imperative in training staff and establishing the TC in a different culture. Personal backgrounds, cultural conditioning, and professional training determine how we interpret the TC treatment philosophy, assign importance to the different aspects of the TC, and select elements that we prefer to adopt. For this reason, there should be a certain consensus on the most basic elements present in a the TC, to fulfill its functions and operate as a treatment community. Different TC experts will attach varying degrees of importance to assorted aspects of the TC as constituting its essential elements. The following list of core elements of the TC is by no means exhaustive:

1. The philosophy, unwritten philosophy, and belief system of the TC.
2. A setting or environment dedicated for the purpose of the TC.
3. An effective method to shape and manage behavior.
4. A proven method to facilitate psychologic change and spiritual healing.
5. Activities that increase self-competence and self-reliance.
6. A system that provides a daily structure with clearly defined member roles within the community.
7. A system of rewards and sanctions.
8. Reliance on self-help as a mode of treatment and the use of community as a social learning environment for healing and personal growth.
9. Peers and staff as role models.
10. A set of community norms, codes of conduct, and a value system that operationalizes the TC philosophy, unwritten philosophy, and belief system.

11. Use of public sharing in interpersonal communication.
12. A treatment process organized by stages designed to prepare the members for social re-integration.
13. A treatment curriculum that teaches the members the elements, processes, and methods of the TC as well as the maintenance of sobriety, health, and a safe lifestyle.

Training Therapeutic Community Staff

How are potential TC workers trained? What skills must an individual acquire to work successfully in the TC environment? What personal attributes must an individual possess to be an effective staff member? There is no guaranteed training guide to meet all the requirements and there are no fool proof tests that predict how anyone does as a TC staff member. One thing is certain: paraprofessionals and professionals are often attracted to working in the TC, not for the financial rewards it offers, because of its "meaning" and the intangible feeling of self-fulfillment it promises, whether to fill a personal void, work on unresolved issues, or live out a meaningful career. A certain level of personal confrontation and accountability in this area is necessary if only to have some clarity on motivation and awareness of potential pitfalls as one interacts with others in the TC.

Staff should be trained to be effective facilitators of the TC, not as the primary source of healing. To fulfill this function, staff must focus on three different levels of operation: (a) the community level, (b) the individual resident's level, and (c) the internal level of emotions and feelings.

The fundamental principle in the concept-based TC is that the community itself is the most effective means of providing treatment. To carry this out, the TC has its work ethic, various group encounters, and its own structure and hierarchy. Operating on this level, it is the main function of staff to determine how the community is functioning as a healing environment. Staff members empower the residents in the hierarchy to develop the therapeutic standards of the community and are expected to use the community structure when dealing with individual residents.

Focusing on the "individual resident's level," staff members work through the senior resident hierarchy and maintain some distance from the younger members of the community. However, staff members need to be fully aware of all the members and must keep track of how they are responding to the environment and the kinds of problems that they encounter or create in the community.

Staff members must have a good grip on their own feelings and should have a healthy self-awareness of their own internal processes. They should know when to seek appropriate help from other staff to maintain their own personal boundaries. Working in the TC involves an intimate process of working with individual issues that trigger, at times, inner and external conflicts requiring the resolution of those conflicts. The emotional challenge to staff members to confront their own feelings and vulnerabilities is always present and tied to their ability to assist the residents in dealing with their own personal vulnerabilities.

Training the staff on the mechanics of the TC and attending to their own emotional issues may fall short in promoting healthy functioning among the TC staff. Formal and informal supervision by seasoned and trained supervisors must be always available and an essential part of the professional development program for all staff. The highly experiential nature of learning TC dynamics and appropriate applications of TC treatment tools require time and proper guidance for neophyte staff by highly experienced leaders. It will take approximately 2 years before a new staff member will be able to grasp the TC processes and integrate with the TC.

Daytop International Training Program

For more than two decades, Daytop has been host to hundreds of foreign visitors ranging from graduate students to all types of professionals and government officials. A particular group of visitors seeks more than just a quick study tour of the Daytop facilities but is interested in learning the TC by undergoing an intensive training on its methods. This group comprises government and private agencies whose primary purpose for coming to Daytop is to learn and to be able to adapt this treatment model to various treatment settings and clientele.

The diverse group of professionals and paraprofessionals who come for this training spend between a month to a year in a carefully designed training curriculum that involves an extended period of immersion in the TC environment. They experience a supervised residential program as TC residents among the regular clients in various Daytop facilities. They go through an accelerated process, rising through the ranks in the TC hierarchy in a highly experiential training experience.

The Daytop on-site training model, coupled with the Daytop International overseas training and consulting activities, is responsible for the successful transfer of the TC technology to different countries with diverse cultures. Even in non-English–speaking countries the TC was adapted and developed through this process. The didactic and experiential approaches of the Daytop on-site training in the United States have helped assure program fidelity in the process of adapting TC to various cultural settings.

Change Process in the Therapeutic Community and the Role of Spirituality

What makes a TC therapeutic lies in how the community is constituted. The term "community" in the TC is qualitatively different from the ordinary village, neighborhood, or housing complex. Affiliation with the TC requires a commitment to its philosophy and a willingness to live by a code of conduct that actualizes the ideals agreed upon by the members of the community. The philosophy and the ideals of the community are statements of what constitutes the "good life" or "right living" that each member aspires to achieve through mutual help and a willingness to learn from others. Implicit in TC participation is the recognition of one's limitations or personal flaws that can be overcome through genuine mutual feedback in a social learning relationship.

Driven by a collective purpose, the community develops its structure for organizing daily life and the sustenance of the system dedicated to serving the needs of the individual members and the community as a whole. Norms and rituals are evolved that embody the ideals and philosophy of the community. Community rituals to deal with transgressions of the norms and a method of redemption, by expressing remorse and offering restitution, both for sins of omission and commission, are developed. In the context of an Islamic TC, how sin, shame, and guilt are to be dealt with are central issues. By taking drugs, the individual has broken the laws of the society and religion, rejected common moral values, and betrayed family and loved ones. This leaves the individual with strong feelings of shame and guilt, constantly haunting the person and making the person vulnerable to negative influences.

The social nature of humans and their development, which is dependent on the reciprocal interactions of their personal traits, their behavior, and their social environment, makes the TC an appropriate setting for personal growth or change. A person's imitative tendency predisposes that person to learn through "role modeling," and an individual's need for social affiliation and affirmation drives the individual to conform to social norms.

Communal living requires a paradigm shift in one's personal identity and locus of identification where one's ego is subsumed to the higher power the community is dedicated to serve. This lifestyle is designed to overcome the natural selfishness of people, which also breeds division and conflict. Compassion and real love, as expressions of spirituality, will not be possible if one fails to sublimate and transcend selfishness. In this community, "responsible love" for one another is an important covenant. This is the way of the spiritual life.

To this ideal community and the healing potential it promises to the "lost" souls of troubled individuals, the TC does trace part of its beginnings. When a person suffers from social or mental maladies, that person finds healing not in isolation but in communion with another human being. This is why therapy heals. Using the contact between two people or a group of people, it brings to bear the social context to alter thinking, feeling, and behavior.

Evaluating Treatment Outcome

Evaluation research serves the important purpose of (a) determining if clients have made improvement, and (b) whether the improvement is truly the result of treatment. Of particular interest to funding agencies and treatment providers about outcome evaluations is to discover if the program is effective enough to justify putting resources there and to determine what aspects of the program work and where changes are needed for improvement.

Some studies focused on determining what variables are predictive of successful client treatment. For example, early studies of the TC found that dynamic variables (e.g., type of treatment, length of treatment, and psychologic profile) are more predictive of treatment outcome than static variables (e.g., race, gender, religion, education).

Most studies of TC treatment outcome comprise posttreatment outcome and psychologic studies of in-treatment changes. Posttreatment studies usually classify the subjects into different groups (e.g., graduates and dropouts, or convicted and nonconvicted clients, or adolescent and adult drug users), comparing them based on a set of outcome measures (e.g., relapse rate, productivity or employment, criminality, or reconviction rates). Most of these studies found that retention is the most significant predictor of positive treatment outcome. However, a study of 255 ex-residents of Odyssey House in Australia found that instead of the length of time spent in treatment as critical to outcome, the amount of progress made in that time is a better predictor. Those residents who made faster progress did better than those who stayed the same amount of time but made slower progress in treatment.

Some studies compared the clients' psychologic functioning and level of social skills at the onset and end of treatment using standard psychologic tests and clinical progress reports. A retrospective study of 2,881 residents who were treated at the Thanyarak TC in Thailand found that residents who relapsed are more likely to experience neurotic symptoms and reflect more introverted personalities, whereas those who remained abstinent have more extroverted personalities. Moreover, relapse cases are likely to exhibit labile mood strains and feel emotionally vulnerable. A retrospective study of residents in a Daytop TC for adolescent boys found that there were significant improvements in educational performance, family/social problems, mental health, and medical status within 6 months of treatment. However, prior to discharge most of the subjects exhibited a marked increase in perceived medical problems and psychologic distress, which indicates possible anticipatory anxiety prior to discharge from treatment.

Conclusion

Therapeutic communities represent an important component of the substance abuse treatment system. Although some are well established and have been in existence for decades, new TC programs open, and expansion into new countries, new settings, and continues, as does targeting new populations. The unique features of the TC provide a mechanism for intervening and changing not just the pattern of drug use by persons who engage in this treatment, but also their lives in a broad, constructive, and fundamental manner.

Suggested Readings

De Leon G. *The therapeutic community: theory, model, and method.* New York: Springer; 2000.

Kressel D, De Leon G, Palij M, et al. Measuring client clinical progress in therapeutic community treatment: client assessment inventory, client assessment summary, and staff assessment summary. *J Subst Abuse Prev.* 2000;19:267–272.

O'Brien WB, Perfas FB. The therapeutic community. In: Lowinson JH, Ruiz P, Millman RB, et al., eds. *Substance abuse: a comprehensive textbook,* 4th ed. Philadelphia: Lippincott Williams & Wilkins; 2005:609–616.

Rawlings B, Yates R, eds. *Therapeutic communities for the treatment of drug users.* London: Jessica Kingsley; 2001.

Smith LA, Gates S, Foxcroft D. Therapeutic communities for substance related disorder. *Cochrane Database Syst Rev.* 2006;(1):CD005338.

30

NETWORK THERAPY

There is a need for innovative techniques to enhance the effectiveness of psychotherapy with abusers of alcohol and other drugs in the office treatment setting in individual practice. Augmentation of treatment by group and family therapy in the multimodality clinic setting has led to considerably more success, and in the clinic these therapies may be supplemented by a variety of social rehabilitation techniques. Groups such as Alcoholics Anonymous (AA) also offer invaluable adjunctive support. Nonetheless, a model for enhancing therapeutic intervention in the context of insight-oriented individual therapy would be of considerable value, given the potential role of the individual practitioner as primary therapist for many patients with addictive problems.

A Learning Theory Approach
Classical Conditioning of Addiction Stimuli

An important explanatory model of drug dependence has been based on his clinical investigations. In an attempt to explain the spontaneous appearance of drug craving in the absence of physiologic withdrawal, certain stimuli may have been conditioned to evoke withdrawal phenomena. It was pointed out that addictive drugs produce counteradaptive responses in the central nervous system (CNS) at the same time that their direct pharmacologic effects are felt, and that these are reflected in certain physiologic events. With alcohol, for example, electroencephalograph (EEG)-evoked response changes characteristic of withdrawal may be observed in the initial phases of intoxication under certain circumstances. With opiates, administration of a narcotic antagonist to an addict who is "high" will precipitate a withdrawal reaction, which may be said to have been present in a latent form. Such responses are overridden by the direct effect of the drug and generally are observed only after the cessation of a prolonged period of administration, when they are perceived as physiologic withdrawal feelings or craving.

Hence, the drug euphoria inevitably is followed by the counteradaptive responses that occur on a physiologic level, shortly after the initial drug administration. The pairing of this administration with stimuli from the environment or with internal subjective stimuli in a consistent manner causes these stimuli to elicit the central counteradaptive response in the absence of prior drug administration. With regard to the issues presented here, however, it should be pointed out that the conditioned stimulus of the drug or the affective state may lead directly to the behavioral response before the addict consciously experiences withdrawal feelings. The addict may therefore automatically act to seek out drugs by virtue of this conditioning upon entry into the addict's old neighborhood, or upon experiencing anxiety or depression, all of which may have become conditioned stimuli. It has been demonstrated that the conditioning of addicts of opiate withdrawal responses to neutral stimuli, such as sound and odor. It was demonstrated that the direct behavioral correlates of such conditioned stimuli in relation to alcohol administration. For the alcoholic, the alcohol dose itself might serve as a conditioned stimulus for enhancing craving, as could the appropriate drinking context.

Learning Theory and the Treatment of Addiction

Systemic research on behavioral variables during intoxication by studying ethanol self-administration among alcoholics has been described. With colleagues, she investigated the effects of a number of variables, including altering the amount of effort necessary to obtain ethanol. It has been undertaken the use of within-subject experimental manipulations to study psychologic factors such as socialization versus isolation and affective state. Such studies gradually have led to a better understanding of the possibility for manipulating an alcoholic's drinking patterns. Further elaboration has been undertaken by behavioral researchers for the therapy of alcoholism.

This experimental work is cited to illustrate a perspective for defining and modifying drinking behavior. Certain conditioned drinking behaviors may be extinguished if the appropriate extinguishing stimulus is interposed in a systematic way. This may be done by using noxious stimuli or by reinforcing constructive behavior patterns.

Cognitive Labeling

A question may then be raised: what would serve as a minimally noxious aversive stimulus that would be both specific for the conditioned stimulus and unlikely to be generalized, thereby yielding a maximal positive learning experience? To answer this, we may look at Wikler's initial conception of the implications of this conditioning theory. He pointed out that the user would become entangled in an interlocking web of self-perpetuating reinforcers, which perhaps explains the persistence of drug abuse, despite disastrous consequences for the user, and the user's imperviousness to psychotherapy that does not take such conditioning factors into account because neither the user nor the therapist is aware of their existence.

Because of the unconscious nature of the conditioned response of drug seeking, the patient's attempt to alter the course of the stimulus–response sequence is generally not viable, even with the aid of a therapist. Neither party is aware that a conditioned sequence is taking place. However, sufficient exploration may reveal the relevant stimuli and their ultimate effect through conditioned sequences of drug-seeking behavior. By means of guided recall in a psychotherapeutic context, the alcoholic or addict can become aware of the sequence of action of conditioned stimuli. The user can then label those stimuli. The therapeutic maneuver consists of applying an aversive stimulus to conditioned responses that are to be extinguished.

At this point, the patient's own distress at the course of the addictive process, generated by the patient's own motivation for escaping the addictive pattern, may be mobilized. This motivational distress then serves as the aversive stimulus. The implicit assumption behind this therapeutic approach is that the patient in question wants to alter his or her pattern of drug use and that the recognition of a particular stimulus as a conditioned component of addiction will allow the patient, in effect, to initiate the extinction process. If a patient is committed to achieving abstinence from an addictive drug such as alcohol or cocaine but is in jeopardy of occasional slips, cognitive labeling can facilitate consolidation of an abstinent adaptation. Such an approach is less valuable in the context of (a) inadequate motivation for abstinence, (b) fragile social supports, or (c) compulsive substance abuse unmanageable by the patient in the patient's usual social settings. Hospitalization or replacement therapy (e.g., methadone) may be necessary here because ambulatory stabilization through psychotherapeutic support is often not feasible. Under any circumstances, cognitive labeling is an adjunct to psychotherapy and not a replacement for group supports such as AA, family counseling, or outpatient therapeutic community programs, where applicable.

Network Therapy Technique

This approach can be useful in addressing a broad range of addicted patients characterized by the following clinical hallmarks of addictive illness. When they initiate consumption of their addictive agent, be it alcohol, cocaine, opiates, or depressant drugs, they frequently cannot limit that consumption to a reasonable and predictable level; this phenomenon has been termed *loss of control* by clinicians who treat persons dependent on alcohol or drugs. Second, they have consistently demonstrated relapse to the agent of abuse; that is, they have attempted to stop using the drug for varying periods of time but have returned to it, despite a specific intent to avoid it.

This treatment approach is not necessary for those abusers who can, in fact, learn to set limits on their use of alcohol or drugs; their abuse may be treated as a behavioral symptom in a more traditional psychotherapeutic fashion. Nor is it directed at those patients for whom the addictive pattern is most unmanageable, such as addicted people with unusual destabilizing circumstances such as homelessness, severe character pathology, or psychosis. These patients may need special supportive care such as inpatient detoxification or long-term residential treatment.

Key Elements

Three key elements are introduced into the network therapy technique. The first is a cognitive–behavioral approach to relapse prevention, independently reported to be valuable in addiction treatment. Emphasis in this approach is placed on triggers to relapse and behavioral techniques for avoiding them, in preference to exploring underlying psychodynamic issues.

Second, support of the patient's natural social network is engaged in treatment. Peer support in AA has long been shown to be an effective vehicle for promoting abstinence, and the idea of the therapist's intervening with family and friends in starting treatment was employed in one of the early ambulatory techniques specific to addiction. The involvement of spouses has since been shown to be effective in enhancing the outcome of professional therapy.

Third, the orchestration of resources to provide community reinforcement suggests a more robust treatment intervention by providing a support for drug-free rehabilitation.

Initial Encounter: Starting a Social Network

The patient should be asked to bring his or her spouse or a close friend to the first session. Alcoholic patients often dislike certain things they hear when they first come for treatment and may deny or rationalize, even if they have voluntarily sought help. Because of their denial of the problem, a significant other is essential to both history taking and to implementing a viable treatment plan. A close relative or spouse can often cut through the denial in a way that an unfamiliar therapist cannot and can therefore be invaluable in setting a standard of realism in dealing with the addiction.

Some patients make clear that they wish to come to the initial session on their own. This is often associated with their desire to preserve the option of continued substance abuse and is born out of the fear that an alliance will be established independent of them to it this. Although a delay may be tolerated for a session or two, it should be stated unambiguously at the outset that effective treatment can be undertaken only on the basis of a therapeutic alliance built around the addiction issue that includes the support of significant others and that it is expected that a network of close friends and/or relatives will be brought in within a session or two at the most.

The weight of clinical experience supports the view that abstinence is the most practical goal to propose to the addicted person for his or her rehabilitation, although as it has been pointed out, patients may sometimes achieve an outcome of limited drinking. For abstinence to be expected, however, the therapist should ensure the provision of necessary social supports for the patient. Let us consider how a long-term support network is initiated for this purpose, beginning with availability of the therapist, significant others, and a self-help group.

In the first place, the therapist should be available for consultation on the phone and should indicate to the patient that the therapist wants to be called if problems arise. This makes the therapist's commitment clear and sets the tone for a "team effort." It begins to undercut one reason for relapse: the patient's sense of being on the patient's own if unable to manage the situation. The astute therapist, however, will ensure that he or she does not spend excessive time on the telephone or in emergency sessions. The patient will therefore develop a support network that can handle the majority of problems involved in day-to-day assistance. This generally will leave the therapist to respond only to occasional questions of interpreting the terms of the understanding among himself or herself, the patient, and support network members. If there is a question about the ability of the patient and network to manage the period between the initial sessions, the first few scheduled sessions may be arranged at intervals of only 1 to 3 days. In any case, frequent appointments should be scheduled at the outset if a pharmacologic detoxification with benzodiazepines is indicated, so that the patient need never manage more than a few days' medication at a time.

What is most essential, however, is that the network be forged into a working group to provide necessary support for the patient between the initial sessions. Membership ranges from one to several persons close to the patient. Contacts between network members at this stage typically include telephone calls (at the therapist's or patient's initiative), dinner arrangements, and social encounters and should be preplanned to a fair extent during the joint session. These encounters are most often undertaken at the time when alcohol or drug use is likely to occur. In planning together, however, it should be made clear to network members that relatively little unusual effort will be required for the long term, and that after the patient is stabilized, their participation will amount to little more than attendance at infrequent meetings with the patient and therapist. This is reassuring to those network members who are unable to make a major time commitment to the patient, as well as to those patients who do not want to be placed in a dependent position.

Defining the Network Membership

Once the patient has come for an appointment, establishing a network is a task undertaken with active collaboration of patient and therapist. The two, aided by those parties who join the network initially, must search for the right balance of members. The therapist must carefully promote the choice of appropriate network members, however, just as the platoon leader selects those who will go into combat. The network will be crucial in determining the balance of the therapy. This process is not without problems, and the therapist must think in a strategic fashion of the interactions that may take place among network members.

Defining the Network Task

As conceived here, the therapist's relationship to the network is like that of a task-oriented team leader, rather than that of a family therapist oriented toward insight. The network is established to implement a straightforward task, that of aiding the therapist in sustaining the patient's abstinence. It must be directed with the same clarity of purpose that a task force is directed in any effective organization. Competing and alternative goals must be suppressed, or at least prevented from interfering with the primary task.

Unlike family members involved in traditional family therapy, network members are not led to expect symptom relief for themselves or self-realization. This prevents the development of competing goals for the network meetings. It also assures the members protection from having their own motives scrutinized and thereby supports their continuing involvement without the threat of an assault on their psychologic defenses. Because network members have—kindly—volunteered to participate, their motives must not be impugned. Their constructive behavior should be commended. It is useful to acknowledge appreciation for the contribution they are making to the therapy. There is always a counterproductive tendency on their part to minimize the value of their contribution. The network must, therefore, be structured as an effective working group with high morale.

Use of Alcoholics Anonymous

Use of self-help modalities is desirable whenever possible. For the alcoholic, certainly, participation in AA is strongly encouraged. Groups such as Narcotics Anonymous, Pills Anonymous, and Cocaine Anonymous are modeled after AA and play a similarly useful role for drug abusers. One approach is to tell the patient that he or she is expected to attend at least two AA meetings a week for at least 1 month so as to become familiar with the program. If after a month the patient is quite reluctant to continue, and other aspects of the treatment are going well, the patient's nonparticipation may have to be accepted.

Some patients are more easily convinced to attend AA meetings; others may be less compliant. The therapist should mobilize the support network, as appropriate, to continue pressure for the patient's involvement with AA for a reasonable trial. It may take a considerable period of time, but ultimately a patient may experience something of a conversion, wherein the patient adopts the group ethos and expresses a deep commitment to abstinence, a measure of commitment rarely observed in patients who undergo psychotherapy alone. When this occurs, the therapist may assume a more passive role in monitoring the patient's abstinence and keep an eye on the patient's ongoing involvement in AA.

Use of Pharmacotherapy in the Network Format

For the alcoholic, disulfiram may be of marginal use in ensuring abstinence when used in a traditional counseling context but becomes much more valuable when carefully integrated into work with the patient and network, particularly when the drug is taken under observation. It is a good idea to use the initial telephone contact to engage the patient's agreement to abstain from alcohol for the day immediately prior to the first session. The therapist then has the option of prescribing or administering disulfiram at that time. For a patient who is earnest about seeking assistance for alcoholism, this is often not difficult, if some time is spent on the phone making plans to avoid a drinking context during that period. If it is not feasible to undertake this on the phone, it may be addressed in the first session. Such planning with the patient almost always involves organizing time with significant others and therefore serves as a basis for developing the patient's support network.

The administration of disulfiram under observation is a treatment option that is easily adapted to work with social networks. A patient who takes disulfiram cannot drink; a patient who agrees to be observed by a responsible party while taking disulfiram will not miss his or her dose without the observer's knowing. This may take a measure of persuasion and, above all, the therapist's commitment that such an approach can be reasonable and helpful.

Disulfiram typically is initiated with a dose of 500 mg, and then reduced to 250 mg daily. It is taken every morning, when the urge to drink is generally least. Particulars of administration in the context of treatment should be reviewed.

As noted previously, individual therapists traditionally have seen the abuser as a patient with poor prognosis. This is largely because in the context of traditional psychotherapy, there are no behavioral controls to prevent the recurrence of drug use, and resources are not available for behavioral intervention if a recurrence takes place—which it usually does. A system of impediments to the emergence of relapse, resting heavily on the actual or symbolic role of the network, must therefore be established. The therapist must have assistance in addressing any minor episode of drinking so that this ever-present problem does not lead to an unmanageable relapse or an unsuccessful termination of therapy.

Format for Medication Observation by the Network

1. Take the medication every morning in front of a network member.
2. Take the pill so that that person can observe the patient swallowing them.
3. Have the observer write down, on a list prepared by the therapist., the time of day the pills were taken.
4. The observer brings the list in to the therapist's office at each network session.

5. The observer leaves a message on the therapist's answering machine on any day that the patient has not taken the pills in a way that ingestion was clearly observed.

Meeting Arrangements

At the outset of therapy, it is important to see the patient with the group on a weekly basis for at least the first month. Unstable circumstances demand more frequent contacts with the network. Sessions can be tapered off to biweekly and then to monthly intervals after a time.

To sustain the continuing commitment of the group, particularly that between the therapist and the network members, network sessions should be held every 3 months or so for the duration of the individual therapy. Once the patient has stabilized, the meetings tend less to address day-to-day issues. They may begin with the patient's recounting of the drug situation. Reflections on the patient's progress and goals, or sometimes on relations among the network members, then may be discussed. In any case, it is essential that network members contact the therapist if they are concerned about the patient's possible use of alcohol or drugs, and that the therapist contact the network members if the therapist becomes concerned about a potential relapse.

Adapting Individual Therapy to the Network Treatment

As noted previously, network sessions are scheduled on a weekly basis at the outset of treatment. This is likely to compromise the number of individual contacts. Indeed, if sessions are held once a week, the patient may not be seen individually for a period of time. The patient may perceive this as a deprivation unless the individual therapy is presented as an opportunity for further growth predicated on achieving stable abstinence ensured through work with the network.

When the individual therapy does begin, the traditional objectives of therapy must be arranged to accommodate the goals of the substance abuse treatment. For insight-oriented therapy, clarification of unconscious motivations is a primary objective; for supportive therapy, the bolstering of established constructive defenses is primary. In the therapeutic context that is described here, however, the following objectives are given precedence.

Of first importance is the need to address exposure to substances of abuse or exposure to cues that might precipitate alcohol or drug use. Both patient and therapist should be sensitive to this matter and explore these situations as they arise. Second, a stable social context in an appropriate social environment—one conducive to abstinence with minimal disruption of life circumstances—should be supported. Considerations of minor disruptions in place of residence, friends, or job need not be a primary issue for the patient with character disorder or neurosis, but they cannot go untended here. For a considerable period of time, the substance abuser is highly vulnerable to exacerbations of the addictive illness and in some respects must be viewed with the considerable caution with which one treats the recently compensated psychotic.

Finally, after these priorities have been attended to, psychologic conflicts that the patient must resolve, relative to his or her own growth, are considered. As the therapy continues, these come to assume a more prominent role. In the earlier phases, they are likely to reflect directly issues associated with previous drug use. Later, however, as the issue of addiction becomes less compelling from day-to-day, the context of the treatment increasingly will come to resemble the traditional psychotherapeutic context. Given the optimism generated by an initial victory over the addictive process, the patient will be in an excellent position to move forward in therapy with a positive view of his or her future.

Treatment by Psychiatry Residents

A network therapy training sequence was developed and implemented at New York University psychiatric residency program and then the clinical outcome of a group of cocaine-dependent patients treated by the residents was evaluated. The psychiatric residency was chosen because of the growing importance of clinical training in the management of addiction in outpatient care in residency programs, in line with the standards set for specialty certification.

A training manual was prepared on the network technique, defining the specifics of the treatment in a manner allowing for uniformity in practice. It was developed for use as a training tool and then as a guide for the residents during the treatment phase. Network therapy tape segments drawn from a library of 130 videotaped sessions were used to illustrate typical therapy situations. A network therapy rating scale was developed to assess the technique's application, with items emphasizing key aspects of treatment. The scale was evaluated for its reliability in distinguishing between two contrasting addiction therapies, network therapy and systemic family therapy, both presented to faculty and residents on videotape. The internal consistency of responses for each of the techniques was high for both the faculty and the resident samples, and both groups consistently distinguished the two modalities. The scale was then used by clinical supervisors as a didactic aid for training and to monitor therapist adherence to the study treatment manual.

Treatment by Addiction Counselors

This study was conducted in a community-based addictions treatment clinic, and the network therapy training sequence was essentially the same as the one applied to the psychiatry residents. A cohort of 10 cocaine-dependent patients received treatment at the community program with a format that included network therapy, along with the clinic's usual package of modalities, and an additional 20 cocaine-dependent patients received treatment as usual and served as control subjects. The network therapy was found to enhance the outcome of the experimental patients. Of 107 urinalyses conducted on the network therapy patients, 88% were negative, but only 66% of the 82 urine samples from the control subjects were negative, a significantly lower proportion. The mean retention in treatment was 13.9 weeks for the network patients, reflecting a trend toward greater retention than the 10.7 weeks for the control subjects.

The results of this study supported the feasibility of transferring the network technology into community-based settings with the potential for enhancing outcomes. Addiction counselors working in a typical outpatient rehabilitation setting were able to learn and then incorporate network therapy into their largely 12-step–oriented treatment regimens without undue difficulty and with improved outcome.

Principles of Network Treatment

Start a Network as Soon as Possible

1. It is important to see the alcohol or drug abuser promptly, because the window of opportunity for openness to treatment is generally brief. Delay of a week can result in a person's reverting back to drunkenness or losing motivation.
2. If the person is married, engage the spouse early on, preferably at the time of the first phone call. Point out that addiction is a family problem. For most drugs, you can enlist the spouse in ensuring that the patient arrives at your office with a day's sobriety.
3. In the initial interview, frame the exchange so that a good case is built for the grave consequences of the patient's addiction, and do this before the patient can introduce his or her system of denial. That way you are not putting the spouse or other network members in the awkward position of having to contradict a close relation.
4. Then make clear that the patient needs to be abstinent, starting now. (A tapered detoxification may be necessary sometimes, as with depressant pills.)
5. When seeing an alcoholic patient for the first time, start the patient on disulfiram treatment as soon as possible, in the office if you can. Have the patient continue taking disulfiram under observation of a network member.
6. Start arranging for a network to be assembled at the first session, generally involving a number of the patient's family or close friends.
7. From the very first meeting you should consider how to ensure sobriety until the next meeting, and plan that with the network. Initially, their immediate company, a plan for daily AA attendance, and planned activities may all be necessary.

Manage the Network with Care

1. Include people who are close to the patient, have a long-standing relationship with the patient, and are trusted. Avoid members with substance problems, because they will let you down when you need their unbiased support. Avoid superiors and subordinates at work, because they have an overriding relationship with the patient independent of friendship.
2. Obtain a balanced group. Avoid a network composed solely of the parental generation, or of younger people, or of people of the opposite sex. Sometimes a nascent network selects itself for a consultation if the patient is reluctant to address his or her own problem. Such a group will later supportively engage the patient in the network, with your careful guidance.
3. Make sure that the mood of meetings is trusting and free of recrimination. Avoid letting the patient or the network members feel guilty or angry in meetings. Explain issues of conflict in terms of the problems presented by addiction; do not get into personality conflicts.
4. The tone should be directive. That is to say, give explicit instructions to support and ensure abstinence. A feeling of teamwork should be promoted, with no psychologizing or impugning members' motives.
5. Meet as frequently as necessary to ensure abstinence, perhaps once a week for a month, every other week for the next few months, and every month or two by the end of a year.
6. The network should have no agenda other than to support the patient's abstinence. But as abstinence is stabilized, the network can help the patient plan for a

new drug-free adaptation. It is not there to work on family relations or help other members with their problems, although it may do this indirectly.

Keep the Network's Agenda Focused

1. Maintaining abstinence. The patient and the network members should report at the outset of each session any exposure of the patient to alcohol and drugs. The patient and network members should be instructed on the nature of relapse and plan with the therapist how to sustain abstinence. Cues to conditioned drug-seeking should be examined.
2. Supporting the network's integrity. Everyone has a role in this. The patient is expected to make sure that network members keep their meeting appointments and stay involved with the treatment. The therapist sets meeting times and summons the network for any emergency, such as relapse; the therapist does whatever is necessary to secure stability of the membership if the patient is having trouble doing so. The Network members' responsibility is to attend network sessions, although they may be asked to undertake other supportive activity with the patient.
3. Securing future behavior. The therapist should combine any and all modalities necessary to ensure the patient's stability, such as a stable, drug-free residence; avoidance of substance-abusing friends; attendance at 12-step meetings; medications such as disulfiram or blocking agents; observed urinalysis; and ancillary psychiatric care. Written agreements may be handy, such as a mutually acceptable contingency contract with penalties for violation of understandings.

Make Use of Alcoholics Anonymous and Other Self-Help Groups

1. Patients should be expected to attend meetings of AA or related groups at least two to three times, with follow-up discussion in therapy.
2. If patients have reservations about these meetings, try to help them understand how to deal with those reservations. Issues such as social anxiety should be explored if they make a patient reluctant to participate. Generally, resistance to AA can be related to other areas of inhibition in a person's life, as well as to the denial of addiction.
3. As with other spiritual involvements, do not probe the patients' motivation or commitment to AA once engaged. Allow them to work out things on their own, but be prepared to listen.

Suggested Readings

Galanter M. Network therapy. In: Lowinson JH, Ruiz P, Millman RB, et al., eds. *Substance abuse: a comprehensive textbook*, 4th ed. Philadelphia: Lippincott Williams & Wilkins; 2005:733–743.

Galanter M. Network therapy for addiction: a model for office practice. *Am J Psychiatry.* 1993;150:28–36.

Galanter M, Dermatis H, Keller D, et al. Network therapy for cocaine abuse: use of family and peer supports. *Am J Addict.* 2002;11:161–166.

Keller D, Galanter M, Dermatis H. Technology transfer of network therapy to community-based addiction counselors. *J Subst Abuse Treat.* 1999;16:183–189.

31

FAITH-BASED APPROACHES

Unlike other established approaches to treating substance abuse, religiously oriented programs are not adequately covered in the professional literature. This chapter examines these approaches in relation to their significance in aiding recovery, maintaining sobriety, and encouraging social re-integration. There appears to be an underestimation of the role of religious treatment modalities on the part of some "secular" professionals and the reverse by religiously oriented practitioners. This dichotomy is further exacerbated by theologic divisions within the religious community.

Clearly, not all substance abusers can be reached, much less successfully treated by way of religiously oriented programs. Nevertheless, faith-based approaches merit serious consideration, because for some individuals with a high degree of religious motivation they have produced positive results, comparable to those of other treatment modalities. For these persons, it is often the treatment of choice.

Varieties of Religious Experience

Pentecostals are important providers of faith-based treatments. Growing out of the holiness movement of the 19th century and the emotion-laden Pentecostal revivals of the early 20th century, Pentecostals take their name from this latter ecstatic religious phenomenon. Pentecostals believe that the gifts of the Holy Spirit are available to modern-day believers. They insist that a spiritual experience of baptism, a "filling by the Holy Spirit," constitutes the mark of the truly authentic Christian. The "gifts of the Spirit" include speaking in tongues and interpretation, the ability to discern the needs and spiritual condition of the brothers and sisters, and divine healing. Holiness in one's personal life is stressed. Secular activities such as dancing, smoking, and social drinking are discouraged. Worship is characterized by singing, clapping, and the spontaneous participation of the congregation. The Church of God in Christ and the Assemblies of God are two of the more familiar Pentecostal denominations.

Although church attendance reportedly is declining in modern, industrialized societies, this is not true in the United States. Growth in this country has been especially noticeable among the Evangelical, Pentecostal, and Charismatic churches, as well as in the emergent New Religious Movements (NRMs). Although this growth is experienced across class and socioeconomic boundaries, expressions of Christianity by these three churches are especially well represented among disadvantaged and low-income people. In cities, particularly, large numbers of Hispanic and African American Christians are active members of these churches.

Mainline Religious Approaches

Most of the early church-related programs were Protestant. Although they stressed religious values and the importance of faith in a god who delivers people from their afflictions, these mainline churches tended to adopt a more secular professional approach to treatment. In essence, they became ecclesiastical social service delivery systems. Religious belief provided the basis and framework for the involvement of these churches, although this was not necessarily emphasized when treating the individual.

The current religious situation is quite a bit different. The Catholic Church, Islam, and Judaism have become increasingly involved in providing treatment and rehabilitation services to substance abusers since the late 1960s. Protestant, Catholic, and Jewish efforts, based primarily in hospitals and other community satellite centers, have been institutionalized and coordinated through organizations such as Catholic Charities, Lutheran Social Services, and Federation of Jewish Philanthropies. For the most part, the participation of local congregations is confined to providing sponsorship and meeting space for Alcoholics and Narcotics Anonymous groups. Some congregations offer a broader range of social services and referrals in conjunction with ministries to the homeless. Others have joined forces with neighboring churches and formally incorporated themselves into community not-for-profit organizations, such as Harlem Churches for Community Improvement in New York City, and Newark Fighting Back in Newark, New Jersey. Islamic groups, particularly the Nation of Islam, have reached out to addicts in the urban ghettos.

Evangelical and Pentecostal Approaches

Evangelical and Pentecostal churches travel a different road. Programs such as Teen Challenge (TC) use religious conversion as the primary step to begin to combat addiction, they believe that there is no other effective way to overcome heroin or cocaine addiction, alcoholism, and other "deviant" behaviors. It is essential, according to their beliefs, that the troubled person, having sinned, be "born again" by accepting Jesus Christ as his or her "personal savior." Ideally, the born-again person will then exhibit a life and personality change that is consistent with scriptural values and behaviors. Ultimately, the converted sinner is brought into the church as a brother or sister in a strong fellowship characterized by love and concern.

Those who come seeking "treatment" are taught to pray and to depend on God's assistance with all their personal problems, including addiction. Ideally, they are entirely freed from the mistakes of their former life, and the desire to continue the old, sinful ways will also fade with the passage of time and spiritual growth. Their interests become largely spiritual rather than "worldly." As individuals relate to a larger reality outside of themselves, their worldview and value system become much less egocentric. Clearly, for Evangelical and Pentecostal Christians, faith is both the starting and end point of recovery. It is the healing power of Jesus Christ, in the Church, and not the intervention of behavioral science, that brings about and maintains the individual's rehabilitation.

Teen Challenge

TC is one of the oldest drug-free religious residential programs for drug abusers. Describing itself as a Christ-centered organization, it is a ministry for people who have "life-controlling problems and are without the necessary resources and opportunities to live productively." TC sees its mission as "helping people become mentally sound, emotionally balanced, socially adjusted, physically well, and spiritually alive," a haven for youth trapped in a world defined by drug and alcohol dependence and immorality. Founded in 1961 by the Rev. David Wilkerson, a minister in the Assemblies of God, the original program was located in the Williamsburg section of Brooklyn, New York.

Most young people who came to the TC center were addicts seeking help. In 1964, Rev. Don Wilkerson, David's brother, assumed the directorship of the center, presiding over its transition to an induction and detoxification center. The group also established a training center on a 200-acre farm in Rehrersburg, Pennsylvania, far away from the "temptations of the city."

As described earlier, the TC grew rapidly during the intervening years. Prizing independence, the program did not accept government funding or assistance. However, residents sign over their welfare checks and food stamps to the program. TC has also expressed an interest in participating in accessing funding through President George W. Bush's faith-based initiative. TC induction centers now exist in most large cities. Referrals and financial contributions come through a vast network of individuals, churches, and other religious organizations. Today, there is a TC induction center in most large cities in the United States, Canada, Puerto Rico, Europe, and Australia. Each local program remains autonomous and is only loosely affiliated with the others.

The TC accepts anyone who has been using drugs and is willing to abide by its rules and practices. However, the program was not prepared to provide services to the "mentally ill." It serves both adolescents and adults of all races and ethnic groups. The racial and ethnic makeup of the program generally reflects its locale. Two thirds of the group come from low-income ghetto backgrounds, and the remainder are middle class. There are facilities for both males and females. The majority of the residents, however, are male.

According to the TC philosophy, individuals using drugs cannot be helped until they "hit rock bottom." They must admit to having a problem and actively seek help. The TC induction centers are crisis centers, accepting people from the streets for immediate help or counseling 24 hours a day. If the individual wishes to enter the residential program, he or she goes through an intake interview to determine whether the program is suitable.

Many of the participants select themselves into the program. Sometimes, however, candidates are referred by a judge, probation officer, minister, or counselor, whereas others find their way through street evangelization efforts or at the urging of relatives and recovering addict friends who are already in the program.

The TC has been successful in re-orienting the lives of some drug users. Future research should focus on cost effectiveness, success rates compared with those of traditional secular approaches, and an analysis of who would appear to benefit from this type of treatment.

Espiritismo

Espiritismo, often referred to as spiritism, is a belief system among Puerto Rican and other Hispanic cultures that transcends both socioeconomic status and national borders. At its core lies the assumption that spirits are able to influence and affect the lives of people existing in the material and tangible world. Spiritists believe that spirits have the ability to make people physically and mentally ill, including by using drugs and other substances of abuse, as well as have the power to cure them.

Perhaps the most significant reason many people seek out folk healing of any type is that it taps into one's reservoir of faith, and that faith, whether in a spirit, God, or oneself, can heal. It is within this latter context that Espiritismo has proved to be an effective support system in substance abuse treatment programs, as well as in other areas. This practice, of course, has been subject to abuse and must be used with caution, and in accordance with the patient's religious belief system. The clinician must be culturally competent, thoroughly conversant with Espiritista principles, as well as with the parallel, psychologic dynamics, and the culture as a whole.

Some of the possible positive clinical aspects and dynamics of faith-based substance abuse treatment can be summarized as the follows:

- Guilt is removed when the addict is "saved," because internalized guilt often causes the individual to continue to self-medicate with illicit or harmful substances.
- The fragmented, dysfunctional family background is replaced by a strongly knitted, cohesive, religious family providing spiritual and emotional support, as well as material/concrete assistance with the necessities of everyday life. The terms "brother" and "sister" illustrate the concept of this newly acquired family.
- An external organized structure is provided, which is internalized in terms of "bad" and "good," or "evil" and "God/Jesus-like" behaviors.
- Forgiveness is central to acceptance by an ideologic father figure "God/Jesus"; hence the addict is once again valued as a worthy human being who was "lost" and now is "found, or born again," thus enhancing the addict's self-concept or self-worth.
- The addict—repented, accepted, and forgiven—uses his or her past life (addiction and sin) to "teach" others, which further enhances and re-inforces the addict's self-concept, ego, and superego by becoming a role model.
- Contrary to the traditional and still-existing therapeutic community approach of a devaluation of the self through harsh confrontation, the addict experiences validation of his or her life as worthy of God/Christ. However, in highly legalistic and abusive religious groups, the individual may also feel and be devalued.
- The support of the religious family continues after the addict finishes treatment and life is centered around the church and his "brothers" and "sisters."

Nonetheless, precautions must be taken when funding faith-based programs. Patients or clients entering such programs may be subjected primarily to its ideologic teachings of the faith-based program, both politically and theologically, and may not receive services or medications that have demonstrated their efficacy. Governmental agencies that fund faith-based programs must not only be evenhanded in their approach, but must also evaluate the teachings of such programs, their past histories, and mission to preclude the funding of fraudulent programs that have the potential to harm participants through brainwashing techniques and by not providing effective treatment. Also, because many faith-based programs will be entering drug treatment initiatives for the first time in their histories, outcome evaluation research must be undertaken to determine their strengths, weaknesses, cost-effectiveness, and appropriateness for treating substance abusers.

New Religious Movements

Since their inception about three decades ago, there has existed controversy about the relationship between NRMs and drugs. Initially, it seemed to many that drugs and new religions were inextricably intertwined and that those involved in new religions were also often involved in drug use. We now know that such a view is overly simplistic, but the apparent co-occurrence of religious experimentation and drug use made such assumptions about the relationship easy to make.

We also now know that both drug use and religious experimentation are anathema to some persons, which contributes to a misunderstanding about the relationship of drug use and religious experimentation among America's youth. Some commentators fail to differentiate fully between these two types of countercultural behavior patterns and, instead, may lump them together. Although religious interventions may be beneficial to some, others have been harmed and require assistance.

Considerable research regarding the relationship between participation in new religions and drug use has now become available. Much of it is based on personality assessment and the effects of participation on psychologic well-being, as well as discussion of specific therapeutic effects of participation in NRMs.

Prevalence of Heavy Prior Drug Use

NRMs are classified into one of three categories—"countercultural," "personal growth," and "neo-Christian"—and compares the values of those individuals from the sample who are attracted to each of the group types on a number of issues, including a few measures of drug-related values and experiences. Those attracted to countercultural groups (such as Transcendental Meditation, Yoga, Zen, Hare Krishna, and Satanism) do have a higher propensity toward having the experience of being "high" on drugs and favoring the legalization of marijuana than those attracted to either personal-growth groups (est, Scientology, Synanon) or neo-Christian groups (Christian World Liberation Front, Children of God, Jews for Jesus, and Campus Crusade for Christ). Personal-growth group participants also usually ranked higher than neo-Christian group participants on these two measures. There was a fairly consistent pattern on the drug-related questions among this sample, suggesting that at least some of the more radical religious groups might be more attractive to those who had been most actively involved with drugs.

New Religious Movements as Halfway Houses: An Alternative Perspective

New religions, including some of the most controversial, have been reported to relieve psychiatric symptoms, psychologic distress, and drug dependence. On the other hand, there exist numerous reports of damage caused by participation in NRMs, suggesting that they "brainwash" people into joining, "destroy families," and create severe psychologic and psychiatric problems. One counterargument that has been made, for example, is that NRMs perform, for some persons, a "halfway house" function. Some NRMs have assisted in the re-integration of a number of young persons into "mainstream" society. They maintain that NRMs re-integrate participants into a more normal existence, while at the same time teaching necessary skills for survival in ordinary society.

Another perspective on the re-integration hypothesis is a social-psychologic model of healing based on similarities between communal practices and the new religions and therapy situations. It was assumed that many participants chose to participate in either modality, seeking to be healed of drug addiction or other problems. Numerous religious groups, as well as many therapies involve common roles of healer (doctor) and healee (patient), and an underlying "deep structure" focused on healing.

It appears that some NRMs may serve a halfway house function for certain participants. This role is needed by those young people who are so disconnected from society that they are unable to access the usual modes of social support. It is also believed that NRM participants are simply exchanging one form of dependency (drugs) for another (religion) when they decide to embrace an NRM. Although there is some truth to this assertion, society in general would tend to agree that "nonpathologic" religious affiliation is usually more acceptable than drug addiction, provided that the religious affiliation does not harm its members.

New Religious Movements as a Support Community

Many who join NRMs do so because their usual social supports are unavailable, either because they have left them voluntarily or because some external agent has alienated those relationships. Individuals may be seeking a surrogate family or simply need food and shelter. Thus, we saw in the 1960s and 1970s a move toward "communalization of religious experience" for many youth as they explored alternatives to a normal lifestyle, for short periods of time.

Religious communal organizations assisted numbers of young people who were at least temporarily dislocated from their usual social moorings. This communal experience would appear to be most useful for those participants who desire to change their lifestyles. These groups typically share a belief system and an ethic built on its religious ideology, and their members support each other in the acting out of these newly acquired beliefs and values. Behavior deemed deviant and negatively sanctioned in previous reference groups may be accepted and encouraged in the new environment of a religious group. The relief effect comes from participation in a human group that is accepting and personal. Participants are often helped with their problems, including drug dependence.

One major reason for contributing to positive response and outcome is self-selection. There is no denying that considerable self-selection occurs by those who enter a program, either because they are under social pressure or because they genuinely want to change their lives. Many participants in NRMs and other faith-based programs act in a manner designed to change themselves. The key to the success at drug rehabilitation of NRMs and other modalities is the volition being exercised by those desiring to use the groups as vehicles of change.

NRM groups, as well as other religiously oriented programs, are not for everyone. This is evidenced by their extremely high attrition rates and small size. Many people who experiment with these groups as possible personal vehicles for change reject them for a variety of reasons. For some, the often quite rigorous and lengthy resocialization methods are simply too difficult to accept. Others find the belief system too strange to accept as a center for their life. Still others may be repulsed by the actions, teachings, or practices of some groups, their leaders, or members, which they regard as abusive, unethical, hypocritical, or illegal.

Some who leave NRMs or other modalities voluntarily after a relatively short period of time have used the experience to become "straightened out" and reoriented. They "move back" to more normal types of existence, establishing families, obtaining and holding jobs, and/or returning to school. For some individuals, the NRM or TC has provided a valuable halfway house function. In assisting participants to avoid the abuse of drugs or other problematic behaviors, participants have been afforded an opportunity to recoup and regroup. The community at large benefits from the capacity of these groups to act as a vehicle for re-integration, by re-inserting individuals into society after having assisted them. Nevertheless, as previously noted, other participants fall victim to abuse in some of these religions or groups.

Final Thoughts Regarding New Religious Movement Approaches

This analysis of participation in NRMs requires some qualification and explication. Much negative attention has been focused on some NRMs, often referred to as "cults" in the media, as well as by many in positions of authority. The issues involved are complex. However, there exists a body of research, published in books and academic journals by psychologists, psychiatrists, and sociologists, that includes data supporting the view that some NRMs and religious approaches serve a valuable role for stopping substance abuse of various kinds. It is important to identify and better understand the essential characteristics of those groups that are critical to producing positive outcomes in this area, but without harming their participants.

Obviously, participation in NRMs is not for everyone as evidenced by the high attrition rates from those organizations. Many people who try out NRMs as vehicles of personal growth do not find them acceptable and simply leave. Some NRMs may not foster personal growth and do not seek to be vehicles of personal change for their participants. Tragedies like those involving the People's Temple, the Branch Davidians, Heaven's Gate, and Aum Shirikyo do occur. Participation in traditional NRMs has not been a positive experience for all involved. Clearly, one size does not fit all, and careful scrutiny must take place to establish that participants are helped and not harmed.

Recent Developments

On January 29, 2001, President George W. Bush established the White House Office of Faith-Based and Community Initiatives by executive order. The purpose of this office was to provide federal support for religiously based social services including substance abuse treatment and prevention. In the area of substance abuse, President Bush asked Congress to allocate $200 million to provide vouchers for persons seeking faith-based treatment. Similar initiatives have been proposed or are being funded in various states.

For example, the University of Nebraska received a $3 million federal grant to develop faith-based behavioral health interventions for that state. In 2003, Governor Jeb Bush of Florida announced the opening of a faith-based prison. He noted that participation would be voluntary, as is said to be the case in relation to all federally funded faith-based substance abuse treatment. In 2003, Americans United for Separation of Church and State expressed concern that there are coercive elements to these proposals because acceptance of religion is socially approved and rejection of this modality including prisons could be viewed negatively and result in possible reprisals. Although secular options, such as Save Our Selves (SOS), SMART Recovery, Women for Sobriety, and Life Ring Secular Recovery, must be made available, this may not always be feasible because of waiting lists or a paucity of such programs in certain geographic areas. This is in addition to the possible reluctance of government to fund or assist such programs under the faith-based initiatives.

A related concern is that the government may fund only those religiously based programs that are in sympathy with its philosophy, political and theologic, as well as its goals and objectives. A concrete example, in terms of the current administration, is preferential funding and support for fundamentalist Pentecostal-type programs, to the exclusion of others. Another area that is a cause for concern relates to qualifications of personnel working in such programs, as opposed to secular programs, regarding employment of professional staff. The White House Office of Faith-Based and Community Initiatives noted that funding of programs sponsored by groups such as WICCA, a neopagan earth-centered religion, would not be acceptable. On the other hand, programs that engage in punitive practices such as "brainwashing" or corporal punishment and that are spiritually abusive might be funded if clear guidelines are not developed. In terms of personnel, staff members of some faith-based programs are expected to be of the same religious faith or, at a minimum, subscribe to the principles of the faith. An example of such could be programs like Roloff Homes or Straight Incorporated, which have been sued for deaths and brutality allegedly occurring there. Religiously based programs are governmentally protected when engaging in these practices. New York State, in response to a decision of the U.S. Court of Appeals for the Second Circuit, is now requiring that all treatment programs receiving funding or accreditation must not coerce individuals into attending Alcoholics Anonymous, a spiritually based program. Opportunities have to be provided for those persons to attend alternative secular treatment, even though it may not be readily available. Nonetheless, this policy of the New York State Office of Alcoholism and Substance Abuse Services (OASAS) is an equitable response to the court's decision. Another concern is that funding may be diverted from existing, well-functioning, accredited secular programs to untried faith-based alternatives, whose staff or facilities may not be required to meet accreditation standards.

This issue is a complex one that is colored by the ideology of whoever is dispensing governmental funds.

Conclusion

Clinicians providing services within ethnic communities need to be culturally attuned to their clients; particularly to the significance of faith and religious expression among Hispanic, African American, and other cultures. Neglect or derision of traditions that do not derive from Western ideology frequently result in individuals being lost to treatment.

From the discussion presented in this chapter, one may conclude that religious commitment and religiously oriented treatment programs can be significant factors that merit consideration and inclusion when planning a mix of appropriate treatment alternatives. There remains a great need for additional rigorous research examining the significance of religious commitment and affiliation, experienced within mainline, fundamentalist, ethnic, and NRM communities, in treatment readiness and outcomes. Researchers also need to reduce emphasis on seeking predictive indicators of delinquency and deviance, steering the analysis toward issues of social re-integration, potentiating recovery, and maintaining sobriety. Finally, religious practitioners and researchers can and should begin to work collaboratively with their secular professional counterparts. At the very least, serious and open communication needs to be attempted. On the other hand, taxpayer funding of sectarian programs raises serious questions regarding the separation of church and state, as well as serious concern that such funding may interfere with the autonomy of religiously based institutions and generally discriminate against the funding of effective programs that may not be politically acceptable at a given time.

Suggested Readings

Arnold RM, Avants SK, Margolin A, et al. Patient attitudes concerning the inclusion of spirituality into addiction treatment. *J Subst Abuse Treat.* 2002;23:319–326.

Hicks DW, Lu FG. Religious and spiritual considerations. In: Fernandez F, Ruiz P, eds. *Psychiatric aspects of HIV/AIDS*. Philadelphia: Lippincott Williams & Wilkins; 2006:347–354.

Langrod JG, Muffler J, Abel J, et al. Faith-based approaches. In: Lowinson JH, Ruiz P, Millman RB, et al., eds. *Substance abuse: a comprehensive textbook*, 4th ed. Philadelphia: Lippincott Williams & Wilkins; 2005:763–772.

Ruiz P, Langrod JG: Hispanic Americans. In: Lowinson JH, Ruiz P, Millman RB, et al., eds. *Substance abuse: a comprehensive textbook*, 4th ed. Philadelphia: Lippincott Williams & Wilkins; 2005:1103–1112.

Ruiz P, Lile B, Matorin AA. Treatment of a dually diagnosed gay male patient: a psychotherapy perspective. *Am J Psychiatry.* 2002;159:209–215.

32

RELAPSE PREVENTION

For many clients, substance use disorders (SUDs) are chronic conditions that must be managed over the course of time. Similar to other chronic or recurrent medical or psychiatric disorders, relapse is a common problem among clients with an SUD. Although many clients evidence significant benefits from treatment, lapses and relapses often occur at some point in time, thus the clinician who is treating clients with SUDs must understand relapse and integrate strategies to prevent or reduce relapse risk.

By reducing the frequency or severity of relapses, the clinician helps clients improve their quality of life, benefiting the family and society at the same time.

Overview of Recovery and Relapse

Recovery

Recovery from an SUD is the process of initiating abstinence from alcohol or other drug use, as well as making intra personal and interpersonal changes to maintain this change over time. Specific changes vary among people with SUDs and occur in any of the following areas of functioning: physical, psychologic, behavioral, interpersonal, family, social, spiritual, and financial. It is generally accepted that recovery tasks are contingent on the stage or phase of recovery the individual is experiencing. Recovery is mediated by the severity and degree of damage caused by the SUD, the presence of a comorbid psychiatric or medical illness, and the individual's perception, motivation, gender, ethnic background, and support system. Although some individuals may achieve full recovery, others achieve a partial recovery, and may experience multiple relapses.

Recovering from an SUD involves gaining information, increasing self-awareness, developing skills for sober living, and following a program of change. This program may involve professional treatment, participation in self-help programs—Alcoholics Anonymous (AA), Narcotics Anonymous (NA), Cocaine Anonymous (CA), Rational or SMART Recovery, Secular Organization for Sobriety, Men or Women for Sobriety, or Dual Recovery Anonymous. In the earlier phases of recovery, individuals typically rely more on external support and professionals, sponsors, or other members of support groups. As recovery progresses, more reliance is placed on themselves to handle problems and challenges of a sober lifestyle. Information and skills learned as part of relapse prevention offer an excellent mechanism to prepare for the maintenance phase of recovery.

Lapse and Relapse

The term *lapse* refers to the initial episode of alcohol or other drug use following a period of abstinence, whereas *relapse* refers to failure to maintain behavior change over time. Relapse can be viewed not only as the event of resumption of substance abuse or dependency, but also as a process in which indicators or warning signs appear prior to the individual's actual substance use.

A lapse may end quickly or lead to a relapse of varying proportions. The effects of the initial lapse are mediated by the person's affective and cognitive reactions. A full-blown relapse is more likely with the individual who has a strong perception of violating the abstinence rule. Although some individuals experience a full-blown relapse and return to pretreatment levels of substance abuse, many use alcohol and drugs problematically, but not at previous levels, thus suffering less-harmful effects. Relapsers vary in the quantity and frequency of substance use, as well as the accompanying medical and psychosocial sequelae.

Treatment Outcome Studies

Numerous reviews of the treatment outcome literature, as well as studies of specific treatment populations, document variable rates of relapse among alcoholics, smokers, and drug abusers. Despite the high relapse rates reported in some studies, treatment has a positive effect on multiple domains of functioning. Outcome can best be viewed in terms of the following: substance use, social, family, and psychologic functioning. SUDs are not unlike other chronic or recurrent medical or psychiatric conditions in that recovery is not a linear process and relapses do occur, yet significant improvements are often made.

Numerous federally sponsored treatment studies found positive outcomes in the following areas: cessation or reduction of substance use; decreases in posttreatment medical care and related costs; decreases in work problems, including absenteeism and working under the influence; decreases in traffic violations and other arrests; and improvement in psychologic, social, and family functioning.

Individuals who relapse do not always return to pretreatment levels of substance use. The actual quantity and frequency of use may vary dramatically. A cocaine or heroin addict who injected large quantities of drugs on a daily basis for years may return to substance use after treatment, but not to daily use. The quantity of drugs used may be significantly less than previously. Because drug and alcohol use is only one outcome measure, an individual may show improvement in other areas of life functioning despite an actual lapse or relapse to substance use.

Relapse Precipitants

Intrapersonal determinants contributing to relapse include negative emotional states, negative physical states, positive emotional states, testing of personal control, and urges and temptations. The category that most frequently contributed to relapse was negative emotional states. In all, 38% of alcoholics, 37% of smokers, and 19% of heroin addicts relapsed in response to a negative affective state that they were unable to manage effectively.

Interpersonal precipitants include relationship conflict, social pressure to use, and positive emotional states associated with some type of interaction with others. Social pressure to use drugs was identified as a contributor by 36% of heroin addicts, 32% of smokers, and 18% of alcoholics.

For opiate addicts, the variables most strongly associated with relapse were degree of impairment caused by drug use, psychiatric impairment, length and modality of treatment, involvement in crime, lack of family and peer support, negative emotional states, and skill deficits. For alcoholics, they were lack of family or peer support, negative emotional states, skill deficits, and negative life events. For smokers, they were negative emotional states and problems in family or peer relationships. Relapse can be understood as resulting from an interaction of factors related to client, family, social, and treatment, including the following variables (e.g., negative or positive mood states): behavioral (e.g., coping skills or social skill deficits, impulsivity), cognitive (e.g., attitudes toward recovery, self-perception of ability to cope with high-risk situations, and level of cognitive functioning), environmental–interpersonal (e.g., lack of social or family stability, social pressures to use substances, lack of productive work or school roles, and lack of involvement in leisure or recreational interests), physiologic (e.g., cravings, protracted withdrawal symptoms, chronic illness or physical pain, or response to medications used for medical or psychiatric disorders), psychiatric (e.g., presence of a comorbid psychiatric illness, sexual trauma, a higher global rating of psychiatric severity), spiritual (e.g., excessive guilt and shame, feelings of emptiness, a sense that life lacks meaning), and treatment-related (e.g., negative attitudes of caregivers, inadequate aftercare services following rehabilitation programs, lack of integrated services for dual-diagnosis clients).

Overview of Relapse Prevention

Relapse prevention emerged as a way of helping the individual with an SUD maintain change over time. Factors associated with achieving initial change (i.e., abstinence) differ from those associated with the maintenance of change over time. Relapse prevention generally refers to two types of treatment strategies. First, relapse prevention may be incorporated in any treatment aimed at helping the substance abuser maintain abstinence once substances are stopped. In a general sense, psychosocial treatments such as individual drug counseling, group drug counseling, 12-step facilitation therapy, cognitive–behavioral therapy, contingency management, and the MATRIX model, as well as pharmacologic treatments such as methadone and naltrexone (Trexan) for opiate addicts, naltrexone (ReVia), or disulfiram (Antabuse) for alcoholics, all aim to help the client remain substance free and prevent relapse or reduce relapse risk. Second, specific coping skills-oriented treatments incorporating the major tenets and interventions discussed below may comprise a specific program referred to as relapse prevention. Although relapse prevention may be offered as a stand-alone program, it often is incorporated as part of a rehabilitation program. The focus of relapse prevention is to reduce the relapse risk by addressing potential precipitants of relapse and high-risk factors associated with SUD.

Some programs offer specific "relapse tracks" that are geared to clients who have relapsed following a period of sustained recovery. The focus of these programs is primarily on problems and issues associated with relapse. Despite their differences, these approaches have much in common. They focus on the need for individuals with an SUD to develop new coping skills for handling high-risk situations and relapse warning signs; to make lifestyle changes to decrease the need for substances; to increase healthy activities; to prepare for interrupting lapses so that they do not end in a full-blown relapse; and to prepare for managing relapses so that adverse consequences may be minimized. All relapse prevention approaches emphasize the need to have a broad repertoire of behavioral, cognitive, and interpersonal coping strategies to help prevent a relapse. Most are time-limited or brief, making them more feasible in the current climate of managed care.

Cognitive and Behavioral Interventions

The literature emphasizes individualizing relapse prevention strategies, taking into account the client's level of motivation, severity of substance use, gender, ego functioning, and sociocultural environment.

The use of experiential learning (e.g., role playing, fantasy, behavioral rehearsal, monodramas, psychodrama, bibliotherapy, use of workbooks, interactive videos, and homework assignments) is recommended to make learning an active experience. Such techniques enhance self-awareness, decrease defensiveness, and encourage behavioral change. In treatment groups, action techniques provide numerous opportunities for the clinician to elicit feedback and support for individual clients, identify common themes and issues related to relapse prevention, and practice specific interpersonal skills.

The use of a daily inventory is also recommended in order to get clients to monitor their lives continuously to identify relapse risk factors, relapse warning signs, or significant contributing life problems that could contribute to a relapse.

Interventions to Reduce Relapse Risk

Help Clients Identify Their High-Risk Relapse Factors and Develop Strategies to Deal with Them

The need to recognize the risk of relapse and high-risk factors is an essential component of relapse prevention. High-risk factors, or critical incidents, typically are those situations in which clients used alcohol or other drugs prior to treatment. They usually involve intrapersonal and interpersonal situations. Because the availability of coping skills is a protective factor the clinician should assess them and help the client develop new ones as needed.

Numerous clinical aids have been developed to help clients identify and prioritize their individual high-risk situations and develop coping strategies. These include Annis's *Inventory of Drinking Situations* and *Inventory of Drug-Taking Situations*; Daley's *Identifying High Risk Situations* inventory; and Washton's *Staying Off Cocaine* workbook.

For some clients, identifying high-risk factors and developing new coping strategies for each are inadequate, because they may identify too many risk factors. Such clients need help in taking a more global approach to facilitate the learning of problem-solving skills. These can consist of behavioral rehearsal, covert modeling, assertiveness training, cognitive reframing including coping imagery, reframing reactions to lapse or relapse, and lifestyle interventions such as meditation, exercise, and relaxation. Numerous behavioral, skill training, and stress management approaches increase the effectiveness of treatment.

Help Clients Understand Relapse as a Process and as an Event

Clients need to be cognizant that relapse occurs within a context and that clues or warning signs typically precede an actual lapse or relapse to substance use. Although a relapse may be the result of an impulsive act on the part of the recovering individual, often attitudinal, emotional, cognitive, and/or behavioral changes manifest themselves prior to the actual ingestion of substances. An individual's clues or warning signs can be conceptualized as links in a relapse chain. Warning signs have appeared days, weeks, or even longer before they used substances.

New clients can benefit from reviewing common relapse warning signs identified by others in recovery. It is helpful to have relapsers review their experiences in great detail so that they can learn the connections among thoughts, feelings, events or situations, and relapse. It was found that "Understanding the Relapse Process" was the topic rated as most useful topic in this endeavor.

Help Clients Understand and Deal with Alcohol or Drug Cues as Well as Cravings

Research suggests that alcoholics', drug addicts', and smokers' desire or craving can be triggered by exposure to environmental cues associated with prior use. These consist of the sight or smell of the substance and may trigger cravings manifested by increased thoughts of using and physiologic (e.g., anxiety) changes.

The advice given in 12-step and other groups to "avoid people, places, and things" associated with their substance abuse was developed to minimize exposure to cues that can be so overwhelming that they contribute to a relapse. Clients should be encouraged to remove drug paraphernalia (pipes, mirrors, needles, etc.) from their homes. This may be more difficult for tobacco smokers, however, because most relapse crises occur in association with food or alcohol consumption.

Cue exposure treatment can help reduce the intensity of the client's reactions to cues. This involved exposing clients to specific cues associated with substance use. Cue exposure also involves teaching or enhancing coping skills such as systematic relaxation, behavioral alternatives, visual imagery, and cognitive interventions to improve confidence in the ability to resist the desire to use.

Because it is impossible for clients to avoid all cues associated with substance use, a variety of practical techniques to manage cravings can be taught. Monitoring and recording cravings, associated thoughts, and outcomes can help clients become more vigilant and prepared to cope with them. Helpful cognitive interventions for managing cravings include changing thoughts about craving or desire to use, challenging euphoric recall, talking oneself through the craving, thinking beyond the high by identifying negative consequences (immediate and delayed) and positive benefits of not using, as well as delaying the decision to use. Behavioral interventions include avoiding, leaving, or changing situations that trigger or worsen a craving, redirecting and getting involved in pleasant activities, getting help or support from others by admitting and talking about cravings and hearing how others have survived them, attending self-help support group meetings, or taking medications such as disulfiram or naltrexone (for alcoholics) or methadone/buprenorphine for opiate addicts.

Help Clients Understand and Deal with Social Pressures to Use Substances

Direct and indirect social pressures often lead to drinking or substance abuse. This involves anxiety regarding one's ability to refuse offers of alcohol or other drugs. The first step is to identify high-risk relationships (e.g., living with or dating an active drug abuser or alcoholic) and situations or events in which the client may be exposed to or offered substances (e.g., places where people smoke cigarettes, drink alcohol, buy or use drugs). The next step is to assess the effects of these social pressures on the client's thoughts, feelings, and behaviors. Planning, practicing, and implementing coping strategies is the next step. These include avoidance and the use of verbal, cognitive, or behavioral skills. Using role playing to rehearse ways to refuse offers of drug or alcohol is a very practical and easy-to-use intervention. The final step of this process involves teaching the client to evaluate the results of a given coping strategy and to modify it as needed.

Pressures to use alcohol or other drugs may result from relationships with active drug users or alcoholics. The client needs to assess his or her social network and learn ways to limit or end relationships that represent a high risk for relapse.

Help Clients Develop and Enhance a Supportive Social Network

Involvement of immediate families or significant others in the recovery process provides them with an opportunity to deal with the impact of substance use on their lives as well as their own issues (e.g., enabling behaviors, preoccupation, feelings of anger, shame, and guilt). Families are then in a much better position to support the recovering member. Family members can sabotage the recovery of the addicted member in a multiplicity of overt and covert ways. This usually indicates that they have not had an opportunity to deal with their own issues or heal from their emotional pain.

Clients can be encouraged to become involved in community-based support groups. Sponsors, other recovery and personal friends, and employers may become part of a relapse prevention network. Attempting recovery in isolation, particularly during the early stages should be avoided.

The following are some suggested steps for helping clients develop a relapse prevention network. First, the client needs to identify whom to involve and whom to exclude from this network. Substance abusers harbor extremely strong negative feelings toward the recovering person, or generally are not supportive of recovery, and usually should be excluded.

The client should then determine how and when to ask for support or help. Behavioral rehearsal can assist in this endeavor. Rehearsal also helps increase confidence as well as clarify thoughts and feelings regarding reaching out for help. Many clients, for example, feel guilty or shameful and question whether or not they deserve support from others, yet others have such strong pride that help seeking is very difficult to accept. Rehearsal may also clarify the client's ambivalence regarding ongoing recovery, and it helps the client to better understand how the person being asked for support may respond, thus preparing the client for dealing with potential negative responses. Clients should be advised to emphasize that recovery is ultimately their own responsibility.

An action plan can then be devised, practiced, implemented, and modified as needed. Some clients find it helpful to put their action plan in writing so that all of those involved have a specific document to refer to.

Help Clients Develop Methods of Coping with Negative Emotional States

Negative affective states are associated with relapse across a range of addictions. Depression and anxiety were major factors in a substantial number of relapses. Two emotional states that constitute high-risk factors for many are anger and loneliness.

Helping clients improve their ability to identify and manage their emotions is a helpful treatment strategy. Interventions in the development of appropriate coping skills for managing negative emotional states vary, depending on their sources, manifestation, and consequences. For example, strategies for dealing with depression that accompanies the realization that addiction caused havoc in one's life may vary from those for dealing with depression that is part of a bipolar or major depressive illness that becomes manifest after the client is substance free and creates significant personal distress.

Interventions to help the client who occasionally gets angry and seeks solace in drugs, tobacco, or alcohol vary from those needed to help the client who is chronically angry at self and others. The former may need help in expressing anger appropriately rather than in suppressing it. The chronically angry individual, on the other hand, may need to learn how not to express anger because it is often expressed impulsively and inappropriately and often is not even justified. In this case, cognitive techniques that teach the individual to challenge and change angry thoughts that are not justified are helpful. The chronically angry person may also benefit from seeing his or her angry disposition as a "character defect." Psychotherapy and use of self-help modalities are appropriate interventions to help modify such an ingrained character trait.

Interventions for clients who report feelings of chronic boredom, emptiness, or joylessness similarly depend on the specific nature of the emotional state. Clients may need help in learning how to use free time or how to have fun without chemicals. Or, clients may need help in developing new values and relationships or in finding new activities that provide a sense of meaning in their life. Many clients need to alter their beliefs regarding fun, excitement, and what is important in life. Many addicts report that living drug free is boring compared with the high provided by the drug or drug-seeking behaviors. In such a case, the client needs to change not only behaviors but also beliefs and attitudes.

Assess Clients for Psychiatric Disorders and Facilitate Treatment If Needed

Relapse prevention strategies can be adapted and tailored to the specific problems and symptoms of the client's psychiatric disorder. Monitoring target moods or behaviors, participating in pleasant activities, developing routine and structure in daily life, learning to cope with persistent psychiatric symptoms associated with chronic or recurrent forms of psychiatric illness, and identifying early warning signs of psychiatric relapse and developing appropriate coping strategies are helpful interventions for dual-diagnosis clients.

Negative mood states that are part of an affective disorder may require pharmacotherapy in addition to psychotherapy and involvement in self-help programs. Clients on medications for these or other psychiatric disorders may also benefit from developing strategies for dealing with "well-meaning" members of self-help programs who encourage them to stop their medications because it is perceived as detrimental to recovery from their SUD. This particularly applies to methadone-maintained patients participating in 12-step groups.

For Clients Completing Residential or Hospital-Based Treatment, Facilitate the Transition to Follow-up Outpatient or Aftercare Treatment

Many clients make significant gains in structured, hospital-based or residential substance abuse treatment only to have these negated as a consequence of failure to adhere to ongoing outpatient or aftercare treatment. Interventions used to enhance treatment entry and adherence that lower the risk of relapse include the provision of a single session of motivational therapy prior to discharge, the use of telephone or mail reminders of initial treatment appointments, integrating motivational interventions in early recovery, and providing reinforcers for appropriate participation in treatment activities including, providing drug-free urine samples. Studies of patients with schizophrenia and an SUD or patients with mood disorders and SUDs show that providing a single motivational therapy session prior to hospital discharge leads to a nearly twofold increase in the show rate for the initial outpatient appointment. Clients who come for their initial appointment and successfully "enter" outpatient treatment have a reduced risk of dropout and psychiatric or substance use relapse.

Help Clients Learn Methods to Cope with Cognitive Distortions

Cognitive distortions or errors in thinking are associated with a wide range of mental health disorders and SUDs, and have also been implicated in relapse to substance use. The 12-step programs refer to cognitive distortions as "stinking thinking" and suggest that recovering individuals need to alter their thinking if they are to remain alcohol and drug free.

Teaching clients to identify their cognitive errors (e.g., black-and-white thinking, "awfulizing," overgeneralizing, selective abstraction, catastrophizing, or jumping to conclusions) and evaluate how these affect the relapse process is often very helpful. Clients can then be taught to use counterthoughts to challenge their faulty beliefs or specific negative thoughts. Sample worksheets can be provided to help clients learn to change and challenge relapse thoughts. This worksheet has three directives: (a) list the relapse-related thought; (b) state what's wrong with it; and (c) create new statements. A list of seven specific thoughts commonly associated with relapse is used to prompt clients in completing this therapeutic task. These examples include "Relapse can't happen to me"; "I'll never use alcohol or drugs again"; "I can control my use of alcohol or other drugs"; "A few drinks, tokes, pills, lines won't hurt"; "Recovery isn't happening fast enough"; "I need alcohol or other drugs to have fun"; and "My problem is cured." Clients seldom have difficulty coming up with additional examples of specific thoughts that can contribute to a relapse.

Some 12-step slogans such as "this, too, will pass" and "one day at a time" often help the chemically dependent individual work through thoughts of using.

Help Clients Work toward a Balanced Lifestyle

The client's lifestyle can be assessed by evaluating patterns of daily activities, sources of stress, stressful life events, daily hassles and uplifts, balance between wants (activities engaged in for pleasure or self-fulfillment) and shoulds (external demands), health and exercise and relaxation patterns, interpersonal activities, and spiritual beliefs. Helping clients develop positive habits or substitute indulgences (e.g., jogging, meditation, relaxation, exercise, hobbies, or creative tasks) for substance abuse can help to balance their lifestyle.

Consider the Use of a Pharmacologic Intervention as an Adjunct to Psychosocial Treatment

Because some clients benefit from pharmacologic interventions to attenuate or reduce cravings for alcohol or other drugs, enhance motivation to stay sober (clean), and increase confidence in their ability to resist relapse, a therapist should consider using a pharmacologic intervention as an adjunct to psychosocial treatment.

Help Clients Develop a Plan to Manage a Lapse or Relapse

The outcome literature shows that most alcoholics, smokers, and drug addicts lapse or relapse at one time or another. Therefore, it is highly recommended that clients have an emergency plan to follow if they lapse, so that a full-blown relapse can be avoided. If a full-blown relapse occurs, however, the client needs to have strategies to stop it. The specific intervention strategies should be based on the severity of the client's lapse or relapse, coping mechanisms, and prior history of relapse.

Developing a relapse contract with clients that outlines specific steps to take in the event of a future relapse has been recommended. The aim of this contract is to formalize or reinforce the client's commitment to change.

Analyzing lapses or relapses is a valuable process that can aid ongoing recovery. This helps to reframe a "failure" as a "learning" experience and can help the individual prepare for future high-risk situations.

Suggested Readings

Center for Substance Abuse Treatment (CSAT). Substance abuse treatment reduces family dysfunction, improves productivity. In: *Substance abuse in brief*. Rockville, Md: Substance Abuse and Mental Health Services Administration, 2000.

Daley D. *Relapse prevention workbook for recovering alcoholics and drug-dependent persons*, 3rd ed. Holmes Beach, Fla.: Learning Publications; 2000.

Daley DC, Marlatt GA. Relapse prevention. In: Lowinson JH, Ruiz P, Millman RB, et al., eds. *Substance abuse: a comprehensive textbook*, 4th ed. Philadelphia: Lippincott Williams & Wilkins; 2005:772–785.

Daley D, Moss HB. *Dual disorders: counseling clients with chemical dependency and mental illness*, 3rd ed. Center City, Minn: Hazelden; 2002.

Miller WR, Rollnick S. *Motivational interviewing: preparing people to change addictive behavior*, 2nd ed. New York: Guilford Press; 2002.

33

TREATMENT IN PRISONS AND JAILS

To understand the context in which correctional substance abuse treatment services are provided, it is important to highlight several key differences between jails and prisons. Prisons are distinct from jails in that they only house inmates who are sentenced for more than 1 year of incarceration, and who have generally committed serious or more frequent offenses in comparison to jail inmates. Inmates confined in jails are either sentenced for a period of less than 1 year or are unsentenced and awaiting trial or sentencing. Jails are typically operated by municipalities or counties, whereas prisons are operated by state or federal governments.

Jail and prison populations in the United States have increased dramatically during the last several decades, in large part as a result of the arrest and incarceration of drug offenders. There are currently 1.3 million adult offenders incarcerated in state and federal prisons, and 631,000 adult offenders incarcerated in jails. There are now more than 250,000 drug offenders in state prisons, up from 19,000 in 1980, and approximately 3% of all U.S. citizens are under some type of correctional supervision.

The costs associated with expanding jail and prison systems are enormous. The average cost for incarcerating a jail or prison inmate ranges from $20,000 to $23,000 per year. Approximately $40 billion was spent on U.S. prisons and jails in 2000, including $24 billion to incarcerate nonviolent offenders, many of whom are drug offenders. An estimated 77% of correctional costs are linked to substance abuse, representing approximately 10 times the amount that states spend on substance abuse treatment, prevention, and research. In response to the high cost of incarcerating drug offenders, states have begun to revise sentencing statutes to provide early release and reduced sanctions for drug offenders. Ballot initiatives passed in a number of states authorize participation in substance abuse treatment in lieu of incarceration for nonviolent drug offenders.

Treatment Needs in Jails and Prisons

With the closing of state mental hospitals, reductions in public treatment services, and the narrowing scope of private insurance coverage, jails and prisons have increasingly served as "public health outposts" and human service providers of "last resort." In recent years, an increasingly greater proportion of jail and prison inmates are homeless, mentally ill, and have substance use disorders and other chronic health problems. For example, between 6% and 12% of jail inmates have a severe mental disorder, and approximately 10% of jail and prison inmates report mental health problems or a history of residential mental health treatment. Jails and prisons have had to adapt new types of services for the growing numbers of inmates with specialized health care needs, including those with human immunodeficiency virus (HIV)/acquired immune deficiency syndrome (AIDS) and those with co-occurring mental health and substance use disorders.

Well over half of jail and prison inmates have significant substance abuse problems, and need treatment services. Within metropolitan jails, 66% of adult arrestees test positive for drugs, and 70% of inmates are either incarcerated for a drug offense or report using drugs on a regular basis.

Historical Trends in Correctional Treatment Services

Correctional substance abuse treatment services have been influenced by a cyclical pattern of political support for either punishment or rehabilitation of offenders. During the 1960s, several states enacted civil commitment statutes that required substance abuse treatment in secure settings. The Narcotic Addict Rehabilitation Act (NARA) passed by Congress in 1966 required in-prison treatment of narcotic addicts who were convicted of federal crimes. The emerging NARA-supported treatment services were essentially residential hospital programs situated in prisons.

A number of correctional therapeutic community (TC) programs were implemented in the 1970s, but it was not until a decade later that TC programs received widespread support through federal initiatives such as Project REFORM and Project RECOVERY. These initiatives led to implementation of TCs in a number of state correctional systems, and supported a variety of training and technical support services. Since this time, the Residential Substance Abuse Treatment (RSAT) formula grant program funded by the U.S. Department of Justice has supported a wide range of treatment programs in state prisons and in local correctional and detention facilities. Additional prevention and treatment services have been funded through block grants provided by the Department of Justice.

Correctional Treatment Environment

Correctional systems have as their primary focus the control and security of inmates, and have not traditionally provided significant attention to the substance abuse needs of incarcerated offenders. Conflicts often arise within jails and prisons between treatment and security staff, who may have different perspectives regarding the importance of treatment and methods for dealing with inmate infractions, "critical incidents," and contraband. Although basic correctional mental health treatment services are mandated by the courts, there are fewer requirements for substance abuse treatment services. Many correctional systems have begun to experiment with privatized, or partially privatized health care services as a way of limiting liability and containing costs. However, unless substance abuse treatment services are specifically listed as deliverables in these contracts, it is unlikely that the private provider would offer these services.

Standards for Substance Abuse Treatment in Prisons and Jails

Legal Standards

Although the courts have consistently rejected a general constitutional right to substance abuse rehabilitation or treatment in correctional facilities, case law indicates that inmates do have limited rights to substance abuse treatment in prisons and jails. If conditions in a correctional facility demonstrate "deliberate indifference" to inmates' serious medical needs (serious medical needs are defined as those diagnosed by a physician as requiring treatment or those that are so obvious that a layperson would easily recognize the necessity for medical attention, then substance abuse treatment might be court ordered to be made available as part of the remedy.

Although there is a limited legal mandate for substance abuse treatment services in jails and prisons, inmates' rights to medical treatment for withdrawal (i.e., detoxification) and other serious medical problems associated with substance abuse have consistently been upheld. Several lawsuits have also supported the need for correctional personnel in jails and prisons to be adequately trained to distinguish between intoxication from substance abuse and serious medical illnesses, which can mimic symptoms of intoxication.

Professional Standards

A number of professional standards have been developed to guide the implementation of correctional substance abuse treatment services. Standards developed by the National Commission on Correctional Health Care (NCCHC) and by the American Correctional Association (ACA). The following substance abuse services are listed as "essential" by the NCCHC for both jails and prisons:

- Management of intoxication and withdrawal, including medical supervision, use of written policies and procedures, and provisions for transferring inmates experiencing severe overdose or withdrawal to a licensed acute care facility.
- A comprehensive health assessment (including substance abuse history) conducted within 7 days after arrival in prison or within 14 days after arrival in jail.
- A mental health evaluation conducted within 14 days of arrival in jail or prison, including an evaluation of substance abuse history (these services are listed as "essential" for prisons and as "important" for jails).

The NCCHC lists the following correctional services as "important" under its "Standards for Inmates with Alcohol or Other Drug Problems" for both jails and prisons:

- Written policies and actual practice to identify, assess, and manage inmates with substance abuse problems.
- Opportunities for counseling provided to all inmates with histories of substance abuse problems.
- Accreditation of counselors who provide substance abuse treatment services.
- Use of existing community resources, including referral to specified community resources on release.

Although similar to the standards developed by the NCCHC, the ACA standards for jail and prison substance abuse treatment give more detail regarding appropriate programmatic elements. The ACA standards also call for mandatory substance abuse screening of inmates during the initial health examination, and offer the following additional recommendations regarding the use of standardized procedures for substance abuse screening and assessment:

- Inclusion of a standardized battery of instruments.
- Screening and sorting procedures, including clinical assessment and reassessment.
- Assessment and referral for substance abuse program assignment that is appropriate to the needs of individual inmates, including a standardized "needs assessment" administered to investigate the inmate's substance abuse history and identification of problem areas.
- Drug testing and monitoring.
- Routine diagnostic assessment.

ACA guidelines for substance abuse treatment in jails and prisons include the following:

- Development of individualized treatment objectives and goals by a multidisciplinary treatment team.
- Addressing counseling and drug education needs.
- Medical exams to determine health needs and/or observational requirements.
- Development of an aftercare discharge plan with the inmate's involvement.
- Use of staff who are trained in substance abuse treatment to design and supervise the program.
- Written treatment philosophy with goals and measurable objectives.
- Inclusion of recovered alcoholics/addicts as employees or volunteers, with appropriate training.
- Inclusion of self-help groups as adjuncts to treatment.
- Efforts to motivate addicts to receive treatment through incentives such as housing and clothing preferences.
- Provision of a range of treatment services.
- Culturally sensitive treatment approaches.
- Prerelease relapse prevention education including risk management.
- Prerelease and transitional services, including coordination with community programs to ensure continuity of supervision and treatment.

Practice Guidelines

In addition to legal and professional standards for substance abuse treatment in correctional settings, practice guidelines have been established by the American Psychiatric Association (APA) that provide detailed recommendations related to clinical treatment for alcohol, cocaine, and opioid use disorders. Although these do not specifically address issues unique to correctional settings, they provide more comprehensive practice guidelines than the standards outlined above by the NCCHC and the ACA. The APA guidelines give an overview of treatment principles and alternative treatments for these disorders, as well as recommendations regarding assessment, psychiatric management, pharmacology, psychosocial treatments, treatment planning and treatment settings, and legal/confidentiality issues.

A more recent set of guidelines focuses on psychiatric services in jails and prisons, and includes brief but useful sections on treatment of substance-involved offenders, including those with co-occurring mental and substance use disorders. These guidelines note that, in jails, acute conditions can be present at the time of detainment, including intoxication and/or mental disorders. These conditions, along with the stress of arrest and confinement, increase the risks of suicidal and violent behavior, underscoring the need for adequate and timely screening and assessment procedures for both mental health and substance use disorders.

APA also calls for the integration of substance abuse services with mental health services in correctional settings, and notes that co-occurring disorders are often undetected in correctional settings because of inadequate screening and assessment procedures. Nondetection of one co-occurring disorder can lead to exacerbation of symptoms in the other type of disorder and increase the risk of suicide, recurrence of psychiatric symptoms, substance use relapse, and criminal recidivism. Treatment of co-occurring disorders must be comprehensive, integrated, and individualized, with adequate follow-up in the community.

Screening and Assessment in Correctional Settings

Screening and assessment procedures are an important part of any substance abuse treatment system in jails and prisons. Accurate screening and assessment can allow offenders to be routed efficiently into an appropriate level of treatment, while screening out those who do not need such treatment. Without adequate screening and assessment, offenders are likely to be released to the community with their substance use and co-occurring disorders untreated, leading to a high likelihood of criminal recidivism and substance relapse.

Screening typically refers to use of brief measures that rapidly identify offenders with a potential need for substance abuse treatment, and thus informs determinations about eligibility for services. Screening also informs decisions regarding referral for more comprehensive assessment. Assessment typically requires more training than screening, and often includes a comprehensive battery of instruments and completion of a psychosocial interview to determine suitability for placement in available levels of treatment.

Motivation and readiness for treatment is useful to examine to match offenders to an appropriate level and intensity of treatment, and to provide specific interventions to address motivational issues. Screening instruments that can be used to identify offenders' motivation and readiness for treatment include the University of Rhode Island Change Assessment Scale, the Stages of Change Readiness and Treatment Eagerness Scale, and the Circumstances, Motivation, Readiness, and Suitability Scale.

Offenders, as well as substance abusers in general, may be more likely than other populations to attempt to conceal or distort information obtained from self-report screening and assessment measures. Malingering in prison settings has been found to range from 15% to 46%. In pretrial jail settings, malingering has been found to range from 8% to 37%. External factors contributing to offender motivation to report inaccurately include malingering substance use problems to obtain treatment for nonclinical reasons. Staff who provide screening and assessment in jails and prisons should be familiar with the potential reasons and motivations for inaccurate reporting of information.

The accuracy of self-report information can be enhanced through the use of effective screening and assessment measures. Several measures are more effective than others in classifying offenders who are suitable for treatment. These include the combined Addiction Severity Index (ASI)–Drug Use Section and the Alcohol Dependence Scale, the Simple Screening Instrument (SSI), and the Texas Christian University Drug Screen (TCUDS).

The accuracy of screening and assessment can be further improved by obtaining collateral information from friends, associates, or family members of offenders, and from review of medical and other correctional records (e.g., to assess the inmate's history of drug screens in institutional and community settings).

Substance Abuse Treatment Approaches in Corrections

Motivational Interviewing

Motivational interviewing (MI), which is also referred to as motivational enhancement therapy (MET), is a counseling approach designed to increase client motivation and readiness to change, and is based in part on the Transtheoretical Model of Stages of Change. MI is designed to help move clients from earlier stages (i.e., precontemplation and contemplation) to later stages of change (i.e., preparation and action) by increasing their motivation, commitment, and readiness for change.

Cognitive Skills Training and Criminal Thinking

Cognitive skills interventions such as rational emotive–behavioral therapy have emerged as significant treatments for a range of psychosocial disorders. These approaches recognize that behavioral problems are often rooted in distorted thought processes, such as rationalizations to engage in criminal or addictive behavior. Cognitive skills interventions provide self-monitoring skills to identify maladaptive thoughts and learn how to replace or restructure them. These interventions have been successfully adapted for use with substance-abusing offenders. Criminal thinking problems are characterized by denial, minimalization, externalization of blame, and self-centeredness—distortions that are similar to those used by substance abusers. Specific treatment strategies include self-assessment exercises, regular self-monitoring through completion of "thinking logs," and identification of different types of criminal thought patterns.

Relapse Prevention

The relapse prevention model was developed to help prevent substance abusers who have become abstinent from returning to full-blown use. Because many substance-abusing offenders have a history of multiple prior relapses and unsuccessful attempts to maintain abstinence, relapse prevention is an important component of treatment in criminal justice settings, and has been implemented effectively in such settings.

Co-occurring Mental Health and Substance Abuse Disorders

An estimated 3% to 11% of jail and prison inmates have co-occurring substance use and major mental disorders. Incarcerated offenders with co-occurring disorders have more pronounced psychosocial problems than do other offenders in areas of employment, social skills and social supports, cognitive functioning, and adjustment to incarceration. Because of the absence of community services for persons with severe and persistent mental illness, and as a result of fragmented mental health and substance abuse service systems, many offenders with co-occurring disorders repeatedly cycle through the criminal justice system.

Co-occurring disorders frequently are undetected in jails and prisons. The resulting lack of treatment for one or both disorders contributes to poor treatment outcomes, which are often misattributed to client resistance, lack of motivation, or to staff or programmatic factors.

The APA has outlined the following treatment strategies for effective treatment of co-occurring disorders in criminal justice settings:

- Treatment should be integrated and focus concurrently on both substance use and mental disorders.
- Both types of disorders must be considered "primary," and treatment activities should provide greater understanding of how the disorders interact.
- Comprehensive assessment should lead to development of an individualized treatment plan, which should include input from the inmate and family members, if available, and should address specific psychosocial problems and skill deficiencies.
- Intensity, length, and types of services should also be tailored to the specific correctional setting.
- Prescribed medications should be administered with caution, due to their potential interaction with substance use. If possible, inmates who have not previously been prescribed psychiatric medications should be provided a reasonable period of detoxification prior to beginning a trial on medication, unless psychotic or suicidal symptoms are present.
- Treatment must be extended into the community, with special attention to discharge/aftercare planning, and should include ways to address ongoing treatment needs, housing and employment needs, reconnection with the family, and development of support networks, including self-help groups.

Several programs have also been developed in recent years to divert inmates with co-occurring disorders from jail. Prebooking jail diversion programs provide coordination between law enforcement and community mental health and substance abuse treatment agencies and often include mobile crisis response teams that intervene in emergency situations when requested by law enforcement. Postbooking jail diversion programs involve arrangements among courts, defenders and prosecutors, probation agencies, and community mental health and substance abuse treatment agencies to identify and refer offenders who are eligible for community treatment as a condition of their sentence.

Therapeutic Communities

The TC approach was developed more than 30 years ago as a long-term residential treatment for individuals with chronic and severe drug problems. TC is based on development of a peer recovery community that promotes behavior change through a variety of social learning experiences.

Within TC programs, substance abuse is viewed as a disorder of the whole person, which affects all areas of functioning. TCs focus on development of basic skills (e.g., social skills) that may have never been fully learned, and recovery is seen as involving major changes in lifestyle, behavior, and identity. Although offenders usually enter TCs under coercion from the criminal justice system, these programs attempt to instill internal commitment to recovery through peer and staff feedback, and through other self-help and social learning experiences.

Correctional Substance Abuse Treatment Programs

Over the past 25 years, a wide range of substance abuse treatment programs have been developed for correctional settings. Such programs are typically more comprehensive in prisons than in jails, as prisons often have more resources, provide longer periods of confinement, and offer a broader range of institutional settings than jails. For example, the Federal Bureau of Prisons (BOP) has a long history of providing substance abuse treatment. The BOP substance abuse treatment services employ a biopsychosocial approach, which focuses on modification of values, attitudes, and cognitive patterns associated with criminal behavior and substance abuse. Substance abuse treatment is provided at different levels of intensity, followed by postrelease transitional services in the community.

The Florida Department of Corrections (FDC) has also provided prison-based substance abuse program services since the 1970s, which are located in major correctional institutions, as well as work and forestry camps, work-release centers, and road prisons.

The Oregon Department of Corrections (ODC) has also developed a linked, computerized tracking system to ensure that inmates are matched to services that meet their needs. Three TCs provide services for inmates with severe substance use disorders and extensive criminal histories.

Structural Challenges

Recruitment of professional staff with training and experience in substance abuse treatment is often difficult in correctional settings. Correctional facilities are often sited in rural, remote areas that are underserved by health care professionals, and that are far from educational institutions. Some correctional systems provide substance abuse treatment services through contract providers, who are sometimes better able to recruit staff to these remote locations. Because of their location and undesirable working conditions, staff turnover is a frequent problem in many prison systems and jails. One general disadvantage to providing treatment in correctional institutions is that inmates are not exposed to the same environment (e.g., stressors, high-risk situations) as they are when they return to the community.

Most jails and prisons were not designed architecturally to address the specific needs of substance abuse treatment services. As a result, many treatment programs must share meeting rooms with educational and other correctional services. Program space is often not "soundproof," and staff offices and meeting rooms are often located outside the main housing unit. Treatment services must fit within the regimented schedule of the institution, including daily "counts," in which all inmates are required to return to their cells.

Transition to the Community

One of the most significant obstacles to effective substance abuse treatment services in correctional settings is the absence of coordinated aftercare and transition services in the community. A national survey of jail treatment programs found that only 44% of programs offered these services on release. Similarly, few prisons provide comprehensive discharge planning and transition services. Although jails and prisons appropriately view their primary mission as ensuring inmate security within the institution, substance-involved offenders are very likely to relapse and return to the justice system if they do not receive ongoing treatment in the community. The most effective correctional treatment programs are those that combine treatment in the institution with treatment for at least 3 months following release to the community.

A related issue is that many inmates are released to the community with no further criminal justice supervision (e.g., probation or parole), and are unlikely to enter and remain in treatment under these conditions. One solution is to provide early release from correctional facilities with treatment involvement required as a condition of probation or parole supervision. Case management services can provide an important bridge to assist in successful re-integration of offenders to the community. These services are often initiated while the inmate is still in jail or prison, with community treatment staff and/or case managers visiting the institution to begin planning for involvement in ongoing treatment, peer support programs, transitional housing, vocational and educational services, and continuation of medications and other health care needs. A recent initiative funded by the U.S. Department of Justice is designed to develop re-entry partnerships to assist drug-involved offenders in the transition to the community. These partnerships will establish links among correctional institutions, courts, community treatment agencies, community supervision services, law enforcement, other faith-based and neighborhood organizations, and other ancillary services.

Maintaining Professional Boundaries

Providing substance abuse services in jails and prisons requires that treatment staff maintain the trust of both inmates and correctional staff and administrators, which can be challenging at times to achieve. Inmate participants in treatment tend to value the advice of staff who have experienced addiction and recovery, and who are willing to talk about these experiences. In contrast, correctional staff frequently express mistrust of former addicts, and are trained not to discuss their own problems, including those related to alcohol and drug abuse. This practice stems in part from the need for correctional staff members to maintain emotional distance between themselves and inmates, so as to ensure objectivity and fairness in dealing with inmates. Taken to the extreme, the need to maintain distance from inmates can lead to coldness, disrespect, and tension between staff and inmates. For treatment staff working in jails and prisons, it is important to assist correctional staff to see addicts as human beings deserving of respect and even empathy. On the other hand, inmates must never doubt that clinicians are corrections employees, and will carry out their responsibilities despite their respect for the inmates they treat.

Inmates sometimes attempt to gain the allegiance of treatment staff, or to compromise or manipulate treatment staff. When an inmate offers to trade information for an absolute promise of confidentiality, the answer should always be "no." Basic guidelines for correctional treatment staff include avoiding lying, avoiding promises that cannot be kept, and ensuring the confidentiality of selected information.

Relationships between Security and Treatment

Conflicts inevitably arise in jails and prisons between security and treatment staff, as a result of different perspectives on institutional safety, rehabilitation, sanctions, and the purpose of incarceration. It is important for staff working in jails and prisons to understand and appreciate these different professional cultures, values, and missions. Unfortunately, security has somehow become synonymous with punishment, and the misuse of this word is unfortunate. Security should mean safety for everyone who lives in, works at, or visits a jail or prison.

Experienced and competent correctional leaders know that correctional facilities are safest when the inmates are productively engaged, and therefore support treatment services. By the same token, experienced clinicians know that little learning or growth takes place unless the inmates are safe, and that institutional safety is the job of all paid staff within the correctional institution.

Conclusion

Prison and jail populations have grown tremendously over the past two decades as a result of an influx of drug-involved offenders to the criminal justice system. Well over half of jail and prison inmates have significant substance abuse problems, although most have never participated in a comprehensive treatment program. Incarceration provides a significant opportunity to initiate treatment services for those with severe alcohol and drug problems. However, the treatment capacity in jails and prisons has not kept pace with the rising number of drug-involved inmates. In fact, our nation's correctional systems are now treating only a small fraction of inmates who need these services.

Many existing correctional treatment programs are limited to self-help and peer support activities (e.g., AA and NA groups), and are inadequate to address the pronounced behavioral, emotional, and psychiatric problems that are common among this population, and often do not provide key skills (e.g., employment, problem-solving, relapse prevention, interpersonal/social) that are necessary to make lifestyle changes and to maintain sobriety in the community. Although evidence-based substance abuse treatment techniques are available for female inmates and inmates with co-occurring mental disorders, few specialized programs in jails and prisons have been developed for these populations. Moreover, few services are available in most correctional systems to assist drug-involved inmates in making the difficult transition back to the community, and to ensure that offenders are enrolled in ongoing services once they are released from custody.

Several existing program models in prisons and jails feature a comprehensive treatment approach and a continuum of services from the correctional institution to the community. Convergent research findings during the past decade indicate that jail and prison treatment of sufficient intensity and duration (e.g., TC programs) can effectively reduce criminal recidivism and substance abuse in the community. An important corollary to these findings is that involvement in community treatment following participation in jail or prison is critical in ensuring the long-term maintenance of positive outcomes related to recidivism and substance abuse. Preliminary evidence suggests that jail and prison treatment programs are cost-effective and pay significant dividends to society.

This chapter highlights the overwhelming need for substance abuse treatment services in correctional settings; the shortfall of services provided compared to need is almost impossible to exaggerate. Furthermore, although the failure to provide substance abuse treatment services may save money in the short term, in the long term it is a wasteful and ineffective public policy.

Suggested Readings

Inciardi J, Martin S, Butzin C, et al. An effective model of prison-based treatment for drug-involved offenders. *J Drug Issues.* 1997;27:261–278.

Leukefeld CG, Tims FM, Farabee D, eds. *Treatment of drug offenders: policies and issues.* New York: Springer Publishing; 2002.

Pelissier B, Wallace S, O'Neil J, et al. Federal prison residential drug treatment reduces substance use and arrests after release. *Am J Drug Alcohol Abuse.* 2001;27:315–337.

Peters RH, Greenbaum PE, Steinberg ML, et al. Effectiveness of screening instruments in detecting substance use disorders among prisoners. *J. Subst Abuse Treat.* 2000;18:349–358.

Peters RH, Matthews CO, Dvoskin JA. Treatment in prisons and jails. In: Lowinson JH, Ruiz P, Millman RB, et al., eds. *Substance abuse: a comprehensive textbook,* 4th ed. Philadelphia: Lippincott Williams & Wilkins; 2005:707–722.

Wanberg KW, Milkman HB. *Criminal conduct and substance abuse treatment.* Thousand Oaks, Calif: Sage; 1998.

Section VI

MANAGEMENT OF ASSOCIATED
MEDICAL CONDITIONS

34

MATERNAL AND NEONATAL EFFECTS OF ALCOHOL AND DRUGS

The most comprehensive study of perinatal drug epidemiology was conducted between late 1992 and mid-1993 in the United States by the National Institute on Drug Abuse. Generating a probability sample of 2,613 women, the National Pregnancy and Health Survey estimated that 5.5%, or 222,000 of the 4 million women who give birth annually, used some illicit drug during their pregnancy. Highest estimates were found for marijuana (119,000; 2.9%), followed by amphetamines, sedatives, tranquilizers, and analgesics in a nonmedical context (61,000; 1.5%), cocaine (45,000; 1.1%), and smaller numbers for methamphetamine, heroin, methadone, hallucinogens, and inhalants. Those numbers were all considerably less, however, than the numbers for alcohol use (757,000; 18.8%) and cigarette use (820,000; 20.4%) during pregnancy.

Medical and Social Aspects Influencing Pregnancy

Medical complications compromise many drug-involved pregnancies. Sexually transmitted diseases, human immunodeficiency virus (HIV), and other infectious illnesses (e.g., hepatitides) are not uncommon. Opioid-abusing women also can show frequent endocrine aberrations, including amenorrhea, anovulation, and infertility. Although women believe that amenorrhea and infertility occur when they are using substantial amounts of heroin, women maintained on methadone have regular menstruation, ovulation, and apparently normal pregnancies. When it occurs, severe dysmenorrhea is most likely caused by pelvic inflammatory disease.

In addition to these potential medical problems, the lifestyle of the pregnant addict is also detrimental to herself and to society. Because most of her day is consumed by either obtaining or using drugs, she spends most of her time unable to function in usual activities of daily living. Because she may fear calling attention to her drug habit, the pregnant addict often does not seek prenatal care, which may be sporadic and inconsistent, or even totally lacking.

Every pregnant woman should be comprehensively assessed, including a detailed health history, physical examination, and a family psychosocial, medical, and substance-using history. Initial laboratory evaluation should include drug screening and blood work. Other indicated tests include cervical cytology, cervical culture for gonorrhea, and chlamydia screen; hemoglobin electrophoresis, as indicated; tuberculin testing; and baseline sonogram. Optional studies, such as human T-lymphotropic virus (HTLV)-1 testing, diabetic screening, maternal serum alpha-fetoprotein, and toxoplasmosis, other infections, rubella, cytomegalovirus, and herpes simplex (TORCH) studies, may also be considered. HIV education and counseling are essential.

The focus of a comprehensive care program for the pregnant drug abuser should be addiction treatment in a setting in which medical and obstetric care, psychosocial counseling, and long-term planning for the mother and her newborn infant are provided. Treatment should seek to reduce illegal drug use, remove the woman from a drug-seeking environment, prevent fluctuations of drug levels throughout the day, improve maternal nutrition, increase the likelihood of prenatal care, enhance the woman's ability to prepare for her baby's birth, reduce obstetric complications, and offer the pregnant addict an opportunity to restructure her life.

Methadone Maintenance and Pregnancy

For the opioid-dependent pregnant woman, most experts advocate the use of methadone treatment. Clinicians tend to use methadone doses that are individually determined and will keep the woman and fetus subjectively comfortable and stable.

Plasma methadone levels during pregnancy show marked intrapatient and interpatient variability and usually are somewhat lower than those prior to pregnancy. This decrease can be explained by an increased fluid space, a large tissue reservoir, and altered drug metabolism by the placenta and fetus. This suggests that pregnant women may need increased methadone doses during gestation and that lowering the dosage in an attempt to minimize complications is medically inappropriate. Treatment with other drugs, such as tranquilizers, are strictly avoided unless the patient is addicted to these medications, in which case the patient should be transferred to a special detoxification ward where she can be safely weaned from such drugs.

During labor, the patient is generally managed like any other parturient. Conduction anesthesia should be started as early as possible to avoid the use of narcotic analgesics. Because administration of naloxone (Narcan) or any other narcotic antagonist to an opiate-dependent woman in labor may result in stillbirth from fetal withdrawal, as well as more severe neonatal symptomatology immediately after birth, its use is contra-indicated except as a last resort to reverse severe narcotic overdose.

Although methadone maintenance during pregnancy is clearly the treatment of choice, a small number of highly motivated women or those facing logistic or geographic barriers to methadone maintenance may be candidates for medical withdrawal during pregnancy. Undertaking a medical withdrawal regimen is most safely accomplished during the second trimester with careful monitoring of fetal welfare by perinatal experts. Opiate withdrawal is best accomplished through stabilization with methadone followed by gradual reduction of the methadone dosage by 2 to 2.5 mg every 7 to 10 days.

Impact of Maternal Narcotic Use on Fetal Welfare

Maternal narcotic withdrawal is associated with the occurrence of stillbirth. Severe maternal withdrawal is associated with increased muscular activity, metabolic rate, and oxygen consumption. At the same time, fetal activity also increases, and the increased oxygen needs of the fetus may not be met if labor contractions coincide with abstinence symptoms in the mother. As the pregnancy proceeds, the fetal metabolic rate and oxygen consumption increase; therefore, a pregnant woman undergoing severe abstinence symptoms during the latter part of pregnancy would be less likely to supply the withdrawing fetus with the oxygen it needs.

Heroin directly causes fetal growth retardation. Although earlier reports did not differentiate between premature infants and term infants who were small for gestational age, it is now evident that many of these low-birth-weight infants were, in fact, small for gestational age. Laboratory and animal studies show that narcotics may have an inhibitory effect on enzymes of oxidative metabolism and oxygen-carrying cytochromes. Narcotics also alter fetal–placental perfusion by constricting the umbilical vessels and decreasing fetal brain oxygenation. These metabolic effects may cause a decrease in oxygen availability to and utilization by the fetus, resulting in fetal hypoxia or acidosis.

Acute Morbidity and Mortality in the Infant Born to the Narcotic-Dependent Woman

Many of the medical complications seen in the neonates of heroin-dependent women are secondary to low birth weight and prematurity. Therefore, in addition to the neonatal abstinence syndrome, conditions such as asphyxia neonatorum, intracranial hemorrhage, nutritional deprivation, hypoglycemia, hypocalcemia, septicemia, and hyperbilirubinemia should be anticipated in opiate-exposed low-birth-weight babies. Because infants born to women who receive methadone maintenance are more apt to have higher birth weights and a decreased incidence of premature birth, medical complications in that group of infants generally reflect (a) the amount of prenatal care that the mother has received; (b) whether she has suffered obstetric or medical complications, such as hypertension or toxemia of pregnancy, placental accidents, or infection; and, (c) multiple-drug use that may produce an unstable intrauterine milieu complicated by withdrawal and overdose.

A study of infants born to heroin-dependent and methadone-dependent mothers (the latter stratified by women having inadequate and adequate prenatal care) revealed an overall mortality rate of 5.4% compared to 1.6% in controls. In low-birth-weight infants, mortality in the drug-dependent population reached 13.3%, compared with 10% in the controls. Within the methadone-dependent group, better outcomes were achieved with adequate prenatal care. Overall mortality in the methadone/inadequate care group was 10%, compared with 3% in the methadone/adequate prenatal care group and 4.8% in the heroin-dependent group. The same trend was found for mortality rates in the low-birth-weight infants. These data show that comprehensive care for pregnant drug-dependent women significantly reduces morbidity and mortality.

Neonatal Narcotic Abstinence Syndrome
Symptomatology

Neonatal narcotic abstinence syndrome is described as a generalized disorder characterized by signs and symptoms of central nervous system hyperirritability, gastrointestinal dysfunction, respiratory distress, and autonomic symptoms including yawning, sneezing, mottling, and fever.

Central Nervous System

Opiate-exposed infants tend initially to develop mild high-frequency, low-amplitude tremors that progress in severity if untreated. High-pitched cry, increased muscle tone, irritability, increased deep tendon reflexes, and an exaggerated Moro reflex can occur. These infants show an exaggerated rooting reflex and a voracious appetite manifested as sucking of fists or thumbs, yet when feedings are administered the infants may have extreme difficulty because of an ineffectual sucking reflex and inco-ordination of the suck–swallow mechanism. Feeding may be so impaired that formula may have to be "milked" into the infant.

Seizures may occur as the most dramatic drug-associated central nervous system abnormality. Reported incidences of seizures vary among published series. The most extensive report on abstinence-associated seizures found that, among 302 neonates passively exposed to narcotics during pregnancy, 18 (5.9%) had seizures that were attributed to withdrawal. Of these 18 infants, 10 were among the 127 infants (7.8%) exposed to methadone, 4 were among the 78 (5.1%) exposed to methadone and heroin, and 3 were among the 14 (21.4%) exposed to "other" drugs taken during pregnancy. There was no apparent relationship between maternal methadone dose (10 to 100 mg/day) and frequency or severity of seizures, and no correlations were found between seizures and birth weight, gestational age, occurrence of other withdrawal symptoms, day of onset of withdrawal symptoms, or the need for specific pharmacologic treat-ment. Seizures occurred at a mean age of 10 days. Generalized motor seizures or rhyth-mic myoclonic jerks were the principal seizure manifestations. Paregoric was more effective than diazepam in controlling both initial and subsequent seizure episodes.

Gastrointestinal

Regurgitation, projectile vomiting, and loose stools may be seen in the course of neonatal abstinence. Dehydration as a consequence of poor intake, coupled with increased losses from the gastrointestinal tract, may cause excessive weight loss, elec-trolyte imbalance, shock, coma, and death. Timely and appropriate pharmacologic control of abstinence, as well as provision of extra fluids and calories to offset both clinically apparent and insensible losses, are important.

Respiratory

The opiate abstinence syndrome may include excessive secretions, nasal stuffiness, sometimes accompanied by retractions, intermittent cyanosis, and apnea. Severe respi-ratory distress occurs most often when the infant regurgitates, aspirates, and develops aspiration pneumonia. Infants with acute heroin withdrawal show increased respira-tory rates, leading to hypocapnia and an increase in blood pH. The incidence of idio-pathic respiratory distress syndrome is decreased in heroin-exposed infants, either as a result of chronic intrauterine stress or of accelerated heroin-mediated maturation of lung function, or perhaps both.

Autonomic Nervous System

Low-birth-weight infants of heroin-addicted mothers can have higher rates of sponta-neous generalized sweating compared to healthy low-birth-weight babies. Other autonomic nervous system signs seen during abstinence include hyperpyrexia and lacrimation, both of which increase water loss.

Determinants and Patterns of Neonatal Abstinence

Not all infants born to drug-dependent mothers show withdrawal symptomatology. Because the biochemical and physiologic processes governing withdrawal are still poorly understood, and because polydrug abuse, erratic drug taking, and vague and inaccurate maternal histories complicate accurate data gathering, it is not surprising to find differing descriptions and experiences in reports from different centers.

The type and amount of drug or drugs used by the mother, the timing of her dose before delivery, and the presence or absence of intrinsic disease in the infant that may affect drug metabolism and excretion, may all play a role in determining the time of withdrawal onset. Withdrawal may be mild and transient, delayed in onset, have a stepwise increase in severity, be intermittently present, or have a biphasic course that includes acute neonatal withdrawal followed by improvement and then an exacerbation of acute withdrawal.

Immediately after birth, if the mother has continued her drug use, most passively dependent infants, whether born to heroin-addicted or methadone-dependent women, seem physically and behaviorally normal. Heroin is not stored by the fetus to any appreciable extent; if the mother has been on heroin alone, the majority (80%) of infants will develop clinical signs of withdrawal between 4 and 24 hours of age. Methadone, however, is stored by the fetus, primarily in the lungs, liver, and spleen. If the mother has been on methadone alone, the baby's symptoms usually appear within the first 24 to 72 hours but may appear somewhat later. Methadone-exposed babies can have their onset of major withdrawal after the first or second week of life.

A simple relationship between the concentration of methadone in maternal plasma and urine of pregnant women on methadone was not found to be related to levels of amniotic fluid, cord blood, fetal urine, and breast milk, or to the intensity of the neonatal withdrawal syndrome. Because of the variable severity of the withdrawal, the duration of symptoms may last anywhere from 6 days to 8 weeks. Although infants are discharged from the hospital after drug therapy is stopped, their symptoms of irritability may persist for more than 3 or 4 months.

Behavioral Studies in the Neonatal Period

In human neonates, the Brazelton Neonatal Assessment Scale assesses habituation to stimuli such as a light or bell sound, responsivity to animate and inanimate stimuli (face, voice, bell, rattle), state (sleep to alertness to crying) and the requirements of state change (such as irritability and consolability), and neurologic and motor development. Methadone-exposed babies have been shown to be restless, in a neurologically irritable condition, cry more often, and are state labile. The infants are also more tremulous and hypertonic, and manifest less motor maturity than do infants in a control group. In addition, although quite available and responsive auditorially, methadone-exposed subjects respond poorly to visual stimuli. It has been found that infants born to methadone-maintained women showed deficiencies in their attention and social responsiveness during the first few days of life; these abnormalities persisted during the infants' course of abstinence and treatment.

Drug-exposed infants show an uncoordinated and ineffectual sucking reflex as a major manifestation of abstinence. Paregoric-treated infants tend to suck more vigorously than infants treated with sedatives such as phenobarbital and are even superior to those who received no therapy at all. Diazepam-treated infants show depressed feeding behavior.

Assessment and Management of Neonatal Abstinence

Unrecognized and untreated neonatal opiate abstinence may result in death as a consequence of factors such as excess fluid losses, hyperpyrexia, seizures, respiratory instability, aspiration, and apnea. With proper management, the neonate's prognosis for recovery from the acute phase of abstinence should be excellent. Because of the nonspecific nature of signs of neonatal abstinence, other potentially serious illnesses such as bacterial sepsis, meningitis, intracranial hemorrhage, and metabolic disorders such as hypoglycemia, hyponatremia, or hypernatremia, which may mimic abstinence, should also be considered in opiate-exposed newborns.

Because not all infants born to drug-dependent women develop abstinence, prophylactic drug therapy is not recommended. The asymptomatic narcotic-exposed infant should be observed in the hospital for at least 4 days. Even if the infant is still symptom free and evaluation of the home and mothering capability has been adequate to permit discharge, observation at close intervals must be continued.

When signs of abstinence do appear, simple nonspecific measures should be instituted. An individualized treatment program using supportive techniques may ameliorate the abstinence in opiate-exposed babies. These techniques include reducing noxious environmental stimuli, positioning that encourages flexion rather than extension, and individualized handling procedures based on the infant's level of tolerance. Gentle swaddling should be used. Demand feeding, sometimes as frequently as every 2 hours, has been found to reduce irritability.

Indications for specific pharmacotherapy, dosage schedules, and duration of treatment courses have varied widely. To improve the objectivity of judging the severity of symptoms, the use of a neonatal abstinence scoring system is strongly recommended. The Finnegan 21-symptom rating scale is most widely used as a research tool and treatment guide. All infants born to drug-dependent mothers are assessed for withdrawal symptomatology by using this scale at regular intervals. Pharmacologic intervention is begun when the total abstinence score is 8 or greater for three consecutive scorings, or when the average of any three consecutive scores is 8 or greater. The total abstinence score also dictates the dosage of the pharmacotherapeutic agent.

A replacement opiate such as paregoric (camphorated tincture of opium) or a nonspecific central nervous system depressant such as phenobarbital appears to be effective in treating neonatal opiate abstinence. Doses should be regulated so that symptoms are minimized without excessive sedation. Paregoric treatment begins with an oral dosage of 0.2 mL every 3 hours. If symptoms are not controlled based on the severity scale, doses are increased by 0.05 mL to a maximum of 0.4 mL every 3 hours. The stabilizing dose is maintained for 5 days, then the dose is slowly reduced by 0.05 mL every other day, maintaining a dosing regimen of every 3 hours.

Despite its record of efficacy and safety, concerns have been raised about the safety of other ingredients found in paregoric. Paregoric contains the isoquinoline derivatives noscapine and papaverine, which are antispasmodics, and it also contains camphor, a potentially dangerous central nervous system stimulant, which is lipid soluble and requires glucuronidation for excretion. In addition, paregoric also contains alcohol, anise oil, and glycerin. Finally, paregoric contains benzoic acid, which may compete for bilirubin binding sites. Its oxidative product, benzyl alcohol, has been reported to cause a syndrome of severe acidosis, central nervous system depression, hypotension, renal failure, seizures, and death in small premature infants who receive large doses of benzyl alcohol. Because of these concerns, the Committee on Drugs of the American Academy of Pediatrics recommends tincture of opium as the treatment of choice for neonatal opioid abstinence. The committee recommends the use of a 25-fold dilution of tincture of opium, which results in an equivalent concentration of morphine as in paregoric. Dosage regimens can therefore be used in the same way as paregoric, using the above regimens. Tincture of opium dosages may be tapered in the same way as with paregoric.

Although opiate abstinence is best treated with another opiate medication, polydrug abuse in which nonopiate use is suspected or confirmed is probably better treated by taking advantage of the wider therapeutic spectrum of phenobarbital. After a loading dose of 5 mg/kg of phenobarbital intramuscularly or intravenously, a maintenance dose of between 3 and 5 mg/kg per day should be started. By using the severity scale, phenobarbital dosages can be increased by 1 mg/kg to a stabilizing dosage that generally should not exceed 10 mg/kg per day. Few controlled studies exist comparing the efficacy of these two therapies. The use of other agents such as chlorpromazine or diazepam to treat neonatal opiate abstinence should be discouraged. Methadone has been used very infrequently because its pharmacology in the human neonate has not been adequately studied.

Later Sequelae of Intrauterine Opiate Exposure—Sudden Infant Death Syndrome

Sudden infant death syndrome (SIDS) is defined as the sudden and unexpected death of an infant between 1 week and 1 year of age, whose death remains unexplained after a complete autopsy examination, full history, and death site investigation. Anecdotal and small population studies have all found increased rates of SIDS in opiate-exposed infants.

The first large population study linking SIDS to maternal drug use found an unadjusted SIDS rate of 8.87 per 1,000 live births, with the highest rate seen with maternal opiate use. The most extensive report studied SIDS rates in 1.21 million live births in New York City. The authors identified 90 SIDS deaths among 16,409 drug-exposed infants (5.48/1,000 live births), about four times the rate in the general population. Maternal opiate use increased the risk of SIDS about sixfold; after control for high-risk variables including race/ethnicity, young maternal age, parity, maternal smoking, and low birth weight, the risk of SIDS was still three times that of the general population.

Long-Term Outcome after *in Utero* Narcotic Exposure

Children born to heroin-using women or to women maintained on methadone appear to function within the normal range of mental and motor development at 5 to 6 years of age. Some data offer the tentative possibility that selected differences in behavioral, adaptive, and perceptual skills may exist between these children and those of comparable backgrounds whose mothers were not involved with drugs. The lack of both a large database and long-term follow-up well into the school years points to an obvious need for comprehensive studies assessing the development of larger populations of opiate-exposed infants. Overall, the data on the effects of prenatal opiate exposure indicate that through 2 years of age, children function well within normal limits and that between 2 and 5 years of age, they do not differ in cognitive abilities from a high-risk comparison group. Data consistently suggest that psychologic demographic factors may have as much, or more, effect on development as maternal opiate use.

Cocaine

Cocaine use in the United States, especially that of "crack," rose rapidly during the 1980s. The number of babies reportedly exposed to drugs (much of it cocaine) in New York City rose from 7.9 per 1,000 births in 1983 to 20.3 per 1,000 live births in 1987. Significant cocaine use persists. The National Pregnancy and Health Survey reported in 1994 that slightly more than 1% of the surveyed pregnancies were complicated by cocaine use.

Detection

Once absorbed, cocaine is metabolized by serum and hepatic cholinesterases to water-soluble inactive compounds, primarily benzoylecgonine, norcaine, and ecgonine methyl ester. Cocaine may be detectable in blood or urine for less than 12 hours, but its water-soluble products may be recovered from urine for up to 1 week, depending on the sensitivity of testing methodology. The use of meconium testing for cocaine metabolites enhances diagnostic accuracy regarding drug exposure over a longer gestational period. By using meconium analysis, a much higher yield of positive cocaine assays was found when compared to urine drug testing. Hair analysis for cocaine metabolites may give a better estimate of gestational exposure to cocaine. Another diagnostic possibility is amniotic fluid sample testing.

Cocaine Effects on Pregnancy and Uteroplacental Function

The low molecular weight and high solubility of cocaine in both water and lipids allow it to cross the placenta easily and enter fetal compartments. This transplacental passage is enhanced with intravenous or freebase use of cocaine. In addition, the relatively low pH of fetal blood (cocaine is a weak base) and the low fetal level of plasma esterases, which usually metabolize this drug, may lead to accumulation of cocaine in the fetus. Furthermore, the "binge" pattern associated with adult cocaine use may lead to higher levels of cocaine in the fetus. Transfer of cocaine appears to be greatest in the first and third trimesters of pregnancy. Because cocaine has potent vasoconstrictive properties, the constriction of uterine, placental, and umbilical vessels may retard the transfer of cocaine from mother to fetus. A deleterious effect of this vasoconstriction, however, is a concomitant fetal deprivation of essential gas and nutrient exchange, resulting in fetal hypoxia. In addition to an acute hypoxic insult, cocaine use of long duration may produce a chronic decrease in transplacental nutrient and oxygen flow, leading to intrauterine growth retardation. Although the relationship of cocaine use to congenital malformations is controversial, a decrease in fetal blood supply during critical periods of morphogenesis and growth may be expected to result in organ malformations.

The course of labor may also be affected by maternal cocaine use. Intravenous administration of a local anesthetic such as cocaine may cause a direct increase in uterine muscle tone. "Crack" also appears to increase uterine contractility directly and may thus precipitate the onset of premature labor. A higher rate of early pregnancy losses appears to be a major complication of maternal cocaine use. In addition, an increased frequency of abruptio placentae and placenta previa has been reported.

Maternal cocaine use leads to both shortened gestation and restriction of fetal growth. Although the mechanism for reduced fetal growth is not established, it is generally assumed to be mediated through reduced fetal nutritional support. An increase in preterm births, a decrease in mean birth weight, and an increase in low birth weight and intrauterine growth retardation has been reported when cocaine is used during the entire pregnancy. Decreases in neonatal head circumference in cocaine-exposed newborns have been noted in multiple studies, even when controlling for associated substance use (marijuana, alcohol, tobacco). These various data sets suggest that maternal cocaine use is associated with symmetric growth retardation in offspring, affecting both birth weight and head circumference.

Teratogenic Effects

Representative animal studies suggest that cocaine has major teratogenic potential. Data on the relationship of cocaine to human malformations can be characterized as inconsistent. At the present time mothers should be apprised that cocaine use *may* increase the risk of congenital malformations in their fetuses, but, confirmatory studies looking at cause and effect have yet to be done.

Neonatal Complications

Reports on neonatal complications associated with cocaine use show considerable variability. Whereas some have reported no complications, others have noted increased irritability, tremulousness, hypertonia, brisk tendon reflexes, and tremors. In addition, abnormal sleep patterns, poor feeding, vomiting, and fever have also been noted in some case series. At least one report found that during the first week of life there was a high rate of electroencephalographic (EEG) abnormalities in cocaine-exposed children, and there also have been reports of central nervous system insults such as ischemic injuries, intraventricular hemorrhages, and perinatal cerebral infarcts found in newborns who were cocaine exposed. Like much of the research in this area, these findings may be complicated by other drug use, complications of the pregnancy or delivery, and the need for carefully selected comparison groups. Still, the findings suggest that use of cocaine during pregnancy can have significant implications for the neonate.

Follow-up Studies

Sudden Infant Death Syndrome

The precise risk of SIDS in cocaine-exposed infants is not known. Discrepancies in the literature may be in part ascribed to confounding variables, such as low birth weight, racial/ethnic considerations, polysubstance use, and cigarette smoking, which are known to increase the incidence of SIDS.

Postnatal Exposure

Postnatal exposure to cocaine represents another potential source of toxicity for children. Ready passage of the drug into breast milk has been established. Case reports suggest infants can exhibit signs of acute cocaine intoxication following exposure to cocaine from mother's breast milk (included irritability, vomiting, diarrhea, increased sucking reflex, hyperactive Moro reflex, increased symmetric deep tendon reflexes, and a marked lability of mood, as well as elevations of the infant's blood pressure, heart rate, and respiratory rate).

Developmental Outcome

Based on multiple biologic and environmental risk factors, much concern has been voiced regarding the ultimate neurobehavioral prognosis of infants following intrauterine exposure to cocaine. The parents may be of poor socioeconomic status, culturally deprived, or lacking appropriate parenting models. The mother may be poorly nourished, may have medical and sexually transmitted diseases, including AIDS, and may have received little or no prenatal care. The infants frequently show suboptimal body and head growth during the intrauterine period. Uterine flow may be compromised because of cocaine-induced vasoconstriction, leading to acute or chronic fetal hypoxia. Stimulation for intellectual growth may be lacking because of prolonged hospital stays, infrequent and inappropriate parental contact, placement in a congregate care facility, or discharge to a home in which intellectual nurturing is lacking.

A systematic review critically examined outcomes in early childhood after prenatal cocaine exposure in five domains: physical growth; cognition; language skill; motor skills; and behavior, attention, and neurophysiology, and concluded that for children 6 years old and younger, there was no convincing evidence that prenatal cocaine exposure is associated with developmental toxic effects that are different in severity, scope, or kind from the sequelae of multiple other risk factors. Because of the multitude of contributory factors that exist within the lifestyle of the pregnant drug-dependent woman, the child is exposed to multifactorial issues that may have an impact on their future health and development. Many findings that were thought to be specific effects of *in utero* cocaine exposure are correlated with other factors, including prenatal exposure to tobacco, marijuana, or alcohol, and the quality of the child's environment.

Amphetamines

There is little literature describing the effects of amphetamines on the fetus, neonate, and young infant. Amphetamine effects are caused by stimulation of the release and blocking of reuptake of the neurotransmitters dopamine, norepinephrine, or serotonin. Acute neuropsychiatric effects of amphetamines include agitation, tremors, hyperreflexia, irritability, confusion, aggressiveness, and panic states, among others. Methamphetamine is structurally similar to amphetamine but has relatively greater central effects and less prominent peripheral actions.

Because cocaine and amphetamines have similar central physiologic effects, their impact on pregnancies should be similar. Both agents cause vasoconstriction and hypertension, which may result in acute or chronic fetal hypoxia. At the present time, although there is need for more data on amphetamine exposure, concern regarding developmental outcome seems appropriate.

Alcohol

Estimates of intrauterine exposure to alcohol vary. The National Pregnancy and Health Survey estimated that 757,000 infants are born annually in the United States following significant exposure to alcohol during pregnancy. The most notable postnatal adverse effect of significant alcohol exposure is the fetal alcohol syndrome (FAS). This syndrome can be identified in approximately 1 in 300 to 1 in 1,000 births; a lesser degree of damage, termed *fetal alcohol effects*, may occur in 1 in 100 live births. Although the amount of alcohol that must be consumed to cause fetal damage is not known, it is generally believed that consumption of more than 3 ounces of absolute alcohol daily, especially in conjunction with "binge drinking," poses special risk to the fetus. Because subtle effects may go unnoticed, no safe level of alcohol intake during pregnancy has been established.

Three series of findings define FAS:

1. One of the most constant features of FAS is fetal growth retardation; weight, length, and head circumference generally fall below the 10th percentile for gestational age.
2. A nearly constant feature of FAS is the characteristic facial dysmorphism of short palpebral fissures, hypoplastic maxilla, short upturned nose, hypoplastic philtrum, thinned upper vermilion border and micrognathia or retrognathia. Less-common associated features include ptosis, strabismus, epicanthal folds, microphthalmia, posteriorly rotated ears, and cleft lip or palate. Other common somatic abnormalities include structural cardiac defects, cutaneous hemangiomas, aberrant palmar creases, and pectus excavatum; less common features include hypospadias, renal abnormalities, joint malformations, and hernias of the diaphragm, umbilicus, and abdominal wall.
3. The most devastating aspect of FAS is severe alcohol-induced central nervous system dysfunction. Irritability, tremulousness, poor sucking, inconsolable crying, and hypertonia have been noted in many infants.

Follow-up examinations tend to reveal mild cerebellar deficits, hypotonicity, hyperactivity, hearing deficits, speech and language problems, sleep disturbances, and behavioral disorders. The most serious neurologic outcome attributed to alcohol exposure is mental retardation, which occurs in approximately 85% of FAS children. FAS is now believed to be the leading known cause of mental retardation in the United States. Although IQ scores vary, children with full-blown FAS rarely show normal mental ability.

Conclusion

Providing comprehensive multidisciplinary prenatal care for addicts offers an opportunity to significantly reduce morbidity and mortality in both drug-dependent mothers and their offspring. The pregnant woman who abuses drugs should be designated as high-risk and be given specialized care in a perinatal center where she can be provided with comprehensive care. Comprehensive care coupled with methadone maintenance for opioid-dependent women has been shown to reduce perinatal morbidity and mortality. Opiate-dependent women are best treated with methadone maintenance although medical withdrawal using tapering doses of methadone may be offered in selected cases. Studies in progress may show the efficacy of buprenorphine for the treatment of pregnant opiate-dependent women. The pregnant woman addicted to barbiturates or major tranquilizers along with opiates should be medically withdrawn from her drugs of dependence during her second trimester in a specialized detoxification center.

Psychosocial counseling should be provided by experienced therapists who are aware of the medical, social, and psychologic needs of substance-using women. Services should include, but not be limited to, provision of housing, nutritional advice, child care, legal services, and counseling about interpersonal relations. Special emphasis should be placed on enhancing parenting skills. Social and medical support should not end with the hospitalization. The ability of the mother to care for the infant after discharge from the hospital should be assessed by frequent observations in the home and clinic settings.

Suggested Readings

Finnegan LP, Kandall SR. Material and neonatal effects of alcohol and drugs. In: Lowinson JH, Ruiz P, Millman RB, et al., eds. *Substance abuse: a comprehensive textbook*, 4th ed. Philadelphia: Lippincott Williams & Wilkins; 2005:805–839.

Floyd RL, O'Connor MJ, Sokol RJ, et al. Recognition and prevention of fetal alcohol syndrome. *Obstet Gynecol.* 2005;106:1059–1064.

Frank D, Augustyn M, Knight WG, et al. Growth, development, and behavior in early childhood following prenatal cocaine exposure. *JAMA.* 2001;285(12):1613–1625.

Lester BM, Abhik S, LaGasse LL, et al. Prenatal cocaine exposure and 7 year outcome: IQ and special education. *Pediatr Res.* 2003;53(4):534A.

McCarthy JJ, Leamon MH, Parr MS, et al. High-dose methadone maintenance in pregnancy: maternal and neonatal outcomes. *Am J Obstet Gynecol.* 2005;193:606–610.

35

MEDICAL COMPLICATIONS OF DRUG USE

Medical illnesses are common among drug users. Most illicit drugs have direct toxicities, which are responsible for a wide variety of medical sequelae (e.g., cocaine-related cardiotoxicity). Certain behaviors associated with drug use (injection, exchanging sex for money or drugs) place drug users at elevated risk for specific conditions such as endocarditis and sexually transmitted diseases (STDs). As many drug users are socioeconomically disadvantaged, life circumstances (e.g., congregate housing) may confer increased environmental risk for infections such as tuberculosis. Finally, diminished access to and effective use of care, and disruption of daily routines by active drug use (thus impeding self-care behaviors such as medication adherence or appointment keeping), may adversely affect clinical outcomes.

General Principles

To succeed in eliciting from the patient the information needed to provide effective care, the relationship between patient and clinician must be grounded in trust. Physicians must avoid disapproving or critical remarks regarding ongoing drug use, as patients will often respond by withholding information that might provoke such reactions in the future. Caregivers who accept relapse as a common clinical presentation of drug use, and who are aware of available treatment options, are likely to remain more successfully engaged with the drug-using patient, thus enhancing the quality and continuity of care provided. The physician must be familiar with the laws governing confidentiality of patients' substance abuse behaviors and treatment. Sensitivity to this issue by the treating clinician will enhance development of trust in the clinician by the patient.

Integrating care improves health care outcomes, and should be a goal of service delivery. The more information the physician has on hand regarding the components of a patient's care, the more successful the physician will be in averting complications from medication interactions or overlapping medical and psychiatric comorbidities. When examining the drug-using patient, attention should be focused on the systems directly affected by the substances the patient is known to use, while not neglecting evidence of use of other drugs. Special attention should be paid to the presence of a variety of signs. Injection ("track") marks may be recent (appearing as fresh punctate marks, often with mild surrounding erythema) or old (linear, hyperpigmented scars representing the confluence of multiple past injection sites). The nasal septum should always be examined for erosion or infection, suggesting intranasal drug use.

Overlapping Symptoms and Syndromes

A challenge that often arises in the course of assessing and caring for the drug-using patient is differentiation of symptoms and signs related to drug use itself from those of comorbid medical and psychiatric conditions. Such overlapping presentations are most commonly seen among patients with constitutional or psychiatric symptoms.

Constitutional symptoms are frequently related to drug use and withdrawal, but may also reflect systemic illness. Weight loss is commonly seen in association with heavy cocaine use, yet must also prompt consideration of systemic infection (e.g., tuberculosis), malignancy, or HIV infection. Dyspnea in the crack smoker may be caused by chronic pulmonary dysfunction related to drug inhalation, or to asthma, or to community-acquired or HIV-related pneumonia. Seizures may occur in the context of drug withdrawal (e.g., from alcohol or benzodiazepines) or as a result of prior trauma or intercurrent infection. The same principles apply to the overlap between many psychiatric syndromes and syndromes of intoxication or withdrawal.

Prevention

Disproportionately greater emphasis is often placed on treatment than prevention. Harm reduction is one component of an approach to preventing medical conditions among drug users. The goal is to minimize adverse consequences associated with the condition—in this case, addiction to injected drugs. Access to condoms, behavioral skills-building interventions, and sterile injection equipment for persons who continue to inject despite offers of or participation in treatment, are important components of comprehensive care for drug users.

Health Care Delivery

Despite often fragmented access to care, drug users are heavy users of medical care when it is accessible. Comprehensive primary medical care must include vaccinations, screening for infectious diseases, including tuberculosis, STDs, viral hepatitis, and HIV; annual health maintenance examinations; and care of comorbid medical and psychiatric conditions.

Adherence

Active drug or alcohol use has been identified as one of the few relatively consistent predictors of poor adherence, and this is particularly true for cocaine users. However, past history of drug or alcohol abuse has not been consistently associated with poor adherence. The measurement of adherence is challenging in both clinical and research settings, and usually relies on self-report, pill counts, pharmacy records, electronic pill bottle monitors, or a combination of these methods.

Pain Management

Drug users have been found to have a high prevalence of pain, as a result of a variety of medical conditions. Medical illnesses predisposing to chronic pain among drug users include musculoskeletal pain (resulting from infections, degenerative joint disease, and trauma), soft-tissue infections, liver disease, venous insufficiency, HIV-related conditions, and peripheral neuropathies associated with alcohol use or nutritional deficiencies. In addition, opioid addicts have been observed in experimental studies to have hyperalgesia and pain intolerance, and chronic opioid therapy, as with methadone, may increase analgesic tolerance.

Despite their high prevalence of chronic pain, drug users are often undertreated for pain, even during serious medical illness. Studies show that physicians are hesitant to treat pain in hospitalized patients with substance abuse problems, fearing deception by patients seeking opioids for addiction rather than pain, and lacking the appropriate knowledge and skills to evaluate and treat pain and opioid withdrawal. In 1998, the U.S. Federation of State Medical Boards (FSMB) outlined a set of treatment guidelines constituting good medical practice when using controlled substances to treat pain.

Viral Hepatitis

Hepatitis A

The hepatitis A virus (HAV) is the leading cause of acute viral hepatitis in the United States, and results in significant morbidity and health care costs. Hepatitis A is a nonenveloped ribonucleic acid (RNA) virus that is excreted in stool and usually transmitted by fecal–oral contact, although transmission through blood is also possible. Most cases of HAV occur during communitywide outbreaks, but a high proportion of these cases occur in persons who report using drugs. Drug use is now recognized as a significant risk factor for transmission of hepatitis A, and antibodies to HAV have been identified in 43% to 66% of injection drug users.

The usual incubation period for HAV is 28 days (range: 15 to 40 days), and most adults are asymptomatic during acute infection. When symptoms occur, they typically include a mild prodromal illness of fever, headache, malaise, and nonspecific gastrointestinal symptoms, followed by dark urine, jaundice, tender hepatosplenomegaly, and postcervical lymphadenopathy. This classic presentation occurs in more than 80% of symptomatic patients and is self-limited, lasting less than 8 weeks. Most patients are treated supportively and experience complete resolution by 3 to 6 months.

The diagnosis of acute HAV is made by detecting anti-HAV antibodies in patients with symptoms consistent with hepatitis. Abnormal liver function tests are not specific for hepatitis A. Immunoglobulin M (IgM) anti-HAV antibodies can be detected 1 to 2 weeks after exposure and persist for 3 to 6 months. Immunoglobulin G (IgG) anti-HAV antibodies can be detected 5 to 6 weeks after exposure and persist for decades, conferring lifelong protection against HAV. The prevalence of anti-HAV antibodies is particularly high among drug users; in one study, the prevalence among injection drug users was twice that in the general population.

There are two currently available HAV vaccines in the United States, both of which are administered intramuscularly as two injections given 6 months apart. Because of the high prevalence of prior infection and anti-HAV antibodies among drug users, HAV serology should be checked before vaccination.

Hepatitis B

More than 300,000 people in the United States are infected with hepatitis B virus (HBV) each year, and 20% of these infections occur among drug users. Unlike hepatitis A, hepatitis B is a deoxyribonucleic acid (DNA) virus that is predominantly acquired through sexual contact (homosexual and heterosexual), but also by injection drug use and occupational exposure.

The outcome of acute HBV infection is variable. Only approximately 40% of patients develop clinical symptoms of acute hepatitis, 25% develop jaundice, and less than 5% are hospitalized. The incubation period, defined by the appearance of clinical symptoms, ranges from 1 to 6 months. Fulminant hepatic failure is a rare complication, affecting 1 in 1,000 patients. Early in infection, circulating HBV surface antigen (HBsAg) can be detected prior to the development of either clinical symptoms or elevated hepatic transaminases. This is followed by the production of hepatitis B e antigen (HBeAg), and then by elevations in transaminases. The first immune response is the production of antibodies to HBV core antigens (anti-HBc), which appear shortly after HBsAg. Anti-HBc plays no role in host defense, but is a reliable marker of HBV infection currently or within the preceding few years. The development of anti-HBe indicates diminished infectivity with a reduction in hepatic inflammation and normalization of transaminases. During clinical recovery, HBsAg disappears with gradual appearance of anti-HBs. Anti-HBs confers immunity to hepatitis B and, along with anti-HBc, persists in the serum after recovery from acute HBV.

Persistent HBeAg is associated with increased infectivity, more severe disease, and eventual cirrhosis. Current treatment options for chronic HBV, which include interferon-α and lamivudine (Epivir), convert 20% to 40% of patients from the replicative phase (HBeAg present) to the nonreplicative phase (anti-HBeAg present, HBeAg and HBV DNA absent) with consequent reduction in the risk of development of progressive liver disease. Chronic HBV is associated with cirrhosis and hepatocellular cancer, and leads to 4,000 deaths from cirrhosis and 800 deaths from hepatocellular carcinoma annually in the United States. The hepatitis B vaccine is immunogenic, effective, and safe, and has been recommended for injection drug users by the U.S. Centers for Disease Control and Prevention (CDC) since 1982.

Hepatitis C

Approximately 4 million people have evidence of exposure to hepatitis C virus (HCV) in the United States, of whom 74% have evidence of chronic infection. Following implementation of progressive enhancements in screening of the blood supply, injection drug use has become the primary route of transmission of HCV infection. Among injectors, there is considerable geographic variation in HCV seroprevalence, ranging from 66% to 93% in major US cities. Differences in seroprevalence between diverse neighborhoods within a single city likely reflect variations in transmission dynamics among distinct networks of injectors.

Sexual transmission of HCV, although much less efficient than injection-related transmission, can also be a risk for infection among drug users. Multiple sex partners and comorbid STDs increase the risk of sexual acquisition of HCV. Noninjection drug users trading sex for money or drugs may be at particularly high risk for sexual acquisition of HCV.

Serologic determination of HCV infection is generally accomplished by testing for the presence of anti-HCV antibodies. Serum levels of HCV RNA are assessed in antibody-positive persons. If absent, the patient is assumed to have cleared the infection.

HCV treatment has evolved rapidly over the past decade. Eligibility is determined primarily by considering the extent of plasma viremia, hepatic fibrosis, and inflammation. The National Institutes of Health *2002 Consensus Development Conference Statement on Management of Hepatitis C* explicitly states that persons should not be excluded from receiving HCV treatment solely on the basis of active drug or alcohol use. Nor is methadone treatment considered a contraindication to treatment.

Currently, best results are obtained with a combination of pegylated interferon, given by subcutaneous injection, and ribavirin, taken orally. Response to treatment is typically evaluated after 12 weeks: If an insufficient drop in HCV viral load is observed, treatment is discontinued.

Side effects from treatment are significant. Major complications of interferon are constitutional symptoms and psychiatric manifestations. Depression, already prevalent among HCV-infected drug users, is often precipitated or worsened by treatment of HCV with interferon. Screening for depression and other psychiatric disorders at baseline and periodically during treatment is an important component of care.

Efforts to prevent HCV transmission and acquisition, often given less attention than diagnosing and treating existing infection, are vitally important. HCV antibody testing should be widely offered to all persons with current or former drug or alcohol dependence. Persons testing negative should receive tailored counseling. If they are injecting drugs, use of sterile sources of injection equipment should be supported. Referral to syringe exchange programs or to pharmacies with permission to dispense syringes to injectors should be encouraged, and safer routes of use (e.g., intranasal) can be suggested, while simultaneously working with the patient to reduce or eliminate drug use. Bleach disinfection of used syringes may also be an effective intervention. Safer sex practices, particularly for persons with multiple partners, should be supported as well. Persons testing positive for HCV, if injecting drugs, should be counseled not to share injecting equipment.

Hepatitis D

Hepatitis D (delta) virus (HDV) is an incomplete RNA virus that requires co-infection with active HBV to become active, is transmitted in the same manner as HBV, and is prevented by HBV vaccination. It is endemic in the Mediterranean region and in parts of Asia, Africa, and South America and appears to have been spread to nonendemic areas such as the United States and Northern Europe by injection drug users. Outbreaks of severe and fulminant hepatitis, primarily as a result of co-infection with HDV and HBV, have been reported in injection drug users and their sexual contacts, and the prevalence of HDV infection in drug users with chronic HBV is 50% to 80%. In a comparison of HDV infection in drug users and nonusers, evidence of more rapid histologic deterioration of the liver was found in drug users.

Other Viral Causes of Hepatitis

Drug users are at high risk of developing infectious diseases and many infectious organisms have the potential to cause hepatic disease. These include viruses such as Epstein–Barr, herpes simplex, and cytomegalovirus, all of which may cause hepatitis-like illnesses. Most often these viruses are spread through direct contact, but they can be spread parenterally as well.

Sexually Transmitted Diseases

STDs are common among drug users, largely as a result of the exchange of sex for money or drugs, but also as a result of increased sexual risk-taking. Frequently seen STDs among drug users are syphilis, gonorrhea, chlamydia, genital herpes simplex virus, human papilloma virus, and trichomoniasis.

Syphilis

Syphilis is a readily curable, bacterial genital ulcer disease caused by *Treponema pallidum*. In 2001, the rate of syphilis increased to 2.2 cases per 100,000 population (6,103 cases). This increase was largely driven by syphilis outbreaks in certain cities among men who have sex with men. Among drug users, rates of incident syphilis are very high, ranging from 2.9 to 26.0 per 1,000 person-years, a more than 100-fold increase over the general population. Risk behaviors consistently associated with syphilis incidence among drug users include crack cocaine use, multiple sex partners, and the exchange of sex for money or drugs.

Patients who have syphilis may seek treatment for clinical signs of primary infection (usually a painless chancre), secondary infection (manifestations that include but are not limited to skin or mucocutaneous lesions), or tertiary infection (cardiac, ophthalmic, or auditory abnormalities). Latent infections, or those lacking clinical manifestations, are detected by serologic testing.

Because of their high prevalence of syphilis exposure, drug users should be screened annually with rapid plasma regain (RPR) or Venereal Disease Research Laboratory (VDRL) nontreponemal tests. Because of the high rate of false-positive nontreponemal tests, positive results should be confirmed with a treponemal antibody test.

Like all other patients, drug users with STDs should be treated with single-dose regimens, if possible. Benzathine penicillin (2.4 million units) is the preferred single-dose regimen for early syphilis (primary, secondary, or early latent), and has been used effectively for more than 50 years to achieve clinical resolution and to prevent sexual transmission and late sequelae. Treatment of late latent or tertiary syphilis, which requires a series of three weekly injections of benzathine penicillin (total of 7.2 million units), usually does not affect transmission and is intended to prevent occurrence or progression of late complications.

Gonorrhea and Chlamydia

Gonorrhea and chlamydia are the most common bacterial STDs in the United States, with an estimated 650,000 cases of gonorrhea (caused by *Neisseria gonorrhoeae*) and 3 million cases of chlamydia (caused by *Chlamydia trachomatis*) each year. In one study of young (18 to 29 years old) women living in low-income neighborhoods in California, the current prevalence of gonorrhea or chlamydia was 3.9%, compared to 0.7% for syphilis. However, as with syphilis, rates of gonorrhea and chlamydia are much higher among drug users.

These bacterial infections are a major cause of urethritis and proctitis in men, and cervicitis and pelvic inflammatory disease (PID) in women. However, because they are often asymptomatic, particularly in women, gonococcal and chlamydial infections must be detected by screening tests. Screening is essential to prevent complications, including ascending infection, infertility, ectopic pregnancy, and chronic pelvic pain. In recent years, screening of women has been facilitated by highly sensitive new tests, which do not require a pelvic exam, but instead amplify nucleic acid obtained from urine using a ligase chain reaction for *C. trachomatis* and *N. gonorrhoeae*. Regular screening for gonorrhea and chlamydia is now recommended by the U.S. Preventive Services Task Force for sexually active patients, and annual screening of all drug-using women should be performed.

Treatment of gonorrhea and chlamydia is generally offered simultaneously, because of the frequency of dual infection. Several antibiotics are effective in the single-dose treatment of gonorrhea, including cefixime (Suprax), ceftriaxone (Cefizox), ciprofloxacin (Cipro), and ofloxacin (Floxin). Efficacious regimens for the treatment of chlamydia include azithromycin (Zithromax) or doxycycline (Vibramycin), but azithromycin is preferred because it can be given in a single, directly observed dose. The prevalence of quinolone-resistant gonorrhea is increasing in the United States, and nonquinolone regimens may be preferred in the future.

Genital Herpes

Genital herpes simplex virus type 2 (HSV-2) infection is the most common infectious cause of genital ulcers in the United States, with a reported seroprevalence rate of 22% among all adults in the early 1990s. A more recent study identified HSV-2 prevalence to be as high as 35% among women in a low-income community. Although most cases of genital herpes are caused by HSV-2, genital infections with herpes simplex virus type 1 (HSV-1) are increasingly recognized. Most persons with HSV-2 are asymptomatic, but shedding occurs even in the absence of lesions, and HSV-2 transmission usually occurs during subclinical or asymptomatic shedding. Serologic evidence of past HSV-2 infection increases with age and number of sexual partners, and is more common among drug users. In recent studies, the prevalence of antibodies to HSV-2 among drug users has ranged from 44% to 58%. The highest prevalence of HSV-2 (73%) has been found among women who exchange sex for money or drugs.

Optimal management of genital herpes includes antiviral therapy with acyclovir (Zovirax), famciclovir (Famvir), or valacyclovir (Valtrex), appropriate counseling on the natural history of infection, risk for sexual and perinatal transmission, and methods to prevent further transmission.

Human Papillomavirus

Human papillomavirus (HPV) infections are the causative agents for genital wart disease and cervical carcinoma, and are transmitted primarily through sexual contact. The prevalence of HPV is as high as 50% among sexually active adolescent and young adult women, and risk factors for HPV include number of sexual partners, early age of first sexual intercourse, drinking and drug use related to sexual behavior, and partner's number of sexual partners.

The two major manifestations of genital HPV infection are external genital warts, usually caused by HPV-6 and HPV-11, and squamous intraepithelial lesions of the cervix, which are detected by cytologic screening. The major types of HPV associated with squamous intraepithelial lesions are HPV-16, -18, -31, and -45. These HPV types also cause squamous cell cancer of the vagina, vulva, anus, and penis. Subclinical genital HPV infection occurs more often than visible genital warts, and may be diagnosed by type-specific HPV tests. Testing for HPV was recently advocated as a strategy for determining which women with low-grade cervical abnormalities require additional evaluation with colposcopy. At present, no therapy has been identified that effectively eradicates persistent subclinical HPV infection.

Trichomoniasis

Trichomonas vaginalis is a protozoan that causes vaginitis in women, and is highly prevalent among drug-using women. In two recent studies of women in residential drug treatment, the prevalence of trichomonas ranged from 22% to 43%. Recent availability of self-administered vaginal swab tests has obviated the need for pelvic exams followed by wet mount microscopy or vaginal culture in screening for trichomonas, and allows for routine screening of a larger number of women. Like other STDs, trichomonal infection is associated with crack cocaine use and exchange of sex for money or drugs. Because it is frequently asymptomatic, screening for trichomoniasis should be routine among drug-using women.

Skin and Soft-Tissue Infections

Skin and soft-tissue infections are common among injection drug users. In a San Francisco–based sample, one third of active injectors examined by a physician had a concurrent abscess (65%), cellulitis (9%), or both (26%). Of injectors, 16% reported a history of abscess in the previous 6 months in a sample from Baltimore, and prevalence rates of 20% to 30% have been reported in several studies of injectors in Europe. In a prospective study of injectors in Amsterdam, the incidence of abscess was 33 per 100 person-years. Necrotizing fasciitis can complicate skin and soft-tissue infections among injectors, conveying a high (10%) risk of mortality in one series.

Risk of abscess has been associated with route of injection, with intramuscular ("muscling") or subcutaneous ("skin popping") injection conveying greater risk for abscess than intravenous injection. HIV infection is associated with abscess in some, but not other, studies. Other risk factors identified include higher injection frequency and injecting a mixture of cocaine and heroin ("speedball"). In addition to injection of illicit drugs, nonprescription use of anabolic steroid injections has been associated with abscess formation. Common sites of abscess are, in order of descending frequency, arm, leg, buttocks, deltoid, and head/neck, in keeping with the "hierarchy" of injection sites reported in the literature.

Treatment of abscess typically requires incision and drainage, with adjunctive antibiotics. Specialized wound clinics targeting drug injectors have proved to be successful in engaging out-of-treatment patients and in substantially reducing use of more expensive emergency room and inpatient resources. In choosing antibiotic therapy, patients should be asked about their possible use of unprescribed ("street") antibiotics prior to presenting for care.

Infective Endocarditis

Endocarditis is the infection most classically associated with injection drug use, particularly in the pre-HIV era. Among active injectors, estimates of incidence range from

1.5 to 20 cases per 1,000 person-years. The risk of endocarditis is higher among HIV-infected injectors (13.8 vs. 3.3 cases/1,000 person-years). Estimates of mortality among persons with injection-associated endocarditis range from 7% to 37%, although rates may be lower (approximately 10%) among those with right-sided endocarditis.

Infective endocarditis among drug users can affect any heart valve. Although native valve endocarditis in the general population is most often left sided, infective endocarditis is most commonly right sided when associated with injection drug use. The tricuspid valve is involved in 40% to 69% of cases among drug injectors.

Tuberculosis

Drug users are at increased risk for tuberculosis infection and disease. The prevalence of latent tuberculosis infection (LTBI) among drug users varies by locale and population studied, but rates of approximately 15% to 25% are typical. The prevalence of tuberculin reactivity among HIV-seropositive drug users is generally lower than among HIV-uninfected persons, reflecting the diminished delayed-type hypersensitivity response associated with more advanced immunosuppression. Drug users are heterogeneous with respect to their risk for LTBI. Several reports suggest that, among drug users, smokers of crack cocaine are at particularly high risk for tuberculosis infection.

Pneumonia

Community-acquired pneumonia is common among drug users, particularly those with HIV infection. Recent studies have determined that the incidence of pneumonia ranges from 4.4 to 14.2 per 1,000 person-years among HIV-negative drug users, and from 47.8 to 90.5 per 1,000 person-years among HIV-positive drug users. Pneumonia is also the most common reason for hospitalizations among drug users.

Many factors contribute to drug users' increased susceptibility to pneumonia, including depression of the gag reflex by alcohol and drugs, leading to aspiration of oropharyngeal and gastric secretions; impaired pulmonary function as a consequence of cigarette smoking; and weakened immunity as a consequence of malnutrition and continuous antigenic stimulation. In addition, HIV-infection is associated with a markedly increased risk of bacterial pneumonia, and recurrent bacterial pneumonia has been included as an AIDS-defining illness since 1993. The risk for pneumonia among HIV-infected drug users is approximately five times that of non-HIV-infected drug users.

Neurologic Complications
Infections

Injection drug users are at increased risk for systemic infections that may affect the central nervous system, including endocarditis, viral hepatitis, and HIV. Endocarditis is associated with neurologic complications in 20% to 40% of patients, including cerebral embolism and infarction, hemorrhage from ruptured mycotic aneurysms, meningitis, encephalopathy, and parenchymal, subdural, or epidural abscesses. Viral hepatitis may also cause encephalopathy, or, less commonly, hemorrhagic stroke a result of abnormal blood clotting. HIV infection may cause neurologic complications either directly or through opportunistic infections that attack the central nervous system.

Focal central nervous system infections occur commonly among drug users, although most focal infections result from embolization of infected vegetations among patients with endocarditis. The most frequent focal infections are brain abscesses, which may also result from local spread of an ear or sinus infection, hematogenous dissemination from a distant focus, such as infection in the lung, skin, bone, or pelvis, or trauma with an open fracture or foreign body injury. Spinal epidural abscesses are also common, and are caused by direct local extension of vertebral osteomyelitis, hematogenous spread from distant infection, or blunt spinal trauma.

Toxin-mediated diseases, including tetanus and botulism, comprise an additional important category of central nervous system infections among injection drug users. These infections usually result from intramuscular or subcutaneous injection of drugs.

Other Neurologic Complications

Painful peripheral neuropathy has been described among several classes of drug users, including inhalant and injection drug users. In case reports, heroin use is associated with myopathy, cerebral and cerebellar spongiform encephalopathy, and sciatic nerve palsy. Many substances are associated with seizures, which typically occur as a result of drug toxicity or withdrawal. Finally, cocaine use may be associated with an increased risk of stroke.

Other Medical Complications

Other medical complications of drug use cannot be properly reviewed here because of space limitations. However, the reader is directed to recent reviews of pulmonary, renal, and other infectious complications among drug users, as well as to the complications from cocaine use and abuse such as cardiovascular, neurologic and cerebrovascular, renal, pulmonary, gastrointestinal, and sexually transmitted diseases.

Suggested Readings

Contoreggi C, Rexroad E, Lange V. Current management of infectious complications in the injecting drug user. *J Subst Abuse Treat.* 1998;15(2):95–106.

Gourevitch MN, Arnstein JH. Medical complications of drug use. In: Lowinson JH, Ruiz P, Millman RB, et al., eds. *Substance abuse: a comprehensive textbook*, 4th ed. Philadelphia: Lippincott Williams & Wilkins; 2005:840–682.

Laine C, Hauck WW, Gourevitch MN, et al. Regular outpatient medical and drug abuse care and subsequent hospitalization of persons who use illicit drugs. *JAMA.* 2001;285(18):2355–2362.

Lange RA, Hillis LD. Cardiovascular complications of cocaine use. *N Engl J Med.* 2001; 345(5): 351–358.

Samet JH, Friedmann P, Saitz R. Benefits of linking primary medical care and substance abuse services: patient, provider, and societal perspectives. *Arch Intern Med.* 2001;161(1):85–91.

Selwyn PA. Pain management in substance abusers. In: Finkelstein R, Ramos SE, eds. *Manual for primary care providers: effectively caring for active substance users.* New York: New York Academy of Medicine; 2002:153–188.

Tashkin DP. Airway effects of marijuana, cocaine, and other inhaled illicit agents. *Curr Opin Pulmon Med.* 2001;7(2):43–61.

36

HIV INFECTION AND AIDS

In many areas, human immunodeficiency virus (HIV) has spread extremely rapidly among injection drug users (IDUs), with the HIV seroprevalence rate increasing from less than 10% to 40% or greater within a period of 1 to 2 years. Several factors are associated with extremely rapid transmission of HIV among IDUs: (a) lack of awareness of HIV and acquired immune deficiency syndrome (AIDS) as a local threat; (b) restrictions on the availability and use of new injection equipment; and (c) mechanisms for rapid, efficient mixing within the local IDU population. There are various types of legal restrictions that can reduce the availability of sterile injection equipment and thus lead to increased multiperson use ("sharing") of drug-injection equipment.

Preventing Epidemics of HIV among Populations of Injection Drug Users

Current programs for reducing HIV transmission among IDUs should be considered highly effective at the individual level because a very large number of IDUs will adopt "safer" injection practices, but not perfect, because a substantial minority of IDUs will continue to engage in injection risk behavior after exposure to the programs. There are a number of cities and countries, such as the United Kingdom and Australia, where HIV infection has been limited to less than 5% of the IDU population and the rates of new HIV infections are less than 1% per year.

HIV-Related Medical Complications and Treatment

Comparative epidemiologic studies indicate that the expression of HIV-related disease and AIDS may vary substantially in different geographic regions.

Tuberculosis

Tuberculosis in the setting of co-existent HIV infection has been reported with increasing frequency in a variety of geographic settings, including not only industrialized countries, but also of particular importance countries in the Caribbean and sub-Saharan Africa, where both HIV infection and tuberculosis are concentrated. Molecular genetic techniques, namely, restriction fragment length polymorphism (RFLP) and polymerase chain reaction (PCR)-based methods, permit the identification of identical strains of *Mycobacterium tuberculosis*, enabling investigators to identify transmission patterns in a specific geographic area.

Current Centers for Disease Control and Prevention (CDC) recommendations suggest that treatment for active tuberculosis should be continued for a minimum of 6 months, although some experts suggest that treatment for HIV-infected patients should include longer courses of therapy, that is, 9 months.

Sexually Transmitted Diseases

HIV infection frequently is associated with the presence of other coexisting sexually transmitted diseases in a variety of patient populations. In addition, however, the presence of anal and genital ulcerations is a strong independent risk factor for HIV infection in both men and women, presumably through the facilitation of viral transmission via nonintact mucosal or dermal layers. IDUs historically have been found to be at increased risk of sexually transmitted disease, presumably related both to sexual behaviors associated with substance use and to the engagement in prostitution as a means of supporting the costs of substance use.

Initial assessment of substance-using patients with known or suspected HIV infection should include a thorough history regarding other sexually transmitted diseases. Syphilis is the most important example in this regard. In addition, human papillomavirus (HPV) infection, which may cause oral, anogenital, and common skin warts—and, less commonly, genital tract malignancies—in non–HIV-infected persons, occurs with increased frequency in HIV-infected patients. Furthermore, HPV infection has been strongly linked with an increased risk of cervical cytologic abnormalities in HIV-infected women, including dysplasia and frank carcinoma; the degree of malignant cytologic change appears to increase as women become more immunosuppressed in the course of their HIV infection. Reports also describe an increased risk of anal cancer in immunosuppressed HIV-infected homosexual men with co-existent HPV infection, further indicating the importance of the latter virus as a potential cause of malignancies in HIV-infected patients.

Other Human T-Lymphotrophic Retroviruses

HIV, previously known as human T-lymphotrophic retrovirus type III (HTLV-III), is one of three HTLVs identified since the late 1970s. Human T-lymphotrophic retrovirus type I (HTLV-I) was the first virus in this group to be discovered, and was identified as the causal agent in adult T-cell leukemia/lymphoma. HTLV-I infection has since been associated with chronic degenerative neurologic diseases designated as tropical spastic paraparesis and HTLV-I–associated myelopathy. Human T-lymphotrophic retrovirus type II (HTLV-II), although originally isolated from a patient with hairy cell leukemia, has not consistently been identified as an etiologic agent for a specific disease, nor has it been found to have a particular geographic distribution.

Hepatitis B Virus and Hepatitis Delta Virus

Long before the AIDS epidemic, IDUs were known to be at high risk for hepatitis B virus (HBV) infection. HBV infection is believed to be an early event in the career of

IDUs usually occurring within the first 1 or 2 years after the initiation of drug injection. Given these considerations, it is probable that in most populations of chronic IDUs into which HIV is introduced, HBV infection is likely to have been a prior event, with serologic evidence of immunity to HBV in most cases.

New developments in the field of therapeutics show combined benefits in the treatment of both HIV infection and hepatitis B. Studies report that the use of the antiretroviral medications lamivudine and tenofovir (Viread) are associated with a significant reduction in the total viral load of HBV when treating chronic hepatitis B. Additionally, interferon-α and adefovir dipivoxil have been successful in the treatment of chronic hepatitis B.

Hepatitis C Virus

Relatively recently identified as the etiologic agent of what was formerly known as non-A non-B hepatitis, hepatitis C virus (HCV) is a worldwide pandemic infecting an estimated 170 million people worldwide, and 3.6 million people in the United States. Infection with HCV is five times more widespread than infection with HIV-1, and it is the leading cause of liver disease, and a main indication for liver transplant in the United States. The morbidity and mortality rates from hepatitis C infection are increasing, and are expected to continue to increase over the next several years. Because HCV is transmitted primarily through the parenteral route, and because blood banks are now screening blood donations with more comprehensive and effective methods, the vast majority of current infections are through the use of shared needles or drug-preparation equipment.

Malignancies

As noted, heterosexual substance users with HIV infection are at low risk for Kaposi sarcoma as compared with homosexual men. However, case reports and hospital-based series from the United States and Europe document the occurrence of malignant lymphomas among HIV-infected substance users, of which certain lymphomas are AIDS-defining. Furthermore, a review of malignant neoplasms reported among HIV-infected IDUs in Italy described the occurrence of a variety of non–AIDS-defining solid tumors, primarily involving the lung, testis, brain, skin, rectum, and oropharynx.

Reported cases of lymphoma among HIV-infected substance users have included Hodgkin and non-Hodgkin types, with a wide variety of phenotypes, showing a high incidence of extranodal involvement and generally poor prognosis. In addition, as already mentioned, the common occurrence of HPV coinfection in HIV-infected drug-using women requires clinical vigilance for cervical dysplasia and carcinoma in such patients.

Neuropsychiatric Aspects of HIV-1–Infection

Clinically, patients suffer from a wide spectrum of cognitive impairments, personality changes, and motor dysfunction that range from subclinical symptoms without impairment of work or daily activities to severe dementia with paraplegia and double incontinence. This extreme syndrome is known as HIV-1–associated cognitive–motor complex and its severity is related to the degree of inflammatory response in the brain. In patients with moderate to severe dementia, multinucleated giant cells (MNGC) are found and are now considered essential for the diagnosis and pathognomonic of HIV-1–infection in the central nervous system (CNS). Microglial and glial changes, along with MNGC, can be found in any part of the CNS, but are more common in deep white matter of the cerebral hemispheres, basal ganglia, and brainstem. White matter pallor with astrogliosis, diffuse or focal vacuolation that can be associated with axonal or myelin loss, and cortical atrophy are changes that are less commonly observed. Rather than a true demyelination process of the oligodendritic myelin sheath, the pallor is a result of an increase in interstitial water content, most likely caused by a leaky blood–brain barrier.

Peripheral Nervous System Pathology and Myopathy in HIV-1–Infection

Patients with HIV-1–infection may present with a wide variety of symptoms involving the peripheral nervous system (PNS) and the skeletal muscles.

Distal symmetric peripheral neuropathy (DSPN) is the most common presentation among patients with generalized neuropathies. Initial symptoms include trophic changes in the lower extremities, paresthesias, edema, and weakness. These symptoms progress slowly to centripetally spread weakness and sensory loss. Medication-induced neuropathies have a clinical presentation that is similar to DSPN except that they present concurrent with the use of antiretrovirals, whereas the DSPN generally presents in the late phases of the HIV-1–infection. Inflammatory demyelinating polyradiculopathy may be acute (AIDP), presenting at the time of seroconversion and the initial manifestation of HIV-1–infection, or chronic (CIDP), presenting as subacute or chronic weakness in upper and lower extremities, decreased to absent deep tendon reflexes, and mild sensory abnormalities. Cranial nerves may also be involved. Mononeuritis multiplex usually presents as an abrupt onset mononeuropathy with periodic additional abrupt mononeuropathies in other distributions. It may present with sensory or motor manifestations and may involve cranial nerves as well. Pain may accompany any of the above-mentioned neuropathies and may be both severe and incapacitating.

Less-common presentations of PNS dysfunction are progressive polyneuroradiculopathy with early impairment of bladder and rectal sphincter control, and autonomic neuropathy with postural hypotension, diarrhea, and sudden arrhythmias with the risk of death.

The pain management regimen for the treatment of neuropathies includes capsaicin cream, amitriptyline, desipramine, anticonvulsants, or narcotics. Still, effective pain control is often difficult. Corticosteroids, plasmapheresis, and intravenous immunoglobulin have been used with success for DSPN, CIDP, and mononeuritis multiplex. Hypotension related to autonomic neuropathy may be controlled with fludrocortisone.

Myopathy associated with HIV-1–infection has three different histologic findings: (a) polymyositis, (b) necrotizing myopathy without inflammatory infiltrates, and (c) nemaline rod myopathy. Clinically, patients present with painless progressive weakness involving the shoulder and pelvic girdle muscles, elevated creatinine kinase (CK), and electromyographic (EMG) abnormalities. Treatment with prednisone alone or in combination with plasmapheresis is usually effective. The most important and common myopathy among HIV-1–infected patients is that related to zidovudine (AZT). It usually develops after 9 months to 1 year of treatment and manifests with leg weakness and wasting of the buttocks muscles. Symptom reversal may be complete with cessation or reduction of therapy. Patients taking AZT must be monitored regularly to detect early increments of CK.

Diagnosis and Management of HIV-1 Secondary Neurologic Complications

HIV-1 CNS involvement may occur at any time, in the absence or presence of indicators of quantifiable immune compromise. Opportunistic infections and HIV-1-related malignancies affecting the nervous system are usually a late manifestation of the HIV-1 infection, occurring in patients with less than 200 CD4 cells/mm^3 indicates the possible range of nervous pathologies that are likely to attack the CNS as a result of HIV-1 infection. No significant differences in the incidence of neurologic disease between IDUs and non-IDUs have been reported.

Toxoplasma gondii infection is extremely prevalent and is the most frequent cause of focal intracerebral lesions in patients with AIDS. Primary infection is usually asymptomatic, however. Headache accompanied by fever is the most common presentation, along with a subacute onset of focal neurologic abnormalities. Seizures affect one third of the patients. When neuroradiologic studies suggest toxoplasmosis, empirical therapy is almost a universal practice. The problem with neuroimaging studies, however, is that they have a low sensitivity when patients have nonfocal symptoms (22% to 74%) and when serum immunoglobulin G (IgG) is negative. If the patient fails to improve, a brain biopsy is necessary for a definitive diagnosis. Primary prophylaxis followed by maintenance treatment with pyrimethamine and sulfadiazine or clindamycin is usually effective and is recommended.

Cryptococcus neoformans is the most common cause of meningitis and the most important CNS fungal infection in patients with AIDS. The typical clinical presentation includes an insidious onset of fever, headache, nausea, vomiting, and altered mental status in a patient with a CD4 count of less than 100 cells/mm^3. If untreated, this is a fatal disorder, but mortality can be reduced to 17% to 20% with amphotericin B, either alone or in combination with flucytosine or with fluconazole therapy. Again, indefinite maintenance therapy with fluconazole is recommended.

Other secondary neurologic infections associated with HIV-1 include progressive multifocal leukoencephalopathy (PML) secondary to papovavirus infection, cytomegalovirus (CMV), encephalitis and polyradiculopathy, herpes simplex virus (HSV), encephalitis, neurosyphilis, and mycobacterial and other fungal infections. PML is an increasingly important source of neurologic complications in HIV-1 disease, and although there is no proven therapy for PML, cytosine arabinoside has been suggested as an efficacious alternative. Ganciclovir and foscarnet are effective in the treatment of CMV infection and as maintenance therapy. HSV encephalitis is a rare but life-threatening complication of HSV infection, especially in patients with advanced HIV-1–infection and other opportunistic infections of the CNS. Brain biopsy is often required for a definitive diagnosis. Treatment options include intravenous acyclovir, foscarnet, and vidarabine. Neurosyphilis has a more aggressive course in patients with AIDS, and its diagnosis may be difficult. Fortunately, intravenous penicillin is a highly effective and definitive treatment. Herpes zoster, mycobacterial, and fungal infections produce CNS complications in HIV-1–infected individuals and generally respond well to multimodal treatment.

Non-Hodgkin lymphoma is a complication of advanced HIV-1 disease that is present in 8% of the AIDS population. It may involve the CNS, causing neurologic, as well as neuropsychiatric, complications that include delirium, seizures, and cognitive impairment. A diagnosis can be made via neuroimaging, but a brain biopsy or evidence of malignant cells in the cerebrospinal fluid (CSF) is usually required prior to initiation of treatment. Multiagent chemotherapeutic treatment induces complete response in 54% of patients, but these responses are usually of short duration and the median survival time is 4 to 7 months after the diagnosis. Patients with AIDS are 100 times more likely than controls to suffer strokes, sometimes resulting in a clinical syndrome of multi-infarct dementia.

PNS may also be affected by secondary complications, such as herpes zoster neuropathy and cytomegalovirus polyradiculopathy. Toxic neuropathies caused by nucleotides—dideoxyinosine (ddI), dideoxycytidine (ddC)—may appear in late phases of the HIV-1–infection with a CD4 count of less than 200 cells/mm^3. A reversible myopathy secondary to AZT may also affect these patients.

Neurobiologic Evaluation in HIV-1–Infection

Mental Status and Neuropsychologic Assessment

Learning about the pathogenicity of HIV-1 is a key factor in its management. The HIV-1–associated cognitive–motor complex consists of a combination of cognitive, motor, behavioral, and affective disturbances that may be severe and sufficient for the diagnosis of AIDS. Several investigators have found that asymptomatic HIV-1–positive patients have an elevated rate of cognitive dysfunction when compared to HIV-1–negative controls. A careful cognitive history can be an extremely useful adjunct in the differential diagnosis of the etiologies of cognitive dysfunction in HIV-1–infected patients with cognitive complaints.

The most significant signs of cognitive impairment related to HIV-1–infection include early, mild problems with abstraction, learning, language, verbal memory, and psychomotor speed that progress to more serious difficulties with attention and concentration, slowing of information processing, slowed psychomotor speed, impaired cognitive flexibility, impairment in nonverbal abilities of problem solving, visuospatial integration and construction, and nonverbal memory in the late phases of the infection. The early stages of cognitive impairment associated with HIV-1 affect psychomotor tasks (such as the Wechsler Adult Intelligence Scale digit symbol and block design, and the trail making test part B from the Halstead–Reitan Neuropsychological Battery), memory tasks (such as the delayed visual reproduction subtest from the Wechsler memory scale); and the delayed recall of the Rey–Osterrieth Complex Figure. Psychomotor and neuromotor tasks may reveal HIV-1–related cognitive dysfunction and are also sensitive measures for the early detection of HIV-1–related cognitive impairment.

The neuropsychologic tests used for assessment of dementia generally appraise complex language-associated functions (such as aphasia and apraxia), higher-level cognitive functions of verbal and nonverbal abstract reasoning and problem solving, and perceptual functioning of the different sensory modalities. However, it has become apparent that these neuropsychologic assessments are not reliably sensitive for the necessary early detection of HIV-1 minor cognitive–motor disorder. These neuropsychologic batteries are most useful for detecting areas of mental dysfunction related to focal disturbances in the CNS, such as abscess created by an HIV-1–related opportunistic infection or tumor. They are not, however, useful for detecting the often subtle impairments of the early stages of HIV-1 effects on the CNS. The Global Deterioration Scale can provide the necessary information to successfully assess the decline of cognitive function clinically as it relates to an HIV-1–infected person's performance of daily activities, even before the patient fulfills the diagnostic criteria for the HIV-1–associated cognitive–motor complex.

Neuroimaging

Computed tomography (CT) and magnetic resonance imaging (MRI) are very useful in the diagnosis of secondary infections and brain tumors. Primary CNS HIV-1 infection can be associated with characteristic imaging features, including cortical atrophy, ventricular enlargement, diffuse or patchy white matter abnormalities particularly in periventricular areas and, in children, calcification of the basal ganglia and delayed myelination. MRI is more sensitive than CT scan in detecting white matter changes and MRI changes correlate with neuropsychologic testing.

Neuroimaging that reflects physiologic functioning of the CNS via positron emission tomography (PET) reveals early regional metabolic abnormalities with hypermetabolism in the basal ganglia, thalamus, and parietal and temporal lobes among nondemented patients with HIV-1 infection.

Magnetic resonance spectroscopy (MRS) has sensitivity in detecting early changes among patients with HIV-associated minor cognitive–motor complex (HMCMC). It differentiates them from seropositive asymptomatic patients and from those with more advanced HIV-associated dementia (HAD). Frontal white matter changes are an early sign of HMCMC, whereas basal ganglia and frontal cortex abnormalities are also found in patients with HAD.

Electrophysiology

The role of electrophysiology in cognitive and neurologic conditions is a key factor in early detection and understanding of these conditions. The percentage of patients with abnormal electroencephalograms appears to increase as the systemic disease progresses and a low amplitude pattern may be found in advanced dementia and atrophy on CT scan. In asymptomatic patients, studies have found conflicting results, with some finding no abnormalities in asymptomatic patients, and others finding frontotemporal theta slowing as a predominant finding. Computerized electroencephalography may be more sensitive in the detection of early changes and may predict subsequent development of HIV-1–related neurologic disease.

Evoked potential studies have also been useful in detecting abnormalities in neurologically and physically asymptomatic HIV-1–seropositive patients. When compared with controls, these patients showed significant delays in latency of response to the brainstem auditory evoked potential, somatosensory evoked potentials from tibial nerve stimulation, and visual evoked potentials.

Cerebrospinal Fluid Studies

The CSF reflects changes consistent with HIV-1 infection, including HIV-1 virions, abnormally elevated IgG levels, HIV-1–specific antibodies, mononuclear cells, and oligoclonal bands. HIV-1 replicates in the brain with independent dynamics from other organs. Therefore, the CSF viral load is specific for the assessment of the severity of the infection in the CNS. It also correlates with the degree of neurocognitive dysfunction and has a role in monitoring the response to antiretroviral medications in the CNS. Although elevation in myelin basic protein (MBP) and its degradation was found in patients with HIV-1–associated cognitive–motor complex and with PML, this was not seen in patients with other opportunistic infections. An abnormally low CD4+:CD8+ ratio that was found in the CSF, which preceded the one in blood, may have importance for treatment considerations.

Neuropsychiatric Symptomatology of HIV-1 Infection

Mental disorders secondary to medical conditions such as delirium, dementia, mood disorders, and anxiety disorders are the most common neuropsychiatric conditions associated with HIV-1 infection. Personality changes with significant variation in the Minnesota Multiphasic Personality Inventory (MMPI), psychotic disorders caused by general medical condition, and substance-induced disorders may also be seen.

Delirium

Delirium is the most common mental disorder observed in general medical conditions associated with HIV-1 infection. Delirium is also a predictor of outcome in hospitalized patients with AIDS. Delirious patients have a higher mortality rate, longer hospitalizations, and greater need for long-term care when discharged alive, as compared to a group of nondelirious patients with AIDS with similar demographics and markers of medical morbidity. Delirium may also be the most frequently undiagnosed of all organic disorders in the outpatient setting. As the treatment of most HIV-1 complications has become more sophisticated, it has also become simpler. Undiagnosed delirium in the ambulatory setting poses a particular danger because of the lost opportunity to diagnose and treat a potentially reversible complication of a medical disorder.

Delirium reflects diffuse cerebral cellular metabolic dysfunction. A common prodromal phase involves patients' complaints of difficulty in thinking, restlessness, irritability, insomnia, or interrupted short periods of sleep containing vivid nightmares. Evidence of this prodromal phase should be regarded seriously and should generate a search for the underlying cause of the delirium process. A brief mental status examination should focus on arousal, attention, short-term memory, and orientation. Diurnal variations in the delirium process are common, with symptoms typically worsening at night. Motor abnormalities, including tremor, picking at clothing, multifocal myoclonus, and asterixis can also be found.

It is important to attempt to determine the particular etiology for each individual patient. These conditions include Wernicke encephalopathy, hypoglycemia, hyperglycemia, hypoxemia, hemodynamic instability with cerebral hypoperfusion, infections, metabolic disturbances, and electrolyte imbalances. Herpes and *Toxoplasma gondii* encephalitis, cryptococcal meningitis, space-occupying lesions from cerebral tumors, progressive multifocal leukoencephalopathy, and neurotoxicities from antiviral agents should also be included in the differential diagnosis of delirium in HIV-1 patients. In the substance abuse population, the detection of alcohol and nonalcohol intoxication or withdrawal is extremely important in the differential diagnostic considerations for the etiology of delirium in HIV-1 disease.

Prompt pharmacologic interventions may help remediate the various behavioral abnormalities associated with the delirium process. High-potency neuroleptics may be used prudently for the control of delirium in HIV-1–infected patients. Haloperidol, especially by oral or intramuscular administration, has been successful in the management of delirium in HIV-1–infected patients, but not without significant treatment-emergent side effects. At low doses, haloperidol and chlorpromazine (a low-potency neuroleptic) have been used effectively and with few side effects in the treatment of delirium in hospitalized patients with AIDS.

Intravenous haloperidol, either alone or in combination with lorazepam and hydromorphone or buprenorphine, appears to be both safe and effective for use with agitated delirious HIV-1–infected patients.

Molindone has also been reported as a safe and efficacious alternative for the treatment of delirious patients who can take oral medications and are sensitive to the side effects of high-potency neuroleptics. Atypical antipsychotics are used now in the treatment of delirium. They are effective and well tolerated, with less emergence of extrapyramidal side effects when compared to traditional neuroleptics.

Lorazepam is useful in the management of agitated delirious HIV-1–infected patients when used in combination with haloperidol. Lorazepam alone, however, appears to be ineffective and is associated with treatment-limiting side effects.

Dementia

Among the neuropsychiatric complications of HIV-1 infection, dementia is commonly seen. It is characterized as an acquired intellectual impairment resulting in persistent deficits in many areas, including memory, language, cognition, visuospatial skills, personality, or emotional functioning. Basic functions such as alertness, arousal, memory, and normal rates of information processing are impaired by HIV-1 involvement of the white matter in the CNS. Thus, HIV-1–associated dementia is characterized as a "subcortical" dementing process. Symptoms closely associated with subcortical disorders, such as Parkinson disease, progressive supranuclear palsy, and multiple sclerosis, are also seen with HIV-1 CNS involvement and the HIV-1–associated cognitive–motor complex. In the early stages, neuropsychologic tests for HIV-1 cognitive impairment should reflect memory registration, storage, and retrieval; psychomotor speed; information processing rate; and fine motor function. These tests reflect the characterization of HIV-1 cognitive impairment as a subcortical process. In the later stages of HIV-1 disease, other traditionally cortical syndromes such as aphasia, agnosia, apraxia, and other sensory–perceptual functions are also manifested, perhaps as a result of some focal opportunistic infection or neoplastic invasion of the CNS or HIV-1 infection itself.

Besides antiviral therapy to recover and prevent cognitive decline associated with HIV-1 infection, improvement of affective and cognitive symptoms have been described with the use of methylphenidate in doses ranging from 10 to 90 mg per day in divided doses. Medications that prevent the toxicity caused by the HIV-1 through the N-methyl-D-aspartic acid (NMDA) receptor are currently under investigation. They include calcium-channel blockers, such as nimodipine or nifedipine, and NMDA-receptor antagonists, such as memantine and nitroglycerin.

Mood Disorders

Mood disorders associated with HIV-1 infection are most frequently depressive, but manic and hypomanic disturbances have also been described. Close to 85% of HIV-1-seropositive individuals will exhibit some evidence of mood disturbance. The diagnostic process for evaluating mood disorders is complex, requiring careful consideration of the interaction of medical conditions, substances, and behavioral factors. A reliable diagnosis ensures that prompt and effective therapeutic intervention will be undertaken.

Depression is commonly observed in patients with HIV-1–related disorders. A wide spectrum of mood disorders may be classified as depression. Patients may report mood disturbances that range from normal sadness to major affective disorder, as well as mood disorders that may be substance induced or a consequence of a general medical condition.

Suicidal thoughts are almost always a symptom of depression and patients need to be assessed carefully. Because of impaired decision-making capacities and likely cognitive inefficiencies associated with HIV-1 disease, it is vital that clinicians respond promptly to any and all reports of suicidal ideation. A thorough assessment of the patient includes a realistic appraisal of the psychosocial situation and of the motivation for completing the suicide, along with a comprehensive neurodiagnostic assessment to rule out a potentially reversible organic mental disorder.

Still today, the treatment of depressed HIV-1–infected patients often comes down to a matter of the clinician's intuition based on the clinician's own relevant clinical experience. The area of pharmacotherapy, in particular, lends itself to individual interpretation of risk and benefit for any given treatment regimen. The specific choice of medication and dose should draw from the physician's knowledge of the pharmacologic side effects of antidepressants and take into consideration the unusual vulnerability of HIV-1–infected patients with respect to their likely excessive disability from drug therapy. One such consideration is that antidepressants with greater affinity for the central muscarinic receptor should be avoided for symptomatic HIV-1–infected patients because of their anticholinergic effects, which can mask or aggravate HIV-1–related cognitive impairment or precipitate delirium. Another adverse side effect of these agents is the possibility of excessive drying of the mucous membranes, which introduces the possibility of oral candidiasis that is often refractory to treatment in HIV-1–infected patients. Antidepressants that are preferable for HIV-1–infected individuals are the tricyclic antidepressants with low anticholinergic affinity, second-generation antidepressants, such as the selective serotonin-reuptake inhibitors (SSRIs), bupropion, venlafaxine, nefazodone, mirtazapine, and the psychomotor stimulants.

Patients who are being treated with lithium carbonate or monoamine oxidase inhibitors prior to their diagnosis with HIV-1 disease usually should continue to take that medication. Increased vigilance in toxicity monitoring with a concomitant dosage alteration may be necessary as HIV-1 disease progresses, especially when infectious complications cause severe diarrhea or any other form of fluid loss, because rapid nephrotoxicity and neurotoxicity may ensue. Manic symptoms secondary to AZT, didanosine, ganciclovir, or antidepressants may also respond to lithium. Likewise, monoamine oxidase inhibitors may be continued for patients who had depression prior to their diagnosis with HIV-1 disease and who previously responded well to these agents. However, it is usually wise to treat a depression that arises after HIV-1 seropositivity with agents other than monoamine oxidase inhibitors because the associated dietary restriction of tyramine-containing foods may exacerbate the nutritional problems associated with advanced HIV-1 disease. Additionally, monoamine oxidase inhibitors are theoretically incompatible with AZT therapy, which is reported to have catechol-O-methyltransferase-inhibiting effects.

Psychostimulants such as methylphenidate and dextroamphetamine may be tried with depressed patients who are symptomatic of HIV-1 infection, with those depressed patients who are cognitively impaired or who suffer from both depression and dementia. Methylphenidate is a very safe and effective treatment for depression. Response usually occurs within hours of the first administration, providing psychomotor activation, appetite stimulation, and qualitative, as well as quantitative, improvement in higher cortical functions. The initial administration of methylphenidate is usually 5 to 10 mg by mouth, feeding tube, or suppository. Its equivalent dose in dextroamphetamine could also be used. After gradually raising the dose to 20 mg or less three times a day, a favorable response is usually achieved. The use of psychostimulants in managing depressive or cognitive symptomatology in drug-abusing patients is questionable.

Common Psychologic Problems in HIV

HIV-infected patients have been described as facing the problems of grief, stigmatization, the demands of a chronic, life-threatening illness, and changes in self-concept and identity. These problems can lead to demoralization, a condition that might be closer to an adjustment disorder with depressed mood, rather than to true major depression, yet with sadness and hopelessness of sufficient severity as to impair functioning. Adjustment to illness may be more difficult for drug users than for other patients with HIV/AIDS because of their reliance on substance use and other forms of avoidance as coping mechanisms. Maladaptive coping is linked to poor adjustment, to HIV disease, and to psychologic distress. Drug users have been found to experience greater distress than nondrug users following HIV antibody testing.

Responding to Psychologic Problems

Identifying and treating the psychologic problems of HIV-infected patients may improve health-related quality of life and possibly reduce use of health services. Counseling interventions that aim to improve coping skills and reduce avoidance and drug use may be helpful. Reducing psychologic problem intensity may also be important to improve the outcome of substance-abuse treatment in these patients.

Guidelines recommend the application of different standards of care for patients with varying levels of HIV severity and psychosocial functioning. This approach also encompasses different expectations of patients regarding substance-abuse treatment outcome.

Social Problems

The problems that accompany HIV infection are social and environmental, not just psychologic. As a group, IDUs with AIDS have few economic or educational resources; many are impoverished and stigmatized. Their relationships, home environment, and neighborhoods are often unhealthy and unsupportive of recovery. HIV/AIDS can lead to role conflict and significant challenges for the patient's caregivers and partners, especially because many have already witnessed AIDS-related deaths.

Treatment professionals need to understand the variations in culture, ethnicity, gender, and sexual orientation that are so integral to understanding HIV/AIDS among substance abusers.

Assessment of Social Problems

Assessment of social problems involves a thorough evaluation of patient sociodemographic characteristics such as age, education, race, ethnic/minority status, level of acculturation, sexual orientation, religion, and employment history. Other areas to explore during intake or counseling sessions may include familial and partner support, prior psychosocial functioning, housing conditions and homelessness, criminal justice involvement, use of community resources, and accessibility to needed medical and social services (e.g., transportation, making appointments). The social context associated with injecting drugs may also hold cultural meanings and relevant information about daily problems encountered by substance abusers with HIV/AIDS. Perceived social norms, beliefs about the disease, and attitudes toward providers vary widely among different social groups. For women, socioeconomic concerns surrounding child care, custody issues, pregnancy, domestic violence, and prostitution are salient factors to assess and intervene.

Counseling and Case Management for Social Problems

In some communities, drug treatment programs may need to become the primary health care providers for their patients because of the shortage of services. Other settings for psychosocial education and brief intervention include emergency rooms, prisons, and shelters. Community-oriented programs, mobile units or vans, street outreach and peer-driven interventions have also demonstrated empirical support for providing services and facilitating treatment entry. Peer education programs may be a key strategy for influencing social norms and conveying information on health behavior and risk management practices.

One innovation is the application of case management, a social service strategy designed to enroll patients in services and coordinate the services patients require for their complex problems.

Counseling for Reducing Drug Use and Other HIV Risk Behaviors

In discussing counseling strategies, it is important to stress that drug abuse treatment itself is clearly an effective means of reducing HIV risk. The evidence is strongest for methadone maintenance treatment, which has been the most thoroughly studied, but there are strong indications that other treatment modalities also reduce HIV risk.

In addition to the benefits of drug abuse treatment *per se*, a recent meta-analysis of studies indicated that many targeted HIV risk-reduction programs are effective. These programs provide risk-reduction skills and change sexual behaviors, knowledge, attitudes, and beliefs. As might be expected, the most effective programs are those that provide the most intensive services. There is also emerging evidence that

HIV counseling and testing has a positive effect as a means of secondary prevention for HIV-positive individuals.

Suggested Readings

Cunningham CO, Selwyn PA. HIV-related medical complications and treatment. In: Lowinson JH, Ruiz P, Millman RB, et al., eds. *Substance abuse: a comprehensive textbook*, 4th ed. Philadelphia: Lippincott Williams & Wilkins; 2005:922–988.

Des Jarlais DD, Hagan H, Friedman SR. Epidemiology and emerging public health perspectives. In: Lowinson JH, Ruiz P, Millman RB, et al., eds. *Substance abuse: a comprehensive textbook*, 4th ed. Philadelphia: Lippincott Williams & Wilkins; 2005:913–922.

Fernandez F, Maldonado J, Ruiz P. Neuropsychiatric aspects of HIV-I infection. In: Lowinson JH, Ruiz P, Millman RB, et al., eds. *Substance abuse: a comprehensive textbook*, 4th ed. Philadelphia: Lippincott Williams & Wilkins; 2005:988–1007.

Fernandez F, Ruiz P. *Psychiatric aspects of HIV/AIDS*. Philadelphia: Lippincott Williams & Wilkins, 2006.

Sorensen JL, Haug NA, Batki SL. Psychosocial issues of HIV/AIDS among drug users in treatment. In: Lowinson JH, Ruiz P, Millman RB, et al., eds. *Substance abuse: a comprehensive textbook*, 4th ed. Philadelphia: Lippincott Williams & Wilkins; 2005:1007–1011.

37

ACUTE AND CHRONIC PAIN

Terminology

The relationship between the medical use and abuse of opioid drugs cannot be clarified without a precise characterization of terms, including tolerance, dependence, abuse, and addiction. *Tolerance* is a pharmacologic property of opioid drugs defined by the need for increasing doses to maintain effects. *Physical dependence* also is a pharmacologic property of opioid drugs, and is defined by the occurrence of an abstinence syndrome (withdrawal) following abrupt dose reduction or administration of an antagonist. Most experts define addiction in a manner that distinguishes it from physical dependence. According to a definition jointly endorsed by professional societies for pain and addiction in the United States:

> Addiction is a primary, chronic, neurobiologic disease, with genetic, psychosocial, and environmental factors influencing its development and manifestations. It is characterized by behaviors that include one or more of the following: impaired control over drug use, compulsive use, continued use despite harm, and craving.

This definition does not reference phenomena related to tolerance or physical dependence, and appropriately focuses on behavior as the relevant assessment for the diagnosis of addiction.

Use despite harm also has been used to define *abuse*, a term that has been applied additionally to any drug use that is outside accepted societal and cultural standards. There is substantial, but not complete, overlap between the terms *addiction* and *abuse*. An individual who uses an illicit drug could be considered an abuser even if compulsive use is absent. Finally, *pseudo-addiction* refers to drug-seeking behavior occasionally observed in the setting of uncontrolled pain, which disappears when analgesic interventions, often including increased doses of an opioid, become effective.

Categories of Patients with Pain

Acute monophasic pain is the most common pain type, and is acute and self-limited. Most such pains are never evaluated by physicians and demand no therapy beyond simple measures taken by the individual. Some are severe or associated with serious underlying pathology, however, and require clinical intervention (e.g., pains associated with surgery, major trauma, burns). A second type, also extremely prevalent, is *recurrent acute pain* (e.g., dysmenorrhea, sickle-cell anemia, inflammatory bowel disease). These pains, too, range in severity and need for clinical intervention.

Opioid therapy is considered to be the major therapeutic approach to patients with *chronic pain associated with cancer*. Like pain caused by cancer, *chronic pain associated with progressive nonmalignant medical diseases* (e.g., sickle-cell anemia, hemophilia, some connective tissue diseases) is associated with poor prognosis. Although psychosocial disturbances are extremely important determinants of the presentation and management of these conditions, the pain in most patients usually is assumed to be largely explained by the organic lesion. Another chronic pain is *pain associated with a nonprogressive organic lesion* (e.g., musculoskeletal pain syndromes such as osteoporosis, postherpetic neuralgia, painful polyneuropathy). Although opioid therapy for these patients can be controversial, the existence of a clear-cut organic process may encourage some physicians to consider this approach. Last are patients who experience *chronic nonmalignant pain* or associated disability perceived by the clinician to be excessive for the degree of organic pathology extant. Most patients with a chronic pain syndrome have both an identifiable organic lesion and sufficient evidence of psychologic disturbance to fulfill criteria for a psychiatric disorder, such as a chronic pain disorder or somatization disorder.

Comprehensive Pain Assessment

All patients with chronic pain should undergo a comprehensive pain assessment, which requires an appropriate history, physical examination, and, often, confirmatory laboratory and radiographic procedures. The patient should be asked to describe the pain (e.g., temporal features, location, severity, quality, factors that provoke or relieve it). Other relevant information includes medical and surgical disorders, prior history of persistent pain, past pain treatments, and previous use of licit and illicit drugs. The patient's level of physical functioning should be detailed and important concurrent symptoms, such as level of energy, sleep disturbance, appetite, and weight, should be elicited. A psychosocial history is essential. In patients with a known history of substance abuse, the interview must clarify both the specific pattern of addictive behaviors and the relationship between these behaviors and the pain. It is important to determine whether or not the patient perceives that pain precipitated or perpetuates the addiction, and similarly, whether or not the patient perceives that drugs that are abused are treating the pain.

Based on clinical observation, pains with a predominating organic contribution are described as either nociceptive or neuropathic. Nociceptive pain is presumed to be commensurate with the degree of ongoing activation of afferent nerves subserving pain perception. Although this judgment oversimplifies complex neurophysiologic processes, it is nevertheless useful clinically. Pain classified in this way (e.g., related to cancer or arthritis) usually can be reduced through interventions that improve the peripheral nociceptive lesion. Neuropathic pain is related to aberrant somatosensory processes induced by an injury to the peripheral or central nervous system. The pains are often dysesthetic (abnormal pain, unfamiliar to the patient) and disproportionate to any nociceptive lesion identified. The diagnosis of a neuropathic pain may suggest the use of selected types of interventions.

Management of Pain

Chronic Cancer Pain

Pain is experienced by more than one third of patients with cancer undergoing active antineoplastic therapy and by up to 90% of those with advanced disease. Opioid drugs should be considered the mainstay therapeutic approach to this problem; opioids can provide adequate pain control for more than three quarters of these patients. Although a history of substance abuse influences the approach to opioid therapy, the general approach to cancer pain is similar to the management of cancer pain in the population without this history. The first consideration is the feasibility of primary therapy directed against an underlying nociceptive lesion. Radiotherapy to tumors associated with pain can provide relief to more than half the patients treated. Other primary anti-neoplastic therapies, including surgical resection of neoplastic lesions and chemother-apy, can also have analgesic consequences.

Selecting a Pharmacologic Approach

The pharmacologic management of cancer pain requires expertise in the use of three broad groups of analgesics: nonsteroidal anti-inflammatory drugs (NSAIDs), opioid analgesics, and the so-called adjuvant analgesics. The World Health Organization developed an approach to drug selection known as the "analgesic ladder," which employs a stepwise selection of analgesics based on pain severity. Patients with mild to moderate pain are first treated with an NSAID. This drug is combined with one or more adjuvant drugs if a specific indication for one exists. Adjuvant drugs include those selected to treat a side effect of the analgesic (e.g., a laxative) and those with analgesic effects (adjuvant analgesics). Patients who present with moderate to severe pain, or who fail to achieve adequate relief after a trial of an NSAID, are treated with an opioid conventionally used for pain of this severity, which typically is combined with an NSAID and may be coadministered with an adjuvant, if indicated. Patients who present with severe pain or fail to achieve adequate relief following appropriate administration of drugs on the second "rung" of the analgesic ladder should receive an opioid conventionally selected for severe pain. This treatment may also be combined with an NSAID or an adjuvant drug, as indicated.

Drugs typically used on the second rung of the analgesic ladder are pure agonists generally used for moderate pain in formulations combined with a nonopioid anal-gesic (aspirin or acetaminophen). Upward dose titration is usually limited by dose tox-icity of the nonopioid. Trials of this analgesic approach suggest that a large majority of patients can achieve adequate cancer pain relief without additional treatments.

Cancer Pharmacotherapy: Nonsteroidal Anti-inflammatory Drugs

The NSAIDs and acetaminophen are characterized by a ceiling dose and analgesia that is additive to that of the opioids. The NSAIDs comprise an extremely diverse group of drugs that reduce the synthesis of prostaglandins and inhibit the enzyme cyclooxyge-nase (COX). There is large individual variation in the effective dose range and the dose associated with toxicity for these drugs. Moreover, the maximal efficacy of the NSAIDs varies across drugs in any individual patient. Sequential trials may demon-strate striking differences in effectiveness.

Clinically important side effects associated with NSAIDs can include adverse gastrointestinal symptoms (including gastric or duodenal ulcers), renal toxicity, and effects on platelet function (such that they should be used cautiously in patients with a bleeding diathesis). It is prudent to initiate NSAID therapy with a relatively low starting dose when patients have mild to moderate pain or an increased risk of toxicity. During therapy, dose escalation can be considered if pain is uncontrolled, side effects are tolerable, and the conventional maximal dose has not been reached. If a maximal dose is reached without achieving satisfactory analgesia, an alternative NSAID trial should be considered. Long-term NSAID therapy should be monitored for adverse effects.

Cancer Pharmacotherapy: Opioid Analgesics

Several factors should be considered in the decision to use one opioid drug rather than another. First is the distinction between the pure agonists and agonist–antagonists. Pure agonist opioids bind to one or more of the opioid receptors and demonstrate no antagonist activity. Morphine is the prototypic pure agonist, but numerous others are available, including hydromorphone, oxycodone, levorphanol, and methadone. The agonist–antagonist opioids (e.g., pentazocine, nalbuphine, butorphanol, and buprenorphine) are characterized by potential antagonism at one or more opioid receptors, a ceiling effect for analgesia, and the capacity to precipitate an abstinence syndrome in patients physically dependent on pure agonist opioids. These properties suggest agonist–antagonist opioids are not generally useful in the management of chronic pain.

The most common approach to the second "rung" of the analgesic ladder involves the administration of a combination product containing acetaminophen or aspirin plus either codeine or oxycodone. The dose of this drug is increased as needed until the maximum safe dose of the aspirin or acetaminophen is reached. Should pain persist, the patient is usually then switched to one of the so-called strong opioids.

The pure agonist drugs that are customarily employed at the third "rung" of the analgesic ladder include morphine, hydromorphone, oxycodone (when not combined with a co-analgesic), levorphanol, and methadone. Fentanyl is available in a formulation for transdermal administration (Duragesic), and oxymorphone is available in a rectal formulation. In the past, morphine was considered the preferred drug, based on extensive clinical experience, relative ease of oral titration, and availability of numerous formulations.

Some caution is appropriate in the use of the drugs that have considerably longer half-lives than other opioids (e.g., methadone has a variable half-life that can range from less than 24 hours to more than 150 hours), and levorphanol and methadone should be considered second-line drugs. However, methadone has become increasingly used by pain specialists. It is relatively inexpensive, has no active metabolites, and there is a large and favorable clinical experience. Methadone appears to be far more potent than indicated on standard equianalgesic tables. A switch to methadone from another opioid is most safely accomplished by reducing the calculated equianalgesic dose by 75% to 90%. The use of methadone as an analgesic typically requires multiple doses per day.

Apply Appropriate Dosing Guidelines

DOSE "BY THE CLOCK"

It is more effective to prevent the recurrence of severe pain than abort it once it appears, and "by-the-clock" dosing is preferred over "as-needed" dosing. "As-needed" dosing still plays a role, however, and should be considered in the nontolerant patient during the initiation of therapy, in the patient with rapidly changing pain, and in patients with intermittent pains. Additionally, clinical experience strongly supports the use of an "as-needed" dose (so-called rescue dose) in combination with a fixed dosing schedule to treat "breakthrough" pains.

TITRATE THE DOSE

Once an opioid and route of administration are selected, the dose should be increased until adequate analgesia occurs or intolerable and unmanageable side effects supervene. There is no ceiling effect to the analgesia provided by the pure agonist opioid drugs and the maximal dose is immaterial as long as the patient attains a favorable balance between analgesia and side effects. In clinical practice, the range of opioid doses required by patients is enormous. Although doses typically stabilize for prolonged periods during long-term management, dose escalation is usually required at intervals to maintain analgesia.

BE AWARE OF RELATIVE POTENCIES

By using morphine as a standard, relative potencies have been determined for most pure agonist drugs in single-dose analgesic assays. Relative potency tables should be consulted when switching from one drug or route of administration to another. These estimates should be viewed as guidelines. A switch should be accompanied by a reduction in the equianalgesic dose of at least one third, in recognition that incomplete cross-tolerance between opioids may result in a potency greater than anticipated for the new drug.

Cancer Pharmacotherapy: Adjuvant Analgesics

Adjuvant analgesics represent numerous drugs in many classes used commonly in the treatment of many malignant and nonmalignant pain syndromes. When used in the management of cancer pain, they are typically added to an optimally titrated opioid regimen. Some, such as the tricyclic antidepressants, are used as primary analgesics for specific nonmalignant pain syndromes. The largest number of adjuvant analgesics is used in the setting of neuropathic pain. These syndromes are believed to be relatively less responsive to opioid drugs than pain syndromes sustained by persistent injury to pain-sensitive tissues (nociceptive pain). Antidepressants, anticonvulsants, oral local anesthetics, and others are commonly administered to patients who continue to experience inadequate analgesia despite opioid dose titration.

Other Analgesic Approaches in Cancer Pain Management

Other approaches can use nonpharmacologic interventions to reduce or even eliminate the opioid requirement. For example, neurostimulatory approaches, most commonly transcutaneous electrical nerve stimulation, typically are implemented in patients with refractory neuropathic pains and those with more acute, transient pains. Experience is limited in patients with cancer. The anecdotal impression is that many patients respond initially, but long-term benefit is rarely achieved with this technology. Other types of neurostimulatory approaches include counterirritation, acupuncture, percutaneous electrical nerve stimulation, dorsal column stimulation, and deep brain stimulation.

Patients with painful musculoskeletal complications of cancer may benefit from physical or occupational therapy, and the use of orthoses or prostheses may have analgesic consequences in other situations. Anesthetic approaches include the use of nitrous oxide for pain in far-advanced disease, myofascial trigger point injection, and a large variety of nerve block procedures that employ either local anesthetics or neurolytic solutions. The technique of continuous epidural local anesthetic is an innovation capable of providing a long-standing neural blockade without inflicting permanent damage on nerves. Surgical neuroablative procedures isolate the painful part from the central nervous system.

Psychologic approaches are underused in cancer pain management. There is a strong association between mood disturbance and persistent pain, and patients with cancer pain benefit from the support provided by staff. Those with evidence of psychiatric disorders should be appropriately referred and treated. Some patients may benefit from specific cognitive approaches, including relaxation training, distraction, hypnosis, and others.

Other Considerations in the Substance Abuser with Cancer Pain

PATIENTS WITH A REMOTE HISTORY OF SUBSTANCE ABUSE

Although clinical experience suggests that patients with a remote history of substance abuse respond appropriately to opioids, empirical data in support of this conclusion are meager. Some patients with cancer with a remote history of substance abuse are poorly compliant with opioid therapy due to a persistent fear of these drugs. Thus, the optimal management of the patient with cancer pain and a remote history of addiction must incorporate careful, ongoing assessment of drug-taking behavior and the recognition that successful treatment may be compromised both by the attitudes of practitioners and the patient. Education of the staff and the patient may limit the adverse consequence of these attitudes and thereby improve pain management.

PATIENTS IN METHADONE MAINTENANCE PROGRAMS

Patients receiving opioid maintenance also are at high risk for undertreatment of cancer pain. If persistent pain reports are interpreted as a manipulative attempt to obtain opioids for purposes other than analgesia, the therapeutic relationship becomes conflicted. If "drug seeking" reflects only the need for pain relief, however, undertreatment will result from the failure to respond. Patients who have not received an opioid for pain before, but have been receiving methadone for some time, may require starting doses substantially higher than those conventionally used at the initiation of cancer pain therapy.

ACTIVE DRUG ABUSERS

There are a small number of patients who develop cancer pain while actively abusing opioids or other drugs. Careful assessment is critical to appropriate management in these cases. In some cases, efforts to implement a simple and effective pharmacologic regimen for pain may have to be sacrificed in lieu of interventions designed to maintain therapeutic control. Some clinicians favor the use of a written agreement that is kept in the medical record and both defines the medication regimen and states the responsibilities of both the patient and clinician. Factitious pain complaints and malingering appear to be rare among patients who are not actively abusing drugs and probably are uncommon among active abusers who develop cancer. Rather, most substance abusers are like other patients with pain, whose symptoms reflect some combination of ongoing nociception and psychologic distress.

Chronic Nonmalignant Pain

Chronic nonmalignant pain comprises an extremely diverse group of syndromes. All patients require a comprehensive assessment to determine the potential for primary therapy directed against any treatable organic contribution to the pain. There is no definitive primary therapy for most patients in chronic pain, however, and the assessment must also provide the information necessary to develop a multimodality approach to symptomatic therapy that can improve comfort and enhance physical and psychosocial function.

Analgesic modalities can be categorized as pharmacologic, anesthetic, neurostimulatory, physiatric, surgical, and psychologic. The number of approaches used in the management of a patient and the specific therapies within each approach vary according to the needs of the patient.

In recent years, attention has focused on the development of multidisciplinary pain programs, which evolved from the recognition that the complex problems posed by some patients with chronic pain exceeded the clinical capabilities of any one practitioner. Thousands of such programs now exist, and they are widely considered to be the state of the art in the management of patients with intractable pain associated with a high level of disability.

The long-term treatment of chronic pain with opioid drugs continues to be controversial. The conventional rejection of this approach in pain patients with no prior history of substance abuse is gradually evolving to a more balanced perspective. In populations with pain and substance abuse, however, there is neither a large and reassuring clinical experience nor empirical data that confirm the safety and efficacy of opioid therapy. Generally, the use of opioid therapy for chronic pain should not be initiated if the patient is currently abusing licit or illicit drugs, and this treatment should be offered to those with a remote history of addiction only by experienced clinicians.

Acute Pain

Acute pain is, by definition, self-limited and usually is readily associated with a specific tissue injury, related to trauma, surgery, or a disease process. The management of acute pain in the addict is not a trivial issue, because addicts experience traumatic injuries and a myriad of medical disorders at a disproportionately higher rate than does the general population.

Pains associated with recent tissue injury may be associated with signs of sympathetic nervous system stimulation, including diaphoresis, pupillary dilation, hypertension, tachycardia, and even nausea. With the knowledge that very diverse symptoms and signs can result either from a direct effect of a drug or from drug withdrawal, clinicians may express doubts about the nature of the pain or about medical comorbidity. For example, the objective physical signs associated with acute pain may also be produced by opioid withdrawal. Although the management of acute pain in the addict may be difficult, it is nonetheless possible to develop guidelines that ensure a careful assessment of the acute pain complaint and provide the best chance of achieving satisfactory pain relief in these circumstances.

Distinguish among Types of Abusers

The management of pain in the patient with a history of opioid abuse may be facilitated by distinguishing addicts who are actively abusing at the time of treatment from those with a remote history of drug abuse and those receiving opioid maintenance. Although the implications of these distinctions have not been clearly substantiated in prospective clinical studies, it is common practice to apply them in the setting of acute pain management.

Patients who are actively abusing either licit or illicit opioids, and those on maintenance, may be assumed to have some degree of tolerance. Furthermore, patients who are actively abusing drugs often manifest psychologic disorders that can influence pain perception and may require intervention.

Apply Appropriate Pharmacologic Principles of Opioid Use

As in the treatment of cancer pain, pure agonist opioids usually are administered for the management of acute pain in these patients. Patients who are actively abusing opioids or who are participating in methadone maintenance may demonstrate a need for higher doses or shorter dosing intervals because of the development of tolerance. Tolerance to opioid analgesics decreases the duration of effective analgesia following a dose.

Clinical experience in the nonaddict population suggests that some patients with acute, severe pain require rapid escalation of opioid doses. Patient-controlled analgesia (PCA), in which the patient self-administers an opioid intravenously, is being used with increasing frequency. In the population without a history of substance abuse, studies indicate that PCA does not lead to excessive self-administration of the opioid. Despite this favorable impression and the lack of empiric data demonstrating different responses among those with and without a history of opioid abuse, many experts believe that the use of PCA in opioid addicts is problematic. If PCA is employed, it must be implemented with due regard for the possibility that the patient with a history of abuse may be opioid tolerant.

Provide Concomitant Nonopioid Therapies When Appropriate

Nonopioid analgesics may be highly efficacious in specific acute pain syndromes, and their use may minimize the need for opioids. Although NSAIDs may be useful even for severe acute pain in some patients, they are most often helpful in combination with opioids when the latter are causing dose-limiting opioid side effects. An NSAID should not be considered an opioid "substitute," and the desire to withhold opioids from suspected or known substance abusers with acute pain should not be viewed as an indication for these drugs.

Other types of nonopioid therapies may be useful in selected cases. For acute focal pain syndromes, regional anesthetic approaches, such as somatic or sympathetic nerve blocks, should be considered. It is well accepted that anesthetic procedures may be more efficacious than systemic opioids in some types of acute pain, such as acute reflex sympathetic dystrophy.

Recognize and Prevent Specific Drug Abuse Behaviors

Some measures can be recommended that may allow the continuation of opioid use for acute severe pain despite the potential for ongoing abuse. First, it is essential to engage the patient in a frank discussion that clearly defines the expectations. Second, simple security measures are advisable, such as the use of drug infusion pumps with locks that prevent changes in the settings. If oral opioid analgesics have been abused, the patient should be told that ingestions will be witnessed and that room searches for hidden pills or signs of hoarding will be done.

Although acute severe pain in a known opioid addict is seldom treated in the outpatient setting, additional guidelines should be followed if this circumstance arises. Guidelines should be written, given to the patient, and filed in the patient's medical record. They should state the absolute requirement that only one physician prescribe opioid medications and should provide procedures for prescription renewals and the response to lost or stolen prescriptions or drugs.

Chronic Opioid Therapy in Patients without Substance Abuse

Efficacy

The most relevant information about the potential efficacy of chronic opioid therapy for nonmalignant pain is provided by controlled trials that describe treatment that extends for 1 or 2 months; none of these studies observed the development of abuse behaviors during therapy, a finding that might be expected given entry criteria that exclude patients with a history of drug abuse. Surveys suggest a spectrum of outcomes associated with opioid therapy. Although treatment can evidently become a problem in some disabled patients, there appears to be a subpopulation of patients with chronic nonmalignant pain that attains at least partial relief from opioid drugs for a prolonged period, without the development of opioid toxicity, clinically significant tolerance, or abuse. Although some patients who experience relief of pain demonstrate improvement in functional status, others do not.

Development of Tolerance

It is apparent that chronic opioid therapy for nonmalignant pain would not be viable if pharmacologic tolerance to analgesia developed at such a rate that effective pain relief was brief or could be maintained only by rapid escalation of doses to unacceptable levels. A diminution in salutary opioid effects with prolonged administration is seldom observed in surveys of patients with cancer and patients with chronic nonmalignant pain. Concern about waning analgesic efficacy primarily as a result of tolerance is overstated.

Goals of Pain Therapy

It is widely accepted that the management of chronic nonmalignant pain must consider two goals simultaneously: improved comfort and functional gains. Published surveys of opioid therapy for nonmalignant pain describe disparate outcomes. Some patients improved function during therapy and others did not. Given the conflicting survey data, the most reasonable hypothesis is that opioids by themselves neither substantially improve nor damage function. For some patients, access to an opioid can contribute to globally impaired function or a tendency to drug abuse, whereas for others, the availability of a strong analgesic allows a degree of function that would otherwise be impossible. The drug has an important role in determining the overall outcome, but the nature of the outcome cannot be attributed to the pharmacology of the drug.

Adverse Pharmacologic Outcomes

Risk of Major Organ Dysfunction

Major organ toxicity following exposure to opioids has not been observed among patients with cancer or those on methadone maintenance. Pulmonary edema has been reported in several dying patients with cancer who were receiving high doses of an opioid, but this phenomenon is not relevant to the routine treatment setting. There is evidence that acute administration of an opioid can alter immune function. There is also evidence, however, that pain itself is immunosuppressive, and this finding, combined with the lack of evidence of clinically relevant impairment of immune function from opioids, provides support for opioid therapy in the setting of severe pain.

Persistent Side Effects

Acute administration of an opioid produces changes in the hypothalamic–pituitary axis, peripheral vasculature, gastrointestinal tract, urinary tract, skin, and immune system. With chronic administration, tolerance develops at different rates to each effect.

The most detailed assessment of this issue has been done in the methadone maintenance population. Studies of these patients have demonstrated persistent constipation, insomnia, and decreased sexual function in 10% to 20% of patients and complaints of excessive sweating in a somewhat higher proportion. Elevated plasma proteins often persist, and occasionally, sustained abnormalities of hypothalamic–pituitary regulation, particularly abnormalities in the level and fluctuation of prolactin, are observed.

Although cognitive impairment and disturbances in psychomotor functioning are commonly observed following either acute administration of opioids to nontolerant patients or dose escalation in those on chronic therapy, these effects typically wane with stable long-term therapy. Surveys of driving records performed in methadone-maintained populations have not revealed an increased rate of infractions or accidents. A systematic review of neuropsychologic studies of opioid-treated patients concluded that there was generally consistent evidence for no impairment of psychomotor abilities of opioid-maintained patients, inconclusive evidence for no impairment on cognitive function, and strong evidence for no greater incidence of motor vehicle violations or accidents, or abnormalities in driving simulators. The potential for cognitive impairment should be evaluated when opioids are employed in the clinical setting.

Risk of Addiction

The perception that opioid consumption may lead to the development of addiction derives largely from clinical experience with street addicts. The observed reactions of addicts following exposure to opioids are often assumed to be merely a more extreme expression of the experience of patients administered these agents for pain. Implicit in this view is the belief that such powerful reinforcements attend the use of these drugs that administration to otherwise normal individuals for appropriate medical reasons may be sufficient to produce addiction. If this were true, chronic opioid therapy for nonmalignant pain should certainly be rejected, except perhaps in patients with life-threatening diseases.

This conclusion is contradicted by extensive experience with pain patients, predominantly those with cancer pain, and numerous clinical investigations. Although it is widely believed that opioids produce the reinforcing experience of euphoria, surveys of patients with cancer, postoperative patients, and normal volunteers indicate that elation is uncommon following administration of an opioid; dysphoria is observed more typically.

Surveys provide evidence that the outcomes of drug abuse and addiction do not commonly occur among patients with no history of abuse who receive opioids for medical indications. Other epidemiologic data similarly contradict the notion that exposure to opioid drugs reliably leads to escalating use and recidivism after detoxification. For example, there is the evidence that a large proportion of soldiers who abused heroin in Vietnam stopped this activity abruptly on return to the United States, and subsequently demonstrated a low rate of relapse.

These findings suggest that opioid exposure by itself is insufficient to produce abuse or addiction. The reinforcing properties of opioid drugs may be experienced differently by the individual predisposed to addiction than by the typical patient with chronic nonmalignant pain. A reasonable hypothesis is that addiction results from the interaction between the reinforcing properties of opioid drugs and any number of characteristics that are specific to the individual. These characteristics, such as the capacity for euphoria from an opioid, are unrelated to the pharmacology of the drug.

In sum, the existing data suggest that patients without a prior history of substance abuse are unlikely to become addicted during long-term opioid treatment of chronic pain. The risk should not be assumed to be nil, however, and the data also suggest that the risk may vary with specific characteristics of the patient. The risk of iatrogenic addiction during long-term opioid therapy is probably greater among those with a prior history of substance abuse, a significant family history of addiction, severe character pathology characterized by impulsivity, or a chaotic home environment.

Clinical Implications

Opioid therapy, like other primary analgesic treatments, may be best conceived as a useful element in a multimodality approach for chronic pain management. Guidelines based on clinical experience have been proposed for the management of opioid therapy in patients with nonmalignant pain. The guidelines indicate that patient selection is empirical at the present time. Opioid therapy is not considered a first-line approach, but might be evaluated against other therapies in terms of its risk:benefit ratio. Because opioid therapy can almost always be discontinued without difficulty after short-term administration, a therapeutic trial can be initiated like any other reversible analgesic approach.

A careful reassessment is needed whenever pain worsens sufficiently to suggest the need for dose escalation. This reassessment should clarify the nature of the pain, record side effects, determine functional status, and affirm the lack of aberrant drug-related behaviors. Finally, it is important to have a clearly defined strategy for the management of aberrant drug-related behaviors, should they occur. Many clinicians have a stereotyped response to these behaviors based on a perception that they invariably represent addiction. This type of inflexibility is not justified given the diversity of these behaviors and the multiple meanings they may reflect.

Conclusion

Principles of opioid therapy for the treatment of pain are well established and generally are believed to provide the capability for adequate pain control in the great majority of patients with acute and chronic pain. Patients with a history of opioid abuse who are evaluated carefully and are determined to be appropriate candidates for opioid therapy, either brief or long term, require ongoing assessment and the skillful adaptation of pharmacologic principles that have proved essential in the optimal management of pain in patients with no such history. In the much larger population with no prior history of substance abuse, the potential for opioid addiction contributes substantially to the pervasive undertreatment of acute pain and chronic cancer pain.

Physicians should be re-assured that aggressive opioid management of acute pain and chronic cancer pain is fully acceptable, and those physicians who choose to employ opioids in the management of chronic nonmalignant pain should not fear reprisals for this decision if it is undertaken with the care that such controversial therapy warrants. All these objectives will be more likely to be acheived if an active dialogue develops between pain specialists and addiction specialists.

Suggested Readings

Kirsh KL, Whitcomb LA, Donaghy K, et al. Abuse and addiction issues in medically ill patients with pain: attempts at clarification of terms and empirical study. *Clin J Pain.* 2002; [4 Suppl]:S52–S60.

Lussier DA, Portenoy RK. Adjuvant analgesics in pain management. In: Doyle D, Hanks GW, MacDonald RN, et al., eds. *Oxford textbook of palliative medicine*, 3rd ed. Oxford: Oxford University Press; 2004:349–377.

Nicholson B. Responsible prescribing of opioids for the management of chronic pain. *Drugs.* 2003;63(1):17–32.

Portenoy RK, Payne R, Passik SD. Acute and chronic pain. In: Lowinson JH, Ruiz P, Millman RB, et al., eds. *Substance abuse: a comprehensive textbook*, 4th ed. Philadelphia: Lippincott Williams & Wilkins; 2005.

Rowbotham MC, Twilling L, Davies PS, et al. Oral opioid therapy for chronic peripheral and central neuropathic pain. *N Engl J Med.* 2003;348(13):1223–1232.

38

SUBSTANCE USE DISORDERS IN INDIVIDUALS WITH CO-OCCURRING PSYCHIATRIC DISORDERS

Use of, and withdrawal from, alcohol and other substances of abuse can cause, mimic, or mask psychiatric symptoms. At one time when an individual presented with a substance use problem and an apparent mental illness, it was common to ascribe all pathology observed to the substance use and to treat the individual accordingly. That is to say, the psychopathology was ignored with the assumption that once the individual was clean and sober, the psychiatric problems would disappear as well. The substance use was easier to see and diagnose.

Once it became obvious there was a population for whom addiction alone was not the problem, the issue of cause and effect became a subject of debate. Arguments arose regarding which came first. Was the person depressed because he was drinking heavily, or did he drink heavily because he was depressed? Was she psychotic because she smoked voluminous quantities of ganja or did she choose to smoke the drug because, as she claimed, it calmed her nerves and helped her rest? Was he anxious because he chronically abused benzodiazepines and felt the rebound effect, or did he use the benzodiazepines because of his chronic state of anxiety?

One camp saw the problem as substance use and all else as an excuse for bad behavior. The more psychologically minded developed the theory that addicted individuals used their drug(s) of choice as a means of treating uncomfortable or unacceptable impulses. This theory became known as the *self-medication* hypothesis of addictive disorders.

Regardless of the cause, many treatment providers refused to treat any other psychopathology until the substance use disorder had been addressed and the individual abstinent, sometimes for many months. Unfortunately, such an approach condemned the individual with an untreated mental illness to a high likelihood of early relapse and an overall poorer long-term prognosis.

It is now clear that many substance misusers suffer from both addiction and substance use disorders. Furthermore, individuals with such comorbid psychopathology do not typically respond well to traditional addiction treatment approaches. Rather, a unique approach is necessary for these complicated patients that is not available within typical programs. The needs of a large and difficult portion of the addicted population have been largely unmet for many years. In the last decade years, however, great strides have been made to correct this lack.

Terminology

Now that the existence of this large population of individuals with both psychiatric and substance use disorders is recognized, how to describe this subgroup, what to call it, is an issue. Some suggest that such individuals be dubbed "substance abusers with mental illnesses (SAMI)" or "mentally ill substance abusers (MISA)," each placing a slightly different spin on the importance of the pathology. Using the same logic, others have argued for "mentally ill chemically addicted (MICA)" or "chemically abusing mentally ill (CAMI)."

A title that has found considerable favor is "dually disordered." Recently, concern has been raised that this too fails to adequately address the true scope of the problem. It is argued that "dual disorders" could be construed as referring to co-existing medical conditions such as human immunodeficiency virus (HIV)/acquired immune deficiency syndrome (AIDS) and hepatitis, or even misunderstood as relating to those with developmental disabilities. It is rare for such individuals to have only two problems. Rather, they suffer from a whole spectrum of difficulties, including social, financial, and psychologic. They prefer the phrase "individuals with co-occurring disorders."

Currently, there does not appear to be a consensus. The Substance Abuse and Mental Health Services Administration (SAMHSA) uses both *dual disorders* and *co-occurring disorders* in their most recent publications. The latter two appear to be the most commonly used descriptors at this time and will be used interchangeably throughout this chapter.

Demographics

According to the National Institute on Drug Abuse and the National Institute on Alcohol Abuse and Alcoholism, abuse of alcohol and other drugs cost the United States $245.7 billion dollars in 1992, more than a 50% increase over the cost in 1985. This number represents the cost of treating the substance user as well as drug-related diseases such as cirrhosis, liver failure, hepatitis, and HIV; decreased employee productivity and premature death; and the cost of police intervention and incarceration of criminals.

Treatment of individuals with mental illnesses also places a heavy burden on economies both here and in other parts of the world. A study published by the National Institute of Mental Health ranks the economic impact of all medical and psychiatric diseases on society. It concludes that the economic burden exerted by mental illnesses, not including alcohol and other drug use, ranks second only to cardiovascular conditions. Adding substance use disorders to all other mental illnesses places the economic cost of all psychiatric conditions well ahead of all physical disorders. Recognizing that substance misuse and co-occurring mental illness place a heavy economic toll on society, it is clear that when such conditions co-occur, as they frequently do, the economic impact is tremendous.

By looking at a community sample, it has been found that individuals with any mental disorder had a lifetime prevalence of 29% for an addictive disorder. In treatment and institutional settings, the prevalence of co-occurring disorders is even higher. According to the Surgeon General, as many as 65% of persons with at least one mental disorder "also have a lifetime history of a least one substance use disorder." The incidence and prevalence of substance misuse is different among the different disorders. For example, among individuals with schizophrenia, from 25% in community samples to 66% of individuals in specialized samples such as Veterans Administration (VA), community mental health, and in-patient samples, are estimated to have comorbid substance use disorders. Bipolar disorder is associated with an even higher rate of substance misuse, with up to 75% of individuals with this diagnosis found to have co-occurring substance use problems according to some estimates. The anxiety disorders, on the other hand, have a much more variable rate of comorbidity, depending upon the specific diagnosis. Nevertheless, substance use disorders co-occur at a much higher rate among individuals with anxiety disorders than among the general population. It is not clear, however, that this is true among individuals with social phobia. Despite recognition of the high cost of comorbidity and it prevalence, surprisingly little attention has been given to this problem until the last decade.

Impact of Co-occurring Disorders

The co-occurrence of psychiatric and substance use disorders has social, economic, and prognostic implications. When substance misuse and mental illness co-occur, the risk is great that, in general, the individual will not do as well as if the individual had not developed such a comorbid problem. Poverty and homelessness are more frequent, as are the risks of being both victim and perpetrator of violent assault. It is important to note that although most violent crimes are not committed by the mentally ill, those that are perpetrated by members of this population are more likely to be committed by those with co-occurring substance use disorders. Furthermore, among the mentally ill, substance use also increases the risk of both accidental and homicide deaths. Finally, individuals with substance use disorders are less compliant with medication and more likely to drop out of treatment.

Comorbidity, in short, is associated with a worsened prognosis overall. Thus, although substance misuse *per se* is a source of significant social and medical morbidity, in the case of the mentally ill, the problems become magnified many times over.

Treatment Strategies

Various models have been proposed for treating substance misusers with co-occurring psychiatric disorders. Three models, in particular—sequential, parallel, and integrated—summarize the approaches that have been used.

In the sequential model, first one, then the other condition is treated. The idea is that one condition must be controlled before the second can be adequately addressed. Of course, determining which condition to treat first presents a significant problem. Addiction treatment programs have not typically been designed to meet the needs of the mentally ill. Treatment providers have rarely been trained to recognize and treat the psychopathology of the dually disordered patient, and rarely have the patients done well with many of the elements of typical treatment programs. Mental health providers, on the other hand, have been reticent to treat intoxicated patients and ill-equipped to handle them. The concern is often voiced of the potential for a lethal interaction between medication and any drug or drugs of abuse the patient might be using. Furthermore, it is believed that patients will fail to respond to psychotropic medications if they continue to use alcohol and other drugs.

It could reasonably be argued that, where one condition is relatively minor compared to the other, such a model could be successful. Where both conditions pose significant or equally severe impairments, however, how to prioritize the sequence of treatment may become a nearly insurmountable problem.

In the parallel model, both conditions are addressed simultaneously, but in different programs with different staff. Poor communication between staff and the potential for the patient to receive mixed messages can be substantial risks here, however. Furthermore, treatment philosophies may clash and goals may be quite different between addiction and mental health treatment programs. Abstinence-only treatment programs have been unwilling, in the past, to encourage patients to comply with prescribed medications. Mental health providers, on the other hand, often strive for rigid adherence to medication regimens. In addition, staff members often do not understand or, more importantly, approve, of each other's approach to treatment. Although more workable than the sequential model, the parallel model, too, can pose serious problems in implementation and execution.

In the integrated model both conditions are treated simultaneously by providers knowledgeable about both conditions. Widespread use of this approach is made difficult because there is an insufficient number of treatment providers trained in both areas available to treat the large numbers of patients who need such help. Furthermore, especially when the patient suffers from a very serious mental illness, much responsibility may fall on the therapist for close supervision and case management, resulting in a high staff burnout rate.

To address some of the deficiencies inherent in existing programs, there has been a major initiative at the national level to educate mental health and addiction treatment providers in each others' specialties. Cross-training is promoted at national, state, and local levels. Special certification programs were developed to standardize and measure necessary levels of knowledge and skills, and to promote quality programming for treating individuals with co-occurring disorders. Where once treatment programs consisted, in many respects, of promoting the principles of Alcoholics Anonymous and other 12-step, self-help programs, it is now accepted that working with the dually disordered is a much more complex task than this. The treatment provider must help the patient gain an understanding of the patient's substance use disorder, of the patient's mental illness, and of the impact one has on the other. The provider must then help the patient develop strategies for recognizing and dealing with each. Strategies often include medication, especially for individuals with psychotic disorders.

Special Issues in Evaluation of the Dually Diagnosed

Evaluation and detoxification of substance misusers are well described in sections IV and V of this book. General issues pertinent to any substance misuser apply to the individual with co-occurring mental disorders as well, and are not covered here. Special considerations that apply primarily to individuals with co-occurring disorders, however, are described in detail.

The treatment provider should be familiar with, and capable of performing, a basic psychiatric evaluation. A comprehensive review of such is beyond the scope of this chapter and can be found in any general textbook of psychiatry. Among other things, however, such an evaluation should include a list of the patient's past diagnoses, if the patient is aware of what they may have been, past hospitalizations for psychiatric reasons, response to treatment, family history of psychiatric problems, and past medications and response to such. Furthermore, the interviewer should ask about suicidal ideation, both current and past, as well as attempts.

Although assuring the safety of the patient must always be a consideration in dealing with the chemically dependent, it is of paramount importance when dealing with the dually disordered individual. Patients in the immediate poststimulant dysphoric state or who are acutely under the influence of depressants such as alcohol are at an increased risk of self-harm, regardless of whether or not they have a comorbid psychiatric condition. Both acute and chronic use of substances of abuse, however, vastly magnify the risk of suicide in individuals with depression and other chronic, severe mental illnesses, including schizophrenia and bipolar illness. Thus, at intake and at frequent intervals throughout the treatment process, the patient's risk of suicide must be assessed.

It is helpful to determine if the psychiatric symptoms predate the onset of the individual's substance misuse. It is also useful to learn if the patient's psychiatric condition improves, disappears, or worsens when the patient is not using the substances. Unfortunately, it is often impossible to determine either of the above. If the patient uses substances daily and has no substantial periods of clean time, it will not be possible to know if the patient's symptoms improve with abstinence. Likewise, if the patient has been using for many years, memory may not prove accurate whether the substance misuse or the psychiatric symptoms came first.

Many treatment providers refuse to provide medication to the substance-misusing psychiatric patient unless the patient is abstinent. This, of course, often leads to deterioration in function. Such worsening is not necessarily a result of the substance use, but often a consequence of the individual requiring the medication that is being withheld. There is much evidence that working with the patient and helping to treat the patient's psychiatric symptoms improves the chances of engaging the patient in addiction treatment, increases the likelihood of decreasing the patient's consumption of alcohol and other drugs, and can be successful in improving the patient's psychiatric symptoms, even if the patient continues to use substances. *As long as the patient can be treated safely, the patient should be treated.* The decision whether or not to medicate often comes down to the clinician's level of comfort and best judgment based on knowledge of the patient, the substance(s) the patient uses, the medication(s) the patient takes, and of the mental illness.

To treat this complicated population adequately, the treatment provider must be prepared to make judgments about the safety of using medications in patients who may be acutely under the influence of a substance, yet also on prescription drugs.

Principles of Treating the Dually Disordered Patient

Comprehensive treatment for the dually disordered individuals demands that programming provide flexibility, repetition, and medication where necessary.

Flexibility

Traditional addiction treatment programs stress abstinence as a contingency for participation, strict participation, and self-disclosure. Such demands may be neither attainable nor desirable when dealing with the dually disordered patient. Permitting the patient to participate only if the patient is abstinent may render the severely ill patient incapable of ever receiving the help the patient so desperately needs. Besides, if the patient could stay clean without the program, why would the patient need the program? Voices may be telling the patient to use, or the patient may need to use in order to tolerate the presence of others in the program. The patient may be at risk of dropping out of the program just when the patient needs it most; for example, if a woman relapses to cocaine use when her nightmares of rape return and abstinence is a requirement of attendance. Programs for the dually disordered must be able to adjust to accommodate the needs of the clientele they serve, and on an individual basis. This is a difficult population, requiring a prolonged period of engagement and a great deal of support in order to succeed.

Repetition

Repetition is necessary not just for the severely chronically mentally ill, but for all individuals with comorbid psychopathology. For the psychotic patient, interference from thought blocking and hallucinations may prevent the patient from comprehending or using skills suggested for decreasing substance use and avoiding high-risk situations. For the anxious individual presented above, as she experiences a resurgence of traumatic memories for which she is not yet adequately prepared to deal, she may forget all the coping skills that have been presented to her and resort to the one she knows best—her drug use. This does not mean she is "unready for treatment," or "not serious about treatment," or "resistive to treatment." This is a characteristic response of the dually disordered patient suffering from both posttraumatic stress disorder and cocaine dependence. As control of one problem appears to be within reach, symptoms of the other take center stage. A constant refocusing of attention and repetition of techniques for avoiding drugs and for dealing with psychiatric symptoms must be presented and practiced.

Medication When Necessary

There is no question that some psychiatric conditions can be treated with psychotherapy, behavioral interventions, and other psychotherapeutic techniques. There has been considerable concern among addiction-treatment providers that jumping in quickly with a pill to treat a patient's discomfort sends a wrong message. That is, it signals that only a substance, not personal learned strengths, can help the individual through hard times. The problem with the latter reasoning, however, is that addicted individuals with a co-occurring psychiatric condition who present for treatment typically have not learned the alternative means of dealing with their anxiety or depression or they would not be there in the first place. Furthermore, psychotherapeutic interventions take time to be learned and rehearsed, and, although effective for some psychiatric conditions, are not as beneficial for others. In addition, the dually disordered are at a high risk of dropout and relapse. Waiting for lengthy interventions to take effect may ensure the patient's early withdrawal from treatment long before a positive response can occur. Finally, especially for the severely mentally ill, medication is typically a first, not a last, choice. Early and vigorous intervention with medication where indicated with nonaddictive agents may help the patient stay in treatment and gain confidence that the patient will be treated so that the patient can learn the techniques needed for dealing with the patient's substance use and psychiatric disorders.

However, when medication is deemed necessary for treating the dually disordered individual, every effort should be made to use medications that (a) do not induce euphoria, (b) do not cause dependence, (c) are effective in the individual who is actively using substances of abuse, and (d) are safe when used by the active user.

Psychiatric Conditions, Medications, and Substances of Abuse

The following is not an exhaustive review of the literature, but an effort to give the reader a fair overview of the information available regarding medications that have proved safe and effective in relieving psychiatric symptoms in patients with psychiatric disorders who continue actively to use substances of abuse.

Depression, Antidepressants, and Mood Stabilizers

Depression and mania can be improved by active treatment with medication even when the patient continues to abuse alcohol, opiates, nicotine, and perhaps marijuana. To date, no medication has been shown to be unequivocally superior in improving such symptoms among individuals abusing psychostimulants.

Tricyclic antidepressants (TCAs), selective serotonin reuptake inhibitors (SSRIs), and nefazodone (Serzone) decrease depressive symptoms in unipolar depression in actively drinking alcoholics. The clinician is advised to make TCAs available in very limited supplies, however, to a member of this population, because of the potential for a lethal interaction with alcohol. Furthermore, recent data regarding hepatotoxicity with nefazodone may limit utility of this agent in this population until further information regarding the cause is available. Concomitant abuse of benzodiazepines, alcohol, cocaine, and marijuana is common among opiate-dependent individuals. This fact, and that much of the research available regarding opiate addicts comes from methadone maintenance patients, makes it necessary to view data on this population with caution. Nevertheless, there is evidence that simply stabilizing opiate-dependent individuals on methadone improves depressive symptoms. Tricyclics, nefazodone, and SSRIs also improve depression in individuals actively using opiates. It should be noted, however, that abuse of TCAs by methadone maintenance patients is a well-known phenomenon in clinics; thus, such drugs should be used only with close supervision and with only small quantities available. Sertraline (Zoloft) may cause an initial rise in methadone levels, but they will normalize after a brief interval. Two brief reports regarding fluvoxamine (Luvox) and methadone, one positive and one negative, make it important for the treatment provider to use this drug with caution. There is some evidence that SSRI medication may case slight improvement in depressive symptoms in individuals actively abusing marijuana. Thus, erring on the side of the patient and offering to treat these symptoms with medication may be reasonable.

Lithium is relatively ineffective in treating substance-dependent individuals with mania. Furthermore, there is an increased risk of toxicity with this medication if the individual is using alcohol or marijuana. Thus, this mood stabilizer should be avoided in the dually disordered individual with bipolar disorder or cyclothymia. Divalproex (Depakote) improves manic symptoms in actively drinking alcoholics with this disorder, although close observation of liver functions is advised. In one study, gabapentin (Neurontin) decreased alcohol abuse in bipolar patients with alcohol problems. Quetiapine (Seroquel) appears to decrease both manic symptoms and cocaine cravings in dually disordered patients with bipolar disorder and substance use problems. Carbamazepine (Tegretol) must be introduced and used with caution among individuals on opiates, because it lowers methadone levels, leading to withdrawal. Data are not currently available with newer anticonvulsants and olanzapine (Zyprexa).

Psychoses and Antipsychotic Medications

Actively treating psychoses improves retention in both addiction and mental health treatment and reduces psychotic symptoms. Despite concern about the possible interaction between antipsychotics and alcohol, there is little in the literature to support this worry. This may, of course, reflect the long-held habit of withholding antipsychotic medications when individuals with psychoses began to imbibe. Nevertheless, there does not appear to be a great deal of need for concern in treating psychotic symptoms with high doses of typical antipsychotics in active drinkers. High doses of typical antipsychotic medications in conjunction with cocaine appear to increase the risk of dystonic reactions and perhaps neuroleptic malignant syndrome. Whether or not this applies to other psychostimulants is not known. Risperidone (Risperdal), fluphenthixol (Fluanxol), olanzapine, and clozapine (Clozaril) improve symptoms and retention among schizophrenic psychostimulant abusers, although there has been a report of an untoward reaction with use of the latter. Nicotine acts in competition with some antipsychotic medications (such drugs as haloperidol, fluphenazine, olanzapine, and clozapine), which may be affected (reduced) by the presence of nicotine. It is important for the treatment provider to keep this in mind in the event that a patient is abruptly forced to discontinue the patient's routine dose of nicotine or to have it drastically reduced. The patient's level of neuroleptic medication may become suddenly far greater than it had been, resulting in greatly increased side effects and discomfort.

Anxiety Disorders

Treating anxiety symptoms in individuals actively using alcohol, psychostimulants, and opiates improves retention in treatment and provides some degree of symptom relief. Benzodiazepines are among the top three most-abused prescription drugs in the United States and may be abused by nearly half of individuals seeking treatment for substance misuse. These facts, and that there is some evidence of a disinhibiting effect of some benzodiazepines when used by alcohol-dependent individuals, serve as relative, not absolute, contra-indications to their use in this population. Alprazolam (Xanax), in particular, has been suggested as having this effect. This is not surprising, as the shorter the half-life, the greater the potential for abuse. If this class of medication is used, it is advisable to use such agents with caution, in the acute situation rather than as a maintenance strategy, under close supervision, and briefly, if at all possible. Furthermore, longer-acting agents should be used. TCAs, SSRIs, and venlafaxine (Effexor) are helpful in relieving anxiety symptoms in individuals with co-existing alcohol and anxiety problems. The existence of so many nondependence-inducing, effective medications begs the question of the necessity of using potentially addictive agents for the treatment of anxiety disorders for any but very short-term problems. However, the cautions regarding the use of these agents mentioned previously must be noted here. Furthermore, venlafaxine undergoes extensive hepatic metabolism, and close observation of liver functions is advised in individuals abusing alcohol. Many cases of fatal reactions have been reported of opiate-dependent individuals using and abusing benzodiazepines. Consequently, use of this class of agents for individuals with this problem is not advised. Rather, a trial of TCAs, nefazodone, or SSRIs, as in depression, is preferable.

Treatment Outcome

How one defines "success" in the treatment of the addicted individual with a co-occurring psychiatric disorder is a source of ongoing discussion. There is a growing consensus that it is naive to believe that the only criterion of "success" is absolute abstinence from nonprescription psychoactive substances. Yet there is a debate whether or not it is a necessary criterion at all. Are individuals with schizophrenia who used their entire disability check on crack cocaine each month and ended up in the hospital immediately thereafter last year, the so-called "revolving-door patients," who pay their rent, have a part-time job, and have not been hospitalized in 14 months, but who now occasionally smoke marijuana, failures? Are individuals a success if they no longer drink alcohol, but remain homeless, depressed, are repeatedly incarcerated, out of work, and make occasional suicidal threats? If this is success, a new "yardstick" by which to measure our treatment outcome is necessary.

Arguably, outcome should be gauged on the basis of a number of prosocial behaviors, including reduction in length and frequency of hospitalization and incarceration where applicable, improved health, being domiciled, being employed, and reduction in amount and frequency of substance use, as well as a reduction in the problems associated with such. Abstinence alone would tell us almost nothing about the individual's level of "success" in terms of the individual's ability to function in society.

There are some tools available that look at multiple levels of functioning. Such instruments as the Addiction Severity Index (ASI), although valuable for research purposes, have limited practical value, however, because of the time they take to administer. Furthermore, in severely mentally ill individuals, there is a question regarding validity. Work remains to be done to develop a more portable instrument for truly measuring the effectiveness of different approaches to the treatment of the dually disordered patient.

Conclusion

Individuals with both substance use and psychiatric disorders constitute a substantial and difficult-to-treat subsection of the addiction population. Addressing only the substance use predicts a poorer outcome for other disorders including early relapse to alcohol and other drug use. Early and vigorous treatment for each condition should be initiated, including use of medications where indicated. In the latter case, care must be taken that medications used should be proved safe in the individual actively abusing alcohol and other substances, effective in treating the psychiatric condition when the individual is actively using, and nonaddictive where at all possible.

Much remains to be done to demonstrate that one therapeutic modality is clearly superior to another for the treatment of specific comorbid conditions, although studies are under way. It is clear, however, that this complicated and diverse population will present challenges for the treatment community for some time to come.

Suggested Readings

Curran GM, Glynn HA, Kirchner J, et al. Depression after alcohol treatment as a risk factor for relapse among male veterans. *J Subst Abuse Treat.* 2000;19(3):259–265.

Dennison SJ. *Handbook of the dually diagnosed patient: psychiatric and substance use disorders.* Baltimore, Md: Lippincott Williams & Wilkins; 2003.

Dennison SJ. Substance use disorders in individuals with co-occurring psychiatric disorders. In: Lowinson JH, Ruiz P, Millman RB, et al., eds. *Substance abuse: a comprehensive textbook,* 4th ed. Philadelphia: Lippincott Williams & Wilkins; 2005:904–913.

Drake RE, Xie H, McHugo GJ, et al. Dual diagnosis: fifteen years of progress. *Psychiatric Serv.* 2000;51(9):1126–1129.

Sciacca K. On co-occurring addictive and mental disorders: a brief history of the origins of dual diagnosis treatment and program development (an invited response). *Am J Orthopsychiatry.* 1996;66:3.

Weiss RD, Najavits LM. Overview of treatment modalities for dual diagnosis patients. In: Kranzler HR, Rounsaville BJ, eds. *Dual diagnosis and treatment: substance abuse and comorbid medical and psychiatric disorders.* New York: Marcel Dekker; 1998:87–105.

Section VII

LIFE CYCLE

39

SUBSTANCE ABUSE AND THE LIFE CYCLE: CHILDREN, ADOLESCENTS, AND ELDERLY INDIVIDUALS

Children

In 1991, the National Household Survey estimated that more than 4.5 million women of childbearing age had used illicit drugs during the previous month. More recently, assessments indicate that nationwide approximately 8.3 million (11%) children live with a parent who is addicted to alcohol or illegal substances. It is estimated that approximately 40% to 80% of all children in the child welfare system have been placed in foster care because of alcohol or other drug use in the home.

Approaches to the Treatment of Addicted Women and Children

Treatment of Children

When a substance-abusing parent has children, it is critical to remedy those problems that have occurred as a result of parental drug use. The symptoms of affected children can manifest as health, behavioral, or learning difficulties; developmental assessments identify lags in individual children. Assessment and treatment of the needs of children must be coordinated so that the full range of necessary services is offered. Collaboration among medical and social services is particularly critical to facilitate recovery, family stability, improved parent–child interactions, and access to appropriate care for the children involved.

Children of substance-abusing parents often lack basic trust and ability to become attached as they hope for parental love and nurturance; as parents live in continually shifting states of intoxication and abstinence, the child learns self-care that interrupts development of intimacy and results in isolation and depression. Positive, supportive, trusting relationships are helpful in improving a child's self-image.

Treatment of the Parents

Women face multiple obstacles to seeking treatment for substance abuse, including child care, financial constraints, and lack of support systems. They must contend with increased stigma as social mores stereotype female addicts as weak-willed, irresponsible, and promiscuous, and they often experience resistance from their partners and children who resent the treatment that disrupts homeostasis. Single parents are further stressed as they often neglect their own well-being, choosing to meet their children's needs at the expense of their own. Assisting parents in their recovery is the optimal means of treating their children.

Family Treatment

Family therapy combined with drug treatment is effective in treatment of substance-abusing families and is recognized as an essential approach to treating the full range of addictive problems in families. Emphasis should be on the present rather than a historical perspective, interruption of behavior patterns, focus on process rather than on content, and restructuring of families.

Parent Support Groups

The goal of the support group is to improve the parents' interactions with their children by developing viable peer networks. Within this context, the parents are able to consider their children's feelings, to understand their behaviors in the context of developmental stages, and to become aware of the dynamics of their interactions with their children. The group eventually becomes an independent mutual support network that helps its members develop self-esteem and empathy.

Parenting Skills Groups

Men and women who are addicted to drugs often have not experienced positive parenting models; many feel inadequate as parents. More than most caregivers, they need to experience self-esteem by being accepted, respected, and educated in the skills of parenting. Although they have difficulties coping with their children, they want to be "good" mothers and fathers. This motivation can be tapped and used to engage parents in skills groups. Parenting skills training is didactic in format.

Summary

The children of substance abusers suffer from the addiction of their parents and they are at risk for social, psychologic, educational, and medical problems. Drug treatment services do well to include services for parents as patients and to address the special needs of the children of patients. Services sensitive to the needs of parents include attention to daycare needs, perinatal services, and parenting skills training. Medical services familiar with the social and psychologic factors associated with drug and alcohol use can be a point of entry to the service system, and children's services, including schools, need to be aware of indicators of family drug or alcohol use.

Adolescents

A significant number of American teenagers use and abuse illicit and addictive substances. An estimated 1 in 5 teenagers (4.3 million) are current alcohol drinkers, 1 in 13 teenagers (1.7 million) are binge alcohol drinkers, and 400,000 adolescents are in need of substance abuse treatment. It is projected that the year 2010 will witness the largest number of adolescents in American history, so there is a clear need to improve our understanding of adolescent substance use disorders (SUDs), and to provide effective prevention and treatment. The initiation and early stages of substance use have their roots in adolescence.

Substance Use Progression

Substance abuse follows a fairly predictable progression, beginning with experimentation and recreational use of alcohol and cigarettes, followed by marijuana and other illicit drugs, especially cocaine or crack in the inner-city population. The risk of using other illicit drugs tends to be low without prior use of marijuana, perhaps with the exclusion of inhalants, which may be another "gateway" to use. After initiation with a gateway substance, individuals might progress to other illicit drugs such as opiates and hallucinogens.

Developmental and Protective Factors

The developmental stage of adolescence is characterized by dramatic change and readjustment new stresses and anxieties, and increased vulnerability to peer pressure. It is a time of consolidating an identity and practicing new roles. During adolescence, the practice of adult roles and behaviors shifts from pretend play to actual behavior. The pre-adolescent begins experimenting with a range of new behaviors, and for many, cigarettes, alcohol, and other drugs have become a normal part of coming of age. Adolescence is also marked by increasing autonomy from parents and increased reliance on peers for validation and direction. Conformity to the peer group increases rapidly to its peak in early adolescence, then gradually declines. Peers are vital to the teenager's emotional and psychologic development; acceptance by peers is critically important and rejection can be devastating.

Sensation seeking and risk taking appear to be related to the surge of pubertal hormone levels, particularly testosterone. Cognitive development may also contribute to increased risk taking, with adolescents wanting to impress their peers, but not yet adept at assessing risks. Adolescents also tend to exaggerate based on immediate experience, which allows risks to be minimized. Finally, adolescents have a sense of invulnerability—an attitude of "it won't happen to me."

Risk Factors

Risk factors can be grouped into five general categories: cognitive and attitudinal; personality and psychopathology; behavioral, social, and environmental; and biologic or genetic.

Cognitive and Attitudinal

Adolescents who use substances are less likely to be aware of the negative consequences of use, have fewer negative attitudes about substances, and believe that substance use is normative. They are also less likely to have personal competence and decision-making skills that allow the adolescent to manage emotional distress. Females with substance abuse disorders have lower levels of constructive thinking and executive function, with these traits also associated with higher levels of antisocial behavior.

Personality and Psychopathology

Personality characteristics linked to substance use include low assertiveness, low self-efficacy or self-esteem, low self-confidence, low social confidence, and external locus of control; additional characteristics are aggressiveness, unconventionality, problems with interpersonal relatedness, and precocious sexuality. Mood disorders, including depression and bipolar disorder, are also highly comorbid with substance abuse disorders in adolescents. In adolescent girls, increased risk for substance abuse has been found among individuals with eating disorders, more so for those with binge symptoms than those with restrictive symptoms, who typically have more ascetic personality traits.

Behavioral, Social, and Environmental

There are behavioral correlates to substance use, including antisocial behavior and poor academic performance. Of the most powerful predictors of substance use are social influences including behavior and attitudes of family and friends. Family influences, such as parenting, parental substance use, permissive or tolerant attitudes of substance use by parents, and the quality of the relationship between parents and adolescents, are implicated in adolescent substance use. Specific family management styles that appear to promote substance use include inconsistent discipline, lack of maternal involvement in child's activities, use of guilt as a motivator, lack of praise for achievement, and unrealistic expectations.

The most powerful of the social influences are peer influences, particularly in terms of initial experimentation with substances and reinforcement of use by continued association with groups who use substances. Other social or environmental factors associated with substance use include deprivation, children who care for themselves after school if parents work, a low socioeconomic status, a history of sexual abuse or dating violence, and employment during the school year. Cultural factors also deserve strong consideration as risk factors for adolescent substance abuse.

Biologic and Genetic

Studies examining concordance rates in monozygotic versus dizygotic twins and adoption studies of twins reared apart show heritability of alcohol use and abuse and differences in transmissibility between males and females. Some studies show a three- to fourfold increase of alcohol and substance abuse disorders with a positive family history, and greater prevalence of use of gateway drugs with a paternal history of substance abuse disorder.

Screening, Assessment, Treatment, and Preventive Approaches

Approximately 10% of all adolescents would benefit from treatment interventions targeting SUDs, but fewer than 10% of adolescents with symptoms of dependence receive treatment, and those who are in the greatest need of treatment may be the least likely to initiate treatment.

Screening and Assessment

Pediatricians are traditionally positioned to have an ongoing relationship with both the adolescent and the family and are able to detect changes over time. On routine visits most adolescents do not present with dramatic or overt signs and symptoms that are easily accounted for by the effects of alcohol or drug use. A basic knowledge of changes related to substance use proves vital to screening: physical findings (such as weight loss, nasal irritation, chronic cough, needle tracks), personal habits (such as altered sleep pattern, new friends or interests, change in dress), academic performance (such as falling grades, truancy, suspension), and behavioral and psychologic symptoms (such as affective dysregulation, risk taking, stealing). Effective evaluation, history taking, and discussion with the adolescent should yield the desired information. Toxicologic screening for substance use should be limited to emergency situations (overdose, trauma), or in the context of a treatment contract.

Evidence-Based Treatment Modalities

Psychoeducational approaches are known to be of some benefit. Motivational enhancing techniques are employed to assist in forming therapeutic alliances and patient-generated goals. Individual and peer-enhanced motivational interviewing can be effective with adolescents.

There is evidence to suggest that cognitive–behavioral therapy (CBT) has significantly greater treatment efficacy with substance-abusing adolescents than do psychoeducational approaches. Individual CBT, family therapy, combined CBT and family therapy, and group interventions improve treatment outcomes. Interpersonal psychotherapy has been used with adolescents diagnosed with SUD. Studies do not clearly demonstrate one treatment superior to the others, or the optimal duration or intensity.

Family-based therapies improve treatment outcomes. Positive family functioning and relationships, especially the extent to which family members are encouraged to be assertive and self-sufficient, are associated with improved patient prognosis. *Multisystemic therapy* (MST) addresses the multiple risk factors for SUD (individual youth characteristics, family functioning, caregiver functioning, peer relations, school performance, indigenous family supports, and neighborhood characteristics) in a highly individualized and strategic fashion.

Therapeutic residential communities and *12-step programs* strongly endorse role modeling, which is of enormous importance for adolescents. Sponsors and peers serve as mentors to model adaptive behaviors and support the same. Adolescent-specific self-help groups are not present in most communities but could be valuable treatment resources. Skills development usually takes place in a group setting and includes relaxation therapy, recreation and various leisure skills, social skills, relationship enhancing, and other coping strategies with extensive opportunities for practice.

Levels of Care (Inpatient, Residential, Community/Outpatient)

The range of levels of care and programs available to the adolescent substance abuser include detoxification (DT), inpatient hospitalization, residential treatment centers, including therapeutic communities (TCs), outpatient programs (OPs), and self-help.

Preventive Approaches

Prevention of adolescent substance abuse must be multidimensional, complex, and dynamic. It must address a number of risk and protective factors, such as life skills and resistance skills, fostering healthy self-esteem, appropriate decision-making paradigms, stress management, communication skills, and assertiveness training. They are rooted in cognitive and affective systems and require a culturally competent approach to be effective with diverse populations.

In summary, future focus on adolescent SUDs should include an improvement of the quality and consistency of undergraduate and graduate medical education in substance abuse; the continued development of systematic and effective screening and assessment techniques and tools; a database of treatment facilities and specialists in substance abuse available to the primary care provider for appropriate referrals; improved targeting of prevention programs to high-risk adolescents; and expanded funding to develop, evaluate, and disseminate further evidence-based modalities and treatment programs.

Elderly Individuals

It is currently estimated that the prevalence of alcoholism alone is between 3% and 15% in community-dwelling elderly individuals, and as high as 18% to 44% in elderly general medical and psychiatric inpatients, respectively. A 1998 report by the Center for Substance Abuse Treatment stated that drug abuse affects up to 17% of adults older than age 60 years and constitutes an invisible epidemic. Of even greater concern, however, is the large number of elderly individuals using a variety of illicit drugs or prescription medications without proper physician direction.

Age-Prevalent Illness

Symptoms of substance abuse are often missed in elderly persons who tend to suffer more commonly from multiple pathologic conditions. Changes in cognition, behavior, or physical functioning may be wrongly blamed on some underlying medical condition. In fact, both the substance abuse and illness may cause the same problem. In the case of alcoholism, it is readily apparent that alcohol abuse may result in both acute and chronic problems.

Alcohol-Specific Problems

Diagnostic Considerations

There appear to be two types of elderly alcohol abusers: those who have a lifelong pattern of drinking, individuals who were probably alcoholic all their lives and are now elderly, and those who become alcoholic in their drinking patterns for the first time late in life. Depression, loneliness, and lack of social support are the most frequently cited antecedents to drinking for both groups.

As with alcoholics of any age, there is a strong tendency for geriatric alcoholics to try to hide their illness. It is not possible to apply all of the usual diagnostic criteria of alcohol abuse to the elderly alcoholic. Elderly individuals may very well experience amnesic periods while drinking, but again, this will almost always require a history from family or acquaintances. The alcoholic is often unaware of the memory lapses or adamantly denies them. Another strong indicator of alcohol abuse is continuation of drinking even after repeated warnings to stop for medical or cognitive reasons. In the presence of any of these signs, there should be a high index of suspicion of serious alcohol abuse.

The difficulty of recognizing substance abuse in older patients cannot be overemphasized. Patients presenting with symptoms of self-neglect, falls, cognitive and affective impairment, and social withdrawal should be carefully screened for substance abuse. Early identification that a substance abuse problem exists is mandatory if proper treatment is to be instituted. Although many argue that elderly persons are less likely to respond to therapy, studies demonstrate that they are as likely as or more likely than their younger counterparts to make a treatment contact, remain in treatment, and to recover. Programs specially tailored to the older person's needs may have an even higher rate of success.

Acute Alcohol Intoxication

Elderly persons are particularly prone to problems from acute alcohol intoxication. With age there is a decline in total body water content, primarily as a result of a change in extracellular fluid volume. Alcohol is rapidly distributed in body water after ingestion. This decrease in the available volume of distribution for alcohol results in an increase in the amount of alcohol reaching the central nervous system.

Clinically, the same amount of alcohol consumed in earlier years with impunity may now cause clinical symptoms such as slurred speech, instability, falls, and confusion. The elderly alcoholic may be mistakenly diagnosed with dementia or tumor, rather than a subdural hematoma resulting from a fall during a bout of drinking or acute alcoholism. Some regions of the brain are more vulnerable to ethanol than others, which is particularly relevant in older alcoholics. The basal ganglion, hippocampus, reticular activating system, and neocortex undergo neuronal loss with aging at a faster rate than do other regions of the brain. These changes result in impaired cognition and motor skills.

Alcohol also has an acute effect on cardiac muscle, leading to increased cardiac rate and output. Systolic blood pressure may be increased and blood shunted from the splanchnic circulation to the periphery. This latter phenomenon results in cutaneous vasodilation and loss of body heat. Alcohol increases acid production by the stomach's parietal cells. Because aging results in a reduction in parietal cell mass, a significant problem may not result unless an abnormal mucosal lining coexists. As the amount of alcohol consumed increases, there is greater risk of hyperemia, increased mucus production, and decreased acid secretion leading to acute gastritis. Resulting nausea and vomiting may lead to electrolyte and fluid imbalance earlier in the elderly person than in a younger person as a consequence of decreased physiologic reserve.

Although less common with age, alcohol may stimulate secretin production by the pancreas, resulting in increased pancreatic enzyme output. These proteolytic enzymes may lead to autodigestion of pancreatic tissue with the potential for producing an acute pancreatitis. Acute alcohol ingestion may result in alcoholic ketoacidosis. Arterial blood pH is reduced with a high anion gap; test results for serum ketones are usually only weakly positive because the predominant ketone is β-hydroxybutyrate, which is not detected by standard tests for ketones. Patients may vary from being alert, but ill, to frankly comatose. Supportive care is necessary until such time as metabolic balance returns. Although administration of bicarbonate is rarely needed, acid–base balance must be followed closely.

Elderly individuals are particularly prone to alcohol-induced hypoglycemia. Usually preceded by a period of starvation, glycogen stores are further impaired by the inhibition by alcohol of hepatic gluconeogenesis. Inhibition by alcohol of antidiuretic hormone (ADH) secretion from the posterior pituitary gland leads to prompt water diuresis. This more frequently results in symptoms of urinary incontinence in elderly persons. Neurologically, acute alcohol ingestion has a tendency to depress the central nervous system. Tendon reflexes may be hyperactive as a result of reduced inhibitory spinal motor neuronal activity.

Effects of Chronic Alcohol Ingestion

Alcohol can affect almost every cell, organ, and tissue in the body. Changes in vitamin D metabolism may result from the inability of the cirrhotic liver to hydroxylate vitamin D_3 at the 25 position to its more active form. This condition may be worsened by a diet deficient in vitamin D, malabsorption of fat, and/or concomitant use of either phenytoin or phenobarbital. The end result may be osteomalacia resulting in bone pain and fractures.

Because the liver is the main site of "binding globulin" production and catabolism of testosterone and conjugation of its metabolites with sulfuric or glucuronic acid, alcoholic changes may result in an increase in the ratio of physiologically free estrogen to free androgen. This may result in clinical manifestations including testicular atrophy, spider angiomata, palmar erythema, and gynecomastia.

An increased rate of conversion of adrenocortical steroid precursors to estrogen has also been reported. This is thought to result from decreased uptake of androstenedione by the diseased liver with a resultant increase in estrone production. Decreased concentrations of plasma testosterone, decreased testosterone production, increased testosterone clearance, and an altered hypothalamic–pituitary axis have all been noted following alcohol ingestion, even in the absence of liver disease. This may result in impotence, often wrongly dismissed as a function of increasing age. Because decreasing alcohol consumption may reverse the problem, intervention is key.

Chronic alcohol ingestion has both a direct and indirect effect on the cardiovascular system. Care must be taken not to blame cardiomyopathy on atherosclerotic disease when, in fact, the condition is alcohol induced. Alcohol is associated with cardiomegaly, cardiac fibrosis, microvascular infarcts and swelling, and altered subcellular myocardial components, glycogen, and lipid deposition. Clinically, chronic alcoholism is associated with reduced myocardial contractibility and output and with tachycardia.

Elderly persons who are chronic users of alcohol have higher rates of glossitis, stomatitis, and parotid gland enlargement. In addition, they have an increased incidence of squamous cell carcinoma of the oral pharynx, which is further exacerbated by chronic tobacco use. Chronic gastritis may lead to an iron-deficiency anemia. Anemia may also result from a deficiency in folate or vitamin B_{12}. Vitamin B_{12} absorption may decline because of a malfunctioning ileum, not a well-understood condition. Sideroblastic and hemolytic anemias are also more common. Anemia must never be attributed to the aging process and a thorough evaluation must be undertaken to delineate reversible causes, especially in the chronic alcohol abuser. Thrombocytopenia and macrocytosis, with or without granulocytopenia may also be noted as a result of direct bone marrow toxicity. In fact, alcohol is the most common cause of thrombocytopenia; failure of these parameters to return to normal within 1 week of abstinence, however, usually indicates another etiologic factor.

Perhaps the best-known complication of chronic alcohol abuse is liver toxicity. A spectrum of illness has been described ranging from fatty metamorphosis to cirrhosis. On examination, although patients may show typical clinical signs, including spider angiomata, icterus, ecchymoses, gynecomastia, testicular atrophy, muscle wasting, palmar erythema, and Dupuytren contracture, these findings may be easily mistaken for other disorders or wrongly blamed on advanced age. Even laboratory testing may be misleading as normal liver function tests may be noted as the liver fails and production of hepatic enzymes is diminished. Doses of medications cleared through the liver must be adjusted; patients must abstain from alcohol while consuming sufficient calories and vitamins; severe disease will require protein and sodium restriction.

Nutritional deficiencies are common in elderly alcoholics and may include protein-calorie malnutrition, select vitamin deficiencies, hypomagnesemia, hypophosphatemia, and hypocalcemia. The Wernicke and Korsakoff syndromes are associated abnormalities that result from a thiamine deficiency commonly found in alcoholics.

Alcohol also is often used to help with sleeping problems, a common complaint among elderly patients. In normal aging, total sleep time decreases to an average of approximately 6 hours per night. The proportion of rapid eye movement (REM) sleep decreases by nearly 25% and phase IV or deep sleep is significantly decreased in advanced age. Compared to younger adults, elderly individuals have an increased sleep latency, or length of time to fall asleep, and more frequent awakenings throughout the night. Regardless of the length of total time asleep, the decrease in deep sleep results in a less restful or effective sleep.

Alcohol does decrease sleep latency. A "nightcap" thus may help the elderly person fall asleep faster. This effect of alcohol can be subjectively perceived as a definite benefit. The other side of the coin, however, is that a significant alcohol-induced decrease in REM and delta sleep in the elderly alcoholic may result in practically no deep sleep at all.

Depression is a major concern in our elderly population, and the neurotransmitter serotonin has been extensively implicated in its development. Chronic alcoholism leads to substantially lower densities of serotonin transporters, which could serve to worsen pre-existing depression, or at least antagonize proper treatment.

Treatment

Many elderly alcoholics are frankly unaware of the effects of aging on the dynamics of alcohol use and do not realize how greatly alcohol affects their cognition. Often, a frank and direct discussion about the interaction of age and alcohol use can be extremely effective in limiting the use of alcohol by many older people.

For those patients whose alcohol use has resulted in dietary deficiencies and vitamin deficiencies, replacement of the vitamins and an adequate diet is essential. Medical support for those with alcohol-related medical illnesses is also of paramount importance. More specific measures include thiamine supplements of 100 mg daily for at least the first week of treatment. In addition, the patient may require hospitalization for the acute stages of detoxification. More specific medical treatments available for alcoholics such as disulfiram (Antabuse) and naltrexone (ReVia) have either not been studied in randomized controlled trials in the elderly population, or have not demonstrated increased abstinence after use. It is reasonable to offer pneumococcal vaccination to elderly abusers because they are prone to respiratory infections.

Many elderly patients benefit from participation in Alcoholics Anonymous, although some will object that the members of many Alcoholics Anonymous groups are much younger than the patient. Above all, the major objective of treatment of alcoholism in the elderly individual is clearly abstinence. As stated previously, programs specially tailored to elderly people appear to have a higher rate of success.

Problems Specific to Substance Abuse

All forms of addiction know no age limitation. In fact, elderly persons are at particularly high risk for addiction because of their more frequent use of medications to treat a variety of acute and chronic medical conditions, and a high prevalence of depression and anxiety disorders. A myriad of drug-related problems may occur at any age. These include dental problems such as root caries, advanced periodontal disease, and acute necrotizing ulcerative gingivitis; bacterial infections including abscess formation, cellulitis, septicemia, lymphangitis, and thrombophlebitis; endocarditis; tetanus; malaria; tuberculosis; osteomyelitis; septic arthritis; hepatitis; venereal disease; AIDS; and pneumonitis.

Neurologic disturbances are perhaps the most frequently encountered problems. These may result from direct effects of the drugs themselves on the central nervous system or from infections or emboli. Drug use should be considered in all cases of stroke, seizure, altered behavior, or change in cognition.

Cocaine and amphetamine abuse, even in low dosage, is associated with a higher rate of intracranial hemorrhage leading to a cerebral vascular accident. Tics, choreiform or athetoid movements, ataxia, and gait disturbances are also more commonly noted in frequent users of these agents.

Perhaps one of the most underreported problems affecting elderly individuals is the all-too-frequent use of sedative–hypnotics, particularly among women. The most commonly misused prescription drug classes among the elderly population are sedative–hypnotics, antianxiety agents, and analgesics. Diazepam (Valium), codeine, meprobamate (Equanil), and flurazepam (Dalmane) are on top with 92% of those abusing these drugs doing so for more than 5 years. The use of triplicate prescriptions may reduce the use of these agents or at least help alert authorities to potential abuses. Unfortunately, these agents, especially those with longer half-lives, often result in unwanted side effects that affect functional capacity and cognition, placing the older person at greater risk of falling and institutionalization.

Conclusion

Elderly persons have many unique characteristics that predispose them to higher rates of substance abuse, particularly alcohol and "prescribed" medications. A thorough understanding of what constitutes normal age-related changes, age-prevalent disease, and the atypical presentation of illness will enable the health professional to better recognize and successfully treat this problem.

Suggested Readings

Gambert SR, Albrecht CR III The elderly. In: Lowinson JH, Ruiz P, Millman RB, et al., eds. *Substance abuse: a comprehensive textbook*, 4th ed. Philadelphia: Lippincott Williams & Wilkins; 2005:1038–1048.

Jaffee SL, Simkin DR. Alcohol and drug abuse in adolescents: In: Lewis M, ed. *Child and adolescent psychiatry: a comprehensive textbook*. Philadelphia: Lippincott Williams & Wilkins; 2002:895–911.

Juliana P, Goodman C. Children of substance-abusing parents. In: Lowinson JH, Ruiz P, Millman RB, et al., eds. *Substance abuse: a comprehensive textbook*, 4th ed. Philadelphia: Lippincott Williams & Wilkins; 2005:1013–1021.

Patterson TL, Jeste DV. The potential impact of the baby-boom generation on substance abuse among elderly persons. *Psychiatr Serv.* 1999; 50(9):1184–1188.

Pumariega AJ, Kilgus MD, Rodriguez L. Adolescents. In: Lowinson JH, Ruiz P, Millman RB, et al., eds. *Substance abuse: a comprehensive textbook*, 4th ed. Philadelphia: Lippincott Williams & Wilkins; 2005:1021–1037.

Uziel-Miller ND, Lyon JS. Specialized substance abuse treatment for women and their children: an analysis of program design. *J Subst Abuse Treat.* 2000;19:355–367.

Section VIII

WOMEN'S ISSUES

40

ALCOHOL AND DRUGS AMONG WOMEN

Pharmacology of Alcohol in Women

Single doses of ethanol produce higher peak blood alcohol concentrations (BACs) in women than in men given equal doses of ethanol per pound of body weight. This may be explained, in part, by the higher average content of body water in men than women (65% vs. 51%, respectively). Because ethanol is distributed in total body water, a standard dose will be less diluted in a woman. However, body water content differences do not fully account for differences in peak BACs, nor can they account for the observation that sex differences emerge after oral but not intravenous ethanol administration. There is substantial first-pass metabolism of ethanol in the human gastric mucosa, through oxidation by alcohol dehydrogenase (ADH). Normal women were found to have much lower levels of gastric ADH and to metabolize only about a quarter as much alcohol as normal men under standard conditions, thus absorbing significantly more consumed alcohol. These gender differences tend to disappear in individuals age 50 years and older.

Women in treatment for alcohol problems frequently relate their drinking to their menstrual cycles. Women who meet diagnostic criteria for premenstrual syndrome have been found to drink more heavily than controls and to have a high rate of alcohol abuse and dependence. In normally cycling nonalcoholic women, there are significantly more negative moods, more drinking to relieve tension or depression, and more solitary drinking during the menstrual period itself, rather than the premenstruum. These findings suggest that increased use correlates with premenstrual symptomatology rather than the menstrual cycle phase itself.

Alcohol Consumption and Women's Health

Heavy drinking has a uniformly negative effect on women's health. There is some evidence, however, for an association between low to moderate levels of alcohol consumption and decreased risk of coronary artery disease and ischemic stroke. Alcohol intake is directly related both to the risk for hypertension and to overall cardiovascular mortality in women. Evidence of a relationship between alcohol consumption and breast cancer has accumulated over a number of years. Meta-analyses of several epidemiologic studies demonstrate a dose–response relationship between alcohol intake and risk in women, although some studies point to a relatively modest association. However, there is evidence suggesting an increased risk with daily ingestion of two or more drinks.

Prolonged heavy drinking is also known to be an etiologic factor in many diseases of the gastrointestinal, neuromuscular, cardiovascular, and other body systems. There is evidence that women may develop many of these problems more rapidly than men. Several studies demonstrate the development of liver cirrhosis at lower levels of alcohol intake (even accounting for differences in body weight) and for shorter periods of time, when compared to men. In addition, alcoholic women develop both myopathy and cardiomyopathy at lower rates of alcohol intake than men and suffer greater declines in cardiac function.

Effects of Drinking on Sexual Functioning and Reproduction in Women

The effects of drinking on women's sexuality and reproduction are complex and not completely understood. Single doses of alcohol seem to have little effect on levels of female sex hormones. However, acute alcohol intoxication produces an increase in plasma testosterone levels in women, whereas the opposite occurs with men. This effect may be relevant to problems such as inhibition of ovulation, decrease in gonadal mass, infertility, and obstetrical, gynecologic, and sexual dysfunctions.

Women who drink during pregnancy risk significant harm to their offspring, including fetal alcohol syndrome (FAS). FAS is the most common nonhereditary cause of birth defects, and can include prenatal and postnatal growth retardation, central nervous system abnormalities, usually with mental retardation, a characteristic facial dysmorphism (e.g., short palpebral fissures, epicanthic folds, and maxillary hypoplasia), and an array of other birth defects such as microcephaly, altered palmar creases, and heart abnormalities, among others. The full syndrome is seen in the offspring of approximately one third of alcoholic women drinking the equivalent of 10 standard drinks daily, but other fetal alcohol effects, such as spontaneous abortion, reduced birth weight, and behavior changes, are associated with lower levels of alcohol intake.

Epidemiology of Alcohol Use in Women

Surveys of drinking have uniformly found that women are less likely to drink than men, whereas women are more frequent users of prescribed psychoactive drugs. In the early 1980s, a US national survey of male and female drinking practices found that the highest rates of alcohol-related problems occurred in the youngest age group (21 to 34 years old), whereas the highest proportion of heavier drinkers was found in the 35 to 49 years age group. Married women had the lowest overall problem rates, whereas those cohabiting in "common law" had the highest. The investigators also noted a strong correlation between the drinking patterns of women and that of their "significant others," more so than for men.

Using DSM-IV-TR criteria, it has been estimated that there were 2,068,000 adult women (age 18 years and older) in the United States who could be diagnosed as suffering from alcohol abuse and 1,950,000 who could be diagnosed as suffering from alcohol dependence during the previous 12 months, for a total of 4,018,000 women affected. This compares with 11,167,000 adult men suffering from alcohol abuse or dependence.

Factors Influencing Alcoholism in Women

Genetic Factors

Twin studies generally demonstrate a stronger genetic influence on drinking practices, as well as on the development of alcoholism, in males than in females. Epidemiologic studies, however, yield similar heritability estimates (e.g., 50% to 60%) across genders, although the sources of genetic influence do not completely overlap.

Psychologic Factors

A 27-year follow-up study of the drinking status of American adults who had taken part in an earlier survey of college drinking practices found women who had scored highest on a "feeling adjustment" scale, which contained items such as drinking to relieve shyness, drinking to get high, drinking to be gay, and drinking to get along better on dates, had the highest level of later drinking problems.

Results from the National Institute of Mental Health Epidemiological Catchment Area study found that the lifetime prevalence of alcohol abuse or dependence was more than three times greater in women who reported a history of sexual assault. A population-based study of adult female twins shows that sexual abuse in childhood has a particularly important impact in the development of substance use disorders in women, with the odds ratio increasing progressively from nongenital to genital contact and, especially, intercourse.

Several studies have found the lifetime prevalence of dual diagnosis higher among alcoholic women than alcoholic men. For example, one study found that 19% of women who fulfilled diagnostic criteria for alcohol abuse or dependence at some time during their lifetime also fulfilled criteria for a lifetime diagnosis of major depression (compared to 5% of men). Other psychiatric diagnoses found in alcohol-dependent or alcohol-abusing women include anxiety disorders, sexual disorders, bulimia, and borderline personality disorder. Men outnumber women in only two diagnostic categories: antisocial personality and pathologic gambling.

Sociocultural Factors

There is little doubt that sociocultural factors significantly influence the drinking patterns of women. The practical result of social stigma applied to alcohol-dependent women is to keep them in hiding. Women tend to drink alone. High rates of alcoholic women drink at home, and married women, employed women, and upper socioeconomic status women are likely to drink alone. Sociocultural factors can also be protective to women. Protective social factors for women can include less social pressure to drink, different drinking customs, for example, drinking primarily in mixed groups (whereas men drink in both mixed and all-male groups), and the relatively limited range of occasions in women's lives in which drinking is expected.

Clinical Features of Alcoholism in Women

1. Despite differences between men and women in the later age of women's onset of drinking and total amount of alcohol consumed by women, female alcoholics appear for treatment at about the same age as male alcoholics and with the same severity of alcohol dependence. This points to a more rapid development or "telescoping" of the course of the illness in women.
2. Alcoholic women drink significantly less than alcoholic men. As the alcoholic woman ages, her tolerance for alcohol falls and she will drink even less than before.
3. Women entering alcoholism treatment are more likely to be married to or living with an alcoholic sexual partner, or to be divorced or separated, whereas men entering treatment are more likely to be married to a nonalcoholic spouse.
4. Alcoholic women are more likely than alcoholic men to date the onset of pathologic drinking to a particular stressful event.
5. Alcohol-dependent women are more likely to report both psychiatric symptoms and dual diagnosis. Depression is especially common.
6. A history of suicide attempts is more frequent in female than male alcohol-dependent patients.
7. Alcohol-dependent women are more likely to be motivated to enter treatment because of health and family problems, whereas for men, job and legal problems, particularly arrests for driving while intoxicated, are more prevalent.
8. Alcoholic women are more likely to reach treatment with a history of other substance abuse along with their alcoholism, particularly tranquilizers, sedatives, and amphetamines, although they are less likely to be abusers of illicit drugs. The drugs these women abuse have usually been prescribed by their physicians.
9. Women who commit homicide have a much higher prevalence of alcohol abuse and dependence than the general population of women, and are particularly likely to meet diagnostic criteria for both alcoholism and personality disorder.

Identification of Alcohol Use Disorders in Women

Women tend to be underrepresented in alcoholism treatment. Alcoholic women may be reached through systematic screening in the doctor's office, in hospitals, and in medical clinics. Instruments that have been used for case finding among women include the Michigan Alcohol Screening Test (MAST), its short version (SMAST), the four CAGE (cut down [on drinking], annoyance, guilt [about drinking], [need for] eyeopener) questions, and the TWEAK (Tolerance, Worry, Eye-opener, Amnesia, Cut-down). Laboratory testing can also be helpful in screening.

Treatment of Alcohol Use Disorders in Women

There is little research to indicate the best way to treat alcoholism in women. However, sensitivity to women's special needs and problems is critical to treatment success. Special attention should be given to a history of physical and sexual abuse. Careful physical and psychiatric diagnoses are critical for treatment success. Evaluation and treatment of family members is also of special value in women patients. Education about alcohol (and other drugs) should include information about the effects of these drugs during pregnancy, about birth control, and about the prevention of AIDS and other infectious diseases transmitted through blood and body fluids.

Parenting education may be particularly important for alcohol-dependent women. Childcare services are a critical factor in allowing many alcohol-dependent women to participate in treatment. The lack of adequate childcare has been identified as a major barrier to treatment for women. Couples' and family therapies have been useful in some cases as an adjunct to self-help and/or other counseling, which focus on the alcohol-dependent woman herself. Female role models, in the form of female treatment staff and recovering alcoholic and other drug-dependent women, are helpful in treatment. Self-help groups, such as Alcoholics Anonymous and Women for Sobriety, are an important source of support. The low self-esteem of the alcohol-dependent woman should be addressed in treatment. Special techniques such as assertiveness training may be employed. Sexism and its consequences (e.g., unequal societal roles, undervaluation of women's contributions to societal and family functioning, underemployment, inadequate pay) should be explored in relationship to the experience of the alcohol-dependent woman.

Special care must be taken to avoid creating iatrogenic drug dependence. Benzodiazepines, other sedatives, and dependence-producing analgesics should be avoided. Special populations of alcohol-dependent women need focused attention. African American, Hispanic, and Native American women have special needs and may suffer from particularly intense stigmatization. Lesbian women are believed to have a high prevalence of alcohol and other drug problems and may profit from treatment in specially oriented groups. Alcohol-dependent women in the criminal justice system are often overlooked, although their need for specific treatment is no less than that of men.

Treatment Outcome for Alcohol Use Disorders in Women

The literature on alcoholism treatment has little to offer in outcome studies of treatment designed specifically for women. However, a number of studies have reported outcome data by sex. These studies conclude that adult males and females treated together for alcoholism in the same programs do about equally well.

Women suffering from alcoholism experience a high rate of mortality, both when compared to the general population of women and to rates of excess mortality in alcoholic men. For example, nearly 4,000 male and 1,000 female patients were followed over periods ranging from 2 to 22 years, after hospital treatment for alcoholism. Excess mortality was higher for the alcoholic women (5.2 times the expected rate) than for the men (3 times the expected rate).

Prevention and Policy Issues

Prevention of alcohol problems in women should be simultaneously addressed by work to combat stigma while preserving the custom of abstinence or moderation for women. The best strategy would seem to be education about the special sensitivity to alcohol in women, the teratogenicity of alcohol, the risk involved in using alcohol to medicate emotional states, the risk of mixing alcohol and sedatives, and other relevant issues.

Removal of barriers that keep alcohol-dependent women from obtaining treatment are needed. A major barrier is the lack of childcare. Many alcoholic women are single parents, or, if married, lack the resources to provide adequate care for their children. Another major barrier to treatment is lack of third-party payment for care. Many women in need of alcoholism treatment are single or divorced and unemployed or underemployed, leaving them without adequate health insurance coverage. Legal definitions of child abuse and neglect may create additional treatment barriers. In parts of the United States, the habitual or addictive use of alcohol or drugs by a parent makes that parent a child abuser or neglecter by definition. This becomes a barrier, particularly for disadvantaged and single mothers who must rely on public social service agencies for childcare in order to enter treatment. Asking for help in such a situation puts them in jeopardy of losing custody of their children. Paradoxically, continuing alcohol dependency without seeking help does not, in general, have this effect. Child abuse laws can be altered in their language, not only to remove this barrier, but also to provide an incentive for the alcoholic parent to accept treatment.

Women and Other Drugs Other Drugs and Women

Epidemiology of Drug Use in Women

In the United States, the National Comorbidity Survey investigated psychiatric diagnoses of a representative sample of Americans ages 15 to 54 years, and found a lifetime prevalence of drug abuse of 3.5% among women and 5.4% among men; the lifetime prevalence of drug dependence was 5.9% among women and 9.2% among men (male to female ratios of 1.5:1 and 1.6:1, respectively). Data from the 2000 U.S. National Household Survey on Drug Abuse confirmed the overall male to female ratio of 1.5:1 regarding current illicit drug use (5.0% for women and 7.7% for men). Current overall rates of tobacco use in the United States show that men still outnumber women, but the difference is small (26.9% vs. 23.1%, respectively). In the year 2000, girls 12 to 17 years of age were somewhat more likely to use prescription drugs not prescribed by a doctor, including pain relievers, tranquilizers, stimulants, and sedatives, than were boys (3.3% vs. 2.7%, respectively). Women, as compared to men, are also more likely to be prescribed benzodiazepines.

Factors Influencing Drug Use in Women

Genetic Factors

A series of twin studies investigated the contributions of genetic and environmental influences to drug use and drug use disorders across genders. Overall, environmental factors seem to be more important than genetic factors in drug use and abuse. However, genetic influences for drug use and abuse/dependence are greater for males than females (heritability of 33% for men and 11% for women), whereas environmental factors are higher for females than for males.

Psychologic Factors

Epidemiologic data document that, excluding comorbid alcohol use disorders, rates of psychiatric comorbidity are higher among women than men with drug use disorders.

Rates of comorbid mood and anxiety disorders are higher among women, whereas rates of comorbid alcohol use disorders and antisocial personality disorder are higher among men. Male addicts are also more likely to be pathologic gamblers and to report attention-deficit–hyperactivity disorder. Tobacco use is strongly associated with clinically relevant depressive symptomatology in women, making it harder for women than for men to quit smoking.

A history of traumatic life events is a risk factor for the development of drug use disorders. The lifetime prevalence of these disorders is more than four times higher in women with a history of sexual assault.

Sociocultural Factors

Social factors that once protected women from initiating drug use are weaker now. However, the social stigma applied to female addicts still prevents many women from accessing appropriate treatment. Depending on the drug, the male to female ratio of addiction treatment admissions varies from 1.5:1 for cocaine to 3.3:1 for cannabis.

Drug use in women is associated with victimization. Trauma and posttraumatic stress disorder are more likely to precede the development of drug use disorders in women than in men. In addition, women's drug use is influenced by drug-using sexual partners, with most women reporting having been first introduced to drug use and drug injection by a male partner.

Evaluation and Diagnosis

Because of stigma, addiction treatment entry and diagnosis are often delayed. Barriers include fear of loss of children, single-parent responsibilities, and opposition or lack of support from an active drug-using partner, among others. Health professionals often do not feel comfortable in asking women about their substance use because they believe that women might feel offended. Women with drug-related problems are less likely to seek specialized help than are men, more often consulting a general practitioner (suggesting screening should be routinely performed as part of any medical consultation). The use of a screening questionnaire (such as the Drug Abuse Screening Test) and laboratory testing of urine or blood may be helpful.

Problematic areas are also different for women, who are less likely to report legal problems and are less often court-ordered to treatment than men, but probably more often than alcohol-dependent women. Drug-dependent women often report domestic violence and sexual abuse, as well as suicide attempts and overdoses. These issues need to be addressed in a safe environment and time is often required to gain sufficient trust to discuss them. Follow-up appointments may provide more information than single-session assessments.

Evaluating and referring to treatment a drug-using partner, and providing orientation to a nondrug-using partner, are crucial in the treatment of drug-dependent women. Involvement of other family members in the recovery process should be considered, as well as assessment of children, coupled with referrals when appropriate. Medical assessment is recommended because of the high prevalence of drug-related illnesses. Psychiatric evaluation is also an integral part of the assessment of drug-dependent women because of high rates of comorbidity.

Cocaine

Pharmacologic Effects

Women seem to respond differently to than men to cocaine, but the direction of the differences and their explanation is not clear. There are menstrual phase differences in cocaine plasma levels (higher in the follicular than in the luteal phase), although not in the subjective response to cocaine in females. This may be related to the nasal mucosa of women in the luteal phase being more viscous, leading to decreased cocaine absorption and decreased plasma levels.

Course of Illness

Data regarding gender differences in the progression to cocaine dependence are confusing. Some studies suggest that women progress from first use to treatment faster than men, whereas other studies do not report such a "telescoped" progression. Similarly, studies of gender differences in the age of onset of cocaine use also provide mixed results, with some suggesting that women start using cocaine earlier than men, whereas others support the opposite or no gender differences.

The age of women entering treatment for crack cocaine abuse has increased significantly over time (women aged 35 years and older comprised only 19% of total US admissions in 1992 vs. 43% in 1998). The same is true of women with long-term use of crack cocaine (in 1992, only 20% of women entering treatment reported crack cocaine use for more than 10 years; this figure rose to 42% in 1998).

Health Consequences

Cocaine use represents a risk factor for human immunodeficiency virus (HIV) infection and other sexually transmitted diseases. Also, it is associated with a variety of health problems, including cardiovascular and central nervous system diseases. Unfortunately, studies of cocaine-related health consequences that take gender into account are rare.

Effects on Sexual Functioning and Reproduction

Cocaine use seems to be associated with a variety of alterations in the menstrual cycle, with amenorrhea and luteal phase dysfunction, as well as galactorrhea and infertility. Hyperprolactinemia induced by cocaine effects on dopaminergic systems is associated with these abnormalities. Also, cocaine use is associated with increased levels of luteinizing hormone in cocaine-abusing women. Although it is difficult to attribute these abnormalities to cocaine use itself because many women report concomitant use of other substances, animal studies seem to corroborate these findings.

Much has been published about the effects of cocaine use on pregnancy and offspring. Cocaine use in the perinatal period, whether or not associated with opiate use, is related to higher rates of medical complications such as syphilis, gonorrhea, and hepatitis. Cocaine use in this period is also associated with increased rates of abruptio placentae, meconium staining, premature rupture of membranes, and low birth weight, as well as genitourinary and abdominal wall abnormalities. These effects are independent of other confounding substance use.

Research and the public reaction to cocaine use during pregnancy are problematic. Earlier reports referred to a so-called crack baby syndrome. Such descriptions, not supported by scientific evidence, led to punishment and stigma for the mothers and children involved. A systematic review of 36 prospective studies concluded that there is no evidence that cocaine alone (independent of other risk factors such as malnutrition and other drug use, including alcohol and tobacco) affects physical and developmental growth in the first 6 years.

Treatment Response

Few studies have analyzed the gender-related differences in treatment response of individuals with cocaine use disorders. The National Institute on Drug Abuse Collaborative Cocaine Treatment Study found no gender differences in the outcome of the four psychosocial treatments evaluated. Other studies, however, have described better outcomes for women than for men, even though the women had more severe cocaine-related problems at baseline.

Cannabis

Pharmacologic Effects

Research with rats suggests that gender differences in the effects of tetrahydrocannabinol in the hypothalamus may exist. Specifically, there are sex-related effects of tetrahydrocannabinol on corticotropin-releasing hormone and pro-opiomelanocortin gene expression in the hypothalamus. Whether these differences also exist in humans is not known.

Course of Illness

Early conduct problems seem to be more strongly associated with initiation of cannabis use among adolescent women than men. Once cannabis use starts, however, no gender differences in patterns of use were described in a large Australian survey of adolescents. Cannabis use, regardless of gender, is strongly associated with depression, conduct problems, and use of alcohol and other drugs. The progression to cannabis dependence is accelerated in women, despite similar age of initiation of regular use. Women in treatment for substance-related disorders present a lower current rate of cannabis use disorders compared to men.

Effects on Sexual Functioning and Reproduction

Acute cannabis use during the luteal phase of the menstrual cycle is associated with a significant decrease in plasma levels of prolactin and luteinizing hormone that may, in turn, be associated with adverse effects on women's reproductive function. Chronic cannabis use, however, does not seem to be associated with altered hormone levels in women.

Tetrahydrocannabinol is highly lipophilic and may remain in fat tissue for weeks. Because it is slowly released, it may exert potentially dangerous effects on pregnancy and the resulting offspring. Weekly cannabis use during pregnancy is associated with abruptio placentae and prematurity. Cannabis use during pregnancy was not significantly related to increased risk of perinatal morbidity and mortality in a large study involving more than 12,000 pregnant women, but it was clearly associated with decreased birth weight.

Regular use of cannabis during pregnancy is significantly associated with long-term cognitive impairments in offspring, particularly in executive functions involving attentional behavior and visual analysis/hypothesis testing. A prospective study documented that effects of prenatal cannabis exposure on children at 10 years of age, controlled for potential confounders, included hyperactivity, impulsivity, and attention deficits leading to delinquent behavior.

Treatment Response

The few studies examining treatment outcome for cannabis use disorder do not report analysis by gender. Factors associated with cessation of cannabis use among adolescents differ by gender. Although reasons for quitting cannabis use among boys vary, among girls the most important reason is becoming pregnant and assuming parenting responsibilities.

Opiates

Pharmacologic Effects

Women report higher rates of nausea and analgesia associated with acute opiate use than do men. Women clear methadone from the bloodstream more slowly than men, and thus have a longer plasma half-life for the drug.

Course of Illness

Opiate-dependent women are more likely to have a substance-using partner and to be initiated into drug injection by a partner than are their male counterparts, although women are more likely to inhale heroin, whereas men are more likely to inject it. A faster progression of opiate dependence has been described among heroin-dependent females in comparison to males.

Health Consequences

Opiate use is associated with higher morbidity and mortality rates among women as compared to men. Female opiate users may combine two important risk factors for acquiring HIV, hepatitis B and C, and other sexually transmitted diseases: sex with an injecting partner and needle sharing.

Effects on Sexual Functioning and Reproduction

Opiate use during pregnancy is associated with a number of complications, with an increased risk of hepatitis and HIV infection that is associated with its injection, and increased relative mortality, probably as a consequence of a combination of opiate effect and chaotic lifestyle.

The recommended treatment for pregnant women with opiate dependence is methadone stabilization, cautioning that methadone-maintained women may need adjustment of dosage when pregnant because of increased body mass. After delivery, the dose should be returned to previously established levels.

Treatment Response

In a study of methadone treatment, women on admission reported more dysfunctional families of origin and greater prior and current psychologic and medical problems, as well as HIV risk behaviors, but higher motivation, fewer legal problems, and less alcohol use than men. Both genders improved with treatment, as evidenced by reduced substance use, criminal involvement, and other health-related risky behaviors, but women needed more interventions for psychologic and crisis issues, employment issues, and medical referrals. Women were also more likely to seek additional treatment following discharge.

Tobacco

Pharmacologic Effects

Even though they smoke similar numbers of cigarettes daily, female heavy smokers exhibit lower nicotine plasma levels, but greater exposure to smoke than male heavy smokers, reflecting more and larger puffs to achieve the same nicotine intake.

Course of Illness

Epidemiologic data suggest that women are particularly at risk for becoming dependent on nicotine as compared to men, having higher rates of dependence, with more symptoms, at the same quantity of nicotine smoked. Among adolescents more girls than boys are now initiating tobacco use; girls are also less likely to quit.

Health Consequences

Gender influences a number of smoking-related health issues with greater effects for female smokers in comparison to male smokers, including immune responses, cardiovascular diseases, and different types of cancer, such as lung and bladder. It is suggested that the gender difference in cancer risks cannot be attributed to differences in baseline exposure, smoking history, or body size alone. Rather, a higher susceptibility to tobacco carcinogens in women is hypothesized. In the United States, smoking-related lung cancer is now the first cause of cancer-related death among women, ahead of breast cancer.

Effects on Sexual Functioning and Reproduction

Associations between smoking and a number of menstrual abnormalities, fertility problems, and early menopause in women have been reported, which are probably caused by nicotine inhibiting luteinizing hormone and prolactin release. Oxytocin stimulation has also been described and may be the basis for the negative effects of tobacco on pregnancy, such as premature delivery. Other problems include fetal growth retardation, obstetric complications, and neonatal mortality. Risks for sudden infant death syndrome, low birth weight and height, and hypertension are increased.

Treatment Response

Female smokers have higher relapse rates following nicotine replacement therapy than do men. High levels of self-perceived stress predict difficulty in quitting smoking among women, but are not related to abstinence in men. For women attempting to quit smoking, the related weight gain is a concern and strategies to deal with this issue are likely to increase the efficacy of smoking-cessation treatments.

Other Drugs

Little work has been done on drugs such as benzodiazepines, sedatives, and amphetamines in relationship to women, despite high rates of nonmedical use of these medications (either prescribed or not). Some facts deserve special attention. For example, the effects of these drugs, particularly the new "designer" drugs, in women, as well as their effects on pregnancy and the neonate, have not been sufficiently studied. Methylenedioxymethamphetamine, present in ecstasy, produces more intense psychoactive effects in women than in men. Also, higher doses are associated with perceptual alterations more strongly in women, indicating an increased susceptibility of women to the serotonin-releasing effects of ecstasy.

Treatment of Drug Use Disorders in Women

1. Women entering treatment for drug use disorders report extremely elevated rates of suicide attempts and suicidal ideation. Detailed psychiatric assessment is essential to determine suicidal risk and depression that may require specific treatment.
2. Personality disorders may be more frequent than Axis I disorders among women with substance use disorders.
3. Screening for HIV, hepatitis B and C, syphilis, and other sexually transmitted diseases is an essential part of the evaluation of women with drug use disorders entering treatment, particularly for those who inject drugs intravenously.
4. Women entering treatment worry about potential weight gain, and those with comorbid eating disorders may decompensate. The opportunity to discuss healthy nutritional choices and exercise should not be missed.
5. All-women treatment groups may be extremely helpful in addressing difficult topics, such as sexual abuse and victimization.
6. Drug-dependent women can be single or living alone with their children, and it is often difficult for them to enter treatment because of a lack of childcare. Facilities that can accommodate both mother and children are particularly attractive to this group.

Suggested Readings

Blume SB, Zilberman ML. Alcohol and women. In Lowinson JH, Ruiz P, Millman RB, Langrod JG (eds.): *Substance Abuse: A Comprehensive Textbook,* Fourth Edition. Philadelphia, Pennsylvania, Lippincott Williams & Wilkins, 2005, 2005:1049–1064.

Compton WM III, Cottler LB, Ben Abdallah A, et al. Substance dependence and other psychiatric disorders among drug dependent subjects: race and gender correlates. *Am J Addict.* 2000;9:113–125.

Kendler KS, Bulik CM, Silberg J, et al. Childhood sexual abuse and adult psychiatric and substance use disorders in women: an epidemiological and cotwin control analysis. *Arch Gen Psychiatry.* 2000;57:953–959.

Rosenbaum M, Murphy S. Women's research and policy issues. In: Lowinson JH, Ruiz P, Millman RB, et al., eds. *Substance abuse: a comprehensive textbook*, 4th ed. Philadelphia: Lippincott Williams & Wilkins; 2005:1075–1092.

Zilberman ML, Blume SB. Drugs and women. In: Lowinson JH, Ruiz P, Millman RB, et al., eds. *Substance abuse: a comprehensive textbook*, 4th ed. Philadelphia: Lippincott Williams & Wilkins; 2005:1064–1075.

Zilberman ML, Tavares H, Andrade AG. Discriminating drug-dependent women from alcoholic women and drug-dependent men. *Addict Behav.* 2003;28(7):1343–1349.

Zilberman ML, Tavares H, Blume SB, et al. Towards best practices in the treatment of women with addictive disorders. *Addict Disord Their Treat.* 2002;1:39–46.

Section IX

SPECIAL GROUPS/SETTINGS

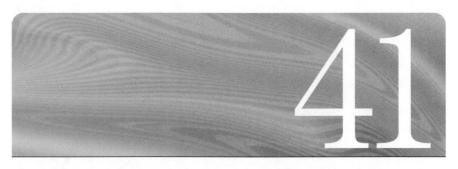

DISABILITY AND REHABILITATION ISSUES

Relationships between Alcohol and Other Drug Abuse and Disability

Substance abuse may be related to disability in several ways. First, it may contribute to the cause of disability, such as driving while intoxicated, sustaining a cocaine-induced stroke, or a gangrenous infection resulting from cocaine or heroin injections. Second, alcohol and other drug abuse may adversely affect the physical rehabilitation process following injury by causing behavioral alterations or by impairing cognition. Because rehabilitation requires the ability to learn, cognitive and learning impairments can limit the benefits of rehabilitation services. Third, physical rehabilitation outcomes may be affected by medical complications resulting from continued substance use. Finally, substance abuse may disrupt vocational rehabilitation and reverse the cost-effectiveness of rehabilitation in persons who continue to abuse alcohol and other drugs.

Patterns of illicit drug use in 1,876 individuals actively involved in vocational rehabilitation services in three midwestern states have been conducted. Prevalence rates of almost all illicit and nonmedical use drug categories were significantly higher in the disability cohort than in the general population. The rates of crack use in the past month and past year were more than three times higher than the prevalence rates in the general population. Factors associated with use included younger age, male gender, low income, having family or friends using illicit drugs, greater feelings of hostility and risk-taking, lower self-esteem, and believing that having a disability entitles one to use substances. Unrelated to substance use rates were disability etiology (congenital vs. acquired), presence of multiple disabilities, chronic pain, and unemployment. Clearly, the extent of alcohol and other drug abuse remains a concern in rehabilitation settings. Fortunately, the frequency with which these problems have been investigated and efforts made to implement assessment, treatment, and prevention programs has increased in the past 20 years.

Factors Associated with Alcohol and Other Drug Use by Persons with Disabilities

Depression, anxiety, social isolation, medical complications, and self-neglect are important factors to consider when alcohol and other drugs are used by persons who incur traumatic injury. One study found that 30% of patients with spinal cord injury (SCI) met diagnostic criteria for a depressive disorder. Longer lengths of stay at a regional trauma center were associated with psychiatric comorbidity, including substance use. The use of alcohol and other substances by persons with traumatic brain injury (TBI) can contribute to greater cognitive and motor skill impairment. The use of substances following TBI is potentially dangerous when combined with prescription medications and may increase the likelihood of seizures. Patterns of substance use postinjury has been examined following recent SCI; they asked patients to report substance use for the 6 months prior to, and for 6 and 18 months following, injury. In particular, alcohol and marijuana use persisted after declining for the initial 6 months following onset of injury; those who used substances for the 6 months prior to injury were more likely to be at risk for use following injury. Substance use following SCI was associated with lower employment rates, lower levels of disability acceptance, and higher levels of depressive symptoms.

A task force sponsored by the National Head Injury Foundation conducted a national survey of alcohol and drug abuse problems among patients with TBI. Approximately 40% of all patients had moderate to severe substance abuse problems before injury, with alcohol the most frequently abused substance. Of the surveyed postacute rehabilitation facilities, only half reported providing substance abuse services. The task force concluded that substance abuse problems are extensive in patients with TBI, service provision is inadequate in rehabilitation facilities, and structured treatment programs are required to meet the multiple needs of such patients.

Blindness and Visual Impairments

Few studies have examined the extent of alcohol and other drug abuse among individuals with visual impairments, including blindness. Risk factors for substance abuse in this population include social isolation, an excess of unstructured time, and underemployment. Individuals with visual loss at adolescence or young adult age resulting from early trauma or genetic etiology probably experience distinct risk factors. Special consideration should be given to even moderate drinking in persons with visual impairments as it can exacerbate underlying health problems for those whose visual loss is related to diabetes and glaucoma. Impaired balance, mobility, and orientation are also special issues. Treatment and prevention programs that use printed materials should consider the communication needs of individuals with visual impairments; talking books and Braille materials may be needed.

Deafness and Hearing Impairments

Etiology has a major influence on the nature and extent of communication problems and consequent social integration for persons with hearing loss. Hearing loss may be the result of a congenital disorder, or may be acquired later in life as the result of injury or disease. People with congenital deafness tend to form communities that give rise to a unique culture. The fluency with which a person communicates with speech reading, vocal training, gesturing, or sign language affects acculturation and assimilation within the hearing community. Insensitivity to communication needs by the general population contributes to social stigma, a major cause of social isolation and a risk factor for substance abuse.

The few studies examining the prevalence of substance abuse among persons with hearing loss and deafness suggest that it is roughly of the same magnitude as in the general population. However, the limited ability of social service agencies, alcohol abuse and drug abuse programs, school and work settings, and the legal system to communicate with persons who are deaf allows some people to avoid the negative consequences of substance abuse. Using telecommunication devices (TDD) to communicate with service agencies, making certified sign language interpreters available, teaching sign language to substance abuse counselors, making cocounseling arrangements with deafness specialists, coordinating outreach efforts to the deaf community, and building contacts with professional organizations that provide substance abuse services to the deaf community are needed. A survey of service providers for deaf individuals and service providers for substance abuse found that substance abuse services are generally inaccessible by telephone to clients who are deaf and that relatively few services are provided to those who are deaf. Few programs contract for sign language interpreters; instead, family members, volunteers, and printed materials are used to communicate with patients who are deaf, often compromising patient confidentiality and violating client rights.

The Minnesota Chemical Dependency Program for Deaf and Hard of Hearing Individuals conducted an outcome study with 100 patients. Patients were asked to complete a pretreatment survey measuring attitudinal, behavioral, and knowledge changes regarding substance abuse; a posttreatment questionnaire; a demographic questionnaire; a client satisfaction survey; and four follow-up surveys. Unfortunately, few people could be contacted at each follow-up point, but each client was contacted at least once. Median age of first use was at 10 years. More than 35% of clients at follow-up reported abstinence and 15% reported using a single drug less than monthly. For those using substances, alcohol was used more often than marijuana and other drugs. Investigators found that employment status, family availability to participate in follow-up, and attendance of Alcoholics and Narcotics Anonymous meetings at follow-up were significant predictors of abstinence. Several individuals had obtained employment at postdischarge follow-up; however, few conclusions could be made because of low follow-up rates. The most salient conclusion was the need for vocational rehabilitation to increase employment for clients posttreatment.

Chronic Pain

Chronic pain is a common problem experienced by millions of individuals. A common intervention for chronic pain is pharmaceutical; however, there have been varying rates of substance abuse in this population. Understandably, many physicians are concerned about the long-term dependence potential of opioid therapy for treating chronic pain given the high rates of prior substance abuse in this population. However, given that the majority of patients with chronic pain undergoing opioid treatment do not have abuse or dependency problems, understanding the characteristics and risk factors for the subset of patients with substance abuse/dependence difficulties is important. For example, it may be necessary to provide coping and recovering skills or a structured therapy to patients with comorbid psychiatric illnesses or histories of abuse to manage opioid treatment adequately. To diagnose addiction in patients with chronic pain accurately, there must be evidence of an inability to fulfill daily life activities because of use of the substance. Obtaining this evidence requires clinicians to look beyond standard diagnostic criteria.

Patients with chronic low back pain form a large subgroup of the chronic pain population. Hesitance to use chronic opioid analgesic therapy has also been noted in this subset of patients; however, some physicians now recommend limited use of opioids for patients who have not responded to other interventions. A subset of patients with severe chronic low back pain may benefit from opioid therapy. Additional measures can be taken to monitor potential abuse and dependence including patient education on possible adverse effects of opioid use; written contracts between patient and physician; regular patient contact, including contact with family members; monitoring pain and functioning parameters; and urine toxicology screenings. Thus, opioid therapy should not be ruled out in many cases and steps can be taken to minimize concerns about abuse and dependence.

The majority of patients with chronic pain receiving opioid treatments do not have current abuse or dependency problems. However, opioid abuse and/or dependency may be prevalent for a subset of patients. Thus, accurate diagnosing, better patient education, and prevention efforts aimed at patients who are at risk for abusing opioid treatments are important steps in managing chronic pain.

Traumatic Brain Injury

TBI is a leading cause of death and disability. An analysis of trends in TBI-related hospitalization rates from 1980 through 1995 using the National Hospital Discharge Survey found a decline in the estimated annual incidence rate of hospitalization associated with TBI from 199 to 98 per 100,000 people. Mild TBI hospitalization rates decreased the most compared to intermediate and severe TBI, declining by 61% from 130 to 51 hospitalizations per 100,000 annually. TBI care has been increasingly shifted to outpatient treatment, emphasizing the need for complete evaluation, including substance use, in both inpatient and outpatient settings.

A study of TBI admissions to a regional trauma center found that substance use was suspected or documented in 49% of all trauma cases and in 66% of motor vehicle traumas. A similar study conducted with a larger sample admitted for head injury found that alcohol was a major factor associated with the injury, with detectable blood alcohol levels (BALs) in 62% of men and 27% of women. In one study, alcohol intoxication was a contributing factor more often for moderate than for mild brain injury. Of 199 patients evaluated for moderate brain injury, 73% were intoxicated, as compared to 53% of 538 patients who sustained mild head injuries. In a sample of 623 patients admitted to an urban trauma center, the odds of brain injury were 1.4 times greater when serum ethanol was detected.

One study followed 257 adults with TBI and found that improvement of Glasgow Coma Scale (GCS) scores was significantly related to BAL at admission; patients with the highest BALs showed the greatest cognitive improvement. Although a common myth is that alcohol protects against injury, drivers who had been drinking were more likely than sober drivers to sustain serious injury or death in one study. The observed improvement in GCS scores for those intoxicated at onset of injury may be misleading when compared to the GCS of sober patients. Alcohol consumption just prior to injury is likely to affect distal outcomes negatively. Intoxication at the time of injury has been shown to be associated with longer lengths of hospital stay, longer periods of agitation, and lower cognitive status at discharge. However, it remains unclear to what extent the actual level of intoxication impairs cognitive outcomes and recovery of injured neurons and cerebral blood vessels.

Young adults are especially at risk for TBI when they have pre-injury histories of substance abuse. One study examined the pre-injury and postinjury alcohol and illicit drug use patterns of 87 individuals who incurred TBIs between 16 and 20 years of age. They found a decline in alcohol use at initial follow-up, but a subsequent increase in alcohol use, with males and individuals with heavy alcohol use histories prior to injury at greatest risk for persistent alcohol abuse following injury.

A study that used the Readiness to Change (RTC) questionnaire for substance use in a sample of persons with TBI found that the questionnaire was able to document individuals' current capacity for change. Measuring readiness to change alcohol use patterns in individuals with TBI has meaningful treatment and outcome implications. Measures with good construct validity, such as the RTC questionnaire, should be used in clinical settings to target subsets of persons with TBI who may respond to substance abuse treatment.

A study was conducted at two treatment programs that provided case management services for persons with TBI who had substance abuse problems ($N = 217$); a comparison group was recruited that did not receive intensive case management ($N = 102$). Self-reported alcohol and illicit drug use was reported at the beginning of services and 9 months later. Although no changes in alcohol or illicit drug use between initial assessment and a 9-month follow-up were found for either group, employment at recruitment and earlier referral for case management were associated with employment 9 months later for those receiving case management. Both groups made significant gains in physical well-being by the 9-month follow-up, as well as in community integration. Life satisfaction increased for the case management group and remained stable for the comparison group. Earlier program referral was associated with larger gains in physical well-being, employment, and community integration. Although the case management group did not report substance use reduction at this early phase of treatment, case management appears to have beneficial effects for adults with concomitant TBI and substance abuse problems.

Given the shift to outpatient treatment for TBI, there is a corresponding increase in the need for comprehensive evaluations of substance abuse issues. There are an increasing number of measures, such as the RTC, that will assist clinicians in assessing the potential for change in substance use patterns. Assessing pre-injury patterns of use is important in understanding the potential for future abuse and/or dependence. Persons with TBI require continued education and monitoring to prevent and to decrease problematic alcohol use and drug use. Despite decreases in TBI rates and increasing quality of care because of technologic advances, persons with TBI still present with complex problems and needs that persist long after the onset of injury.

Spinal Cord Injury

It is estimated that between 183,000 and 230,000 individuals in the United States have SCIs with approximately 11,000 new cases of SCI diagnosed annually. As a traumatic life event, SCI has biologic, psychologic, and social implications. Alcohol and/or drug intoxication is a frequent contributor to SCI onset. Intoxication estimates for persons incurring traumatic injury range from 17% to 49%. Impaired judgment resulting from alcohol and drug use contributes to many of these injuries. High rates of substance abuse are detectable with toxicology screens immediately following injury and can be used to provide substance abuse education and prevention during rehabilitation.

The prevalence of alcohol use and abuse following initial rehabilitation may also be high. Studies of persons with recent SCI estimate rates of alcohol-dependence symptomatology ranging from 49% to 62% in vocational rehabilitation clients. One study of an SCI sample of adults age 25 years and younger reported significantly greater rates of exposure and recent use of amphetamines, marijuana, cocaine, and hallucinogens than did a like-aged national sample. In contrast, an SCI group 26 years of age and older reported significantly greater exposure to narcotic analgesics and tranquilizers than did a national sample, and reported rates of recent use of tobacco, alcohol, amphetamines, and marijuana that exceeded rates in a national sample by 10%. Intoxication at the time of injury served as a marker of pre-injury substance use with the 39% who reported intoxication at the time of injury.

A study examined the relationship between medical complications (pressure ulcers and urinary tract infections) and substance abuse following SCI in 71 inpatient subjects. Abstainers with long histories of alcohol abuse prior to SCI were at increased risk for urinary tract infections 7 to 12 months following injury and for longer inpatient lengths of stay, suggesting poor self-care and coping mechanisms in newly abstinent patients. Illicit substance use 12 to 18 months following SCI was also related to increased incidence of pressure ulcers 19 to 30 months following injury. The relationship between alcohol and drug use and medical complications in patients with SCI is complex, but has important implications for rehabilitative care. A study examined the occurrence of pressure ulcers (decubitus ulcers or "bed sores") in individuals with recent-onset SCI (within 1 year) admitted to an inpatient medical rehabilitation program. Results indicated that pressure ulcers were 2.5 times more likely to occur in patients with severe alcohol use compared to those with no alcohol problems. Thus, patients with SCI with alcohol abuse histories or potentials are at risk for pressure ulcer occurrence during the first 3 years following SCI onset.

Substance use and abuse is a concern for this population because it occurs frequently, increases the risk for medical complications, may complicate medical and vocational rehabilitation, and reduces the capacity for independent living. It is important to remember that substance use is not necessarily abuse or dependence, nor does use necessarily result in specific problems, making it imperative that chemical dependence and rehabilitation professionals understand the context, expectancies, and motives for use. It is important to assess substance use and its consequences in this population routinely.

Health Implications of Substance Abuse for Persons with Disabilities

Alcohol and other drug abuse can affect the health of persons with disabilities in direct and indirect ways. Direct effects of drugs include gout, increased spasticity, increased tolerance and potentiation of medication effects, and reduced coordination and concentration. These effects can have adverse consequences for persons with arthritis, SCI, and brain injury, among other conditions. Indirect effects result primarily from neglected self-care. For persons with SCI, the failure to relieve skin pressure regularly increases the risk of pressure ulcers. The consequences of forgetting to take prescription medications as prescribed reflect the nature of the condition being treated; for example, a person who fails to take a prescribed antihypertensive medication following a stroke increases the risk of recurrent stroke. Thus, health professionals are encouraged to inquire about missed appointments, recurring medical problems and injury because alcohol and drug abuse is a frequently concealed cause of these problems.

Alcohol and Other Drug Abuse Treatment Issues for Persons with Disabilities

Etiologic Considerations

A physical disability can either precede or follow the onset of substance abuse. Persons who are primary substance abusers are at increased risk of injury that may result in permanent disability. Risks faced by individuals with substance abuse problems may limit rehabilitation outcomes, including insufficient social resources, low socioeconomic status, and multiple disabilities.

A study examined the rate of self-reported alcohol use, consequent problems, perceived need for treatment, and receipt of treatment in a sample of 75 persons with recent SCI. Subjects reported alcohol use information at three time periods from 6 months prior to injury to 18 months following injury. Drinking on three or more occasions was reported by 93% of respondents at least once during the follow-up assessments, 71% reported at least one drinking-related problem. However, only 15% reported a need for alcohol abuse treatment and only 11% received treatment. The risk of alcohol abuse following injury in those without abuse was low, with 65% reporting drinking problems before injury and only 6% reporting drinking problems for the first time following injury. Issues of dual disability in individuals with histories of substance abuse who also sustain SCI are important topics for rehabilitation and chemical dependence treatment programs.

Representative Treatment Approaches

Systematic Motivational Counseling

Systematic motivational counseling (SMC) is a useful and promising intervention for adults with substance abuse problems and its use has been extended from inpatient substance abuse programs to adults with TBI. SMC is based on the hypothesis that the common route to substance use is individual motivation, despite the complex biologic, psychologic, and environmental influences affecting substance use. Variables affecting alcohol and other drug use do so as they contribute to expectations of emotional change resulting from use. Thus, an individual's decision to use is based on the expectation that the positive emotional consequences of using will outweigh those of not using.

Studies examining the effects of SMC in TBI populations have yielded positive results. The SMC treatment model was evaluated in 60 patients with TBI during a 12-week rehabilitation program. At a 1-year follow-up, 40% maintained abstinence, 14% became abstinent, 38% continued using, and 8% began using. Additional details for a subset of 40 participants receiving SMC and 54 control cases showed that from baseline to follow-up, the SMC group demonstrated significant increases on indices of Appetitive Action, Active Role, Joy, Sorrow/No Success, and Time Available, and a significant decrease on the scale of Unhappiness, with no corresponding changes in the control group. Substance abuse assessments showed lower rates of substance use at follow-up than at baseline for the SMC group, with an approximately 50% decrease in use by SMC participants compared to an increase in use for the control group; however, between-group differences narrowed from posttreatment to follow-up, indicating a need for continued support and perhaps for SMC booster sessions. Overall, the data yielded evidence for a shift to a more adaptive motivational structure in SMC participants. An integrated treatment emphasizing problem solving, such as SMC, holds significant promise not only for addressing substance abuse problems, but also for more global issues including increasing independence and life satisfaction.

Skills-Based Substance Abuse Prevention Counseling

Skills-based counseling (SBC) was developed specifically for persons experiencing cognitive deficits resulting from a brain injury. The model uses a skills acquisition sequence in which clients are taught to recognize high-risk situations related to their pre-injury lifestyle or the consequences of their brain injury. Strategies are role-played and practiced in clinical and field settings. Alcohol use and the consequences of brain injury are viewed as transactional in SBC, with each exacerbating problem originating from the other, and each contributing to both problem realms. Efforts to reduce substance abuse must be integrated carefully with physical and cognitive rehabilitation because alcohol and other drugs can be used both as a means of coping with frustrations and as a reinforcer of poor coping mechanisms. SBC aims to develop an alternative lifestyle in which substance use is no longer central.

An evaluation of SBC with a sample of 40 adults with TBI was conducted. All subjects had sustained moderate to severe TBI and were receiving supported employment services. A comparison group of 103 adults received no treatment. History of substance abuse was reported in 56% of the SBC group. The SBC group had significant increases on measures of skillfulness from initial to follow-up assessment, whereas no change was observed in the no-treatment comparison group. Members of the SBC group also changed their drinking patterns from before to 1 year after the commencement of counseling such that 24% became abstinent, compared to only 9% of the no-treatment control group; in fact, 40% of the control group continued to drink, as compared to 21% of the SBC group. These results support the potential effectiveness of SBC in preventing substance abuse in TBI patients with cognitive impairments.

Prevention of Alcohol and Other Drug Abuse for Persons with Disabilities

Rehabilitation specialists often feel unprepared to confront alcohol and drug use because of their limited educational background in substance abuse assessment and treatment. Few graduate programs address substance abuse as integral to the training of a rehabilitation specialist. Similarly, no accreditation standards address substance abuse prevention as an area of competence for a rehabilitation specialist. Thus, there are no accepted standards of performance.

In addition, interdisciplinary training is limited. Rehabilitation specialists include, among others, psychiatrists, speech–language pathologists, physical and occupational therapists, and counseling and clinical psychologists. Because training programs fail to address substance abuse prevention for each rehabilitation discipline, clinicians frequently fail to detect, and consequently do not address, alcohol and drug problems in their practice. Therefore, teams of professionals may not deliver care in a coordinated manner.

An absence of quantifiable research data that limits knowledge about the extent and consequences of substance use problems in rehabilitative populations is another difficulty. Although the body of research data is growing, studies of substance abuse and disability are relatively few, with little uniformity on sampling, data collection, and criteria for abuse and dependence. There are few long-term evaluations of the relationship between alcohol and other drug use and rehabilitation outcomes. Today, the vast majority of rehabilitation professionals have begun to recognize substance abuse as a clear and persisting problem for their clients, even though they may not feel qualified to address these problems.

Labeling substance abuse as a secondary disability may lead to a perception that it is less important than a physical disability or that it is a condition that can be addressed following medical rehabilitation and by another service provider. Gaps in service delivery also contribute to a perpetuation of alcohol and other drug abuse problems, such as the lack of private or government insurance reimbursement for substance abuse intervention services. Thus, many rehabilitation programs ignore the substance abuse problems or offer collateral services at patients' expense through an outside provider. Unfortunately, the large gaps in community health delivery systems mean that most persons with disabilities never receive treatment or prevention services. Finally, most substance abuse professionals are unaccustomed to working with persons with disabilities, so fully accessible programs are rare.

Preservice Education

Rehabilitation and chemical dependency professionals play vital roles in understanding, recognizing, and addressing the substance abuse problems of people with disabilities; therefore, training for these professionals regarding substance abuse problems in disabled populations is vitally important. Information designed to change the attitudes and knowledge of professionals is likely to lead to a change in rehabilitation practices. Rehabilitation educators are implementing innovative programs to address the need for enhanced training on substance abuse issues in persons with disabilities.

In-service Education

National needs for alcohol abuse and other drug abuse education for rehabilitation professionals were investigated among members of the American Congress on Rehabilitation Medicine. A survey was conducted assessing members' knowledge of substance abuse, attitudes toward patients' substance use, and referral practices for patients with substance abuse problems. Respondents suspected that 29% of their patients with traumatic injuries had substance abuse problems. Only 30% reported routine screening for alcohol and drug problems at their facilities. Substance abuse education for staff was reported by 50% of respondents and patient education regarding substance abuse was reported by 59%. Although 79% of respondents reported having procedures at their facilities for making substance abuse services referrals, only 44% reported actually making referrals, with the majority of referrals made to Alcoholics Anonymous. Thus, there is a need for enhanced in-service education regarding substance abuse assessment and treatment, facility policies, and referral procedures.

Consumer Education

In the past several years, a variety of organizations have emerged and resources have been developed that address alcohol abuse and other drug abuse issues for persons with disabilities. A resource guide for persons with SCI and their families was developed entitled, *Inform Yourself: Alcohol, Drugs and Spinal Cord Injury*. The guide provides personal stories of addiction and recovery, a self-assessment tool, organizational contact for additional information, along with an extensive glossary and bibliography. Sam Maddox's *Spinal Network* covers medical, sports and recreation, travel, media, technology, sex, disability rights, legal and financial issues, and resource information in the United States and Canada. Substance abuse issues are addressed in two sections of a "featured page" chapter. For persons who have sustained TBI, Robert Karol and Frank Sparadeo's booklet, *Alcohol, Drugs and Brain Injury*, provides an overview of alcohol and other drug effects, reproduces assessment tools, and helps consumers create an action plan for dealing with substance use and urges to use.

Rehabilitation Setting Issues

Agency Policies

Rehabilitation agency policy issues regarding possession and use of alcohol and drugs, including recreational or socialization programs that incorporate alcohol use, need to be clearly formulated in light of studies examining controlled drinking outcomes. Although moderate alcohol use is likely to pose a few problems for many persons, those with histories of substance abuse are at risk of relapse as a consequence of policies and programs that provide opportunities for alcohol consumption; persons with cognitive impairment resulting from brain trauma or other neurologic injury are at particular risk. Policies that provide for monitoring of psychoactive prescription medications obtained during or after hospitalization should also be considered. In short, the opportunity for abuse of prescribed medications and histories of alcohol or illicit drug use requires case-by-case assessment of each patient's history as rehabilitation plans are made.

Staff Education

In-Service Education

Several educators and rehabilitation practitioners have advocated for the need for enhanced education on substance abuse issues. Several clinical issues have not been addressed sufficiently in medical rehabilitation settings, with one of the most important medication prescription misuse. Continued monitoring of long-term prescription use in all disability populations, not only the chronic pain population, is necessary. Clinicians should attend to depression and poor psychologic adjustment, which may underlie medical complications and may be associated with substance use. Physician, nursing, and allied health staff education should focus on recognizing prescription medication misuse and the reasons for misuse.

Recommendations

Relatively few persons who sustain traumatic injury may realize a need for substance abuse treatment. Such a perception may reflect individuals who are at relatively early stages of readiness for change. For some persons intoxicated at injury, the injury may illustrate the extent and consequences of their substance use problems and motivate them to initiate action. The belief that one does not need treatment, despite major trauma, can be understood as an aspect of denial or rationalization about the severity of drinking or drug problems. The importance of external agents, such as employers, courts, family, and physicians, in encouraging treatment is evident in findings that these agents were most often cited as a reason for pursuing treatment. Clearly, the process of acknowledging substance abuse problems is developmental in nature; major injury does no more to cure drinking or other drug problems for some persons than does job loss, divorce, or other traumatic events.

Knowing the etiology of substance abuse and whether it preceded or followed disability is an important issue, as is assessing alcohol and drug use in the context of coping skills, in rehabilitation settings because of the evidence that predisability substance abuse places individuals at high risk for abuse after disability. Traumatic onset disability may provide an opportunity for some persons to recognize the gravity of their substance abuse patterns and to make changes. Although some persons may make changes on their own, others will continue to use and experience consequences of their use. The pernicious quality of addiction is illustrated by continued use after injury related to substance use. The success of rehabilitation interventions will probably be enhanced when familial and personal substance use histories are considered.

Several implications for enhancing medical rehabilitation are evident. First, alcohol use and other drug use assessment should be a routine component of all admissions to acute care and rehabilitation programs for persons incurring traumatic injury. Second, training team members to recognize alcohol and other drug abuse is critical in enabling them to provide competent assessments. Substance abuse treatment program professionals should consult with physical medicine and rehabilitation providers to acquire this knowledge. Third, referral networks to substance abuse treatment programs are necessary if a potential dual disability is to be identified and treated in a timely fashion. Adequate communication links must be established so that chemical dependence treatment programs and counselors learn about the special needs of persons with disabilities. Accessibility needs, functional abilities, and attitudes toward persons with disabling conditions are some of the topics that could be addressed in training substance abuse treatment personnel.

Chemical Dependence Treatment Setting Issues

Chemical dependence professionals are often uninformed about the unique risks and needs of people with disabilities; consequently, they may be ill prepared to provide appropriate treatment. Moreover, attitudes of professionals regarding what constitutes a primary and secondary disability influence treatment provision. If substance abuse is viewed as a secondary disability, then it may be considered less important than the primary disability. Thus, it may be left untreated. Chemical dependence and rehabilitation professionals need to appreciate the value of treating primary and secondary disabilities concurrently.

Implications of the Americans with Disabilities Act

The Americans with Disabilities Act of 1990 (ADA; Public Law 101–336) is one of the major civil rights laws passed since 1964. It addresses the severe disadvantages persons with disabilities experience in daily life. These include intentional exclusion, overly protective policies and rules, segregation, exclusionary standards, and architectural, transportation, and communication barriers. The ADA is important for alcohol and other drug prevention programs because public accommodations, along with other social service, health care, and educational programs, must allow people with disabilities to participate fully.

Summary

Knowledge about the extent of substance abuse problems and the consequences of substance abuse in persons with disabilities has grown remarkably in the past two decades. Promising treatment and prevention programs have been evaluated. Professional education and program accessibility has increased. Continuing efforts are required in the next decade to ensure that alcohol abuse and other drug abuse services are made available to persons with disabilities in both rehabilitation and chemical dependence settings.

Suggested Readings

Basford J, Rohe D, Barnes C, et al. Substance abuse attitudes and policies in U.S. rehabilitation training programs: a comparison of 1985 and 2000. *Arch Phys Med Rehabil.* 2002; 83: 517–522.

Elliott T, Kurylo M, Chen Y, et al. Alcohol abuse history and adjustment following spinal cord injury. *Rehabil Psychol.* 2002;47:278–290.

Guthmann D, Blozis S. Unique issues faced by deaf individuals entering substance abuse treatment and following discharge. *Am Ann Deaf.* 2001;146:294–303.

Heinemann AW, Rawal PH. Disability and rehabilitation issues. In: Lowinson JH, Ruiz P, Millman RB, et al., eds. *Substance abuse: a comprehensive textbook*, 4th ed. Philadelphia: Lippincott Williams & Wilkins; 2005:1169–1187.

Heinemann AW, Corrigan JD, Moore D. Case management for TBI survivors with alcohol problems. *Rehabil Psychol.* 2004;49(2):156–166.

42

THE WORKPLACE AND METHADONE ADVOCACY

The Workplace

There are two basic groups of recovering substance abusers in the treatment setting: those who, as a consequence of their abuse or other environmental or family factors, have never worked, and those who have worked and been suspended from their jobs or fired as a consequence of substance abuse. The first group is looking to enter the workforce for the first time and the second group is looking to return. Although there are similarities between the two, care must be taken to understand fully the unique dynamics influencing each group's movement toward work.

Recovering substance abusers entering the labor force for the first time may be confronted with poor, inadequate, or unrealistic concepts of what work is and who they are and can be as workers. Individuals who grew up in disadvantaged or unstable homes because of poverty, generational substance abuse, or family conflict may never have worked formally or been raised with close "worker" role models. Employment may be seen by recovering substance abusers as foreign and unknown, creating feelings of inadequacy and fear. Many of their lifestyle patterns and habits are maladaptive and not conducive to work. Adolescents and young adults whose lives have focused on drug or alcohol addiction have not experienced many of the stresses and fears that most people gradually confront in high school educational programs or their first part-time or summer jobs.

In addition to not experiencing these feelings early on, substance abusers may have missed the opportunities to develop effective coping skills and strengths, to make mistakes in less-significant vocational responsibilities, and to learn from these mistakes, integrating healthy social and personal management skills into their sense of self.

These individuals arrive at the job market overwhelmed by the enormity of the task of entering the "straight" world and meeting employers' expectations to have already completed the more basic vocational development tasks. Still, a position in the labor force is attractive, because it offers to place them into a recognized position in society for the first time in their lives.

Other individuals coming from the mainstream with an intact background may have come to accept their chemical addiction only when their substance abuse destroyed their ability to work. They were removed from the labor market for one or more periods of unemployment. Paradoxically, they may now question their ability to handle work demands sober and drug free. They face discrimination because of employment gaps and poor previous work references. They may lack a career plan because of the unstable and interrupted patterns of their prior employment. Employment for these people is a sign of their restored health and a return to their place in society.

Vocational Rehabilitation

The process for many who are characterized by a late onset of substance abuse, or who have worked before and are returning to competitive employment, may appropriately be termed vocational "rehabilitation." These individuals are being restored to a former level of functioning. However, for those recovering people who have lived on the fringe of society, never having worked before, vocational "habilitation" provides a more accurate understanding of their need to learn what work is about and to establish for the first time effective work behaviors. Having made this distinction, the term *rehabilitation* is used in this chapter to refer to both concepts.

There are three basic vocational rehabilitation strategies. The first and most desirable strategy is to remedy the cause of the person's disability by restoring or developing functional ability. The second strategy is to enhance the individual's other vocational/educational attributes so that the person can compensate for the disability.

The first and most crucial component of vocational rehabilitation for any disabled group is assessment. A vocational inventory needs to be undertaken by recovering individuals to develop their vocational plans. They must be evaluated in four key areas: Is the recovering substance abuser ready to begin work or return to work? If so, for which specific employment position is the individual best suited? If not, what is the client lacking to effectively obtain and maintain a job? And, finally, where and how can these needs be addressed?

Motivation is a crucial ingredient and, unless properly assessed and addressed, will lead to resistance from the client and frustration for the counselor later in the process. If the client is not able to progress to a point where the client is keeping appointments on time and demonstrating initiative and choice in selecting from available vocational options, then the client's motivation is questionable.

Another area to evaluate is the client's social readiness in view of the facts that a significant percentage of recovering substance abusers have been living in a "subculture" with limited exposure to the work environment. Can the client communicate effectively, talking as well as listening? Does the client know how to dress appropriately for a specific job environment? Has the client evidenced the ability to interact appropriately with co-workers and supervisors? Does the client possess sufficient self-management and planning skills to ask questions when unclear about instructions and to notify an employer when unable to meet a commitment?

Finally, the client needs to be evaluated in relation to job-finding skills. Can the client complete a job application or resume? Is the client capable of presenting marketable job qualities and a positive work attitude in an employment interview? Is the client able to address an employer's possible questions about work gaps, conviction history, or possibly past substance abuse, in a way that will relieve the employer's fears about hiring that person?

Counseling and Referral

Vocational counseling has four classic elements: developing a positive self-concept, obtaining occupational information, expressing the self in occupational terms, and learning job-seeking skills.

A fundamental task for rehabilitation counselors is to help clients remove the stigma of disability that many have internalized. Many of these clients believe the label that society has assigned them, more convinced of what they cannot do than confident of what they can do.

Recovering substance abusers in vocational counseling will generally present one of four major needs. The first group possesses no occupational goals and will therefore need assistance in establishing them. The second group has inappropriate or unrealistic goals and will need help in developing more achievable goals. The third group has appropriate goals, but needs support in planning the steps and obtaining the resources needed to achieve the goals. The fourth group sees no value in working.

Impediments to Vocational Rehabilitation Service

The federal government has joined with state and local governments in endorsing the connection between work and recovery. This is evident in its policy developments and antidiscrimination legislation. This extends to funding provisions for training and job opportunities for recovering substance abusers. Certainly the Rehabilitation Act of 1973 serves as a cornerstone for the legal rights and public opportunities available to individuals with disabilities.

However, it is naive to believe that this support alone guarantees vocational rehabilitation services to those who need and desire it. There are three major categories of hindrances to effective provision and use of these services by recovering substance abusers: the clients themselves, the programs that treat them, and the society to which they return.

Treatment program obstacles can be examined in terms of the themes of philosophy and staffing. There is a significant lack of research addressing the vocational rehabilitation of substance abusers. This is indicative of the low priority and concern that treatment professionals in general have for this component of treatment. In most residential facilities, the last few weeks or last few months at best are devoted to job placement referrals. In methadone and other outpatient treatment modalities, there are usually no vocational rehabilitation services onsite and only limited contact with educational/vocational resource agencies, due to limited funding and heavy caseload.

The drug and alcohol treatment field in general suffers from staff shortages and high turnover. Faced with this reality, treatment program administrators knowingly or unknowingly diminish the status of vocational rehabilitation services.

Societal obstacles are probably the most difficult to overcome because of the prevalent ignorance and fear which are at their roots. Recovering substance abusers suffer from the same degrees of employment discrimination as many other disabled individuals and ex-offenders. The fear about acquired immune deficiency syndrome (AIDS) has been generalized to label all substance abusers and increase the stigma.

Regretfully, they are also frequently faced with discrimination and misunderstanding by social service agencies which supposedly exist to help them. A similar, if not more extreme, situation exists for physically disabled substance abusers who are often rejected by substance abuse treatment programs who cannot accommodate some of their special needs and are uneasy about how to treat these clients.

Employee Assistance Programs

Standards for Employee Assistance Programs (EAPs) defines EAPs as worksite-based programs that are designed to assist in the identification and resolution of productivity problems associated with employees impaired by personal concerns that may adversely affect employee job performance. Personal concerns may include, but are not be limited to, health, marital, family, financial, alcohol, drug, legal, emotional, stress, or other personal concerns. EAPs are worksite-based intervention programs designed to help employees identify and address personal concerns that may be affecting job performance.

Critical to effective EAPs is the development and implementation of a clear policy. This policy should be developed by an advisory committee representing different levels of management and labor groups in the company. "Program acceptance and utilization is directly related to the amount of support from top management and involvement by employees, supervisors, management and unions."

EAP services may be provided through a variety of delivery systems. Some companies have internal programs where services are delivered by EAP professionals employed by the company. In external programs, EAP services are delivered by EAP professionals under contract with the organization. Some companies combine a core internal EAP program with contracts with external EAP vendors for certain services. Consortia of smaller companies may contract with an independent EAP vendor to provide services.

A primary responsibility of the EAP professional is to make accurate assessments to identify employee or family member problems and then make appropriate referrals to resources in the community that are most likely to resolve the problem. The EAP identifies, fosters, and evaluates community resources to determine which provide the best quality care at the most reasonable cost. The EAP professional provides short-term counseling or problem resolution (as opposed to referral to community resources for long-term counseling) when this is assessed as the best response for timely and effective help. Crisis intervention is also within the purview of the EAP professional who is responsive with intervention services for employees, family members, or the organization when acute crises surface.

Drug-Free Workplace Act

A critical cornerstone for employment policies regarding drug abuse was laid by the federal government in 1988 with passage of the Federal Drug-Free Workplace Act, which mandates that publicly funded employers provide worker education about illegal drug abuse and monitor and discipline such activity.

The Act requires employers who have a contract with the federal government for at least $25,000 to maintain a drug-free workplace. First, these employers must establish a company substance abuse policy and inform all employees of its existence. They must also educate employees about drug abuse and the availability of drug counseling and treatment programs, and specify the penalties for violating the company's substance abuse policy.

Union Programs

Although joint labor–management programs are in operation and growing, there is a history of differing philosophies between labor and management; generally unions prefer to run their own programs. Although both labor and management address deteriorating job performance and confront troubled employees, there is a distinction in their priorities. Unions have perceived the well-being of their members as coming first and have resisted management's last-resort strategy of firing an employee whose job performance does not improve. Since World War II, the AFL-CIO Community Services Network has provided counseling services for its members.

Drug Testing Programs

In recent years, a variety of drug testing programs have developed, including pre-employment, random, incident, probable cause, and scheduled drug testing. Pre-employment testing, in which urinalysis is used to screen job applicants for drug use, is increasingly used by the nation's largest employers, including major corporations, manufacturers, public utilities, transportation, and some smaller employers. Pre-employment testing is primarily viewed as a deterrent for drug-abusing job applicants. Interestingly, the most abused drug, alcohol, is rarely included in these testing programs.

Postemployment drug testing programs have been implemented, especially by federal employers and companies employing workers in safety-sensitive positions. Some companies that have EAP capabilities view drug testing as a means of early identification and treatment of substance-abusing employees.

Future Concerns

Managed health care has and will continue to have a strong impact on EAPs. Health maintenance and preferred provider organizations have flourished as employers have been forced to identify alternatives to rapidly increasing health insurance premiums. Catastrophic claims for ailments such as AIDS and substance abuse treatment expenses, along with advanced medical technology and drug therapies, have fueled increases in health costs. EAPs also will need to continue addressing concerns raised by the AIDS-diagnosed employee.

Federal government employers and the general public are also expressing growing concern about creating drug-free work environments. Although more EAPs in industry are broad-brush programs addressing a wide range of employee problems, it is critical that they continue to recognize and target services to substance-abusing employees. EAPs will also need to address the growing concerns of employees who do not have drug problems themselves but who have family members who do.

Methadone Advocacy

New Era for Methadone Advocacy

The National Alliance of Methadone Advocates (NAMA) is now 15 years old. In spite of sparse funding and support, NAMA has never lost sight of its primary mandate to advocate for the patient in treatment. During these years NAMA has also acquired experience and expertise that has been invaluable to understanding methadone treatment, both in the United States and abroad.

From the start NAMA received minimal funding, especially from the methadone community, and often has had to endure hostile attacks from those who would discourage advocacy. Today, NAMA exists solely through the membership fees from patients and enlightened professionals. This also means that no one is paid a salary at

NAMA. Many patient groups abroad that are funded by their governments look to NAMA for leadership. Currently, NAMA has more than 45 chapters and 12 international affiliates. On May 17, 2001, the Center for Substance Abuse Treatment began a 3-year transition period during which all programs must be accredited.

The new rule includes patient participation in program policy. Now methadone programs must have some mechanism for patients to be involved in program policy. This can be a single patient representative or a patient counsel depending on the size of the program or even a committee of patients and staff. Some states have also begun to set up patient consumer groups that are involved in policy-making committees.

The Grievance Process

When NAMA was conceived, resolving individual patient grievances was not considered. However, that very quickly changed as patients began asking for assistance. It was decided to acknowledge when programs or professionals do something that is exceptional in helping patients. Thus, the concept of a compliment report was included and today the form is called the "Grievance/Compliment Report."

A NAMA Grievance Report can involve programs, state agencies, hospitals, the criminal justice system, employment, and other services that patients use and can have trouble with. The most common complaint is the patient being discharged for invalid reasons, including opiate drug use. The New York State Office of Alcoholism and Substance Abuse Service (OASAS) has an advocacy unit that handles thousands of complaints a year. Outside of New York it is another matter and depends on that state's authority.

NAMA believes that a grievance against any program or agency in the methadone treatment system means that a failure has occurred somewhere. Whether the failure is the fault of the treatment provider, regulatory authority, or advocate does not really matter. If the situation degenerates to the point where outside help is needed, the patient has been failed. In NAMA experience, very few patients want to "rock the boat" by asserting their rights. It is not unusual for patients to feel as though any efforts to change things will be futile. Thus, when patients finally file a grievance it usually means that they have been frustrated in their own attempts to resolve problems and literally see NAMA as a last resort. The methadone treatment system is a bureaucracy and can be confusing to the average patient. We have found that the best approach to grievance resolution is to coach the patient to contact the appropriate parties and to provide support and counseling throughout the process.

Methadone program grievances fall into two basic categories. The largest number of complaints is by individual patients regarding a specific problem, such as not receiving any take-home medication or being discharged without due process. A broader category of complaints involves a program policy that affects the entire patient population. These complaints although filed by an individual patient are handled at the program level. Usually the grievance coordinator begins by contacting the program to validate the program policy. If the policy contravenes federal or state regulations, the program is contacted and informed. If the program does not cease the policy, then NAMA will contact the proper authorities. This can be accomplished at a variety of levels, as program staff members may not realize that they are violating the patients' right.

The Greatest Barrier: Stigma

Stigma, prejudice, and discrimination constitute the greatest barrier to recovery. Employment and maintenance of a stable, responsible lifestyle are critical aspects of treatment and recovery. The employed methadone patient lives with the constant fear of discovery. Despite the fact that they are protected by the Americans with Disabilities Act (ADA), patients lose their jobs merely for being enrolled in a methadone program. Many of these patients do not challenge their employers because they do not realize that it is against the law, indeed against the U.S. Constitution. Nor do they know how to proceed with such a case.

Not only are methadone patients confronted with employment discrimination, but many schools, training opportunities, and service programs exclude them, thus compounding the problem. On the other hand, the abstinence-oriented former addict who is cared for in a protected residential environment with all the needs being met receives most of the accolades. Methadone patients from the day they enter treatment face opposition and discrimination virtually every step of the way. It is only because of their determination and strong character that the majority of methadone patients succeed as accomplished and productive taxpaying citizens. They support themselves and their family, while very often having to pay $250 to $300 a month for their treatment. Methadone patients do not have the cheering squads or community support that recipients of abstinence-oriented treatment do; instead they make their contributions quietly, fearful that their secret will be discovered and that they and their family will lose everything.

Stigma is also a major barrier for the dysfunctional methadone patients who need special services. Too often, the mental health community refuses to accept methadone patients for treatment of depressive and affective disorders and typically tells patients that they must withdraw from methadone treatment in order to be considered for their services. Patients with a secondary drug problem, such as cocaine and alcoholism, are also refused services unless they, too, withdraw from methadone. If it is discovered that they are enrolled in a methadone program, homeless methadone patients are denied housing and the ones with housing are evicted.

Methaphobia and the Medical Profession

Obtaining health and medical care has become a serious problem for many methadone patients, especially because most methadone programs, for budgetary reasons, have had to eliminate the primary medical care that they provided in the past. Prejudice and hatred toward methadone treatment, patients, and the medication itself has been given a name—*methaphobia*. Methaphobia has become critical during the past decade, especially because of the large number of human immunodeficiency virus (HIV)-infected drug users admitted to methadone programs and the increasing number of former drug users being diagnosed with hepatitis C.

The prejudice that methadone patients experience in health care settings is an extension of the bias of the medical profession against heroin addicts in general. The Harrison Narcotic Act removed the problem of opiate addiction from the medical profession and placed it under the control of the criminal justice agencies. The first group actually to be prosecuted under the Harrison Narcotic Act was medical professionals, resulting in the arrests of approximately 38,000 physicians and the imprisonment of more than 5,000. Medical schools began to advise their students to stay away from addicts, viewing addiction as a law enforcement problem, a message that continues to this day. Today, the average medical student receives about 1 hour of training in addiction that includes alcohol use; thus, methadone is rarely mentioned except for its use to withdraw from opiates.

Certification of Methadone Advocates

As accreditation moves forward, programs are forced to learn that patients will have to be treated as consumers. The new rule (42 CFR 8) stresses the concept of individualized treatment. It is imperative during this period for NAMA methadone advocates to be active in order to combat myths and half-truths being spread by those who are not properly trained and mentored.

In an effort to rectify what many, both inside and outside of NAMA, see as a serious problem, the board of directors created the NAMA Training and Certification Committee. The committee's role is to encourage the growth of responsible methadone advocacy. The committee's goals are as follows:

1. The establishment of an ethical code for patient advocates.
2. The creation of standards for individual advocates.
3. The establishment of a certification procedure for advocates.
4. The provision of training for advocates and mentoring of less-experienced advocates.

The committee is also responsible for the establishment of a mechanism so that once advocates are trained and certified, they will receive ongoing supervision and ongoing training.

What Is a Methadone Advocate?

A major purpose of methadone advocacy is education. Some advocates mistakenly believe that advocates only handle grievances and complaints. This is a reductionist view of what methadone advocacy should be about. As discussed above, a grievance means that a failure has occurred and only education, monitoring, and advocacy can prevent it.

Everyone who works in the methadone field should be a methadone advocate. Stigma affects methadone treatment on every level. It is the reason programs are unable to open in a community, thus leaving opiate-dependent individuals in the area without any access to treatment. More directly, it reduces a patient's opportunities, making recovery all the more difficult for methadone patients. Stigma also affects professionals working in the field and it is not unusual for a counselor to spend an entire day trying to find somewhere to place a homeless patient when the counselor's time would be better spent counseling the patient or other patients. It is not unusual to hear about a professional who was embarrassed to admit at a social gathering that he or she works in methadone treatment. It has been a primary mission for NAMA to end the ignorance that drives stigma, and the certification of advocates will give NAMA the opportunity to be able to reach out and galvanize the entire methadone community to end the stigma that reduces the effectiveness of treatment.

It is not uncommon for some professionals to feel threatened by advocacy because it is new and there are unknowns. But methadone advocacy does not mean the relinquishment of power for professionals; instead, the result will be an elevation for the entire field. This is the goal of the responsible methadone advocate.

The Power of Advocacy: Patients and Counselors

NAMA has come to realize that the most powerful advocates for methadone are patients and counselors because they bring firsthand experiences to their advocacy.

Provider representatives have acknowledged that when talking to legislators and interested citizens they are often interrupted with, "We would expect you to say that. You represent the providers, or a manufacturer, or the program."

On the other hand, when responsible patients and their families speak, there is often interest, because their experience is firsthand and sometimes because patients have no economic stake in methadone treatment. Patients and their families are not the only credible advocates; counselors are just as powerful because they know first-hand the effectiveness of treatment. Treatment is not just effective for a few and nearly every patient can benefit.

The Primary Problem Is Stigma

As methadone treatment expanded, patients took less of a role in methadone treat-ment. The early program employed successful patients as counselors and role models. However, as treatment expanded, typical counselors came from social work and social science backgrounds. They trained that opiate addiction was a behavioral prob-lem. This was partly due to ever-increasing credentialing requirements. Because these counselors had never confronted the problem of addiction directly, there began puni-tive programs and the us-versus-them mentality in methadone programs.

The way to end stigma is to educate patients about methadone, their rights, and their treatment. Educating and organizing both patients and counselors and organizing coun-selors to work together as advocates is critical. Advocates are essential in the process.

A New Era Is Emerging

The majority of the public still does not understand opiate addiction and it will take a tremendous educational effort to correct this misperception. The best messengers in teaching that opiate addiction is a medical condition that can be treated effec-tively are the patients themselves in conjunction with the community.

As the national advocacy organization for methadone treatment, NAMA will con-tinue to respond actively to the issues that affect the quality of treatment and that affect the daily lives of patients. The objective of NAMA has always been to work toward the day when all methadone patients can publicly come forward to celebrate and state with pride their numerous achievements. Only through the empowerment of patients with everyone working together will methadone treatment begin to gain the respect it so rightly deserves.

Suggested Readings

Engelhart PF, Barlow L. The workplace. In: Lowinson JH, Ruiz P, Millman RB, et al., eds. *Substance abuse: a comprehensive textbook*, 4th ed. Philadelphia: Lippincott Williams & Wilkins; 2005:1331–1346.

2002 NADAP Placement Statistics. New York: National Association of Drug Abuse Problems, 2003.

Woods J, Ginter W, Scro T. A new era for methadone advocacy. In: Lowinson JH, Ruiz P, Millman RB, et al., eds. *Substance abuse: a comprehensive textbook*, 4th ed. Philadelphia: Lippincott Williams & Wilkins; 2005:1325–1330.

43

PHYSICIANS AND OTHER HEALTH PROFESSIONALS

Physicians have the moral responsibility to care for their patients not only by direct care and precept, but also by the example of their lives and personal conduct. The misuse of alcohol and drugs by a member of the medical profession is an occupational, social, and personal problem that demands action to ensure early detection, treatment, and rehabilitation.

This chapter focuses primarily on physician impairment caused by chemical dependency. It identifies assumptions underlying the concept of physician impairment; outlines the characteristics of an impaired physician; describes the identification, intervention, treatment, rehabilitation, outcome monitoring, and the effectiveness of treatment; presents the evolution, progress, and policies that link organized concern for sick doctors to social, legal, and political pressures of professional accountability; and documents the practice of medical supervision of problem doctors in terms of its compatibilities with professional values and interests.

Prevalence

The literature from the United States related to physician alcohol and drug problems from the mid-1950s to the mid-1980s consistently documented an apparent excess prevalence of these disorders. Several major surveys in the United States and internationally have assessed the prevalence of substance abuse and dependence disorders within the general population. One of the largest surveys measuring psychiatric and substance use epidemiology is the National Institute of Mental Health Epidemiologic Catchment Area program (ECA).

Currently, there are more than 700,000 physicians in the United States. Based on ECA data, an estimated 100,000 physicians will have alcohol disorders during their lifetime. Physicians are believed to have essentially the same incidence and prevalence rates for alcohol and drug abuse and dependence disorders as the general population. There are no published scientific studies that measure the damage done by physician substance abuse and dependence. However, chemical dependency does appear to be the single most frequent disabling illness for the medical professional and poses a major problem for the profession and society alike.

Etiology

There is no evidence to support the existence of a premorbid "professional" personality type that predisposes a physician to addiction. Physicians whose childhood and adolescence were unstable also appear to have excess risk of addiction. A narcissistic personality type, non-Jewish ancestry and lack of religious affiliation, nicotine dependence of more than one pack per day, the regular use of alcohol, the history of alcohol-related difficulties, and a family history of alcoholism, substance dependence, and/or mental illness are risk factors. It has also been found that certain specialty groups and physicians in academic medicine appear to have risk for addiction. By comparison with controls, physicians are five times more likely to take sedatives and minor tranquilizers without medical supervision, and self-prescribing and (self-treatment with prescription drugs) is a risk factor for chemical dependents.

Potential risk factors are (a) access to pharmaceuticals, (b) family history of substance abuse, (c) emotional problems, (d) stress at work or at home, (e) thrill seeking, (f) self-treatment of pain and emotional problems, and (g) chronic fatigue.

Physicians may be no more at risk for addiction than the general population. No study has specially looked at the genetic predisposition, the psychobiology of craving, the relationship of classically conditioned factors, brain reward mechanisms, psychodynamic factors, and sociocultural determinants of addiction in physicians by comparison with nonphysician peers.

Identification

Detection of the chemically dependent physician is often delayed by the ability of physician-patients to protect job performance at the expense every other dimension of their lives. Identifiable signs and symptoms can be listed as follows.

Family: Withdrawal from family activities, unexplained absences; spouse becomes a solicitous caretaker; fights, dysfunctional anger, spouse tries to control physician's substance abuse; disease of "spousaholics": isolated, angry, physically and emotionally unable to meet the demands of the addict's illness, the grieving loner; child abuse; children attempt to maintain normal family functioning; children develop abnormal, antisocial behavior (depression, promiscuity, runaways, substance abuse); sexual problems: impotence, extramarital affairs; spouse disengages, abuses drugs and alcohol, or enters recovery.

Community: Isolation and withdrawal from community activities, church, friends, leisure, hobbies, and peers; embarrassing behavior at clubs or parties; driving under the influence of alcohol (DUI), legal problems, role-discordant behaviors; unreliable and unpredictable in community and social activities; unpredictable behavior: excessive spending, risk-taking behaviors.

Staff and Employment Applications: If any three of these items are present on a job application, suspicion index is high. Numerous job changes in past 5 years; frequently relocated geographically for unexplained reasons; frequent hospitalizations; complicated and elaborate medical history; unexplained time lapse between jobs; indefinite or inappropriate medical references and vague letter of reference; working in an inappropriate job for individual's qualifications; decline of professional productivity.

Physical Status: Personal hygiene deteriorating; clothing and dressing habits deteriorate; multiple physical signs and complaints; numerous prescriptions and drugs; frequent hospitalizations; frequent visits to physicians and dentists; accidents and trauma; serious emotional crisis.

Office: Appointments and schedule become disorganized, progressively late; behavior to staff and patients hostile, withdrawn, unreasonable; "locked door" syndrome; ordering excessive supply of drugs from local druggists or by mail order; patients begin to complain to staff about doctor's behavior; absence from office: unexplained or frequently sick.

Hospital: Making late rounds or inappropriate abnormal behavior; decreasing quality of performance in staff presentations, writing in charts, and the like; inappropriate orders or overprescribing medications; nurses, secretaries, orderlies, licensed practical nurses (LPNs) reporting behavioral changes: "hospital gossip"; involved in malpractice suits and legal sanctions against the physician or hospital; emergency room staff reports: unavailability or inappropriate responses to telephone calls; failure or prolonged response to paging; reluctance to undergo immediate physical examination or do urine drug screens on request; heavy drinking at staff functions.

Early identification and diagnosis are critical. Barriers to early diagnosis are the conspiracy of silence and denial by family, friends, peers, and even the patients. It is significantly more difficult to identify and diagnose female physicians than male physicians. Gender attitudes, female metabolism, and cultural factors concerning females account for some of these difficulties.

Intervention

Chemically dependent individuals rationalize their avoidance of treatment. Denial is an almost universal characteristic of the disease of addiction. Denial absolves the physician-patient of personal accountability. At the same time, denial (both the deliberate, conscious deception and the unconscious defense mechanism) fills the addicted physician with guilt, shame, and remorse, so that most addicted physicians cannot reach out for help. It is the nature of the disease for the denial system to progress as the addiction gains control over the individual's functioning. This distortion of the truth is an unconscious defense stand that the illness is treatable. An intervention should never be done alone.

Trained and Experienced Intervention Leader

Proper preparation for an intervention is essential. The interventionist must select individuals to do the intervention, train the interveners to present relevant information to the physician-patient, set goals for the intervention, and expedite the prompt referral for recommended treatment.

Selection of the Intervention Site

The site of the intervention needs to be nonthreatening and quiet. Time and experience have taught that an early morning intervention prior to the intake of alcohol or other drugs by the physician is best accomplished in the patient's home with the cooperation of the spouse and children. Occasionally, guilt and shame are present to such a degree that intervention needs to be away from the home at some neutral site. Some spouses believe that their participation in an intervention will result in divorce. If the spouse is not convinced that addiction is a progressive, potentially fatal, but treatable illness affecting the entire family, it may be wise to exclude the spouse from the intervention. It is necessary that all members of the intervention team present a strong cohesive explanation of the problem.

Intervention Goals Must Be Established

This needs to be done in advance, understood, and accepted by all intervention team members. Interveners must decide what choices they will give the physician-patient and what they will commit to if the physician-patient refuses all offers of help. Frequently, the perception of reality is grossly distorted by the effects of alcohol and drugs on the brain. Interveners need to review the pain and consequences they have experienced as a result of the addict's substance abuse. No attempt at intervention is a failure because the seed has been planted. The impaired physician may reject, refuse, or even elope from the intervention, but the physician will recognize that his or her support systems are aware of the impairment and concerned about the physician.

Factual Data

It is critical that the data be factual and documented. Previous gossips or innuendoes may reduce the chances of having a successful intervention. The intervention team members should write down and present to the physician-addict their experiences of the addiction-influenced behaviors. The addicts should be told why the intervention is necessary, along with the legal, social, personal, health-related, and professional implications of their illness. The team needs to also consider presenting the advocacy/immunity regulations within the state, should the individual voluntary seek the appropriate treatment as a result of the intervention.

Adequate Intervention Time

Intervention sometimes must be repeated. Extremely important is the fact that the individual not feel rushed during the intervention and that adequate time is allowed. The doctor should not be intoxicated. An intervention done after an addiction-precipitated crisis frequently is likely to be successful. If the physician-patient refuses recommended help, the interventionist may negotiate a behavioral contract, so that with the next relapse or crisis, another intervention can be swiftly initiated.

Rehearsals

Careful planning including rehearsal is critical. All individuals of the intervention team must know and practice their roles and what they will say during their intervention. Anticipation of the doctor-patient's reaction including hostility and flight needs to be anticipated and plans for this complication provided. Some interventions fail. A cohesive team can develop an action plan for the next time the addicted doctor is in an addiction-precipitated crisis.

At the conclusion of the successful intervention, the physician-patient will follow the recommended assessment, treatment, or both. Referral options, transportation, and an action plan should be in place before the intervention is begun. More than one intervention has seemed successful, but the doctor negotiated his or her own arrangements that enabled suicide.

Assessment

Interventionists, most state medical society impaired-physician committees, and many state licensing boards recommend a comprehensive assessment in a specified treatment facility for impaired physicians to determine the extent of illness and the individual's treatment needs. Physicians who voluntarily seek the recommended treatment after assessment, successfully complete their treatment, and enter into their state medical society–sponsored monitoring program frequently receive advocacy in lieu of punitive sanctions. Ideally, recovering physicians will allow the experienced treatment team to make the best choices about their recovery, rather than to treat themselves or undertreat their illness. The four teams required for the assessment are the addiction medicine team, the psychiatric team, the neuropsychologic team, and the family therapy team.

Addiction Medicine Team

This team is headed by a certified addiction medicine specialist. Trained to diagnose and recommend a range of addiction medicine services, these individuals provide needed detoxification services after a comprehensive addictive disease assessment is obtained. They evaluate the psychologic behavioral effects of the drugs that have been used by the patient, assess addiction severity from a biopsychosocial perspective, and collect information from the individual support system members (including intervention team members) to validate the physician-patient's history. A rapid data acquisition effort, followed by presentation of the information the physician-patient and family, is often critical for rapidly decompressing the impaired physician's denial system.

Psychiatric Team

Events of recent years have made it apparent that the disciplines of addiction medicine and psychiatry must work in concert for the benefit of the addicted physician. Addicted patients frequently manifest multiple addictions and psychiatric problems simultaneously. Consequently, a comprehensive psychiatric assessment is a critical component of any assessment of an alcohol-addicted and/or drug-addicted individual. It is necessary to determine if a definitive psychiatric diagnosis is present, or if there is a working differential diagnosis, contingent upon further evidence and re-evaluation. Treatment evaluation research documents that untreated dual-diagnosed patients are more likely to relapse after treatment than addictive patients without psychiatric comorbidity.

Neuropsychologic Team

The addicted physician may appear cognitively unimpaired in the clinical interview. However, neuropsychologic testing will often reveal significant deficits in reasoning memory. After focused clinical interviews, psychologic test should involve the Halstead-Reitan Neuropsychological Battery (HRNB) test, which can include the Booklet Category Test, Tactile Performance Test, Reitan-Indiana Aphasia Screening Test, the Trailmaking Test, Reitan-Klove Sensory Examination, and the Seashore Rhythm Test. Useful adjuncts to the HRNB test include the Wechsler Adult Intelligence Scale (WAIS), Wechsler Memory Scale Revised (WMS-R), the Graham-Kendal Memory for Design Test, Minnesota Multiphasic Personality Inventory (MMPI), the Millon Clinical Multiaxial Inventory (MCMI), and the Rorschach test. Often missed in standard evaluations or in less-robust specific psychologic testing, neuropsychologic deficits may become apparent with more-sensitive evaluation techniques.

Family Therapy Team

The family is critical to the treatment and monitoring of addicted patient by the program. Interviews with the main significant other, children, parents, and siblings are diagnostically very helpful. Enlistment of these individuals in the treatment and recovery program is coordinated by the family therapists. Assessments are done ideally in the hospital or partial hospitalization programs where close and constant observation allows documentation of withdrawal symptoms, medical symptoms, and complications. Obviously, informed consent must be obtained from the patient to gain this information. Finally, a primary Axis I diagnosis, as well as subdiagnoses, are arrived at by team members. A detailed plan of treatment is then recommended.

The team then meets with the patient. It is useful to have the referral source or family members available for the diagnostic therapeutic recommendations of the assessment team.

If treatment is indicated, adequate time should be provided for questions and answers from the patient and the patient's family. Often the patient and the patient's family are given a choice of two or three facilities for treatment. Similarly, various alternatives for treatment should be discussed, as well as the problems that may be anticipated if the patient refuses treatment. Assurance of patient confidentiality is of the highest priority.

Treatment

Commonly accepted goals of treatment include (a) abstinence from alcohol and other nonprescribed psychoactive substances and (b) identification of the biopsychosocial treatment modality to which the patient's severity of illness will be matched. Treatment centers specialized in the care of chemically dependent physicians provide levels of care based on the American Society of Addiction Medicine (ASAM) patient placement criteria. These levels are labeled to be descriptive of the intensity of services provided: Level I, outpatient treatment; Level II, intensive outpatient/partial hospitalization; Level III, medically monitored inpatient treatment; and Level IV, medically managed inpatient treatment.

Identification of the Trigger Mechanisms

By appreciating that abuse plus genetic predisposition will produce the disease, identification of triggers that produce abuse is critical to recovery. Such triggers can involve a variety of emotional, personal, physical, and situational stresses. Each impaired physician must, over a period of time, with education and counseling identify his or her own triggers.

Nonchemical Coping

Chemically impaired health professionals have become dependent on coping with emotional, situational, and physical pain by using mood-altering drugs. Basic to the recovery process is the development and use of a nonchemical way of coping with life that includes social, environmental, dietary, and lifestyle practices.

Impaired health professionals must develop a multitude of nonchemical coping skills and capabilities that will allow them to deal with these crisis situations. For all of their professional lives, physicians have been taught that drugs and chemicals are a powerful part of their therapeutic armamentarium, so this requires "extended unlearning" procedures and practices on their part.

Balance in Changing Priorities

By virtue of their selection of their life work and their training, many impaired physicians put their professional lives and their physician's work as a priority before everything else. Almost by definition, they are both workaholics and perfectionists. For many, this behavior becomes a major "trigger" for substance abuse to relieve their stress. If the biogenetic predisposition is there in the face of this abuse, then disease is likely to occur. Recovery depends on medical, emotional, and spiritual growth.

Family Involvement

The family is critical in the diagnostic process, as well as in the recovery and therapeutic processes. Most often the family knows of the disease long before peers, friends, or individuals in the professional's office or in the hospital. Coming from a diagnostic standpoint, the signs and symptoms of individual health professionals, impairment must be familiar to the family. It is important to initiate family therapy, couples therapy, and educational workshops as soon as possible in the treatment process. Families should be encouraged to participate in 12-step self-help groups designed to help family members.

Mutual Help Groups

Successful health professionals' programs have demonstrated the use of 12-step programs. Careful study and acceptance of each of the 12 steps and then translating that into elements of the recovery program have proved particularly successful in health professionals. A frequent major barrier to recovery is the health professional's difficulty in understanding the dynamics of the 12-step program. This is not purely an intellectual process. By attending numerous programs with their peers, health professionals will accept the effectiveness of the 12-step program.

Aftercare and Monitoring

The planning of aftercare and monitoring should start from the first day of treatment and should involve the family and all other support systems of the impaired physician.

Treatment team members should be experienced in setting firm limits and boundaries, and they need to be experienced with the specific needs (both legal and professional) in treating the impaired physician. They should be familiar with the National Practitioner Data Bank, malpractice insurance, Drug Enforcement Administration (DEA) certification, and issues of state medical licensures. These professionals also need to be experienced with specific drug therapies, such as naltrexone and disulfiram (Antabuse). They need to be skilled at helping to solve re-entry problems once the patient returns to work, and they need to be available for frequent consultation.

Treatment Outcome

The primary goal of treatment is to help the physician-patient achieve and maintain long-term remission of his or her addictive disease. Recovery rates vary considerably, with reported rates for complete abstinence from mood-altering substances ranging from 27% to 92%.

Physicians appear to have better treatment outcomes than the general population when long-term aftercare and monitoring are done. There are also sufficient data to conclude that most physicians can be successfully rehabilitated and are able to re-enter medical practice with reasonable skill and safety for their patients.

Aftercare and Monitoring

Because substance abuse is a chronic illness, treatment is but the beginning of recovery. Most treatment centers have developed structured aftercare programs so that patients can continue to work on issues identified during their treatment program. Initially, many recovering physicians regard aftercare as punitive, hostile, or intrusive. However, when the patient understands and accepts the relapsing nature of the disease, and when aftercare monitoring is presented as a legal and licensing advocacy issue, compliance, acceptance, and gratitude usually result.

Stages of Recovery

A thorough recognition of the stages through which the recovering physician must pass and ways to overcome "stuck points" in the journey of recovery is essential. The recovery stages are as follows:

1. *Transition:* Starts when individuals begin to believe they have a problem with alcohol or drugs. It ends when the individual becomes willing to reach out for help.
2. *Stabilization:* The patient completes the physical withdrawal and acute withdrawal. Both physical and emotional healing begin. The obsession from drug or alcohol use subsides. The physician-patient begins to feel hope and to develop motivation for recovery.
3. *Early Recovery:* A time of internal change when the recovering physician begins to let go of painful feelings about his or her disease (guilt shame, fear,

resentment, etc.). The compulsion to use alcohol and drugs vanishes. The reliance on nonchemical coping skills to address problems and situations, which previously triggered chemical use, strengthens.

4. *Middle Recovery:* Balance begins to be restored. The wreckage of the past is cleared. Relationships are developed that positively reinforce learned skills that ensure continued personal growth.
5. *Late Recovery:* Resolution of painful events and issues related to growing up in a dysfunctional family must occur.
6. *Maintenance:* The recovering physician begins to practice the principles of successful recovery in all daily activities.

Prevention

The American Medical Association (AMA) has provided leadership in the prevention of chemical dependence and early rehabilitation for physicians with addiction. Every medical society now has a stated policy and a committee on physician impairment. The Federation of State Medical Boards (FSMB) has suggested guidelines for the relationship between the impaired physician health programs (PHPs) and the regulatory entity.

It is the responsibility of every physician to become involved in the prevention of alcohol, tobacco, and other drug problems. Through the treatment of their own illness, recovering physicians have a heightened awareness of the disease of chemical dependence. Traditionally, physicians in recovery have played a primary role in prevention as practitioners, as educators, as consultants to policy makers, and as concerned citizens. Through their recovery, there is a positive "ripple effect" of prevention into their families, patients, colleagues, and within the communities they serve.

Regulatory Issues and Ethical Considerations

The FSMB has proposed guidelines to promote uniformity in rules and regulations regarding impaired physicians. The goal of the federation is to protect the public. Efforts to educate citizens and the dissemination of information to the public about physician impairment have been initiated. The federation also communicates with the AMA, state medical hoards, state medical societies, and administrators in medicine. When appropriate, the federation pursues federal and state legislative initiatives to provide improved powers to state medical boards for the supervision of impaired physicians.

Conclusion

In recent years, many stakeholders who guard public safety and the practice of medicine (the AMA, FSMB, medical and specialty societies, ASAM, regulatory agencies, Federation of State Physician Health Programs, and others) joined forces to find solutions to the "challenging" issues of physician substance abuse. Changes in the landscape of health care delivery have diverted the attention of many practitioners away from compassionate concern for colleagues who have become impaired by chemical dependence. In spite of significant improvements in identification, intervention, assessment, treatment, and aftercare and monitoring, much is still unknown about the nature of chemical dependence.

Suggested Readings

Centrella M. Physician addiction and impairment—current thinking: a review. *J Addict Dis.* 1994;13:91–105.

Gallegos K, Lubin B, Bowers C, et al. Relapse and recovery: five to ten year follow study of chemically dependent physicians—the Georgia experience. *Md Med J.* 1992;41:315–319.

Reading E. Nine years experience with chemically dependent physicians: the New Jersey experience. *Md Med J.* 1992;41:325–329.

Richman JA. Occupational stress, psychological vulnerability and alcohol-related problems over time in future physicians. *Alcohol Clin Exp Res.* 1992;16(2):166–171.

Talbott G. Reducing relapse in health providers and professionals. *Psychiatr Ann.* 1995;25(11):669–672.

Talbott GD, Wilson PO. Physicians and other health professionals. In: Lowinson JH, Ruiz P, Millman RB, et al., eds. *Substance abuse: a comprehensive textbook*, 4th ed. Philadelphia: Lippincott Williams & Wilkins; 2005:1187–1202.

Section X

MODELS OF PREVENTION

44

PUBLIC HEALTH APPROACH TO THE PREVENTION OF SUBSTANCE ABUSE

For the several recreational mood-altering drugs and the laws applied to their distribution, sale, possession, and use, the differences in how the laws are actually implemented are defined as follows:

- For whom, which drugs, are illegal
- Which criminal drug laws are *de facto* decriminalized in which jurisdictions
- Which drug laws are enforced and against whom they are enforced

In practice, only a narrow band of the criminal drug laws is enforced employing the criminal sanction, primarily against certain selected elements of the population. By using the criminal law, nonwhites are selectively punished for violations for which the white user majority on the whole is not held either civilly or criminally accountable.

In practice, therefore, under the law as it is actually implemented, drug categorization differs rather markedly from the commonly held legal–illegal dichotomy. Rather, defined both by the laws themselves and how they are enforced, there are three categories, none distinguished from the others by a simple legal or illegal label.

- *Category I:* Tobacco and alcoholic beverages (the so-called legal drugs). The distribution by, sale to, and use of these drugs are illegal for persons younger than age 18 to 21 years (the age varying by state and drug). In practice, however, the enforcement of the relevant laws is effectively decriminalized in most jurisdictions.
- *Category II:* Prescription psychoactive drugs. The distribution, sale, possession, and use of these drugs, on a nonprescription basis, are illegal for persons of all ages. The enforcement of these laws, too, is either effectively decriminalized or simply not undertaken at all in most jurisdictions. Ironically, depending on how one counts, there are between 1.7 and 2.7 times more regular users of the prescription psychoactives on a nonprescription basis than there are regular users of cocaine and heroin added together.
- *Category III:* Marijuana, heroin, cocaine, and other illicit drugs. Like the category II drugs, their distribution, sale, possession, and use are *de jure* illegal for persons of all ages. In most jurisdictions in the United States, the criminal laws concerning these drugs are enforced, but they are enforced selectively. For the most part, general enforcement occurs only in geographic areas in which sellers and users are found in open or otherwise easily accessible spaces: poor, minority neighborhoods.

Defects in Current Policy

Before considering the principles and components of the public health approach (PHA) for the prevention of substance use/abuse in detail, we must first answer the question: Why is it necessary to develop and implement a new policy? What's wrong with the current national policy for dealing with drug abuse? From the public health perspective, at least 10 defects can be identified.

Artificial Bimodality/Lack of Comprehensiveness

The most prominent feature of national policy is that it is based on an artificial bimodality that, in turn, is based on the fallacious legal–illegal dichotomy discussed above. We have already seen that the true picture is quite different; the drug problem, in medical, public health, and epidemiologic terms, is a unity. Because national policy approaches category I drugs in one way, category III drugs in another, and category II drugs hardly at all, it is by definition totally lacking in comprehensiveness.

Lack of Focus on the Real Drug Problems

Because it has no basis in medical/public health science, the most serious defect in current national policy is that it directs the bulk of its attention to the least of the drug-related health harms. For example, in 1990, there were about 500,000 deaths associated with the use of alcohol and tobacco. By 1995, it could be estimated that that figure had risen to at least 590,000.

Conflict over the Role of Education

In current policy, there is a conflict over the role of education in dealing with the drug problem. For category I drugs, the major emphasis of national policy is on education. *De facto*, the law plays a secondary role, for example, banning cigarette smoking in many public places, making some effort to enforce laws against the sale of both tobacco products and alcoholic beverages to underage persons, cracking down on drunk drivers. There is no program of any kind for dealing with category II drugs. For category III drugs, although criminal law enforcement aimed at nonwhites is widely employed, some attempts at education are also made. But they are warped by the artificial bimodality of current policy.

Contradiction in Drug-Use Goals

Although the National Drug Control Strategy does not address the issue of the currently legal drugs, another federal document does. Healthy People 2010 lays out national objectives for disease prevention and health promotion. Objectives are set for reduced prevalence for the use of the two major drugs as well as for marijuana and cocaine. There are also goals for significant reductions in alcohol- and tobacco-related negative health outcomes. Recognizing reality, "drug free" is not on this national health agenda for any of the drugs.

However, the 1988 White House Conference for a Drug Free America, which laid the political groundwork for current national category III drug policy, called for just that: "drug free." Thus, the true drug use goal of current national policy remains unclear. Is it drug free, or drug use reduction? Or is it drug free for certain users of the minor drugs, drug use reduction for all users of the major ones, tobacco and alcohol, and ignoring all other categories of drugs (like category II) and subcategories of uses?

Futility of Criminal Law Enforcement Aimed at Simple Use

Studies indicate that the perceived certainty and severity of punishment are insignificant factors in deterring use. In the late 1980s and early 1990s, what apparently was more important in reversing the trend of increasing illicit drug use that marked the 1970s was the growth in perceived harmfulness of the activity, which, in turn, likely augmented social disapproval of drug use behavior. Among users, in any weighing of legal and health risks of drug use, concerns about health predominated. There is no evidence that this situation has changed.

These events occurred in the context of rapidly rising imprisonment levels for drug-related crimes by nonwhites. But if imprisonment or threat of it had a real impact on illicit drug use, as noted one would expect it to be much lower among nonwhites than whites because the former are imprisoned for drug offenses at a much higher rate than are the latter. But that is not the case.

Implementing a Pseudo "Demand-Side" Strategy

In 1990, a law enforcement–based "demand-reduction," "user-accountability" strategy was introduced to national policy for illicit drugs. It remains with the program. Ostensibly, this strategy recognized the limitations of the traditional "supply-side" approach. However, it did not focus on the causes of demand, such as the drug culture and the gateway drug effect. Rather, it simply targeted the "casual user" for the imposition of criminal sanctions. As if those "casual users," entirely on their own, were the major, indeed the only, factor in creating demand; as if they existed in a society that was either neutral or negative on drug use, in general.

Failure to Acknowledge the US Drug Culture

Demand and demand creation are, of course, very important factors in the drug problem. In fact, the way category I drugs are promoted and sold has a major impact on their use. This impact is mediated through the drug culture and the gateway drug effect. Current national policy fails to recognize that there is a drug culture in the United States that directly and indirectly promotes the use of all drugs.

To compound the problem, the "do drugs" messages of the drug culture extend well beyond the world of the recreational mood-altering drugs. Over-the-counter medications are sold as instant problem solvers: if you have a headache, take this pill; if you overate, swallow this liquid; if you can't get to sleep, take this other pill. The message never is "to avoid feeling overstuffed from eating too much pizza, why not try eating less pizza next time?" Since the mid-1990s, an antacid called Pepcid AC actually has been promoted as a medication to take before eating some food that you know will give you heartburn, so that you can eat the food anyway and not suffer the heartburn.

Furthermore, although vitamins are not drugs, they come in pill form and to many people look like drugs. And how are they promoted and sold? As an easy, painless means of self-improvement, in pill form, even for children. Is it any wonder that some of those children a few years later experiment with other kinds of pills that are promoted as easy, painless ways to a better you?

Finally, in America, medicine is practiced with an inordinate emphasis on treatment using pharmaceutical drugs as contrasted to personal health promotion and disease prevention by lifestyle modification. From the late 1990s onward, even the use of the prescription drugs has been heavily promoted to the general public by their makers, as are a bewildering variety of herbal remedies and dietary supplements. All pills. All painless ways to self-improvement of one sort or another.

And then there is gambling. Compulsive gambling is coming to be recognized as an addictive behavior. Gambling has been described as "an exploding entertainment industry starring cash." "Exploding," "addictive," and governments, especially at the state level, heavily promote it through lottery advertising, and do nothing even to warn people against the dangers of the many other forms of—totally legal—gambling.

Gateway Drug Effect

In most drug abusers the problem starts in childhood or the early teenage years. As Healthy People 2010 noted, tobacco use and addiction usually begin in adolescence. For almost all youngsters it is the "OK" drugs, tobacco and alcohol, that form the "gateway" to the use of the "not-OK" drugs, which are all of the others. One study, for example, found that a teenaged user of marijuana is eight times more likely also to be a cigarette smoker than is a teenager who does not use marijuana.

On Simple Availability and Drug Use

The most common argument against ending the Drug War has consistently been that to do so would lead directly to vastly increased use. Several responses to that argument can be made. First, it is not the case that a regulated, taxed supply of drugs, being sold only through controlled retail outlets, would necessarily lead to any relative increase in supply. In the present drug marketplace, there is almost always an excess of supply over demand for any of the drugs, including the illicits.

Second and more important, it happens that there is no historical evidence to support the notion that simple availability, without significant advertising and promotion, leads to use or that simple increase in availability leads to increase in use. Consider the following. Since World War II the greatest success achieved in the United States in drug use reduction has been for cigarette smoking among adults. This was accomplished in the face of unlimited supply, low price, and extensive prodrug use advertising and promotion.

If the drug problem were caused simply by the presence of a drug or drugs, the Andean countries themselves would be awash in cocaine addicts, which they are not, and neither tobacco nor alcohol use would have declined in the United States, which they have. The drug problem is caused primarily by demand for drugs and those factors that create demand, not simple supply.

The Drug War Does Not Work

The most serious defect of the Drug War is that it simply does not work, either in its own very narrow purview of category III drugs alone, or on the true drug problem, caused primarily by the still widespread use of tobacco products and alcoholic beverages. By its own admission, the programs of the Office of National Drug Control Policy (ONDCP), and the Drug War, have had little impact on illicit drug use. Alcohol use and its consequences remain a very serious health problem, and cigarette smoking is still widespread. It had been declining since the publication of the first *Surgeon General's Report on Smoking and Health* in 1964, but that decline leveled out in the mid-1990s.

Nevertheless, there is no indication that the proponents of the Drug War are considering either broadening their purview to cover all three categories of drugs of abuse or changing their tactics, ranging from attempts at source control to imprisoning otherwise noncriminal users, tactics that have no effect on illicit drug use.

Principles of the Public Health Approach

The Public Health Approach in Brief

The *primary goal* of the PHA as herein described is to:

> Reduce the use and abuse of all the recreational mood-altering drugs, to provide, when, as, and if possible, for their safe, pleasurable use, consistent with centuries' old human experience, while minimizing to the greatest degree possible the harmful effects of their use on individuals, the family, and society as a whole.

The PHA uses epidemiologic, pharmacologic, toxicologic, and medical science to define the drug abuse problem and to create the program components. It does not use predilections, politics, or prejudice. It identifies the real causes of the drug problem and then develops interventions directed at those causes, not imaginary ones. Some of the interventions are of a classically "public health" nature, as they appear, for example, in the "Statement and Resolution on Tobacco and Health" of the Committee on Public Health of The New York Academy of Medicine. Others are drawn from a broader perspective.

The PHA is a comprehensive national policy and program for dealing with the use and abuse of all the commonly used recreational mood-altering drugs, regardless of category. It is based on tried-and-true public health principles. In its details, it has a few new wrinkles here and there. However, it is constructed largely of ideas, programs, and recommendations that have been in the marketplace of ideas for some time now.

The Drug Problem Is a Unity

As shown above, the drug problem presents as a seamless web. The evidence of the interrelatedness of its various components is clear. If one's true goal is the reduction in overall drug use, it is fruitless, as present experience shows, to attempt to deal with only one part of the problem, or to deal with one part one way and another part another way. Biologic, medical, and epidemiologic science all tell us that a recreational mood-altering drug is a drug, regardless of its current status in the criminal law.

Single National Policy

Perhaps the most important element of the PHA is that there will be a single national policy for controlling the abuse of all the recreational mood-altering drugs. Among other things, this approach will end the current "OK"/ "not-OK" drug/person dichotomies.

Drug Abuse Is a Problem with a Natural History

Suffering from a drug abuse problem is not like having a common cold. It is not something a person catches one day that shows up in its clinical form the next. Furthermore, unlike the common cold, drug abuse in adults manifests itself over time differently in different persons and varies widely in breadth and depth from person to person and drug to drug. For example, most users of cigarettes are habituated to them, but a few are not. All cigarette smokers are at much higher risk for a number of serious diseases than are nonsmokers for the same diseases. But most cigarette smokers contract only one of those diseases, if they contract any at all.

Most users of alcohol do not become alcoholics. Most cocaine users do not become abusers. Some do. The PHA recognizes and provides for the reality that drug abuse in adults has no consistent natural history. However, the PHA also recognizes that in children there is a common natural history: for most drug abusers, the problem starts in childhood or the early teenage years, with the use of tobacco, alcohol, or both. Thus, the PHA pays a great deal of attention to preventing the use of those two drugs by young people.

The Universally Harmful Drug Form Is Tobacco

As noted previously, there is one drug form that, when used as intended, increases the risk of negative health outcomes for most users, as well as for all of those in the vicinity of use. That is, of course, tobacco. That fact, in addition to the centrality of tobacco to the gateway drug effect, makes tobacco use prevention in children central to the PHA.

The Spectrum of Harmfulness and the Concept of Safe Use

All the commonly used recreational mood-altering drugs other than tobacco increase the risk of health harms for only some of those who use them and for only some of those in the vicinity of use. The primary risk incurred by the use of drugs other than tobacco is that one might eventually use them to that level at which the risk of health harm appears. Thus, for drugs other than tobacco, there is a "spectrum of harmfulness" from none to severe.

Some of these harms are a result of the actions of the drugs on the body. Others are the result of drug-induced behaviors in the user. Of course, any use of any drug makes the user susceptible to the possibility of incurring health-harmful risk. But apparently for each commonly used drug other than tobacco, safe use is possible. For no recreational mood-altering drug has this spectrum been fully defined or clearly understood.

Law Enforcement Can Be Used Intelligently

History has taught us that criminal law enforcement works poorly to reinforce moral sanctions against personal behaviors such as the use of recreational mood-altering drugs. However, selectively applied criminal and civil law enforcement is an important tool in implementing many programs for improving the public's health.

The PHA respects the belief that the raising of moral considerations and the invocation of moral sanctions may be useful for some people in diminishing drug use. At the same time, the PHA recognizes that in dealing with this kind of highly personal behavior, our historical experience demonstrates the futility and waste of attempting to invoke or reinforce the moral sanction through the use of the criminal law. Doing the latter often produces a "cure" that is worse than the disease at which it is aimed.

Legalization Is Not the Focus; Solving the Drug Problem Is

Distinguishing the PHA from what is known as the "drug policy reform movement" is that for the latter, the target is the Drug War. For the PHA, the target is drug abuse, in all of its forms. Thus, the PHA is neither for nor against what is called "legalization." However, it recognizes the great health harms the Drug War brings to the nonwhite communities in which it is waged, harms probably more injurious to the public's health than the use of any of the drug forms other than alcohol and tobacco. Thus, it sees as a direct and very important benefit of its own implementation the opportunity to end the Drug War.

The Public Health Approach

The PHA to the prevention of drug abuse has a number of components. Some are of a classically "public health" nature; for example, improved school and public health education, strengthened regulatory approaches, such as limitations on the advertising and promotion of all recreational mood-altering drugs, and the legal prohibition of cigarette vending machines. Other measures are political, such as shifting the national leadership emphasis of the drug abuse control program from one that focuses on punishment for bad behavior to one that focuses on health. All these measures stress helping people to change their behavior in a positive way. Certainly not every element in the list below need be included for a PHA to be effective. As well, there may be other elements inadvertently left off the list that should be added.

Components

National Policy Education Campaign

The top national political and health leadership will be called on to educate the public on the new policy and stimulate its participation and cooperation. The educational campaign will recognize the drug culture and the gateway drug effect as significant causes of the total drug abuse problem and thus will focus major emphasis on dealing with them. To be effective, this campaign must be very carefully thought out, because the American people have been trained by present national policy (which tolerates the promotion of recreational mood-altering drug use) not to think of alcohol and tobacco as "drugs."

Rational Drug Classification System

A rational system for classifying all of the recreational mood-altering drugs (including tobacco and alcohol) by their potential dangers and benefits would be developed. This system would be based on these five major criteria: addictive potential, short-term personal hazards, long-term personal hazards, personal benefits (if any), and potential harmfulness to other individuals and society. Pharmacologic, toxicologic, pathologic, medical, epidemiologic, and sociologic data would be used to develop the system.

Responsible Use/Safe Use

As part of this effort, the highly controversial "safe use" and "responsible use" issues would be dealt with. To define safe use and responsible use for each of the major recreational mood-altering drugs is no mean feat. There are several starting points on which agreement could be reached fairly easily.

CHILDREN

For children there is no such thing as responsible use of any drug. This is based on the fact that most regular and addictive drug use begins before the age of 21 years.

ADULTS

There is responsible use of certain drugs for adults. For example, most consumers of alcohol in the United States are light to moderate users. There is some evidence that this is also true for the major illicit drugs. Certainly, any effective program to reduce the use and abuse of all recreational mood-altering drugs must deal with the reality of safe alcohol use by many American adults. At the same time, the majority of Americans appear to have recognized that there is no such thing as responsible use of cigarettes, at least in public.

The Regulated Sale Model

The regulated sale model for tobacco products would be developed for all drugs. They might be sold only in "drug stores," either state-run or licensed to private interests. Or there could be "drug sections" in general retail stores, with access permitted only for adults. The regulated sale model would be supported by the other elements of the PHA, below. As shown above, there is a significant difference between "simple availability" versus "availability with promotion." There would be controls on the places and hours of availability and sale of all the recreational mood-altering drugs.

Rational Price/Tax Structure

A rational price structure and tax policy for all drugs would be implemented. It would be aimed both at raising funds to pay for the program and at reducing consumption. It could be modeled on the British approach to alcohol beverage taxation and availability control. To assist in the overall public health campaign against drug abuse, the taxes should not be referred to as "sin" taxes, but rather as "risk-reduction" taxes or some similar appellation.

Assault on the Drug Culture

A clear assault would be made on the drug culture. This is a critical part of the program. The public must be educated to understand the interrelatedness of the use and abuse of all the recreational mood-altering drugs. They must also be educated to understand that the atmosphere created by the promotion of legal drugs, over-the-counter medications, and vitamins, and the way medicine itself is practiced, contributes to the drug abuse problem.

Advertising Policy

In the PHA there would be no future expansion of drug advertising beyond that which is at present permitted: no re-introduction of radio and television cigarette advertising, no advertising of spirits on radio and television, and no advertising of any kind for any currently illicit drug for which the legal status might change in the future. Also, a complete ban on pro-drug use advertising could be undertaken.

If it were to be concluded that a complete advertising ban were not desirable or not constitutional, pro-drug advertising could be taxed.

Public Education Campaign

There would be a comprehensive public education campaign against drug use *per se*, beyond the national leadership education program outlined in the section on National Policy Education Campaign. It would be much more comprehensive than the modest anticigarette smoking program of the last 20 years.

School Health Education

A comprehensive school health education program dealing with all of the recreational drugs in a unified manner should be implemented.

Research shows that successful prevention programs must not only involve schools, but entire communities. As students develop refusal skills, their commitment to nonuse must be reinforced and supported by parents, churches, businesses, and community leaders. To sustain this commitment, communitywide changes in attitudes must be made.

Treatment

Comprehensive treatment, rehabilitation, and job-training programs for those who are addicted to or who are abusers of any of the recreational mood-altering drugs would be made available. The matters of the appropriateness of "on-demand" treatment, the role of the law enforcement system in placing drug abusers in treatment, and who would pay for what would have to be worked out.

Assistance for Displaced Drug Workers and Farmers

Subsidies, relocation assistance, and retraining opportunities for the tens of thousands of workers and small farmers who would be put out of work in the United States by a significant decline in the legal recreational drug trade and/or the ending of various crop subsidy programs would be provided.

National Domestic Spending

The very important programs of national domestic spending to deal with the identified political, economic, and social causes of the illegal drug trade in those inner-city neighborhoods that are scarred by both legal and illegal drug use and the War on Drugs would be implemented.

Focused Law Enforcement

Finally, the focus of drug-related law enforcement would be on punishing criminal behavior resulting from drug use, not simply punishing drug use, although the required effort to enforce the laws against traffic in illicit drugs would be maintained.

Current law enforcement efforts would be continued until the use and abuse of all recreational mood-altering drugs are significantly reduced. However, the current emphasis on the incarceration of "casual users" would be brought to an end as counterproductive and wasteful of law enforcement time, money, and personnel. The drug traffic focus would be returned to the major dealers, as well as to corrupted law enforcement officials and "illegitimate" business activity, such as money laundering.

Conclusion

Solving the drug problem requires (a) recognition that it is a continuum occupied by all three drug categories; (b) setting rational, achievable goals for its control, goals that are consistent with human experience with the mood-altering drugs, achievable by the methods to be used in the program, and separate from the goal of crime reduction; (c) clearly understanding that its causes in this country go far beyond the simple availability of drugs upon which current policy focuses so much of its attention; (d) recognizing that the Drug War has not only consistently failed to meet its own stated objectives but also by its very nature cannot in any way be successful in dealing with the drug problem because of its totally distorted focus; and (e) therefore turning major attention from the supply side to the demand side, to the drug culture, the gateway drug effect, the centrality of tobacco product and alcoholic beverage use to the drug problem, and the specific causes of the inner-city drug trade: unemployment, poor housing, poor education, and hopelessness.

This program would markedly reduce the use and abuse of all the recreational drugs; reduce the tremendous pressure on and corruption of the criminal justice and law enforcement systems created by the present approach, freeing them to focus on other criminal behaviors, and would largely pay for itself through taxes on recreational drug sales, use, advertising, and profits. Its major political downside is that it requires a major assault on the tobacco and alcohol industries and the abandonment of the Drug War as an instrument of social oppression and a political weapon. But it can be done. Based on the record achieved by public health so far, it would meet with success.

Suggested Readings

Goldstein A. *Addiction: from biology to drug policy*, 2nd ed. Sect. II. New York: Oxford University Press; 2001.

Holden C. "Behavioral" addictions: do they exist? *Science.* 2001;294:980–982.

Jonas S. The public health approach to the prevention of substance abuse. In: Lowinson JH, Ruiz P, Millman RB, et al., eds. *Substance abuse: a comprehensive textbook*, 4th ed. Philadelphia: Lippincott Williams & Wilkins; 2005:1255–1267.

Kandel DB, Jessor R. The gateway hypothesis revisited. In: Kandel DB, ed. *Stages and pathways of drug involvement: examining the gateway hypothesis*. Cambridge, U.K.: Cambridge University Press; 2002.

King RS, Mauer M. *Distorted priorities: drug offenders in state prisons*. Washington, DC: Sentencing Project; 2002:11–13.

Section XI

TRAINING AND EDUCATION

45

MEDICAL EDUCATION AND CLINICAL PERSONNEL TRAINING

It is impossible to present a single prescription for the treatment of drug abusers and addicts. It is also impossible to present a single set of recommendations about the training of clinical personnel. In light of the progress achieved in the development and evaluation of effective substance abuse treatments, it is distressing that the training provided for clinical professionals to deliver these treatments has not kept pace.

Treatment Issues

Because of the strong convictions that both medical and nonmedical personnel bring to the arena, training in this field needs to be particularly sensitive. This sensitivity can be successfully negotiated by presenting a historical overview in a training setting, including review of some of the cultural, political, and religious features of drug use. This history is best presented in terms of its effect on treatment choices.

History of Treatment Challenges and Struggles

Drug abuse treatment has frustrated and perplexed people for decades. From the 1920s to the early 1940s, the cultural view of the drug abuser was reflected as a person with weak character and morals. In response to that cultural belief, jail was the common remedy and the only treatment choice was to detoxify addicts. Invariably, however, detoxified people returned to drugs, giving rise to the conviction that "once an addict, always an addict."

After World War II, the problem slowly but steadily grew worse, and there was an increase in criminal penalties for those found guilty of using drugs. By the early 1950s, there were stirrings in the Public Health Service of a more enlightened response to the problem of drug addiction. This expressed itself in an attempt to treat addicts by using what little was known at the time about social casework, vocational training, and some aspects of group therapy. The thinking was that if these activities kept the addict away from drugs long enough, restored the addict to physical health, and gave the possibility of insight or job skills or social casework support, there was hope that the individual could or would return to the community, no longer requiring drugs. To some extent, these efforts were successful.

By 1960, heroin use had expanded greatly and, with it, criminal behavior. Substance abuse professionals became discouraged: It seemed that psychiatry had not paid off, social work had not paid off, jail in and of itself had not paid off, and pure vocational training had not paid off. Furthermore, in the community and at large, there was little reimbursement to professionals, and practitioners often did not even experience the gratification of knowing that they were making an impact on the problem.

As the scope of drug abuse threatened to overwhelm the United States, two major new paradigms came into being. One was the therapeutic community (TC) movement. The TC approach was primarily conducted by people who had been afflicted with the problem, claiming that they alone, because of their affliction, could work successfully with this population. Cure could result, they felt, only in a rigorously honest disclosure of self and a challenging demand for new behavior, conducted in large measure by those who knew the addict's world from the inside.

The second major breakthrough was the development of methadone. Initially, methadone maintenance was resisted by those in drug enforcement, the mental health community, and by most workers in drug-free treatment communities. It slowly gained in use and credibility. Its use fit into the medical model, in that it was a medication. As such, it lent itself to a wide variety of studies in the academic and medical communities. These studies tended to verify its promise.

The New "Professionals" (Paraprofessionals and Others)

Despite the discovery of the ability of methadone to inhibit some heroin use, it soon proved evident that the medication itself was not enough to "cure" drug addiction. People who claimed that personal experience with addiction was a route toward successfully engaging users became more prominent. These ex-addicts became the first nonacademically trained, nonprofessional drug rehabilitation workers. They became known as "paraprofessionals." Their tough, pragmatic, sometimes brutally honest, empathetic approach to the problems of addiction, along with their intimate knowledge of the workings of an addict's life, gave the field a much-needed push in the direction of understanding and creating change in lives that seemed hopeless.

The Middle Class Enters the Picture

The majority of treatments for drug addiction in the second half of the 20th century were aimed at the bewildering problem of heroin addiction. However, during the late 1960s and early 1970s there was a slow, but ever-expanding, use of other drugs, particularly marijuana and psychedelics. Because these "new" drugs were used in large part by children of the middle class, some of the previous criminal sanctions surrounding drug abusers were called into question. Middle-class parents did not want their children to go to jail. Confusion reigned about how destructive these new drugs were, primarily because the many youthful users of these drugs seemed to demonstrate to their parents that they could use the drugs without problems, and because criminal penalties for the possession and use of these drugs were disproportionate to problems created by them.

The Government Steps In

By 1970 the first "War on Drugs" began in the form of the Special Action Office for Drug Abuse Prevention (SAODAP). Shortly thereafter came the birth of the National

Institute on Drug Abuse (NIDA). SAODAP, with the help of NIDA, mounted a national strategy meant to diminish the problem of drug abuse in America. The goal was to create a treatment system that could accomplish the following outcomes: (a) reduce crime in the streets; (b) reduce tax-consumptive behavior (i.e., any activity that costs the public money such as welfare, unemployment, public hospitals); (c) reduce illicit drug use; (d) increase tax-productive behavior (i.e., any activity that restores individuals so they can work and earn money); and (e) enhance personal well-being.

At that point, one of the tasks of these new agencies was to develop a pool of person-power that could address the treatment of this pervasive problem. This indicated a clear switch, both in overt policy and in mentality. The addict would no longer be exclusively a criminal; instead, the addict was also to become a "patient." In light of this new view, "treatment systems" were the way to deal with the drug user. This new approach called for a network of national treatment agencies and experts who could devote the time and research necessary to become career practitioners and teachers in the field, and training became paramount. Although this expansion created fresh enthusiasm, it also created a certain amount of chaos. How were various treatments to be tracked? How would efficacy be verified? To answer these questions, systems of reporting, patient tracking, and program management were instituted.

Some Gains, Some Losses

This interest attracted new professionals to the field. They merged with the paraprofessionals who had already been working in the field. Short-term treatment planning and short-term counseling systems, more in line with conventional psychologic counseling and social work counseling, took some precedence over TC approaches and work done by the earlier paraprofessionals in the treatment of heroin addicts. Some crossover of approaches did occur, but there were definite demands on the paraprofessional treater to adopt and adapt. Although there were benefits for the street paraprofessionals and TCs in establishing treatment and tracking plans, some of the unique methodologic breakthroughs, skills, and approaches pioneered by TCs and methadone maintenance were neglected.

Treatment systems across the country attempted to expand in light of the new public funds available and a resurgence of interest in the field. In the mid-1970s, however, these public funds were cut back just as the field began to mount a national effort against drug abuse, and just as these systems began to show positive outcomes. The field lost career teachers and the more-trained practitioners. Public funds and support eroded even further during the 1980s. During these same years of funding reductions, however, services grew in two quarters. The first was in public sector methadone maintenance programs and TCs, and the second included private for-profit insurance reimbursement approaches.

Within the public sector, heroin users continued to seek help from methadone maintenance clinics. TCs expanded to meet an increase in demand as well. The TC had realized that the methods originally intended to aid heroin addicts were equally effective with multidrug users and ever-younger users. Both methadone clinics and TCs responded strongly during the years of government cutbacks, despite the decrease in public money available to them.

A second expansion that took place in the 1980s consisted of privately funded, for-profit drug programs operating chiefly in hospitals. This new direction in treatment germinated from the incorporation of Alcoholics Anonymous (AA) and 12-step programs into hospital settings under the umbrella of doctors and other allied health providers. Because the first of these programs began at Willmar State Hospital in Minnesota and was further refined at Hazelden and the Johnson Institute in Minnesota, these programs are often referred to as the "Minnesota Model."

Two-Tier Treatment System

By the end of the 1980s, a two-tier response system existed, with the public nonprofit groups (stretched thin as a result of diminished public funding and with massive waiting lists) and the private for-profit groups competing with each other. Both tiers required training either to respond to demand or to improve the attractiveness of their services. Despite the multiplicity of these public sector and private sector programs that now exist in explicit response to drug abuse, training had not kept pace in its ability to prepare those who work in the field.

Training Issues

How Bias Affects Treatment and Training

Those who come to drug abuse training programs often do so with strong biases that result from prior education, as well as personal experience, and they have a significant impact on the way in which people approach training. If people are convinced that their treatment ideas are the "only" correct ideas, they tend to herd people through a rigid set of interventions that simply are not flexible enough to bend to individual needs. Cultural beliefs further complicate these practitioner biases. Some of the biases in basic thinking about substance abuse are as follows:

1. Drug abuse and drug dependence are phases of a disease process.
2. Working with a client who is actively using drugs is "enabling."
3. If clients do not think of drug abuse as an out-of-control disease, they are in denial.
4. If a client does admit to having a "disease," a 12-step program is the only concrete, long-lasting solution.
5. Psychotherapy is ineffective.
6. Psychotherapy is necessary to produce long-term recovery.
7. Medical intervention in the form of medication is destructive or impedes recovery.
8. The only real, cost-effective help lies in a medicopharmacologic response.
9. Drug-dependent people most likely have substance-dependent parents.
10. The TC approach is the only long-lasting rehabilitation that is drug free.
11. TC approaches work with only a small segment of the drug-using population.
12. Regardless of original drug use patterns, all "recovering" people must abstain from any drug use (e.g., alcohol, medications) for the rest of their lives.

Obviously, these divergent convictions can create a chaos of misunderstanding in both treatment and training programs. No one approach is right. The goal of drug abuse training should be to create an atmosphere in which people are able to listen openly to new ideas and to offer a range of care options broad enough to encompass many kinds of addicts, at many stages of addiction.

Attitudinal Changes

The social science and psychiatric literature suggests the following techniques of training for behavior that counteracts social norms:

1. A message has more attitudinal impact if its *source has credibility and perceived expertise.* This means *role models* who are from their own clinical discipline.
2. Yielding occurs when *the recipient agrees with the presented attitude.* Cognitive yielding probably precedes affective and conative yielding and may occur in classroom settings in response to didactic presentations.
3. Retention is enhanced by *repetitions of experience over time.* The effects of short courses die quickly if reinforcement and support are not present. *Active participation in the learning experience and subsequent practice* contribute to the persistence of attitudinal changes. Retention or attitude change is greatly enhanced by a supportive group of peers and faculty.
4. *Overt behavior reflecting the new positive attitudes.* Requiring the desired behavior *in conjunction with close supervision* usually results in maintenance of the behavior. This likelihood of change is enhanced if the behavior is accompanied by favorable results such as a positive outcome.

The educational research suggests that the best results, in terms of positive attitudes and skills, occur when trainees rotate through addiction treatment units and are supervised by experts in addictions.

Gap between Science and Clinical Services

Researchers perceive that many science-developed innovations have improved the treatment of drug abuse. For example, methadone maintenance treatment began as a research effort, relapse-prevention techniques were honed by research investigations, the stages and processes of behavioral change were studied in depth, and, recently, motivational enhancement techniques have improved retention in treatment. Studies have found that treatment intensity and systematic follow-up improve treatment outcomes, yet few of these findings have been incorporated into standard treatment settings.

The treatment practitioners are on the other side of the gap. Faced with the challenges of providing services on a daily basis, they are frustrated by what they see as the failure of research to provide them with specific answers to their day-to-day questions. They perceive that current policy, including funding, provides little opportunity or incentive for treatment programs to implement new scientific findings. The barriers between the science and the practice are multiple, but the insufficient training on evidence-based practices is one of the most prominent and disturbing. Furthermore, just as research findings have been underused by the treatment community, there are treatment approaches that have been understudied by the research community. Even when studies document that a treatment can be successfully implemented in a clinical setting, the challenges in the final stage of transfer to treatment programs are the provision of additional training for staff in delivering the new treatment, changing the attitudes of the providers, and providing evidence that the new treatment is effective in the local clinical environment. Each of these components of training poses problems for the treatment programs.

Basic Concepts of Training

Successful training in drug abuse treatment is predicated on certain fundamental theories. These basic ideas permeate any and all specific parts of the curriculum. They serve the dual purpose of being both immediately applicable to the training setting and to the workplace.

1. Personal responsibility: Methods that help mobilize the individual impulse toward health, despite personal and environmental obstacles
2. Self-help: Technology whereby both individuals and groups can become effective in coping and problem solving on an ongoing basis
3. Social systems perspective: Information that stresses practitioners' awareness of the interdependence of individuals and their social environment
4. Social support: Methods for creating or using helping networks that can enhance the functioning of individuals and help maintain change
5. Transdisciplinary practice: Skills and attitudes that prepare disciplines to collaborate toward "whole person" responses in planning, goal setting, and problem solving
6. Systematic problem solving: Goal-oriented perspective that recognizes a common systemic and empirical process of stages and strategies that can be applied in assessing and treating problems at the individual, family, community, and societal levels
7. Interorganizational relations: Concepts and perspectives relevant to understanding the forces that shape service-delivery systems
8. Cooperative learning: Concepts and techniques to enhance self-esteem, acquisition of knowledge, and prevention of drug use

Skill Enhancement

Although inclusion of general information about the context of drug abuse treatment and models is essential to training, it must be accompanied by skill development—pragmatic techniques that help practitioners perform their jobs better. For those people fighting in the trenches of drug abuse treatment programs on a day-to-day basis, skill development becomes of the utmost importance. Skill enhancement for drug treatment personnel essentially can be divided into two categories. The first category concerns skills demanded by the funding and oversight agencies, which require ever more accurate and specific reporting mechanisms and management systems. Practitioners who are overwhelmed by paperwork simply cannot perform as effectively with clients. In light of this, many training candidates need specific organizational information, such as how to keep clinical records and how to track client and management activities.

The second category of skills needed by treatment personnel in the field includes the art of specific case-management skills, including treatment planning, case notemaking, and assessment skills. These skills are all part of the practitioner's main concern: How do I improve my ability to do the required paperwork while successfully treating this client?

Training Populations

Within any particular training model, there should be unique program training approaches. These programs must be relevant not only to emerging problems (such as AIDS, child abuse, sexuality, homelessness, and needs of women with children), but must accommodate particular populations likely to seek training, such as workers in mental health, social welfare, drug and alcohol treatment, health, corrections, and education. Each of these populations needs basic substance abuse treatment information, as well as job-specific information.

Curricula for substance abuse training programs should cover a broad spectrum, from law enforcement, prevention, education, intervention, and after-school programs to day-care programs and family care programs. This information should cover the following topics: theories of drug dependence and addiction; historical, cultural, social, and biologic implications; what types of treatment are available; the pros and cons of each type of treatment; how to care for clients without bias; and how to determine the most suitable treatment for each client. Training in the treatment needs of special populations is of great importance.

Social welfare curriculum should include information about child and family welfare, poverty, aging, community-based care, and community development. Health workers who directly address the emotional and living needs of people with serious medical and degenerative conditions require knowledge about death and dying, coping with chronic disabilities, maintaining extrainstitutional relationships, and providing opportunities for continuing social contributions. Participants from public and private institutions that treat drug and alcohol abuse need material about engagement, recruitment, retention, assessment, inpatient and outpatient treatment, and differentiation between adult and adolescent treatment, as well as school and community prevention programs.

Training Philosophy

Training Adult Learners

The best approach to teaching adults is to view training as a planned, sequential process designed to provide the self-awareness, skills, knowledge, and attitudes needed to perform particular tasks. Whenever possible, trainees should be responsible for suggestions regarding training content and design. This increases feelings of "ownership" and fosters personal engagement with the training. The most effective training for adults is designed with the following points in mind:

1. A climate of mutual respect must exist between trainer and trainees.
2. An open, friendly, and casual atmosphere facilitates the exchange of differing viewpoints and ideas.
3. Trainees should be aided in diagnosing their own skills and growth needs, as well as in analyzing the specific training elements needed by their agency.
4. Adult learners learn best that which is relevant and useful to them. Whenever possible, training ideas should be applied to current work situations.

Creating a Receptive Training Climate

Several considerations go into creating an open-minded, fruitful training setting: overall tone and climate, geographic location, and class composition. To begin with, the tone and climate of training sessions are crucial. People hear information in different ways and at different points in their lives, depending on its relevance to their own experience. The first challenge of training is to elicit an investment in the training itself, both from those undergoing training and the managers, directors, and administrators in the environments from which the trainees come. One way to accomplish this is to discuss the different perspectives among the trainees at the beginning of the training. It is then possible to create a desire to think about the potential benefits of differing perspectives.

From a training point of view, this early intellectual activity has the effect of engaging people. Requiring active participation in the training increases the emotional readiness for new experiences and reduces anxiety so that absorption can occur. Much depends on the group itself—how it defines what it needs to improve its competence. This activity models tactics and procedures that are useful in treatment: negotiating differences, making an investment, and determining options. Learning is drastically increased when trainees feel that they have control over what and how they learn.

To foster an active learning atmosphere, work is done to establish the sharing of information, in terms of both talking and listening. Ensuring a balance between receiving and giving information permits learners to share without fear of failure. It also increases their skills as both dispensers and collectors of information. With information flowing in both directions, no one can take a passive stance. This promotes a dynamic learning environment.

Logistics and Atmosphere

In any training plan, the site location—such as geography—can influence outcome. For some, instruction seems to be most effective when it is done physically close to home or their worksite. For others, leaving the normal work environment and traveling to unfamiliar surroundings for training has a bracing effect. In the absence of supervisors and peers, these individuals may feel less inhibited about disclosing certain problems and questions and more free to receive new information and ideas. Needs assessment prior to training can help determine what might work for a particular trainee or group of trainees.

Composition

Finally, class composition is a determining factor in the creation of a successful training climate. There are advantages to both homogeneous and heterogeneous groupings. People from similar disciplines have the following advantages when training together:

1. They can practice skills relevant to their particular methodology, because they are familiar with the treatment model and its context.
2. They can offer feedback and problem-solving ideas appropriate to their unique setting.
3. If the trainees already work together every day, problems characteristic of their system can be addressed in training in ways that are impossible in a day-to-day setting.
4. People who already know and work with each other can study, practice skills, and work together as teams in ways that they can carry directly to the workplace.

Trainees from different backgrounds, on the other hand, can benefit greatly from a classroom situation in which people come from various disciplines, as follows:

1. They may feel freer to ask questions.
2. They may feel important because they can offer a unique perspective from their setting.
3. They can hear how others handle similar problems in different settings.
4. Work problems will not cloud their ability to learn.
5. They may bypass power struggles that exist in a homogeneous group that works together.

Successful Training Methods

It is important for training sessions to include a mix of methods. This counters boredom and acknowledges that people learn in different ways. Several methods may be used in successful training: (a) didactic presentations, (b) small groups, (c) large groups, (d) simulation and role playing, (e) task groups, and (f) videotaping.

Physician Training in Addictions

Medical education excels in the development of skill acquisition. The process begins in the basic science years and continues throughout training and practice with continuing knowledge acquisition. Attitudes are acquired more often by example than by discussion. As the field of addiction medicine has matured, there has developed a much greater clarity about the type of skills needed by any physician in this field. Core competencies in addiction medicine have been identified for physicians:

Level I

All physicians who see patients should be able to do the following:

1. **Perform age, gender, and culturally appropriate substance abuse screening.** This is part of basic medical interviewing and should be taught in the introduction to clinical medicine courses in the first years of medical school. Reinforcement should occur in the clerkships and residency years. A key skill in the screening area is the ability to inquire about the use of addicting drugs: tobacco, alcohol, prescription, and illicit drugs. Screening questions can help the physician decide whether a more extensive assessment is needed.
2. **Provide brief interventions to patients with substance use disorders (SUD).** A growing body of evidence indicates that brief interventions by practicing clinicians are effective in reducing hazardous or harmful drinking. Brief interventions take less than 10 to 15 minutes. They can be manual-guided or as simple as communicating concern and putting the patient in contact with a treatment clinician.
3. **Use effective methods of counseling patients to help prevent SUD.** There is little known about the efficacy of physician efforts in primary prevention. However, establishing a therapeutic alliance with the patient will help at all levels of primary, secondary, and tertiary prevention.
4. **Refer patients with SUD to treatment settings that provide pharmacotherapy and psychosocial therapy for relapse prevention.** Once abstinence is

established there is a high risk of relapse. Research has highlighted the value of pharmacotherapy and psychosocial therapy in reducing the rate of relapse.

5. **Recognize and treat or refer comorbid medical and psychiatric conditions in patients with SUD.** High rates of comorbid disorders have been reported in patients with SUD. The available data and clinical experience indicate that better outcomes occur when the SUD and medical/psychiatric conditions are treated concurrently rather than consecutively.

6. **Refer patients with SUD to appropriate treatment and supportive services.** Referral to treatment programs should be done when there is evidence of alcohol or other drug dependence, especially when the patient continues to drink or use other drugs despite the physician's attempts at interventions. Referral works best when a referral appointment is scheduled while the patient is in the office. A direct link to the referral source at that time increases patient compliance.

7. **Describe the ethical and legal issues around physician impairment from SUD and of the resources for referring potential impaired colleagues.** Physicians are as vulnerable as the general population to alcohol abuse and dependence and have a much greater access to other addicting drugs. Every practicing physician should be aware of the fundamentals of physician impairment. This is especially important if the physician works in a group practice, practices in a hospital setting, or has a responsible position on the medical staff of a hospital or clinic.

8. **Identify the legal and ethical issues involved in the care of patients with SUD.** Legal complications are common in patients with more severe SUD. Arrests for driving under the influence, drunk and disorderly, possession, and the like may result in sentencing involving probation or parole. This coercive pressure can be very helpful in keeping patients in treatment for their SUD and enforcing abstinence long enough for recovery to begin to occur.

Level II

All physicians coordinating care for patients with SUD in addition should:

1. **Use effective methods to assess patients with SUD.** Training for the development of *assessment skills* is diagnostic training. The skills necessary to diagnose substance abuse or substance dependence are best acquired in clinical settings. This includes skill in taking a history from the patient and acquiring information from other sources, including family members. The level II physician will be very familiar with drug testing.

2. **Provide pharmacologic withdrawal to patients with SUD.** Withdrawal from addicting drugs can be done safely in inpatient or office settings. In all instances, withdrawal should be done in conjunction with psychosocial treatment for addiction.

Level III

All physicians providing specialty services to patients with SUD should:

1. **Provide pharmacotherapy for relapse prevention in patients with SUD.** One of the principles of addiction treatment outlined in the NIDA research-based guide is that "[m]edications are an important element of treatment for many patients, especially when combined with counseling and other behavioral therapies."

2. **Provide or refer for psychosocial counseling for relapse prevention in patients with SUD.** Research in the psychosocial therapies in the last decade demonstrates the effectiveness of this aspect of treatment. Researchers from the NIDA Collaborative Cocaine Treatment Study commented on "the importance of 12-step involvement as a primary or adjunctive aspect of substance dependence treatment."

Teaching Methods and Evaluation for Physicians

Teaching methods are being addressed more frequently in the substance abuse literature. The lecture is the best-known method of passing on the knowledge base. Lectures have little influence on attitudes or skills, but can serve as an introduction to be followed by clinical experience. Recovering AA or Narcotics Anonymous (NA) members can also be very useful in the classroom, in small-group discussions, and in taking medical students to open meetings.

In the clinical clerkship years students need exposure to addiction treatment programs. This experience has the greatest impact if there is continuity in following patients and exposure to residents working in these programs. In residency training, supervised clinical experience on addiction treatment units appears to be essential for the development of positive attitudes and clinical skills.

There is a need for faculty role models. These are most likely to come from physicians who have taken training in addiction medicine in fellowships. Most of these fellowships require completion of postgraduate training in an accredited specialty. The development of a certification exam by the American Society of Addiction Medicine (ASAM) and the Certificate of Added Qualification in Addiction Psychiatry by the American Board of Psychiatry and Neurology provide recognized roots for the development of competent faculty and teaching clinicians.

Conclusion

As with many endeavors in education and professional training, substance abuse treatment and training began as apprenticeship training—learning by doing. Gradually, more formal training emerged: first, by treatment agencies themselves; next, by government agencies with hopes of expanding resources; then, by groups or agencies with similar operating philosophies; next, by groups allied with certain agencies who offer certification; and, finally, by schools granting credit for specific courses at the college or university level.

At the present time there is a shortage of subspecialists to teach addiction medicine in each of the medical specialties. This means that clinical departments may have to look for teachers from other clinical specialties, for example, psychiatry and family medicine, until they can develop their own. The last two decades have produced a cadre of experienced clinicians who can materially upgrade medical education in addiction medicine. These specialists in addiction medicine can serve as supervisors and role models to medical students and residents.

When it comes to specific techniques of treatment or prevention, more extensive and specialized training is required. Such exposure aimed at drug abuse practitioners faces many challenges. Certainly, the interplay of client needs, available funds, community agency operating philosophies and goals, as well as diverse trainee beliefs and assumptions can, and often do, cause conflict. In this light, training should be viewed as a growth process that occurs within the context of a facilitative relationship and information exchange.

Suggested Readings

Chappel JN. Medical education in substance abuse: the acquisition of knowledge, attitudes, and skills. In: Lowinson JH, Ruiz P, Millman RB, et al., eds. *Substance abuse: a comprehensive textbook*, 4th ed. Philadelphia: Lippincott Williams & Wilkins; 2005:1269–1286.

Deitch DA, Koutsenok I, Marsolais K. Education and training of clinical personnel. In: Lowinson JH, Ruiz P, Millman RB, et al., eds. *Substance abuse: a comprehensive textbook*, 4th ed. Philadelphia: Lippincott Williams & Wilkins; 2005:1286–1300.

Fiellin DA, Butler R, D'Onofrio G, et al. The physician's role in caring for patients with substance use disorders: implications for medical education and training. *Subst Abuse*. 2002;23(3):207–222.

Miller NS, Sheppard LM, Colenda CC, et al. Why physicians are unprepared to treat patients who have alcohol and drug related disorders. *Acad Med*. 2001;76:410–418.

Saitz R, Friedman PD, Sullivan LM, et al. Professional satisfaction experienced when caring for substance abusing patients. *J Gen Intern Med*. 2002;17:373–376.

46

FORENSICS

This chapter is an introduction and practical guide to *criminal* forensic practice for the specialist in addiction medicine. The discussion is necessarily a synoptic overview. A comprehensive analysis of the relevant legal rules, doctrines, and principles; the evolution of the insanity defense; a detailed medicolegal discussion of significant cases; and a comparative analysis of the relevant federal and state laws are clearly beyond the scope of this chapter. The urgent conceptual problems arising from the interaction between the law and addiction medicine are highlighted throughout the discussion.

The Addiction Medicine Specialist as a Forensic Expert

Clinical Experts in the Criminal Law

The participation of specialists in addiction medicine as experts in forensic matters is a development that reflects the growth of the accredited specialty of addiction medicine over the past two decades and the courts' long-standing disenchantment with the testimony of traditional mental health experts in these matters.

Qualification as an Expert

Determining who should be an expert witness for "psychologic" matters has been a difficult task for the courts. Although there are federal and state standards that govern expert testimony, there is little consistency between and within jurisdictions about the qualifications of expert witnesses. Often, decisions regarding who qualifies as an "expert" are made on pragmatic rather than jurisprudential grounds.

Rationale for the Admission of Expert Testimony

Most states have a rule of evidence that parallels Federal Rule of Evidence 702, which provides that "if scientific, technical, or other specialized knowledge will assist the trier of fact [judge or jury] to understand the evidence or to determine a fact in issue, a witness qualified as an expert by knowledge, skill, experience, training, or education, may testify thereto in the form of an opinion or otherwise." But a few states have adopted different and confusing rules on this point. The states also have tended to follow Federal Rule of Evidence 704, which limits expert testimony to an explanation of the defendant's diagnosis and the characteristics of the disease or defect. This rule specifically precludes expert opinion on "whether the defendant did or did not have the mental state or condition constituting an element of the crime charged or of a defense thereto."

How the Law Views Expert Testimony

Under prevailing rules of evidence, the testimony of expert witnesses is presented to the court in the form of expert opinion, and as such it does not enjoy the same privileged status as "fact" testimony. It remains for the trier of fact (judge or jury) to evaluate the credibility, reliability, relevance, and applicability of any expert testimony introduced. What an expert in addiction medicine may know to be an accepted medical "fact" is nonetheless considered to be only "opinion" when expressed in expert testimony. As opinion, such information may be accepted, discounted, or rejected in whole or in part by the trier of fact. When testifying, any lapse of awareness of this crucial distinction may result in the expert being perceived as argumentative, defensive, sanctimonious, condescending, or hostile. This always compromises credibility, undermines the power of testimony as evidence, and may prove fatal to the client's case.

Role of the Expert in Addiction Medicine

The following discussion may seem to express a defense bias, but bear in mind that it rarely serves the interest of the prosecution case to introduce expert testimony in support of exculpating or mitigating mental defenses. Of course, the prosecution may call experts to rebut testimony introduced by defense experts. Although an expert is more likely to be engaged by the defense, the expert should be willing to appear for either side. Remember that an expert witness is not an advocate. The professional mandate is to assist the court.

Pretrial Phase

In the pretrial phase, the addiction specialist can assist the attorney by reviewing the initial discovery materials (e.g., police reports, arrest forms, affidavits of investigating agencies, waivers of rights, medical examiner reports, toxicology screens, statements of witnesses and the accused, confessions, the formal complaint, information, or indictment) to identify any immediate or potential issues related to intoxicants. Attorneys also may seek assistance in managing a difficult, compromised, or dangerous client. It may be necessary to evaluate and refer the client immediately for primary treatment or stabilization so that the client can adequately assist counsel in the preparation of the case. Determination of competency to stand trial is a separate matter, both clinically and legally.

Once prospective witnesses have been identified, the addiction specialist should make a preliminary assessment of all available background materials to identify any possible clinical (i.e., medical, neuropsychiatric, or addiction) issues that require investigation. The specialist can also help the attorney to prepare for depositions by (a) drafting specific questions to be posed, (b) doing content and psycholinguistic analyses of taped or written evidence (e.g., statements or depositions made by the defendant or witnesses), and (c) suggesting strategies and tactics for conducting interviews or depositions. It is often important to interview family members, friends, former teachers, or others who may have particular knowledge or a different perspective of the defendant or witness.

The cornerstone of an addiction specialist's evaluation of the defendant is a comprehensive addiction history. The specialist must aggressively inquire about every aspect of use and experience with intoxicants of all classes, and all of the addictive processes. Also necessary is a lifetime neuropsychiatric history, exploring every sign or symptom reported, suggested, implied, or suspected. Of course, complete medical (including all responses to prescription and over-the-counter medications), psychosocial, developmental, educational, relational, and vocational histories must be taken. History or indicia of psychologic, sexual, or physical abuse also must be aggressively sought and explored.

If the other side will be calling an addiction expert, the addiction specialist can assist the attorney by (a) evaluating that expert's credentials, (b) anticipating the nature of the testimony, (c) analyzing the strengths and weaknesses of both expert positions, and (d) drafting appropriate questions for the attorney to ask in cross-examination.

Trial Phase

The two most common types of cases in which an addiction specialist will be engaged are those in which a person either is accused of having committed a crime while drug involved (i.e., while experiencing the acute, subacute, chronic, or residual effects of previous intoxicant use, dependence, or withdrawal) or is on trial as the result of statements made to law enforcement officers or testimony given by witnesses who themselves are or have been drug involved. The first type of case typically requires testimony about the nature and effects of intoxicant use on the defendant. Common issues here include the impact of specific intoxicants on (a) the physical and mental ability to have committed the crime, (b) the state of mind required for the offense charged, or (c) the formation of the requisite intent. Other potential questions may involve the special issues of diminished capacity or insanity. The second type of case typically involves testimony about the effects of acute and chronic intoxicant use on cognition and memory, and how such use might affect the credibility of witnesses.

Postconviction Phase

It is difficult to accept that defenses involving intoxicants usually do not prevail—even in cases where one believes that any colleague in the field would find the clinical evidence supportive of the defense position. It is always painful to lose a case in which one strongly believes. Long-standing biases in the criminal law, public opinion, and political factors often have greater influence on the outcome of a case than does the clinical evidence. Realize that most clients will be convicted. But also realize that, as the result of one's testimony, the conviction may be for a lesser offense, which carries a lesser penalty. Try to remember that testimony in every case can make a meaningful difference to what eventually happens to the defendant.

Often, the most valuable contribution to a case will be made in the postconviction phase, that is, at sentencing. Most jurisdictions permit the defense to present evidence (including expert testimony) in support of mitigation during the sentencing process.

Criminal Responsibility and Intoxicants

Although the connection between the use of intoxicants and crime has been universally recognized, the explosive increase in drug-related crime over the past two decades has had only minimal impact on substantive criminal law. The recognition (albeit equivocal) of substance use disorders as "diseases" and the growth of a professional field and industry around the field has had significant social and professional consequences and instructive (although surprisingly limited) effects on the legal rules.

Conceptual Problems

Definition, Description, and the Problem of DSM-IV-TR

Because the criminal law has a long history of difficulty defining the concepts of "mental disease" and "mental defect," it is perhaps not surprising that the American Psychiatric Association's DSM-IV-TR has been adopted by the courts as a Rosetta Stone for recognizing a defendant's alleged "mental" problems as true diseases or defects.

Disease, Disorder, Defect, and Dysfunction

Moving beyond the hurdle of DSM-IV-TR, one must be prepared to confront the distinctions between "disease," "disorder," and "dysfunction." The first two terms have long and tortuous histories in the law of every jurisdiction, whereas the concept of cerebral "dysfunction" has virtually none. And yet, it is precisely in terms of cognitive, emotional, and behavioral dysfunction that one can best explain (and even quantify) the effects of acute, subacute, and chronic intoxicant use. Most defendants seeking to avail themselves of an intoxicant-based defense will have grossly normal findings on objective neuropsychiatric diagnostic tests as the electroencephalogram (EEG), computed axial tomography (CAT) scan, or magnetic resonance imaging (MRI) scan. Even when administered using the latest enhanced techniques, these modalities are of limited value in demonstrating cerebral dysfunction. Although the newer brain imaging technologies, such as the quantitative EEG, single-photon emission computed tomography (SPECT), and brain electrical activity mapping (BEAM), promise considerable future utility, at present, valid norms for these modalities are still in the earliest stages of development.

Use, Misuse, Abuse, Dependence, Addiction

Terminology in the field of addictive disease remains an unsettled area. Within DSM-IV-TR, for example, there is no formal definition or use of the word "addiction." That term as it is often used is referred to instead as "dependence," a word less likely to have pejorative connotations within the courtroom. One might argue that substance dependence is a medical disease whereas substance addiction is a social issue. Use of a substance does not establish the presence of a disease, but it does establish the presence of potentially intoxicating effects. Finally, if appropriate, one may need to educate participants regarding use of the "substance-induced" category as it applies to alteration of mood or perception.

Elements of the Offense

Definitions of both common law and statutory crimes require the voluntary commission of a bad act or harmful omission (*actus reus*) in conjunction with a bad state of mind (*mens rea*). However, these fundamental concepts have resisted enduring definition. Most older common law crimes have been redefined in modern criminal statutes. Criminal codifications often use adverbial qualifiers such as "knowingly," "willfully," or "intentionally" to designate as voluntary an act performed consciously as the result of effort or determination.

Exculpatory Doctrine in Common Law

Over time, scientific views of human behavior gradually supplanted moral ones. Concurrently, there was a substantial increase in the consumption of alcohol in all social and economic strata. In response to these societal changes, the common law evolved what came to be known as "the exculpatory doctrine." This doctrine permitted the presentation of evidence of specified mental conditions (including intoxication) in legal proceedings as a means of mitigating culpability, liability, or responsibility. Such evidence could be introduced in the form of an assertion of a defendant's insanity or lack of the "specific" intent required as an element of the offense charged. New and more difficult problems arose almost immediately.

Enduring Problematic Concept of "Intent"

The early cases in which the exculpatory doctrine was applied involved alcohol intoxication. The courts gradually realized that "common sense" suggested that a distinction should be made between a crime committed by an intoxicated as opposed to a sober person. But traditional moral attitudes stigmatizing intoxication as a vice indicated the impropriety of complete exculpation. The criminal rules on "intent" provided an expedient, if inadequate, means of mediation.

These doctrines, which were the foundation of the exculpatory rule, imply that "specific intent" is distinguishable from "general intent." These also signify that certain crimes require only "general intent," whereas other offenses require certain "specific" intents.

Intoxication as a Defense

Today, the effect of intoxication on criminal responsibility is well established, but only precariously settled. At law, intoxication can be either (a) involuntary, where the intoxicant is ingested as the result of force or duress, deceit or trickery, medical advice, or lack of awareness of a susceptibility to a recognized atypical reaction to that substance, as in pathologic intoxication; or (b) voluntary, where the intoxicant is ingested for effect, as in recreational drug use. Many jurisdictions have recognized involuntary intoxication as a complete defense to criminal behavior in appropriate circumstances. Most jurisdictions, however, adhere to the view that voluntary intoxication does not excuse a criminal act unless the actor, because of his intoxication, could not form the intent required by the statutory definition of the crime.

Dependence as a Defense

Dependence on an intoxicant or active intoxication, absent more, does not provide a complete defense in any jurisdiction. The nature, course, and effects of dependence on specific substances on cognition, emotion, or behavior have not been recognized by the law.

Interestingly, opioid intoxication (but not dependence) may be of such extent as to negate the "knowingly" element of criminal intent. But neither opioid intoxication nor dependence has been held to negate the "willfully" element of criminal intent. Intoxication (but not dependence) induced by any substance may be sufficient to render a person incapable of the "deliberation" or "premeditation" required as an element of a specific degree of an offense, as in first-degree murder. In no jurisdiction has dependence on specific intoxicants been differentiated from that of alcohol, thereby warranting special consideration.

Withdrawal as a Defense

Defenses based on the argument that the criminal act at issue was the direct or indirect product of withdrawal from an intoxicant have not prevailed, except in the limited and infrequent circumstance where a defendant in withdrawal commits an act while semiconscious or unconscious. An action that, while purposive, is not spontaneous, and therefore is not voluntary, is defined at law as an "automatism" and does not incur criminal responsibility.

Intoxicant-Induced Insanity as a Defense

An insanity defense asserts that at the time the accused committed the act for which he or she is charged, a mental illness precluded the person from having the required bad state of mind to be convicted of the act.

Insanity that arises from either acute or chronic intoxicant use has not been distinguished from insanity produced by other causes. Thus, whether temporary insanity caused by voluntary intoxication will be exculpatory largely depends on the legal test for insanity used in that jurisdiction. Several states have statutorily excluded this defense.

Concept of Partial Responsibility

Partial responsibility, or diminished capacity, is a difficult and muddled concept in the law, with little coherence or consistency. Many courts appear to reject or not understand it.

Insanity of the legal type is considered a complete defense to criminal acts in most jurisdictions. A mental disorder that constitutes "something less than insanity" is not considered a complete defense to a crime, but is widely thought to lessen the degree of criminal responsibility, at least for crimes where there is a lesser degree of responsibility or severity available (as in murder, which might be reducible from first degree to second or a lesser degree).

Intoxicant Use and Effects as Mitigating Factors

Although many states now require judges to adhere to legislatively prescribed sentencing guidelines, in some jurisdictions judges have retained limited discretion to consider a convicted defendant's complete drug history (including intoxication and dependence) as a mitigating factor. However, it is a general rule that the nature, extent, and effects of the intoxicant history must be introduced into evidence before being eligible for consideration at sentencing.

Addictive Processes

The concept of behaviors involving addictive processes, rather than intoxicating substances, as in "compulsive" or "pathologic" gambling, is of exceptional theoretical importance for the criminal law and the addictions field. The concept has required a re-examination of many fundamental legal postulates, precedents, and assumptions about criminal responsibility and intentionality. If viewed as addictive disorders (as in "compulsive gambling") in which no exogenous intoxicating substance is ingested, such processes raise profound questions about the paradigms that inform research, theory, and practice in the addictions field. If viewed as impulse control disorders (as in "pathologic gambling"), these processes raise difficult questions about the causal and temporal relationships between a person's impulses and the acts issuing therefrom. Unfortunately, in recent years, addiction terminology has been used to refer to everything from Internet usage ("Internet addiction") to dedication to one's career ("workaholic"), thus lessening its applicability and meaning with respect to physiologic addictive disease.

Pathologic Gambling

One critical step toward the resolution of the conceptual problems associated with pathologic gambling would be for the field to formulate a classification of pathologic gamblers and the situations relevant to their behavior(s) that would be defensible empirically and relevant to the issue of criminal responsibility.

What we find in the fact patterns of cases involving pathologic gambling is not a total or even substantial incapacity to carry out simple (or even complex) acts that can be reasonably attributed to the "disease." Nor do we find such a compromise of intellectual function as to entirely exclude purposeful conduct. Instead, we observe an apparent blunting of ethical sensitivity sufficient to destroy the understanding, appreciation, or regard for the moral quality of the criminal act, combined with a drastic, often protracted, lapse of inhibition.

Clinical and Forensic Distinctions

It is recognized clinically that at least some compulsive gamblers who commit crimes are impaired physically and psychologically, and thus may be only partially responsible for their misconduct. In this sense, at law they resemble the inebriate, whose reason has been temporarily compromised; and for them the rules governing intoxication often seem more applicable than do those for insanity. Although they are only very rarely psychotic, and only a few may even be neurotic, they are nonetheless considered abnormal by many clinicians, albeit in ways of questionable relevance. Hence, for this subgroup of "impaired" compulsive gamblers, neither complete exculpation nor full responsibility seems appropriate.

Sexual Addiction

In recent years, the diagnosis of "compulsive sexuality" or "sexual addiction" has been offered as the basis for exculpation or mitigation in cases involving sexual, as well as less obviously related, offenses. Some few courts have admitted expert testimony about this controversial condition.

Eating Disorders

There have been a few cases involving shoplifting and petty theft from groceries where an eating disorder (bulimia) was advanced as a defense. In none of these cases did the defense exculpate the accused.

Compulsive Spending or Shopping

Recently, support groups based on 12-step principles and other self-help models have emerged for persons with the "diseases" of "compulsive spending" and "compulsive shopping." Advocates in these movements have adopted or endorsed addiction-derived explanations, language, and treatment approaches for these problems. The application of an addiction paradigm to these behaviors is of dubious validity, and neither problem has been widely recognized as an addictive disorder by professionals in the field.

Effects of Intoxicants on Memory

Expert Testimony about the Memory of Witnesses

In cases where the defendant has been accused by persons who are or have been drug involved, an expert must assess the potential impact of their intoxicant use on their credibility as witnesses. The focus must be on the effect of the relevant intoxicant(s) on memory and its constituent cognitive processes.

Cocaine-Related Memory Dysfunction in Criminal Proceedings

Although any of the intoxicants can have potentially deleterious effects on selected memory functions, the effects of cocaine raise the most serious and frequent concerns. A significant number of today's large-scale cocaine trafficking cases are founded principally or solely on the testimony of alleged or self-styled coconspirators, who, more often than not, were themselves using large amounts of cocaine (and usually other intoxicants as well) during the period about which they will testify in great detail as to time, place, person, sequence, and events. In evaluating the credibility of such witnesses, it is critical to look for any possible effects of intoxicant use on their memory functions.

Phenomenon of Confabulation

Confabulation is a neuropsychiatric symptom that is characteristic of diffuse organic brain disease and/or dysfunction. It refers to the unconscious filling in of memory gaps by imagined experiences, fabricated stories, or grossly distorted accounts of recent or remote events. It is absolutely distinct from lying, which implies both motive and awareness of the distortion or untruth. Confabulatory recall is inconsistent; it may change from moment to moment; and it may be induced unwittingly by suggestion. Confabulation is never a consistent finding in any clinical condition. It is most frequently seen in cases of severe, nutrition-deficient alcoholism, head trauma, cerebral hypoxia, certain heavy metal poisonings, certain infections of the central nervous system (e.g., herpes or HIV encephalitis), or high-dose psychostimulant use.

Cocaine-Induced Confabulation

Confabulation may be seen in two phases of high-dose cocaine use. During the acute intoxication phase, the profound confusion, grandiosity, emotional lability, false sense of mastery, illusions, delusions, and hallucinations occasionally can induce certain users to confabulate "in real time." During the convalescent phase, after a period of abstinence from cocaine, the person gradually recalls fragments of past experience (many of which may have been originally misperceived) in a distorted way. In an attempt to preserve logical consistency, these may be linked with confabulated material. The more often such confabulated material is ratified by the social setting and in particular by authority figures (e.g., physicians, attorneys, or law enforcement officers), the more likely it is to become a fully integrated and unquestioned part of that person's self-history. It even may go on to become the basis for future thoughts, conclusions, and actions.

Although the U.S. Court of Appeals for the Sixth Circuit upheld the disallowance of such testimony in *United States v. Ramirez*, finding that such testimony went to the credibility, not the competence, of a witness, the exclusion of such testimony by a qualified addiction expert has been the rare exception, not the rule.

Regulatory and Administrative Proceedings

Members of licensed, regulated, or otherwise supervised professions (e.g., health care professionals, attorneys, airline pilots, interstate truckers) can find their licenses at risk for a number of reasons involving intoxicants. Two, however, are of exceptional importance and are discussed here: (a) allegations of "impairment" consequent to intoxicant use, and (b) for physicians, allegations of the "inappropriate" prescribing of opioids for the long-term management of chronic nonmalignant pain. In cases involving professional impairment, two fundamental and very serious medicolegal issues have been identified: (a) the common presumption that "use equals abuse equals addiction equals impairment," and (b) that only a few regulatory agencies (e.g., the Federal Aviation Administration for pilots and the Department of Transportation for interstate truck drivers) have normative data defining the cognitive, sensory, or motor skills required of a normal, that is, a "nonimpaired" practitioner. With the exception of the blood alcohol concentration, which, as a matter of public policy, has been adopted in every state as an objective, affirmative indicium of impairment for the operation of a motorized vehicle, there are no similarly established norms for any other intoxicants, nor for alcohol-mediated impairment in other contexts.

Professional Impairment

In the assessment of professional impairment, regulatory policies do not reflect the clinically significant, specific differences between intoxicants in terms of their effects, patterns of use, routes of administration, nature of the dependence and/or withdrawal syndromes (if applicable), or resultant substance-related disabilities. Although there are a few regulatory and legal cases where (limited) consideration was given to these crucial distinctions, such deliberations are clearly the exception, not the rule.

Prescribing Opioids for Pain in Private Practice

Each year the prescribing profiles for controlled substances (class II opioids, in particular) of thousands of physicians are routinely (often automatically) monitored, sampled, or otherwise scanned, and evaluated by state regulatory bodies. Despite the dubious ethics and questionable purposes/efficacy of such monitoring programs, these practices increasingly are being "justified" by state regulatory bodies in the name of public health and safety, which are (presumptively) privileged over issues of individual privacy and confidentiality. The legal authority for these actions and the regulation of opioid prescribing for pain is provided by health (medical) practice acts legislated at the state level and by federal and state acts governing the use of controlled substances.

The two most frequent bases upon which regulators found allegations that a physician's use of long-term opioid therapy for chronic, nonmalignant pain is inappropriate are that such therapy "creates addicts" and that opioid therapy is contraindicated in any patient with a history of substance abuse. Both assertions are highly controversial, and the underlying assumptions, concerns, and issues of both have been comprehensively examined and challenged by specialists in pain management and addiction medicine.

For even the most-knowledgeable, best-intentioned, and best-prepared practitioner accused of opioid prescribing violations, exculpation is by no means assured, and ultimate vindication should never be assumed. However, documentation of the following material in the medical record often has proved to be the pivotal element in the successful defense of such cases:

1. A comprehensive evaluation and assessment of the etiology, history, and character of the patient's pain.
2. Clinical records or summaries from the specialists or subspecialists who have diagnosed and treated the primary medical or surgical conditions thought to be producing the patient's pain.
3. An appropriately executed (signed, witnessed, and notarized) document of the patient's "Informed Consent to Treatment with Opioid Drugs." Because the law on informed consent varies substantially from state to state and is subject to increasingly frequent review and revision, this critical document must be drafted in close consultation with an attorney who is experienced, and absolutely up-to-date in this area of the law. Moreover, the trend in the law of informed consent is in the direction of requiring increased specificity about alternatives and risks, broader comprehensiveness, and clearer evidence of the patient's practical understanding of both the proposed treatment and the meaning of the signed document of consent.

4. Frequent multidimensional assessment and documentation of the efficacy of opioid therapy, the absence of drug toxicity, and the absence of indicia of "addiction" (including periodic urine toxicology screening). Multidimensional assessment of the frequency and distress illuminates the impact of symptoms and the efficacy of treatment on a patient's quality of life.

5. Annual (or more frequent if indicated) "Letters of Indemnification" from an appropriate surgical or medical specialist stating that the specialist has re-examined the patient, found that the underlying medical or surgical condition is still present and/or unchanged, that there have been no treatment innovations or technologic breakthroughs from which the patient might be expected to benefit, and that therefore continued management of the patient's pain is clinically justifiable.

6. If the physician prescribing the opioids is not a credentialed expert or specialist in either pain management or addiction medicine, letters of consultation from a specialist in both of these areas are essential. Moreover, even if the prescribing physician is an expert in one of these two areas, a consultation letter from an expert in the other area is critical. These consultative reports should be updated at intervals appropriate to the patient's underlying diseases and/or reflective of the results of the regular multidimensional assessments described previously. Thus, patients who have exhibited behaviors that might be construed as "drug-seeking behavior" will need to be more frequently assessed by an addiction medicine specialist. Patients whose response to opioid therapy is untoward or inadequate (in terms of enhanced function and comfort) will require more frequent evaluation by a pain specialist.

It is early yet to determine whether the availability of buprenorphine for the office-based practitioner will lead to significant legal difficulties. However, given the strict supervision being administered in terms of specialized Drug Enforcement Agency (DEA) certification, specialized training requirements, and limitations on patient quantity, it is certainly likely to be a closely examined process.

Administrative Proceedings

The effects of intoxicants of different classes have not been differentiated in administrative hearings or other proceedings involving employment eligibility, benefits, restriction, discrimination, supervision, discipline, or termination. In these venues, as in professional regulatory contexts, the prevailing presumption reflects the false and dangerous syllogism that "use equals abuse equals addiction equals impairment." Moreover, routine screening for intoxicant use in the workplace is technically problematic as well as legally and ethically questionable. Well-established principles of administrative law procedure are often violated, and fundamental legal rights (e.g., due process) often ignored. Despite their being treated like criminal "defendants," the accused in these proceedings are neither guaranteed adequate legal representation nor provided with the funds and resources (e.g., expert witnesses) necessary to present an adequate defense.

Given the cultural prejudices about intoxicant use and the pressures on employers to maintain a "drug-free workplace," an employee who is accused of intoxicant use cannot safely assume that he or she will get a fair hearing or receive an equitable disposition. Addiction medicine specialists must be aware of these prevailing inequities. The need and opportunities for professional involvement in intoxicant-related matters of administrative law are great.

Conclusion

There can be no doubt that there are many serious conceptual problems and resultant inequities in the modern criminal law. History has shown that "the engine of the law doth indeed grind slowly." Now more than ever, the practice of law and the science of jurisprudence are in need of consultation and collaboration with other professions, intellectual disciplines, and fields of knowledge. The challenge to the medical, biologic, and cognitive sciences is clear. The response remains to be seen.

Doubtless, working in the forensic arena is not for everyone. For many addiction medicine professionals, the intense adversarial nature and constricting rules of criminal proceedings are personally offensive and professionally intolerable. For some others, ethical concerns, opinions and values, or personal experiences make them reluctant or unwilling to participate in what they perceive to be the shielding of an intoxicant user from the full consequences of his or her actions. For a few others, their understanding or personal history of addiction may lead them to interpret and condemn any such involvement as a form of professional "enabling" of a patient's addiction. But for those addictionists who do choose to participate in the judicial process, to make a contribution to the cause of justice, and to work to illuminate this vital medical–legal interface, the rewards from the intellectual challenge, professional enrichment, and personal fulfillment can be substantial.

Suggested Readings

Ackerman TF. Chemically dependent physicians and informed consent disclosure. *J Addict Dis.* 1996;15(2):25–42.

Beatty WW, Katzung VM, Moreland VJ, et al. Neuropsychological performance of recently abstinent alcoholics and cocaine abusers. *Drug Alcohol Depend.* 1995;37:247–253.

Burglass ME, Gitlow S. Forensics. In: Lowinson JH, Ruiz P, Millman RB, et al., eds. *Substance abuse: a comprehensive textbook*, 4th ed. Philadelphia: Lippincott Williams & Wilkins; 2005:1300–1316.

Duffy JD. The neurology of alcoholic denial: implications for assessment and treatment. *Can J Psychiatry.* 1995;40(5):257–263.

Savage SR. Opioid use in the management of chronic pain. *Med Clin North Am.* 1999;83(3):761–786.

Index

507